P9-EAI-853

THERAPEUTIC EXERCISE

THIRD EDITION

This volume is one of the series,
Rehabilitation Medicine Library,
Edited by John V. Basmajian,
Originally published as the Physical Medicine Library,
Edited by Sidney Licht.

Therapeutic Exercise

Third Edition

Edited by

JOHN V. BASMAJIAN,

M.D., F.A.C.A.

Rehabilitation Centre, Chedoke Hospitals
and McMaster University
Hamilton, Ontario

 WILLIAMS & WILKINS
Baltimore/London

Copyright 1978 by The Williams & Wilkins Co.
First edition, 1958
Second edition revised and enlarged 1961 and 1965
Second Printing, 1969
Third Printing, 1976
Reprinted 1978
Third Edition, 1978
Reprinted August 1978
Reprinted November 1978
Reprinted November 1979
Reprinted June 1980
All Rights Reserved

The text of this publication or any part thereof may not be reproduced in any manner whatsoever without permission in writing from the publisher.

Library of Congress Cataloging in Publication Data

Main entry under title:

Therapeutic exercise.

  (Rehabilitation medicine library)
  First-2d ed. edited by S. H. Licht.
  Bibliography:
  Includes index.
  1. Exercise therapy. I. Basmajian, John V., 1921– II. Licht, Sidney Herman, 1907 – ed. Therapeutic exercise. III. Series. [DNLM: 1. Exercise therapy. WB541 T398]
RM725.L5 1978   615'.824   77-11071
ISBN 0-683-00433-6

Waverly Press, Incorporated
Baltimore, Maryland
Printed in the United States of America

Foreword by Series Editor

When I accepted the mantle as Editor of the Rehabilitation Medicine Series from the incomparable Sidney Licht, I had not planned to become book editor of any individual volume. Only a Licht could edit all the books with equal authority. However, it became clear that this pivotal volume required special attention and expertise both of which I could provide. This, then, is the only volume in the series where the series editor is also the book editor.

Plans for the future of all the other books in the Rehabilitation Library are solid. While several books are being either phased out or perpetuated unchanged, most of the volumes will appear as new editions with new editors (all appointed and at work). Several volumes will appear in the same year (and perhaps the same month) as this book. Through 1978–1981, most of the rest will have reappeared as vigorous new editions edited by leaders in their fields. Two at least are so revived and altered that they are new books with new titles, rising like the Phoenix out of the ashes of earlier volumes. In addition, some four editors for new volumes are under contract and these books too will appear over the next two years to augment the resources of the rehabilitation team.

JOHN V. BASMAJIAN

Preface to the Third Edition

Therapeutic Exercise was clearly a unique book throughout most of the long lives of its first and second editions. Only in the late 1960s did a satisfactory complement appear: the proceedings of NUSTEP, the classic month-long conference at Northwestern University in 1966 (also published by The Williams & Wilkins Company). Both books began to get shadowed by a creeping obsolescence through the 1970s, although NUSTEP contains excellent long sections written by authoritative expositors describing specific techniques. Those sections still represent the state of the art and alone appear to justify the continued life of *that* book; but *this* book has needed complete overhauling and renewal for several years.

How has this book changed? A major change is a rather ruthless elimination of chapters and topics that presented material generally unavailable in earlier decades, but now either freely available elsewhere or inappropriate here. Another major change is the addition of fresh chapters written to meet the needs of the physical rehabilitation team in the late 1970s and 1980s. The chapter on the morphological and functional basis is not only specially tailored by Dr. Wolf to the exact subject of therapeutic exercise, it also provides a comprehensive bibliography of great value. Dr. de Lateur's short chapter gives an additional lift to the scientific end. Dr. Harris's authoritative chapter on the specific methods of therapeutic exercise manages for the first time to critique them well, and the new chapter (by the editor) on biofeedback puts into perspective the application of that supportive therapy that was quite unknown in the past.

Other completely new chapters which cover areas dealt with in earlier editions are those by Dr. Sarno (Therapeutic Exercise for Back Pain), Dr. Swenson (Therapeutic Exercise in Hemiplegia), Dr. Gilbert (Exercise for the Heart), Dr. Cailliet (Exercises for Scoliosis), Dr. Allman (Exercise in Sports Medicine), Dr. Corcoran (Gait and Gait Retraining), and Dr. Halpern (Therapeutic Exercises for Cerebral Palsy).

Other authors (Drs. Abramson, Cailliet (on Multiple Sclerosis), Hoberman, Kite, Knapp, Liberson, Licht, Moore, Russek, Schram, Sinclair, Stewart, Wynn Parry, and Wilson) have modified and modernized valuable chapters previously found in the book. Their work has not necessarily been easier; in some cases it has taken more time and effort than writing a fresh new chapter. A massive re-arranging of the chapter order has permitted bringing more order to the book and in particular Dr. Licht's revised chapter to the beginning of the book where this tour-de-force on history belongs.

The result of all this work restores this book once more to its position as the unique publication on this topic addressed to the whole medical rehabilitation community. Now smaller in size, it still embraces all the important aspects of the subject and is the only book that even attempts to do this. The editor wholeheartedly thanks all the contributing authors for their excellent contributions and also Miss Arlene De Bevoise for her extra efforts in helping to edit the book. Arlene, my trusted assistant at the Emory University Rehabilitation Research and Training Center, was much more involved in this book than could be expected of an executive secretary to the director. I hope she enjoys the results of her work. Emory University also deserves a note of sincere thanks for it was there that this book was started well along on its way. The Williams & Wilkins Company represented by Sara Finnegan and James Sheets continued to provide the editor with gracious assistance and complete editorial freedom and deserves a special thank-you.

Hamilton, Ontario   JOHN V. BASMAJIAN
1978

From the Preface to the First Edition

Before the Second World War a physical therapy prescription was often considered complete when it mentioned heat, massage and electricity. When exercise was prescribed, it was often listed vaguely; most physicians counted on the therapist to do the right thing in that department. A rapid and great change has occurred. Physicians have become increasingly aware of the need for exercise; indeed, for some physical medicine specialists the pendulum has swung so far from the old regime that they have virtually excluded previously practiced methods in favor of exercise. We have the assurance of history that a proper balance will one day prevail. All this is another way of saying that a book was needed to which the physician, therapist and student could refer for information on all aspects of the subject.

The organization of this book posed several problems: What aspects are too irrelevant to include? In what order shall the components be placed? What shall be the order for basic subjects and methods? Perhaps the reader will not agree with our choice, placement or emphasis. This is of small consequence if he finds useful information in the book, and we think he will.

It is easy to measure size. By count of words or pages this is the largest single volume on therapeutic exercise in any language. Quality cannot be measured in numbers; it must be experienced. An editor must read each contribution at least four times: original typescript, final typed copy, galley proof and page proof. Each time we read the chapters offered by the contributors to this book we experienced that deep warmth of snug confidence, the feeling that here was a book which would fill a need well, for this is many books in one. It is the kind of document which will give the enclave of therapeutic exercise its sovereignty. In behalf of the readers and the patients who will benefit from this collection of gifts to medical literature, we say thank you to the contributors who gave of their time and themselves to make the book possible.

New Haven, Connecticut   SIDNEY LICHT, M.D.
April 1, 1958.

The Contributors

Arthur S. Abramson, M.D.
> Professor and Chairman, Department of Rehabilitation Medicine, Albert Einstein College of Medicine, Yeshiva University; Director, Physical Medicine and Rehabilitation Service, Bronx Municipal Hospital Center, and Lubin Rehabilitation Center, New York City.

Fred L. Allman, M.D.
> Director, Sports Medicine Clinic, Atlanta, Georgia

John V. Basmajian, M.D., F.A.C.A.
> Professor of Medicine, McMaster University; Director, Rehabilitation Centre, Chedoke Hospitals, Hamilton, Ontario.

René Cailliet, M.D.
> Professor and Chairman, Department of Rehabilitative Medicine, University of Southern California School of Medicine; Director, Department of Rehabilitation Medicine, Los Angeles County-University of Southern California Medical Center, Los Angeles, California.

Paul J. Corcoran, M.D.
> Acting Chief, Department of Physical and Rehabilitation Medicine, Tufts University School of Medicine, New England Medical Center Hospital, Rehabilitation Institute, Boston, Massachusetts

Barbara J. de Lateur, M.D.
> Professor, Department of Rehabilitation Medicine, University of Washington School of Medicine, Seattle, Washington 98195

Alfred Ebel, M.D., F.A.C.P.
> Chief, Clinical Services, Department of Rehabilitation Medicine, Montefiore Hospital and Medical Center, Bronx; Professor Emeritus of Rehabilitation Medicine, Albert Einstein College of Medicine, Yeshiva University, New York City

Charles A. Gilbert, M.D.
> Professor of Medicine (Cardiology), Emory University School of Medicine, Atlanta, Georgia

Daniel Halpern, M.D.
Professor, University of Minnesota Medical School, Department of Physical Medicine and Rehabilitation, Minneapolis, Minnesota

F. A. Harris, M.D.
Research Assistant Professor, Physiology and Biophysics, University of Washington School of Medicine, Seattle, Washington

Morton Hoberman, M.D.
Clinical Professor, Physical Medicine and Rehabilitation, College of Physicians and Surgeons, Columbia University (Retired); Director, Physical Medicine and Rehabilitation, Yonkers General Hospital, Yonkers, N.Y.; Consultant, Physical Medicine & Rehabilitation, Nyack, New York; Central Suffolk Hospital, Riverhead, New York

Joseph H. Kite, M.D.
Former Surgeon-in-Chief, Scottish Rite Hospital for Sick Children, Decatur; Associate Professor, Orthopedic Surgery, Emory University School of Medicine, Atlanta, Georgia

Miland E. Knapp, M.D.
Emeritus Clinical Professor Physical Medicine, School of Medicine, University of Minnesota; Former Director of Treatment and Training, Elizabeth Kenney Institute, Minneapolis; Former Area Consultant, Physical Medicine and Rehabilitation, Veterans Administration

W. T. Liberson, M.D., Ph.D.
Chief, Rehabilitation Medicine, Brooklyn-Cumberland Medical Center, Brooklyn, New York; Director, Rehabilitation Services, Grynolds Park Rehabilitation Center, Miami, Florida; Physician-in-Residence, Veterans Administration, Washington, D.C.; Senior Lecturer, Downstate Medical School, Brooklyn, New York; Formerly at the University of Illinois and Loyola University, Chicago, Illinois

Sidney Licht, M.D.
Honorary Curator, Physical Medicine Collections, Yale Medical Library, New Haven, Connecticut; Clinical Professor, University of Miami School of Medicine, Miami, Florida

Margaret L. Moore, B.S., R.P.T., M.S., Ed.D.
Professor of Physical Therapy, Department of Medical Allied Health Professions, School of Medicine, University of North Carolina at Chapel Hill, Chapel Hill, North Carolina.

Mieczyslaw Peszczynski, M.D.
Professor Emeritus and Former Chairman, Department of Physical Medicine, Emory University, Atlanta, Georgia

Allen S. Russek, M.D.
Former Professor of Clinical Rehabilitation Medicine, New York University School of Medicine.

John E. Sarno, M.D.
Professor, Clinical Rehabilitation Medicine, New York University School of Medicine

Duane A. Schram, M.D.
Chief, Physical Medicine and Rehabilitation, Memorial Medical Center, Williamson, West Virginia

J. D. Sinclair, M.D., F.R.A.C.P., B. Med. Sc.
Professor of Physiology, Auckland University School of Medicine, Auckland, New Zealand

J. B. Stewart
Former Consultant in Physical Medicine, Cirencester, Swindon and Pewsey Hospital Management Committees, Oxford Regional Hospital Board, England

James R. Swenson, M.D.
Chairman, Division of Physical Medicine and Rehabilitation, University of Utah Medical Center, Salt Lake City, Utah

Colon H. Wilson, Jr.
Professor, Rheumatology-Immunology, Emory University School of Medicine, Atlanta, Georgia

Steven L. Wolf, Ph.D.
Assistant Professor, Rehabilitation Medicine, Assistant Professor, Allied Health Professions, Assistant Professor, Anatomy; Emory University School of Medicine, Atlanta, Georgia

C. B. Wynn Parry, M.B.E., M.A., D.M. (Oxon.), F.R.C.P., D. Phys. Med.
Director, Rehabilitation and Consultant Rheumatologist, Royal National Orthopaedic Hospital, Stanmore and London.

CONTENTS

1

History

SIDNEY LICHT

Therapeutic exercise is motion of the body or its parts to relieve symptoms or to improve function. Since the earliest known writings on this subject describe relatively elaborate procedures we must assume that therapeutic exercises were used in prehistoric times. MacAuliffe (88) wrote that the *Cong Fou*[1] of ancient China is the earliest known writing on therapeutic exercise. The *Cong Fou* was a series of ritualistic postures and motions prescribed by the priests for the relief of pain and other symptoms. The ancient Hindus[2] also used positioning and movements in a somewhat less empiric manner. Megasthenes, a Greek historian of the third century B.C., wrote about an order of Brahman physicians who relied chiefly on natural (physical) therapeutics, including individual exercises for different parts of the body (131). But the medicine and therapeutic exercise of mainstream occidental practice was of Greek origin.

Ancient Greece

The ancient Greeks believed that medicine began with Aesculapius, a mythical person deified before the advent of Homer. The shrines to this god were Temples of Health called Asclepia. Since they were religious institutions they were directed by priests,[3] at first, but eventually lay practition-

---

[1] The *Cong Fou* was conducted by the Taoist priests for more than a thousand years before Christ. It consists of body positioning and breathing routines. The exercises had relatively little motion and most were entirely unrelated to modern concepts of exercise. For example, the subject pulled on his toes to counteract bad dreams. A full description of *Cong Fou* was brought back to France from China by the great eighteenth-century missionary, Father Amiot. Amiot, J. M. *Memoires Concernant l'Histoire, les Sciences et les Arts des Chinois*. Paris, 1779, Vol. IV.

According to Chancerel (30), the ancient Chinese Emperor Yin-Kang-Chi made his subjects engage in military exercises to prevent the diseases caused by the almost continuous rains. He also invented the dance called "turnings" to combat miasmatic fevers.

[2] The fourth volume of *Atharva-Veda* of ancient India is *Ayur-Veda*, an anatomy book which recommends exercise and massage in chronic rheumatism. The date of this work is about 800 B.C. according to D. Guthrie in *A History of Medicine*. London, 1945.

[3] According to Littré (83), there were three classes of medical practitioners in ancient Greece: 1) priest-physicians, 2) philosophers, and 3) gymnasts, who studied the effects of diet and exercise.

1

ers also became associated with the Temples. Although much of Temple treatment was concerned with spiritual matters and the interpretation of dreams, medicinal and physical agents were also used. Gymnasia were annexed to several of the Temples and prescribed exercises were performed in them. The antiquity and importance of therapeutic exercise[4] are clear from Galen's remark that Aesculapius himself recommended equitation as a health restorative (77).

What little is known about medicine before Hippocrates the Great is to be found in his writings and the writings of those who succeeded him. Among the earliest physicians to recommend remedial gymnastics were Iccus of Tarento and Medea (77). There is general agreement that Herodicus[5] was the first to write on the subject. LeClerc (77) said that many physicians accepted part of the system[6] of Herodicus. Hippocrates, one of his students, declared that the master went too far sometimes. "He killed

---

[4] The general term for exercise among the Greeks was *ascesis* (35). An ascete was a man who exercised his mind and body, which he regarded as inseparable; he considered the whole man (*l'homme tout entier*), as Dally expressed it. Those who exercised only to win a prize (*athlon*) were called athletes. Most exercises were done in a state of complete undress. The Greek work for nude is *gymnos*, hence the exercises performed in the nude were gymnastics. The derivation of the work "exercise" is less well understood. The prefix *ex* means out; the component *erc* is derived from *arcere*, to lock. Thus exercise means to unlock, or to free a part to move.

The Greeks had many exercises, and, at one time or another, almost every one of them was recommended by some physician. Hippocrates (83) recommended *achrocheirismos* for weight reduction. It was a form of finger wrestling in which "a man taking hold of his antagonist's fingers, strove to break them, and did not give up until he compelled him to yield." A favorite type of equipment was *halteres* (weights which resemble modern dumbbells). They were made of different substances in different shapes, of which the ellipsoid was possibly the most popular. Some had holes and other thongs for easier grasping. They could be weighted with lead in different quantities and used in progression.

One of the most frequently mentioned exercise prescriptions was the *haiora* or gestation. The patient rode, sitting or lying, in a horse-drawn carriage over rough roads. Equitation or horseback riding was said to have been prescribed by Aesculapius himself for the restoration of health.

Exercises were usually performed in a covered area called a *palestra* (gymnasium), under the supervision of gymnasts and trainers. The palestra became a fairly elaborate edifice with steam baths and swimming pools in addition to exercise and games areas.

[5] Herodicus, called Prodicus by some, was born in Lentini, Sicily (88), at about the time of the 88th Olympiad (480 B.C.). Some authors gave his birthplace as Selymbria in Thrace. He claimed to have cured himself of an incurable illness with exercise. Herodicus started life as an instructor and noted that the weakest among his students could be brought to greater strength by wrestling and boxing. He developed a rather elaborate system of exercises (*Ars Gymnastica*) which, according to Pliny, could not be understood without a knowledge of geometry. In fact, Pliny claimed that the students of Herodicus left him because the method was so difficult. Plato condemned Herodicus for his excessive use of exercise, saying that a twenty-mile walk without rest was too much for patients; in *Timaeus* he reversed his opinion.

[6] Galen indicated that the following advocated some form of medical gymnastics as proposed by Herodicus: Diocles, walking exercises; Erasistratus, walking for dropsy; Themison, passive and active exercises; also Praxagoras, Philotinus and Theon (77).

the febrile with walking, too much wrestling and fomentation. There is nothing more pernicious for the febrile than wrestling, walking and massage. It is like treating a disturbance with a disturbance" (83).

The word exercise appears often in the works of Hippocrates.[7] Although most references are to the hygienic aspect of general exercise, Hippocrates recognized its value in strengthening weakened muscles[8] in hastening convalescence and in improving mental attitudes. The three books *On Regimen* are attributed by some to Hippocrates but the third book contains so many statements on exercise in relation to health and disease that LeClerc (77) ascribed the book to Herodicus, considered by some the father of therapeutic exercise.

In his book *On Articulations* (2), Hippocrates demonstrated his deep insight into the relationship between motion and muscle (which he called flesh). "In dislocation inward of the hip joint, whether from birth or childhood, the fleshy parts are much more atrophied than those of the hand because the patient cannot exercise the leg. The wasting of the fleshy parts is greatest in those cases in which the patient keeps the limb up and does not exercise it. Those who practice walking have the least atrophy."

In Littré's translation (83) of the works attributed to Hippocrates, there are more than a dozen references to the medical uses of exercise. Frequent and rapid walks were recommended to reduce obesity. On the other hand caution was advised in the resumption of strenuous exercises after prolonged rest.

The pathogenesis of mental disease baffled the ancients even as it does some today. Hippocrates attributed mental aberration to an improper combination of humidity and heat and based his treatment on this concept. In other words, his therapy was rational in relation to the supposed pathology. To rid the body of excess humidity, or to increase the heat in it, he advocated exercise.

The most remarkable words written by him on the subject of exercise were those on medical rehabilitation, for the Greeks not only believed in it but also had a word for it—*analepsis*. The following stirring remarks appear in *On Articulations*. "One might say that such matters (strengthening weakened limbs by exercise) are outside the healing art. Why, forsooth, trouble one's mind further about cases which have become incurable? This is far from the right attitude. The investigation of these

---

[7] Soranus fixed the time of Hippocrates' birth as the first year of the 80th Olympiad (460 B.C.). He is said by different authors to have died between the ages of 85 and 109. Few things about his life are known with certainty, but there is little doubt that he was born on the Island of Cos, a descendant of a long line of priest-physicians with the name Hippocrates, a fact which lends confusion to matters concerning his writings. Thus of 60 or more books attributed to Hippocrates, only 13 are accepted by scholars as genuine (83).

[8] Hippocrates was ignorant of the function of muscle fiber. The important discovery that animal motions were performed by the muscles is attributed by John Hunter (68) to Lycus of Macedonia; Bastholm credits it to Alcmaeon of Crotona.

matters belongs to the same science (that is, medicine); it is impossible to separate them from one another . . . Generally speaking, all parts of the body which have a function, if used in moderation, and exercised in labors to which each is accustomed, become thereby healthy and well developed, and age slowly; but if unused and left idle, they become liable to disease, defective in growth, and age quickly. This is especially the case with joints and ligaments, if one does not use them. In those who are neglected and never use the leg to walk with but keep it up in the air, the bones are more atrophied than in those who do use it; and the tissues are much more atrophied than in those who use the leg" (134).

Therapeutic exercise, then as now, was prescribed by physicians and gymnasts. Daremberg (39) shares the bitterness of physicians of all eras in such matters when he says, "The gymnasts offered the physicians the most lively competition in the care of the wounded just as do our bone setters who meddle in the treatment of diseases and just as our gymnastic teachers today."

Few writings of Greek physicians who followed Hippocrates have been preserved. Polybus, the son-in-law of Hippocrates, indicated in his treatise *On the Nature of Man* that he prescribed exercises (83). Erasistratus, who taught at the famed medical school of Alexandria, about a century later, was so opposed to excessive exercise that he is sometimes misquoted as being against all exercises. For example, Paulus Aegineta states that he taught that "exercise is not at all necessary for the health of the animal frame." Herophilus,[9] who taught at Alexandria about the same time as Erasistratus, shared his views on the value of moderate exercise.

Ancient Rome

According to MacAuliffe (88), many Romans thought that gymnastics was the cause of the decline of Greece. Gymnastics came to Rome late,[10] but its acceptance by the masses was rapid. Soon the people were not satisfied with ordinary athletic exhibitions; public spectacles turned into staged slaughter and planned murder. The coming of Christianity accentuated the decadence of physical exercise, and Theodosius put an end to popular exhibitions of athletics by abolishing the Olympic games in 394. For more than a thousand years which followed, there was virtually no organized exercise in Europe. Most people in Ancient Rome recognized the value of moderate exercise.[11] Asclepiades[12] recommended walking and

[9] "To Herophilus belongs the honor of having first discovered in the nerves, the organs of sensation and of voluntary movement" (68).

[10] The first athletes did not appear in Rome until 186 B.C., when M. Fulvius ordered public games to acquit himself of a vow made in the Aetolian War, but regular gymnastic games did not begin until later.

[11] Seneca (88) believed in short simple exercises but found exercise for the sake of pleasure "not decent." Cicero loved to walk while dictating his speeches to his secretaries (who had to walk along with him). Cicero's desire for moderate exercise was probably influenced by his association with Asclepiades, whom he mentioned in his senate speech, "De Senectute."

[12] Asclepiades, one of the first great Greek physicians to practice in Rome, was born in

running for dropsy (9). Themison, most famous pupil of Asclepiades, recommended strenuous exercises in many acute diseases, according to Chancerel (30), for example, equitation in gout.

A. Cornelius Celsus[13] wrote much on exercise. In fact, the first chapter of his first book (29) discusses hygiene and advises frequent exercise. In discussing hemiplegia and other paralyses, he noted that although "a perfect cure is rare . . . gradual exercise and walking as much as possible" are necessary. He suggested exercise and amusing games for the demented, vigorous exercises for those with dropsy and, in comsumption, increase in exercise as the disease diminishes.

The greatest name in Roman medicine was Galen.[14] In his book *On Hygiene* (52), he classified exercises according to their vigor, duration, frequency, use of apparatus and the part of the body involved. As in most other writings, his approach to exercise was moderate. "The attention should be closely applied to the exercising body, and it should be stopped at once when any adverse signs appear . . . suspend the completion of the exercise and order him to stop." Galen deprecated the intemperate pursuit of gymnastics as not only injurious to health but also illiberal. Moreover, out of these practices arose a large class of quasi-medical *iatroleiptes* (anointers after the bath), who brought their craft into much disrepute and antagonized most of the better physicians, above all, Galen.

Galen reserved his highest praise for the game of the small ball (53), which corresponds roughly with our game of handball. "The best exercises of all are those which cannot only train the body but also delight the mind. For so much in them can move the mind that many have been delivered from diseases solely by delight . . . but even this game is not to be considered without dangers to which others are liable. For fast running has injured many by breaking an important blood vessel . . . So not to

the Bithynian town of Prusa about 174 B.C. He is regarded by Pagel (103) as the father of physical medicine for his espousal of natural or physical agents in treatment. Celsus attributed to him the doctrine, "The best medicine is none." Pliny informs us that in the book *On Common Aids* Asclepiades set down five rules for preserving health, one of which was walking. Asclepiades was one of the ancients was condemned immoderate exercise.

[13] Little is known about Celsus. He may have been born in what is now Narbonne, France, about 25 B.C. Celsus was an encyclopedist rather than a medical practitioner. Among his many writings was *De Medicina*, lost until the fifteenth century, when it was rediscovered by Pope Nicholas V. It was printed in 1478 at Florence as one of the first medical books to come off the newly invented printing press (60).

[14] Galen was born in Pergamus, a city of Asis Minor, about 131 A.D. He studied medicine at almost all of the scattered teaching centers of his time. He was one of the most prolific writers of all times. He wrote about 500 books (some of chapter length) and, in fact, devoted two books to his own bibliography. His renown was such that a century after his death, according to Eusebius, veneration for him resulted in a religious cult for his worship (77). His writings constituted the principal medical text for students for more than a thousand years.

The ruler of Pergamus entrusted the care of gladiators to him and in that capacity he developed a knowledge of traumatic surgery and the musculoskeletal system, a sound basis for his writings on exercise. The second book of his *On Hygiene* is titled *Exercise and Massage*.

incur danger would be the best qualification of all exercises taken for the benefit of the body."

Culpeper (36) found scattered in the works of Galen the following attributes of moderate exercise: "It stirs up natural heat, equally distributes the spirits, opens the pores, strengthens the members, and profits nature much."

Aretaeus[15] (1) was also a firm believer in therapeutic exercise. In discussing headache he said, "If the symptoms progress gradually, patients are to take exercises in the erect position for the benefit of the chest and shoulders." He also recommended long walks and other exercises for vertigo and epilepsy.

In Rome as in Greece, priest-physicians appreciated the value of exercise in disease. An *ex-voto* tablet of the second century was found (4) with an inscription concerning a young dyspeptic patient in whose incubation the god gave directions concerning exercise, among other remedies.

Antyllus[16] was one of the first to write on the abuse of rest. "Acutely ill patients should be put to bed because when they are in that condition they must avoid fatigue; those who are chronically ill need to go to bed only during exacerbations; during the intervals nothing should prevent them from moving about, because they require movement and varied stimuli." He recommended jumping for patients with weak legs and ball games for strengthening all weakened limbs. He graduated exercises according to the strength of the parts to be exercised. Thus, the punching bag (*corycos*) for weak arms was filled with cereal grains and that for stronger arms filled with grains of sand (102).

Philostratus[17] (106) listed the values of therapeutic exercise: "To purge the humors, to evacuate superfluous matters, to soften harder parts, to fatten, to transform or warm some part; these are in the realm of the gymnast. The *pedotribe* (physical trainer) either will not know these things, or if he does he will use them poorly. Physicians treat all diseases which we call fluxions, hydropsy, phthisis, and all of the sacred diseases, with affusions, potions and topical applications. Gymnastics, on the other hand, repress these affections by a regimen of exercise and friction. When a part is torn or wounded, when the vision is disturbed or if some joint is sprained, athletes should be sent to a physician, for the gymnast has no business to treat such conditions."

---

[15] Aretaeus, called the Cappadocian, was probably a contemporary of Galen. (This is assumed from the fact that neither mentioned the work of the other, an indication of smallness among supposedly big people of all eras.)

[16] Antyllus lived in the second century. His works are known through the writings of Oribasius (102).

[17] Although Herodicus wrote an entire book on medical gymnastics 400 years before Christ, it and any other books which may have been written on the subject during the next 600 years have been lost. Flavius Philostratus (170–245 A.D.) wrote *Gymnasticon* early in the third century. Although he was not a physician, his book touched on therapeutic exercise.

Caelius Aurelianus[18] has listed some amazingly modern concepts held by the ancients on physical treatment, including hydrogymnastics, suspension and kinesitherapy with pulleys and weights. Even more important was his insistence on the practice of *analepsis* (medical rehabilitation as proposed by Hippocrates). The first section of his second book *On Chronic Diseases* (10) discusses paralysis of different parts of the body and its treatment. It emphasizes the intelligent, purposeful use of exercise more clearly than any writer for more than a thousand years before or after him. "If the patient must lie on his back, a bandage is placed around the paralyzed leg. The loose end of the bandage is passed over a suspended pulley and is given to the patient or an attendant to hold. A demonstration of the twofold motion of the device is given; both patient and attendant being shown how to raise and lower the leg by alternately pulling and relaxing the cord. But since we desire not only to raise and lower but also to stretch and bend the paralyzed parts, we must tie two bandages, one around the knee and the other around the ankle. The ends are then passed as before, over the pulley, and given to the patient or attendant to pull alternately. Thus, when the end connected with the ankle is pulled and that connected with the knee remains slack, the resultant motion is a stretching of the leg. And if the patient can sit up, the middle of the bandage may be passed under the sole of the foot and the ends given to him to hold. He is thus required to impart motion to his leg by his own efforts, alternately pulling and slackening the ends of the bandage. And it is clear that the arm, when paralyzed, can be similarly exercised. . . . When the paralyzed parts have been moved and exercised as indicated, have the patient sit in a barber's chair which has arms at the sides. Let him try to lift himself by supporting himself on these arms. Again let him try to walk, either propped up under his arms by attendants on either side of him or resting on a staff. He may also lean on a carriage which is easily moved by hand, a device of the kind often used to teach children to walk, but built up to the patient's height. Then when the amount of walking which the patient does with the help of supports has been increased sufficiently, arrange wooden hurdles and have him try to step over them. Also add leaden weights to his shoes, at first only a small amount, say an ounce, then gradually more and more, up to a pound. Then have him increase the speed of walking, for this will require the use of more effort. . . . Then give him restorative treatment and have the patient use natural waters, especially the warm springs. . . . Also prescribe swimming in the sea or in the

---

[18] It is not known where Aurelianus was born or died, or even where he lived. From the style of his writing and the authors he quotes, it is believed that he lived toward the end of the fifth century, and that he practiced in Sicca, a town in the north of Africa. His writings have preserved for us much of the best in the works of physicians who preceded him and are especially valuable since so many of the original texts no longer exist. The first complete translation of his works into English was that of Drabkin in 1950 (10).

warm springs; at first however, an inflated bladder should be attached to the paralyzed parts to reduce the effort required in swimming."

In the section on wound surgery, Aurelianus advocates postoperative exercises, "For the little additional motion cannot cause the wound to open again; on the contrary, it will aid in building up the patient's strength during the period of recovery."

For arthritis, Aurelianus suggested kneading of wax with the fingers and later the use of progressively heavier dumbbells. He advised rest during periods of exacerbation, "And in the intervals of remission, strengthen the body and then apply metasyncritic (eliminative) therapy. Thus, first prescribe passive exercise with due regard to the patient's strength, then walking on ground strewn evenly with soft straw."

Drabkin (10) found more than 60 references to exercise in the works of Aurelianus, of every type and for every part of the body, from the raising of the eyebrows in facial paralysis to the use of irritating suppositories in paralysis of the anus. The remarkable catalogue of exercises listed in Aurelianus is not original with him but is a selection from his predecessors (to whom he gave full credit).

Paulus Aegineta, last of the Greek eclectics, compiled a synopsis of medicine in seven books toward the middle of the seventh century in which there are chapters on exercise (3). He defined exercise as violent motion which renders the body organs fit for their functional action. For the most part, Paulus followed the writings of Galen.

The Middle Ages

Christianity reacted to the gymnastic spectacles of the ancients by discontinuing exercise. All forms of public exhibition under the Romans had become increasingly un-Christian. The Christian disciples were taught to renouce material things—preservation of body strength and beauty were abandoned.[19]

After the fall of the Roman Empire, Greek and Roman medicine was kept alive by the Arabs through Syrian and Hebrew translations. It was only toward the tenth century that the Califs accepted science and permitted foreigners to have status. As schools multiplied, the ancient Greek writings were translated directly into Arabic (60). Rhazes was the first Arab physician to write a book on hygiene. In it he stated, "Health is preserved by a just measure of exercise and the other non-naturals; and also by the cleanliness of the place in which we live." Avicenna (60) wrote that for each organ there is an exercise, and that "if men exercised their bodies by motion and work at appropriate times, they would need neither physicians nor remedies."

---

[19] Until the ninth century, exercises were virtually forgotten except by the lords and knights. In their heavy armor, even they could do little exercise. Exercise reappeared in the fifteenth century, primarily as sports. The word "sport" came from the word *desports*, from the old French *des porter*, which meant to play at games. At the time of the French Revolution, emigrés took the word with them to England, where it caught on (97).

Puschmann (111) tells of the great Mansurian Hospital in Cairo in the eleventh century where "a large pavillion was erected in the garden, where the patients could take walking exercise in the shade."

There are two versions of how Greek and Roman medical writings returned to Europe. According to one, when the medical school at Salerno was formed in the ninth century, one of the founders was an Arab who brought translations of Hippocrates and Galen with him. According to another view, Constantine the African returned from a tour of the Orient in the eleventh century with translations from the Arab works that began a medical era in which Avicenna and Haly Abbas[20] were for a while more important than Hippocrates and Galen, from which they derived their writings.

Isaac Judaeus (54) wrote, in the tenth century, that "nothing is more harmful to the regulation of health than idleness." Johannes Actuarius, in the thirteenth century, prescribed a system of cure by diet and exercises, especially in mental diseases (4). One of the early masters of the medical school established in Montpellier was the Catalan, Arnold of Villanova, who wrote at the beginning of the fourteenth century, "Among other things . . . there is a need of convenient medicines, exercise and gladness" (7). Later that century, Petrarch (105) espoused the cause of natural remedies (including exercise) in place of drugs.

The Fifteenth Century

The great impetus to the reintroduction of physical education in the educational program came from Pietro Vergerio (1349–1428), who wrote a long letter on the subject which was reprinted many times (80). The letter had a strong influence on Vittorino da Feltra, a comtemporary physician turned educator, who started a school for young noblemen in Mantua in 1423, in which the schedule was divided between mental and physical education.[21]

---

[20] According to Haly Abbas (a Persian who died in 994), exercise was useful in rousing the natural heat, opening the pores, and improving strength of the animal actions.

[21] Although the Mantuan school did not enjoy a long life, this pioneering work (69), based on the classical concept of the ancients, aroused another physican, John Locke, to write an essay on the subject in 1693 (*Thoughts Concerning Education*). In 1572, Michel de Montaigne (98) had also proposed the idea of a balanced education. But it was not until two centuries later that Rousseau (104), influenced by all these writers, sparked the revolution in education. "It is a sad error to think that exercise of the body is bad for the operation of the mind, as if these two could not proceed simultaneously . . . Exercise the body continually, render it robust and healthy to render it wise and reasonable." At last the world was ready for the important change to the dual educational program as related in the popular novel, *Émile*. In 1771, Prince Friedrich-Leopold-Franz of Anhalt called on J. B. Basedow to put Rousseau's ideas into practice. In 1774 there opened at Dessau the *Philanthropinum*, a model training school, where for the first time in the Christian Era physical and mental education were fully integrated. Christian Salzmann, a pastor connected with the school, left there in 1784 to establish a similar school at Schnepfenthal, where physical education was placed under Johann Friedrich Guts Muths, who in 1793 wrote the very influential book *Gymnastik für die Jugend*, which became the text for the rapidly spreading movement. The

The second half of the fifteenth century witnessed a remarkable stimulus to intellectual activity, for which the invention of the printing press must be given major credit. It was introduced at almost the same moment as the siege of Constantinople, during which, it has been reported, the Greeks escaped westward and took with them manuscripts of ancient Greek writings, those of Hippocrates and Galen presumably included. Although some scholars deny the validity of this story, it fits into history very conveniently, for soon thereafter the Greek classics began to appear in print and were read. Almost at once, an ancient practice was resumed — that of writing books based almost entirely on the works of predecessors, without necessarily giving deserved credit. Antonius Gazius of Padua published an encyclopedia (54) of hygiene under the title of *Florida Corona*, "a crown of the most beautiful flowers in the works of Hippocrates and Galen," in 1492. Symphorien Champier, physician to Charles VIII and Louis XII, plucked some of the flowers from Gazio's crown and called his book *Rosa Gallica* (88), without acknowledgment. Both books mention the hygienic value of exercise.

The Sixteenth Century

Leonard Fuchs, professor at Tübingen from 1535 until his death in 1566, was one of the first physicians to abandon the teachings of the Arabs for that of the ancients. His *Institutiones Medicae* (50) contained a resumé of the art of exercise. The first chapter of Book Two of *On Motion and Rest* discusses types of motion. "There are two kinds of exercise; the first is simply exercise; the second is both exercise and work" — in other words, gymnastics and occupational motions (perhaps the first suggestion in medical literature of kinetic occupational therapy).

All medical books up to this time had been written in Latin. Jean Canape (27), physician to Francis I, broke tradition by translating important works into French. Ambroise Paré, the famous surgeon, followed the example by translating Vesalius into French and writing the first book in French on hygiene. In the introduction to his *Surgery* (104) he dealt in detail with motion and rest. He believed that exercise of the limbs following fractures was indispensable. Laurent Joubert of Montpellier (70) attached great importance to daily exercises and insisted that physicians and not teachers prescribe them.

The first printed book on exercise by a physician was the *Libro del Exercicio* of Christobal Mendez of Jaen (Fig. 1.1). In keeping with the tradition of previous writings on the subject, it dealt largely with the subject of hygiene and personal reminiscences.

The first important book in modern times on therapeutic exercise was *De Arte Gymnastica* (96) by Hieronymus Mercurialis.[22] The book was trans-

---

book was republished in Denmark (1799), Bavaria (1800), the United States (1802), France (1803), Austria (1805), Holland (1806) and Sweden (1813). Each new appearance of the book made converts, many of whom had a considerable influence on therapeutic exercise.

[22] Mercurialis of Forli, a professor at Padua, searched the library of the Vatican, during a

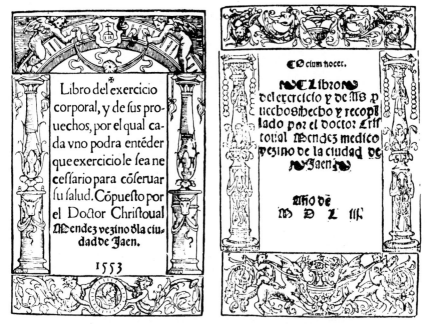

Fig. 1.1. First and second title pages of the first printed book on exercise by a physician, Dr. Christobal Mendez of Jaen in Spain. One unusual feature of this book was its appearance in a modern language. Only three copies of this book are known: two in the Biblioteca Nacionál in Madrid; the other, from which these reproductions were photographed, is in the important physical medicine collection of the Yale Medical Library. This book, with translation and facsimile reproduction, was published by Elizabeth Licht, Publisher, in 1960.

lated into Italian, but no English rendition was available until 1864 when Blundell (14) interspersed a partial translation of it with his own comments. Mercurialis set the following principles for medical gymnastics: 1) Each exercise should preserve the existing healthy state; 2) exercise should not disturb the harmony among the principal humors; 3) exercises should be suited to each part of the body; 4) all healthy people should take exercise regularly; 5) sick people should not be given exercises which might exacerbate existing conditions; 6) special exercises should be prescribed for convalescent patients on an individual basis; 7) persons who lead a sedentary life

7-year stay in Rome, for ancient references to exercise, especially those related to medicine. In 1569, he published at Venice (96) a book on gymnastics which was reprinted five times during the following century. The most popular book after his was that containing the three dialogues of Tuccaro (69). Tuccaro, a famous Neapolitan physical educator, devoted his third discourse to hygienic exercises. The Mendez book on exercise (Fig. 1.1) was so poorly circulated that it did not come to the attention of Mercurialis or his successors.

Marcellus Cagnatus of Verona (26) agreed with Socrates that dancing is a good exercise and stressed the importance to the physician "to know what properties exercises have for the entire body . . . in order to properly prescribe this exercise or that movement in a given case."

urgently need exercise. He advised mountain climbing for weak legs and discus throwing for the wrists of arthritics, and advised pregnant women to avoid jumping exercises (69).

Most of the books on medical and other gymnastics which followed were based on the scholarly researches of Mercurialis; and there were many. Timothy Bright, for example wrote two books (20) on hygiene and therapeutics in which he stressed the importance of exercise in the preservation of health, as laid down by Mercurialis.

The Seventeenth Century

In the sixteenth century Vesalius lead the rebellion against ancient dogma in anatomy. In the seventeenth century there began a revolt against entrenched opinions in clinical practice.

Joseph Duchesne (45), physician to Henry IV, one of the first to popularize the new doctrines of Paracelsus, wrote a treatise on hygiene in which he said, "Exercise is a salutory thing which guarantees the human body from many infirmities and diseases to which idleness and rest render it subject . . . it renders the body agile, strengthens the nerves and joints."

Sanctorius Sanctorius (117) wrote seven books on medicine, the fifth of which was on exercise and rest. "Moderate exercise gives the body lightness and vigor; it cleanses the muscles and ligaments of their waste products and prepares the matter for dissipation through the sweat. . . . Walking is a better exercise to bring on perspiration than motion on the litter or boat. Nevertheless, even these exercises continued for some time will improve the body perspiration. The best indoor exercises are handball, shuttlecock, dancing and fencing; outdoors, they are walking, bowling, equitation and riding in a carriage. When perspiration is low, the individual should exercise; it is the most important remedy."

Martin Luther[23] preached the value of exercise. "Music chases chagrin and melancholy; gymnastics produces a strong robust body and keeps it in a state of health. It can keep young people from idleness, debauchery and drink" (88).

Giovanni Borelli of Naples, a mathematician, became interested in the mechanics of muscle as a result of his friendship with Malpighi. He wrote a two-volume treatise (19) on muscle motion,[24] the second of which was devoted to the mechanics of motion. This book had much to do with the birth of iatrophysics, which culminated later in the work of Friedrich Hoffmann, the leading proponent of hygienic exercise in his century.

---

[23] Several religious leaders have been outspoken on matters of health and medicine. Moses promulgated laws of hygiene. Mahomet applied the cautery, Wesley wrote on electrotherapy and Mary Baker Eddy established a system of healing.

[24] *De Motu Animalium*, published a year after the author's death, is beautifully illustrated with precise drawings and formulae on the "laws" of motion. Borelli was a pupil of Galileo and a contemporary of Isaac Newton. His book is divided into two parts. In the first, Borelli said that when muscles contract, even against light resistance, they use great force. The insertion of each muscle is always close to the center of motion. Borelli believed that a

Toward the end of the seventeenth century, the most important physician in England was Thomas Sydenham. He had been a captain of calvalry during the Civil War, and it was only natural for him to become an advocate of horseback riding, which "strengthens the blood and spirits." He put his theory into practice by lending his own horses for poor patients to ride. Sydenham introduced horseback riding for the tuberculous.[25] His influence was felt for many years. It may be found in the writings of Benjamin Rush (37) and Trudeau, three centuries later. His most important immediate influence was on Francis Fuller, who wrote the first book on medical gymnastics in the eighteenth century.

The Eighteenth Century

Francis Fuller suffered from hypochondriasis, which he believed he cured by horseback riding (and emetics). His book, *Medicina Gymnastica*, based on his own experiences, went through nine editions and was translated into German.

Cheyne[26] was one of a long line of writers on the subject of living long (31). He included exercise, as did the others, in the hygienic regime. "Of all the exercises that are, or may be used for health, walking is the most natural, as it would also be the most useful, if it did not spend too much of the spirits of the weakly. . . . Using any organ frequently and forcibly, makes it grow plump and brawny. . . . Therefore, to the asthmatic, and those with weak lungs, I should recommend talking much and aloud. . . .To those that have weak arms or legs, playing two or three hours at tennis, or at football, every day."

Physicians who freed themselves from the dogma of ancient authorities sought new systems to explain and treat diseases. Paracelsus lived in the age of alchemy and saw in chemistry the basis of a system of healing. Borelli lead the way to the iatromechanical or physiatric school and influenced the triumvirate of Stahl, Hoffmann and Boerhaave, who saw in motion the most immediate expression of life (38). Of these, Hoffmann[27] did

---

man jumped because of the elasticity of the earth, an error caused by relying on mathematics alone to explain motion in man. Barthez (11) took credit for showing that jumping resulted from muscle contraction. In his book on motion in man and animals, Barthez gives good analyses of walking, running and posture.

[25] "The best thing I know to fortify and animate the blood and mind is to ride a horse every day and to take long rides in a carriage in the fresh air" (61). Stahl of Halle, one of Sydenham's contemporaries, also recommended exercise for the tuberculous. In France, Burette, another important physician of the period, wrote in 1707 on the importance of exercise in inducing perspiration.

[26] George Cheyne, a native of Scotland, enjoyed the good life so well that he grew to a weight of 445 pounds, which he finally decided was too many. He went to Bath to lose weight through diet, waters and exercise. In his *An Essay on Health and Long Life*, first published in London in 1724 (and which exhausted three printings that year), he devoted the fourth chapter to *Exercise and Quiet* (31). In spite of his weight he lived to the age of 72.

[27] Hoffmann was born in Halle in 1660 and at the age of 34 was named first professor at the University there, where he continued to teach for 48 years. His reputation was such that

most to establish the importance of exercise in hygiene and treatment. In 1708 he published *Dissertationes Physico-Medicae*, the sixth chapter of which is entitled *On Movement Considered as the Best Medicine for the Body*. He wrote, "We must distinguish with the ancients among movement, exercise, and work (*kinesis, gymnasion*, and *ponos*).

"Nothing favors the circulation more than motion of the muscles. While the muscles contract with a lively expansive action under the control of the will, there is a prompt contraction of the vessels, especially the veins, which accelerates the circulation and reduces the thickness in certain parts. We cannot afford to prefer other forms of treatment to exercise.

"We are reminded of visits to medicinal spas and believe that the movement which the patient executes in preparing to drink the water does more good than the waters themselves.

"There is no better remedy for biliary colic than exercise. Sydenham recommends riding on a horse or in a carriage for people whose condition has become chronic. 'I do not hesitate to state that in this way I have more than once cured this type of illness radically, something I have not been able to do with other methods.'"

One of the most interesting observations made by Hoffmann was that "Exercise improves the action of many medications, to such an extent that without it the desired effect cannot be obtained." He also quoted Galen as saying, "Exercise prevents gout."

One of the earliest discussions of kinetic occupational therapy (a genuine step forward from Fuchs), and one that possibly influenced Tissot later in the century, is Hoffmann's classification of occupational movements as exercise. "We shall place among the exercises, the occupational movements of workers and farmers—such work as threshing wheat, cutting wood, fishing and other agricultural tasks. The strength and good health which peasants enjoy prove to us how much these occupations contribute to the prolongation of life and the prevention of disease."

Hoffmann contributed very little to the advancement of exercise technique, but his name was so prominent in European medicine that the emphasis he placed on natural treatment, including exercise, did much to re-establish the role of physical exercise in daily life as extolled by the ancients.

The man who took the first real step forward in relating exercise to the musculoskeletal system was Nicolas Andry.[28] On March 4, 1723, he read a paper (38) before the Medical Faculty of Paris entitled, "Is Exercise the

when Friedrich Wilhelm, King of Prussia, asked Boerhaave for a medical consultation, the Dutch Sydenham replied that the best advice he could give was to send for Hoffmann.

[28] Nicolas Andry was born in Lyons in 1658. He was ordained a priest but renounced the cloth in 1690 to study medicine at Reims and Paris. In 1712 he became professor at the medical school in Paris, and its dean in 1724. He began to quarrel with so many people at the Faculty that he soon lost the (elective) position. At the age of 83, he gave the world the word "orthopedics" in the first book on that subject. He died in the following year. (Mauclaire, M.: *Bull. Soc. Franç. Hist. Méd.*, 27: 345, 1933.)

Best Means of Preserving Health?" Its first sentence was the key to his beliefs. "Of all the methods of alleviating and even curing many infirmities to which the body is subject, there is nothing to equal exercise."

In this talk he gave early evidence of his later work in corrective exercise. "It acts to halt rachitic disease in children." He suggested specific exercises and sports for reducing weight, increasing mobility and strengthening the spine. Almost a century before Ling, he said, "Fencing is one of the few exercises which contributes greatly to the development of all muscles, especially those of the arms and legs. . . . The right hand is stronger than the left because it does more work. . . . It is well known that those who have lost their right arm conpensate by increased strength and agility in the left arm and hand.

"Rest has its advantages. It repairs dissipated spirits and refreshes the fatigued body. It helps to cure many diseases, but under this pretext, to abstain from all exercise is a great error. . . . Let us remember that the abuse of rest is more dangerous than that of exercise. . . . There is in the space where the bones articulate a thick, slippery humor called the synovial fluid, which helps the movement of the parts. When this humor becomes to abundant or viscous it is more of an obstacle than an aid to motion . . . This abundance and thickness are the ordinary consequences of prolonged rest."

Andry's work was comsummated in his book *L'Orthopédie*, published in 1741, and translated into English 2 years later. He gave simple rules for correcting postural deformities. "It is likewise a good expedient for helping rickety children, sometimes to tickle the soles of their feet, on their sides. This throws them into such motions as they could not make without it, and these motions are so effectual, that sometimes they are sufficient, without any other assistance, to make the body recover its natural shape."

In 1699, Stahl, the forerunner of modern animistic medicine, encouraged the use of horseback riding in tuberculosis (124) and in the last year of his life wrote again on the therapeutic value of exercise (125). In 1748, two books on medical gymnastics were published in the city of Helmstadt (16, 57). Three years later, Richard Mead, who enjoyed the most lucrative practice in London, wrote (94), "It is obvious that exercise must be necessary to health . . . we see every day that the active are stronger than the sedentary." A few years later, MacKenzie (89), who along with most of his contemporaries regarded sweating as most healthful, urged that "When the perspiration is defective, the remedy is exercise."

Théodore Tronchin of Geneva studied under Boerhaave in Leyden where he later became president of the college of medicine. He became famous for his introduction of inoculation into Holland and Switzerland. The Duke of Chartres called him to Paris to inoculate the royal children in 1756. Soon after he was installed at the Palace, the idle rich of Paris came to him with their complaints, for most of which the custom of the day demanded blood letting, purges and emetics. Tronchin persuaded them instead to take long walks in the fresh air and other exercises. His success was rapid and dramatic; exercise became a fad among the nobility.[29]

It was during the second quarter of this century that increasing attention was paid to exercise equipment. Samuel Quelmalz described a suspened rocking horse (112) in 1735, for which he claimed the same therapeutic benefits as the living horse, which few could afford to ride. Pierre Chirac, physician to Louis XV, recommended the ancient exercise of riding in a carriage over cobblestones. The Abbé St. Pierre, inspired by Chirac, invented a vibrating chair in 1734, which he called a *trémoussoir*.[30] It was praised by physicians, by the encyclopedist Denis Diderot and by Voltaire, who insisted that it relieved his constipation (91).

In 1766, Nenci of Siena published a book on medical gymnastics (100) which emphasized the importance of exercise in preventing blood stagnation and increasing the all-important perspiration.

Chronic ulcers of the legs have always posed a problem for physicians: to treat with rest or motion? It is interesting to note that an entire book was written on the subject in 1770. Rowley (116) advised not only exercise but also vigorous motion, since "it must appear very rational, that where the cure of an ulcer is effected without rest, there will be no possibility of its being afterward affected by exercise."

The last quarter of the eighteenth century witnessed amazing strides in human thought and action. There were revolutions in political life and education and accelerated evolutions in the sciences. It is no wonder that in such provocative times there appeared the first book on therapeutic exercise as we know it today. In 1780, Joseph-Clément Tissot[31] produced a work so far advanced in its thinking and comprehension that its full importance was not recognized or implemented for many years to come. He broke with the tradition of the ancients by recommending mobilization in

---

[29] "Posterity will scarcely believe that a foreign physican could have such great success" in France with such unusual methods, wrote Chanel. (*Essai sur l'Histoire de la Médecine en France*. Paris, 1762.)

[30] Other exercise machines invented during this century included one by Tiphaine, mentioned in *Mercure* (113) for 1772, and the highly secret device which gained Pugh (110) many patients and medical endorsements. This century also witnessed the opening of the first Orthopedic Institute under Vesel in Switzerland in 1780.

[31] Tissot was born on June 4, 1747, in Ornans (51). His father was a cousin of the celebrated Swiss physician of the same name who 2 years earlier had published a very popular book on hygiene at Lausanne. Tissot obtained his medical degree at Reims in 1776 and soon after became secretary to Tronchin, who had Tissot added to the Palace staff. During the Reign of Terror, Tissot was thrown into prison for his affiliation with the Royal household but was soon released to rejoin the army, in which he had been appointed a surgeon-major of light cavalry in 1779. Ironically, he was later jailed for siding with the revolutionaries and again rapidly released. He campaigned in Austria, Prussia and Poland, and was made Surgeon-in-Chief of the army in Italy in 1808. While in Italy he was recalled because of a scandal concerning a woman who was reported to be more than the servant he reported her to be. His book, *Gymnastique Médicinale et Chirurgicale*, was translated into German, Italian, Swedish and Norwegian. (Information furnished by Colonel Hassenforder, Chief of the Museum Service of the Ministry of National Defense of France.)

surgical patients. Dally (38), a fellow countryman, who wrote the longest book on medical gymnastics almost a century later, dismissed Tissot's book as unimportant. The chief reason for this seeming slight is that during the century following Tissot, medical exercises continued to be prescribed more for their general effects than for strengthening weakened muscles or moving stiff joints. Tissot insisted that a knowledge of anatomy was essential in prescribing orthopedic exercises. He analyzed the motions involved in many manual and craft activities and improved upon the beginnings made by Fuchs and Hoffmann by advising the disabled to exercise through the motions of craft work. In addition to founding occupational therapy, he began the use of recreational therapy and adapted sports. Although Ling is credited with having introduced fencing as a curative exercise, Tissot wrote about it a quarter of a century earlier. (Andry, of course, had anticipated both.) "Of all the gymnastic exercises, fencing is not only the most active but gives the greatest number of stimuli to the whole body mechanism and sets all the muscles of the extremities into action.

"In fencing, almost all the muscles of the thighs, legs and arms are constantly contracting. The arm which holds the foil is in frequent pronation and supination and the ligaments of the moving joints are forced to stretch and protect them against all violent motions. This activity furnishes medicine and surgery a salutory means of strengthening the extremities, increasing the range of the joints as well as the circulation of the viscera."

His belief in the use of arts, crafts and occupations as kinesitherapy is repeated throughout *Gymnastique Médicinale et Chirurgicale*. "Most craft activities place the muscles of the upper extremities in almost continual contraction. According to their use, some activate certain muscles more than others. Anatomical analysis tells us which exercises to choose in the cure of certain diseases where motion is indicated. For example, if we wish to re-establish motion of the humerus and scapula, or the elbow and wrists, we may use the handle of the printing press, the axe, the action of rowing, the bowing of the violin, the drums, and those exercises (as indicated by the symptoms) which gymnastics offer to the surgeon . . . If the arms are shortened because the forearm flexors are stiff, the action of drawing water from a well will greatly stretch the biceps brachii and the internal brachial muscles. If supination and pronation are needed, such activities as making holes with a drill or beating a tambourine will often set into motion the pronator teres and internal radial muscles."

His ideas on respiratory exercises were most advanced. "If it is necessary to develop chest capacity, use those exercises which contract the pectoral muscles and thereby move the cartilages of the true ribs, which they pull each time the arms are extended or elevated . . . From the daily continuation of these exercises we will obtain a gradual lengthening of the ligaments of the shoulder joint and the muscles in this region will continue to grow stronger as will the thoracic organs and the thorax itself. We should add that the use of some of these exercises is good for the correction of spinal deformities in young children."

Tissot insisted that the surgeon regard exercise as much a part of treatment as anything else he prescribed or did. "If for example after a wound, felon or sprain has healed, there is a residual difficulty of joint motion, or if the difficulty of motion is related to a stiffness of the flexor and extensor muscles, it is up to the surgeon to choose the most suitable exercise indicated and if he can find none among those listed, it is up to him to devise one, for this is never impossible if a sufficiently profound study of the disability is made."

He was a vigorous opponent of prolonged bed rest. "To better demonstrate the abuse of prolonged bed rest we make the comparison with iron which rusts when not used. Motion has never rendered the limbs useless but very long periods of rest have done just that many times. It must be considered an absolute necessity to get the wounded out of bed and on their feet, especially when the lesion is in the upper extremities and the healing is slow."

Tissot's discussion of decubitus ulcers sounds almost contemporary. "The weight of the body pressing on the side on which the patient lies, results in changes in those parts which are prominent, especially at the coccyx. The pressure which these parts suffer soon results in inflammation and gangrene unless care is exercised. These changes come from poorly arranged bed linen, from moisture of putrid discharges which irritate and erode the skin... The remedy for these conditions we have borrowed from Dr. Stephen Hales.[32] It is to change the position of the patient often to avoid the formation of kidney stones,[33] to minimize compression of the parts, to change the linen often and to avoid the bad effects of perspiration and putrid discharges. Ambroise Paré, who noted this condition often, used the last two methods during the treatment of fractures . . . All these methods will not suffice to restore strength to the wounded . . . It is also necessary to get them off their beds."

It is difficult to understand why Tissot's recommendations for the management of hemiplegics remained ignored for so long. "The important point in the treatment of stroke consists in reawakening the weakened control of the brain by bringing into play all those body elements that sustain wakefulness. Motion can help in this urgent indication. Apoplectics must not be kept in bed. This position increases the propensity for complete rest and sleep . . . The horizontal position will serve them as a continuous incentive to remain inactive. We must try to recall sensation and motion . . . by tickling the soles of the feet . . . We are obliged to keep him occupied, even to the point of annoying him . . . When the patient's understanding has returned, he should be given exercise.

---

[32] An English clergyman who made outstanding contributions to physiology and medicine as well as to other sciences.

[33] Another example of an old idea rediscovered in the twentieth century.

"Apoplexy, especially when caused by a hemorrhage, is a tyrant whose sword is always held over the head of the patient he has menaced. That is why it is necessary to use different exercises during convalescence and for a long time after . . . Experience has shown that continued exercises taken for a certain period each day have been more useful to these patients than all the meaningless remedies which they have taken while stretched out on an easy chair or bed."

To conclude our case for Tissot's singularity, we quote from his recommendations on arthritis. "There is fever, swelling and pain in some parts of the body; sometimes in all the joints at the same time, in violent attacks of rheumatism. The condition of the patient is awesome. The action of his muscles is suspended, for the least movement will increase his suffering. He fears the approach of all who would help him. He cannot bear the weight of covers and the very motion imparted to the floor of the room by people walking on it doubles his pain.

"This condition is the same as that of acute diseases and requires the prescription of complete rest . . . Nevertheless, it is not proper to leave the patient totally immobilized, for there will soon result a loss of limb motion if we do not move him from time to time.

"Once the great severity of the disease has partly diminished, even though there is still pain and difficulty on motion, we must use motion, which is the best remedy. It is absolutely necessary to start motion to hasten return of strength in the weakened parts. Start with dry massage and follow with moderate passive motions . . . The greatest reward to be gained from assiduously continued exercise is the prevention of invalidism, which some have experienced after one or two prolonged attacks."

Across the channel, John Hunter was teaching anatomy before Tissot was born; nevertheless, for a period of almost 20 years they were contemporary. Hunter was the first surgeon equally at home in the basic sciences and the operating room. He appreciated the agonist-antagonist relationship of muscles, knew the importance of early mobilization following disease or injury and preferred voluntary to passive exercise. In his Croonian Lecture on muscular motion (68) he said, "Muscles are capable of being improved and increased in different ways by exercise, or employing the muscle much in its natural functions." He was the leading endorser of the system of therapeutic exercise (110) developed by Pugh.[34]

---

[34] In 1794, there appeared in London a book entitled *A Physiological, Theoretic and Practical Treatise on the Utility of the Science of Muscular Action for Restoring the Power of the Limbs*, by John Pugh, Anatomist. The book is possibly the most beautifully illustrated of any dealing with exercises. The anatomical plates are well labeled, and the kinesiology of each muscle is given. The author gives quotations on the virtues of exercise in hygiene and disease from Hippocrates to his own time and reproduces letters from some of the leading surgeons of his day, endorsing his work. There is no illustration or description of the machine, about which there was much secrecy. The machine was probably a treadle and pulley device with which it was possible for one set of extremities to give assistive motion to

In his lectures on the *Principles of Surgery*, Hunter discussed the use and value of exercise following fracture. "When union is formed, it would be proper to give some passive motion; but voluntary motion is always better, because the will is always sensible how far the powers of a part extend, and will attempt no more; but if force is used to extend a part ,all of the muscles of which have not their due power, may be thrown into such a situation as to give an improper action to a weak muscle; the will alone is to perform those actions she has determined on herself."

Hunter's successor and favorite pupil, John Abernethy, was a strong believer in the value of exercise. He is alleged to have told a gouty gentleman (41), "The best remedy is to live on sixpence a day and to earn them."

In 1779, Jean David of Rouen won the French Academy of Surgery Prize for the best essay (40) on the use of motion and rest in surgery. He advocated the use of early motion following fracture and other disabilities to prevent joint ankylosis. He credited Watson of the Westminister Hospital for introducing early mobilization in traumatic surgical disorders, "one of the most certain curative methods, the efficacy of which is established by experience."

The Nineteenth Century

Much of the credit for the rapid growth of the gymnastic movement in the nineteenth century is given to Ling,[35] whose thesis was "physical and

---

the others.

Pugh may have been influenced by the earlier success of another inhabitant of London, Buzaglo (25), who, a dozen years before, made extravagant claims for his secret exercises in the "cure" of gout. Buzaglo warned that unless Parliament or some other group of persons would repay him for the time and money he spent developing his methods, his secret would die with him. It did. He claimed that his patients gained immediate relief from the exercises which they performed themselves and which were superior to those recommended by Sydenham (horseback riding) in that they did not cause jolting.

[35] Pehr Henrik Ling was born in 1776 in the parish of Lingery, from which his forbears took their name. Little is known about his life before 1799, and much about his life after that year has been called "legendary" by one of his most accurate biographers, Carl A. Westerblad (131), from whose works (but not opinions) we have borrowed.

Franz Nachtegall opened the first private gymnasium in Europe at Copenhagen in 1799 with the help of King Frederic VI, whose interest in gymnastics was military. Soon after, by command of the King, Nachtegall was made Professor of Gymnastics at the University, where Ling was one of his students.

As a result of the French Revolution, noblemen escaped to other countries, where they tried to earn a living doing the few things they had mastered, and these often included fencing. Ling had had an excellent training in languages, particularly in French, and possibly through an interest in practicing the language, he attended the Copenhagen fencing school organized by Chevalier de Montrichard, where after 3 years he became sufficiently proficient with the foil to win an instructor's certificate in the art. Shortly thereafter, the aging fencing master at his old University of Lund sought retirement, and Ling's application to succeed him was approved. Ling believed that a good fencer should be a good athlete as well, and he imported and arranged exercise equipment. This widened interest lead him to formulate a combination of *fencing and gymnastics* which in time moral perfection" of the citizen through physical exercise (and epic poetry). Ling's great contribution was the introduction of system into exercise: dosage, counting, detailed directions. He classified starting positions and degrees of activity. He labeled certain exercises specific (even though they were not specific in a scientific sense). His system was empiric and sometimes bordered on the esoteric.

An even greater contribution, however, was the stimulation he gave to exercise for all. He had the backing of a king and the support of many loyal propagandists. Most of his ideas on the educational values of exercise[36] can be found in the education of *Gargantua*, written by a physician, Rabelais, in the sixteenth century.

Ling taught that all voluntary motion is produced by an agonist group of muscles moderated by an antagonist group. Although the moderating influence is necessary for ordinary motion, the antagonist action must be eliminated to obtain isolated motion of a muscle. To do this he replaced the action of the antagonist with a resistance placed on the bony lever in the direction of movement. This resistance varies according to certain "laws" set down by Ling and may be provided by the gymnast or patient. In flexion of the knee, the gymnast opposes the motion the first time, the patient offers his own resistance the second time. To the exercise in which

---

changes to *gymnastics and fencing* and finally to *gymnastics*. Ling learned that Nachtegall had opened a school for training gymnastics teachers in Copenhagen and wanted to do the same in Stockholm (80). He addressed himself to the Minister of Public Instruction. The Minister replied, "We have enough jugglers and mountebanks without increasing their numbers by state training" (88). But Ling was persistent and finally reached King Charles XIII, who, through the bitter experience of his country's reverses in the Napoleonic wars, favored any method designed to make better soldiers. By royal command, the Central Institute of Gymnastics of Stockholm was created in 1813. In the following year, Marshall Bernadotte succeeded to the throne as Charles XIV and was happy to lend his support to the Institute and the military aspects of exercise.

Soon after the Institute was opened, Ling began to develop medical gymnastics. Many patients and a few physicians were attracted by the glowing reports they heard.

Ling published two small manuals on gymnastics during his lifetime but nothing on medical exercise. After his death in 1839, his students published books on medical gymnastics, presumably based on notes that Ling had left. One such book was written by Augustus Georgii (56) in 1847 and by its title coined a new word—kinesitherapy.

During his lifetime, Ling was unpopular with organized medicine in Sweden, and, during the decade following his death, fierce arguments took place between the gymnasts at the Institute and the physicians at the two local orthopedic centers (which were patterned on those of France and Germany). It was not until 1864 that a physician, Truls Hartelius (81), was placed in charge of the Institute.

[36] Ling was neither alone nor the first to develop physical education in the early nineteenth century. Among others were Jahn in Berlin, Clias at Berne, Amoros in Paris and Walker in England. Jahn, who was born in Lanz in 1778 and died at Fribourg in 1852, was a great patriot who espoused gymnastics as the method of strengthening Germany for freedom through war. So successful did he become in arousing a warlike attitude among the German people that the Prussian government forced the closure in 1819 of all gymnasia in the country, only nine years after Jahn had opened the first one. They remained closed until 1828, when a government more sympathetic to Jahn's ideas reopened them.

the gymnast gave the resistance, he gave the name semi-active; to the other, semi-passive. To both he gave the name double or synergic movements. The two types of contraction which resulted he called concentric and eccentric.

Opinion on Ling's work varied from virtual worship by some of his followers to vilification by a few.[37] The movement of Swedish exercise spread throughout Europe and the United States.[38]

Charles Londe was the first French physician in the nineteenth century to publish a book (84) on medical exercise. It was concerned almost exclusively with hygiene. In keeping with the established pattern, it discussed exercises for the body as a whole, not the motions of diseased tissues.[39]

The interest in gymnastics during the Napoleonic era was naturally weighted on the side of the military and the traumatic. When the world settled down to peace again, there was a great resurrection of interest in civilian therapeutic exercise, especially in scoliosis.[40] The new movement was lead by John Shaw (121), who believed that curvature of the column was caused by weakness of the spinal muscles. Except for Andry, Portal and a few others in France, the treatment of scoliosis had been immobilization—in bed, in a brace, in suspension or in traction. Shaw noted that such treatment was ineffective, but that patients who fell into the hands of

---

[37] DuBois-Reymond, one of the masters of physiology of the nineteenth century, was also a master of invective. Schreiber (119) quotes him as saying, "A mere glance at the writings of Ling is enough to show that they are a product of that miserable 'natural philisophy' which for a quarter of a century made a laughing stock of German science. His arbitrary constructions, his empty-sounding symbolism, his meaningless schematizations, and pedantic terminology no doubt impose on such semieducated minds which, unable to detect the nonsense, accept a few scraps of anatomy and physiology as evidences of profound learning. For him who has any conception at all of scientific aims, it will require no little resolution to wade through writings in which one might reasonably expect to find at least a few valuable facts deposed by this well meaning though misled individual whose whole life was devoted to but this one pursuit. But here too we are doomed to disappointment. What there is in the book is laid down in a trivial, dogmatic way, and might, the principles being given, have been deduced by anyone. Nothing whatever in Ling's writings indicates a truly physiologically conceived explanation of the underlying facts."

Pichery (107) accused Ling of using obscure words and metaphysical generalities such as, "Every movement is a thought expressed by the body." Such statements "appall the French intelligence."

[38] The first physician to introduce the Ling system to America was George Taylor (126), who became medical director of the Remedial Hygienic Institute of New York City shortly before the Civil War.

[39] Londe's book was preceded two years earlier by that of P. Clias (32), a Swiss military officer, who presented his manuscript to the Medical Society of Paris prior to publication. The Society named a committee to review it. The medical committee under Bally had much praise for the work (88). They agreed that "among the lesions which, it seems to us, yield to methodical exercise of the legs and thighs, we place lumbago and sciatica which are difficult to relieve" and many other conditions such as rheumatism, paresis and imminent gout. The book also described tests with the dynamometer for measuring the strength of the fingers, arms and trunk.

[40] In 1822, Bampfield won the Hunter prize for an essay on the subject. In 1825, Charles Bell, Jarrold, Dodds and Ward also wrote on the subject.

professional rubbers sometimes improved. He advocated a treatment program of graduated exercises, massage and alternate rest periods. "From a conviction that the muscles are the natural supports of the spine, I never permit patients to go through fatiguing exercises unless they can take complete rest immediately afterwards, and in such positions as would facilitate the growth of the bones and ligaments in the manner desired.

"In the case where some of the vertebrae have become anchylosed or firmly united by bone, violent exertions would not only be of no avail in restoring the figure, but they would be actually dangerous. The opinion that the spine is strongest where it is anchylosed is founded in ignorance of its structure; for it has been proven, by various experiments, that the strength of the spine mainly depends on the elasticity of the peculiar matter by which the vertebrae are united."

Shaw's principles of exercise in spinal deformity were simple and direct. "First, to act upon the spine so as to alter the false position of the vertebrae, and consequently of the ribs and shoulders. Secondly, to keep the vertebrae in their new and improved position. The third and most essential object is to bring the muscles of the back into such a condition, that they will after a certain time, be capable of retaining the spine in its natural position, without the aid of any artificial support."

Shortly after the appearance of Shaw's work, interest in France was resumed. In 1827, Pravaz (109) wrote of exercise machines to use in correcting scoliosis. He described a shoulder wheel with an adjustable handle. "If the arm exercised, corresponds to the side of the dorsal concavity of the spine, it is evident that the scapula, drawn by the muscles which attach it to the humerus, will react on the column to efface its curves." He devised a teeter board with overhead pulleys and ropes for which he claimed great success. He considered this an advance over the "ingenious machine of Delacroix by which one can imitate the act of rowing through a series of weights and pulleys."

Delpech[41] became so interested in the subject of spinal curvature that he established near Montpellier (where he distinguished himself as professor of surgery) a remarkable school for scoliotic girls. In his book (44) on posture correction he describes the center and includes unusually fine drawings of exercise apparatus. He relied heavily on many devices to obtain suspension. "The advantages of suspension of the body by the hands from very elastic objects have seemed so great to us that we have incorporated it into most of our sports and have pursued this thought completely." He also espoused swimming, for, "When the body floats in the horizontal position, the weight is no longer placed on the vertebral column. The density and temperature of water are more desirable than those of air . . .

---

[41] Jacques M. Delpech was born in 1777 in Toulouse. In 1832, while driving to his orthopedic center, an assassin shot him through the heart. As his servant rose to prevent his fall another shot rang out from the bushes and the servant fell dead. The mystery of the double murder was never solved.

With the oarlike action of the arms, there is a genuine although light pull on the vertebral column along its axis. With this in mind, a swimming pool was built in the park of our Institute of Montpellier."

Delpech critically reviewed the approach to scoliosis recommended by others. He found the prescription of unequal weights to balance curvature unjustified, since "such a procedure will aggravate one or both of the curves as a direct result of the weights carried . . . It is easy to make conjectures; it is not as easy to support them; only a study of the facts will teach us something solid. We can now guarantee that nothing has as powerful an effect on tonus as well directed and well graded exercises, and that nothing is less objectionable."

Tissot had advocated motion following arthritis, but this suggestion was not widely accepted. In 1853, Bonnet wrote a very advanced text on the treatment of arthritis (17) in which he started that "absolute rest for diseased joints must be temporary. After a variable period, depending upon the acuteness or needs of the illness, we must give functional exercise . . . something between immobilization and full exercise. This intermediary we find in non-weight bearing passive motion. We could call this branch of medicine functional therapy . . . destined to take its place alongside the other branches of medicine."

The system of exercise proposed by Ling required the continuous personal attention of a gymnast. This could be tiring to the gymnast and expensive to the patient since a gymnast could work with only one patient at a time. Gustav Zander[42] gave this problem of economics much thought. He decided that with levers, wheels and weights, he could offer both assistance and resistance and eliminate the gymnast except for getting the patient started and infrequent supervision. With this thesis he won his Licentiate from the Medical Faculty of Stockholm in 1864. On December 20 of that year he demonstrated his machines at the meeting of the Swedish Doctors of Medicine and a month later opened his Medico-Mechanical Institute with 27 machines (81). Before his death, he had developed 71 different types of apparatus for active, assistive and resisted exercise and massage. Zander institutes were opened throughout the Continent and the United States. In many orthopedic hospitals, large areas were devoted to Zander apparatus. At first, machines were powered by the patient, later by steam engines, and still later by electric motors. For more than a half-century Zander machines enjoyed great popularity, but, with the advent of

---

[42] The work of Zander was carried to Argentina by Ernesto Aberg, who settled there and in 1884 published *Mechanotherapy of Zander*, the earliest book on therapeutic exercise in South America. Aberg's work was carried on by Argentina's first woman physician, Cecilia Grierson, who wrote *Practical Massage with Complementary Exercises*, in 1897. She was followed by Nicanor Palacios Costa, who founded a School of Kinesiology at Buenos Aires (1937), since directed by Juan Manuel Nágera and his foremost pupil, Claudia Olga Ceci. Under their leadership, a series of 25 monographs in five volumes, the largest work on therapeutic exercise ever published, was completed in 1958.

The Zander system was introduced into Chile by Cabezas. In Uruguay, therapeutic exercise was promoted by Rivero Arrarte and Bado (99).

the First World War and the establishment of many new hospitals, exercise programs had to be developed rapidly and with makeshift and minimal equipment. Further, most Zander apparatus had been made in the German city of Wiesbaden, and thus was not available to the Allies. During the war, emphasis was placed on exercise with little or no equipment. Soon after the war, Zander equipment went into storage or the dust bin or, in some instances, remained set up but seldom if ever used. This is unfortunate, since many Zander devices could be converted easily and profitably into devices in keeping with current concepts, for, basically, the ideas of Zander and his apparatus remain quite sound.

Zander made "dosage" more exact by using weights of known size and levers with graduated rules. He stressed "localization" of action by mechanical positioning. Lagrange was so impressed with the accuracy of expression in exercise made possible by the work of Zander that he wrote (76) of "medication by exercise." His limit of maximum dosage was fatigue. "By the daily execution of an exercise we see each day a postponement of the fatigue limit because the functional capacity of the organ exercised increases each day."

Zander's interest in exercise started with his attempt to cure scoliosis[43] (136). As he became more and more involved in exercise, he widened his fields of application with the invention of many machines. The introduction of mechanotherapy swept the imagination of physicians as no other exercise apparatus had before. By 1893 there were fully equipped Zander Institutes in seven countries, and Zander apparatus found its way into far off Egypt and Argentina. Zander had accomplished what his compatriot had failed to achieve—the acceptance of therapeutic gymnastics by physicians, at home in Sweden and abroad.

The year that Zander opened his therapeutic gymnasium saw the publication of a book on medical exercise (24) in Spain which was remarkable for its use of the word "rehabilitation" in its present-day sense, possibly the first such use. "It has been demonstrated in the anatomy and study of movements of the locomotor system that exercise may be limited to a single joint and even to just one of its motions, to the exclusion of all others. These constitute the special exercises referred to as orthopedic gymnastics. Based on this proposition we have established the general rule of insisting on such movements as may directly rehabilitate the muscle groups which are weak, and at the same time calling attention to the fact that the failure to use such special exercises is the cause of alterations in alignments and even of deformities."

Many discoveries have been made accidentally or incidentally. What distinguishes the innovator from his neighbor is the ability to recognize,

---

[43] Zander was born in Stockholm in 1835 (81). He took his first medical degree at Uppsala in 1856 and in the following year conducted gymnastic exercises for his sisters at a boarding school for girls that they established in Bararp. It was during that year that the idea of mechanotherapy occurred to him. "The insufficiency of my strength gave me the idea to substitute for it with mechanical agents."

appreciate and pursue the novelty. In 1867, Lucas-Championnière saw a woman who had failed to have treatment for a fractured radius. He noted that in spite of her failure to observe the accepted method of treating fractures — immobilization — she ended with a better result than most patients who kept their broken bones at rest. After years of trying this incidentally discovered method on certain fractures he wrote (87), "there is much evidence that early motion for the muscles and joints in the course of treatment of a fracture maintains flexibility and increases the circulation and nutrition of the part . . . In fracture of the radius, I have not used immobilization for many years . . . not only did I omit the use of apparatus, but I prescribed regular motions . . . The most striking result at first was the rapid disappearance of pain and the ability of the limb to regain part of its function very rapidly." The work of Lucas-Championnière was continued in the twentieth century through the efforts of Mennell (95) and Lorenz Böhler, among others.

As early as 1854, William Stokes of Dublin advised regulated exercises and planned walks for patients with heart disease (127). In 1875, Oertel (101) of Munich was told that he had a fatty heart, which he set about to cure by mountain climbing. He proposed a comprehensive regime for others with this disease, in which walking for several hours a day over a planned terrain was featured. The Schott brothers (118) enlarged further on the idea of exercise in heart disease. They devised a series of 19 exercises, involving one limb at a time, to be used by patients in early convalescence as a preparation for the "aftercure" of walking increased periods of time daily on increased gradients.

In 1874, S. Weir Mitchell (90) had proposed a "rest treatment," which he soon modified to include graduated exercise and massage. Mitchell did much to popularize physical therapy on both sides of the Atlantic during an era when physical education was beginning to assume new importance in schools and colleges in the United States. Chiefly responsible for the new movement were the exponents of the "Swedish System" and the "German System," who brought them along to America from their native lands. Their efforts would not have been as fruitful if it had not been for the concomitant work of two American physicians, Dudley A. Sargent of Cambridge and R. Tait McKenzie of Philadelphia. Sargent, whose major interest was in physical education, designed many of the exercise devices now found in American gymnasia, notably the modifications of Chiosso's pulley weights. McKenzie introduced physical education into medical practice and during the first quarter of the twentieth century was its greatest proponent in the United States.

As the nineteenth century was closing, neurologists began to pay more attention to the treatment of hemiplegia. Todd was the first to describe the posture of the newly erect hemiplegic. Erben recommended the use of short steps with flexion of all joints to improve ambulation. Hirschberg (65) distinguished three periods in hemiplegia: the first, immediately following the attack, in which he recommended absolute rest; the second (end of the first week), in which passive motion was begun to avoid ankylosis. "The third period is the time for muscle re-education.[44] The most important symptom is contracture, which sets in rather rapidly . . . Active motion is necessary in the third period. We ask the patient to move some part of his body and oppose it with resistance.

"The patient is not able to dorsiflex his foot, or does it only feebly. We ask him to try it while we place a restraining hand on the dorsum. The patient makes an effort at motion and if it is not completely paralyzed, there comes from the force of the often repeated exercises an amelioration of the paresis of the dorsiflexors. To complement this action we will plantar-flex the foot in opposition. The objective of this last motion is to excite function in the antagonists. If the paralysis is not complete, we will see the muscles of the anterior lateral leg contract while the foot is trying to overcome the resistance.

"The second motion which is in default in the lower extremity is flexion of the leg on the thigh. We ask the patient to flex while we offer light resistance. As in the previous instance, if there is not complete paralysis, the exercise will soon show results . . . During this period we see the other foot move. Sometimes the associated motion is in the same direction, at others in the opposite. Re-education can use associated movements to advantage. Thus, to stimulate extension of the paralyzed fingers, ask the patient to extend the non-paralyzed fingers, then the two simultaneously, and finally the paralyzed side alone."

Hirschberg (65) recommended methods of ambulation and exercises to prepare for them. "Advance the good foot a short step with the weight on that side. Then transfer the weight to the poor side and place the good foot next to the bad. Repeat. As a variation, carry the good leg back a step with the weight on it and return it to the side of the bad leg. March backwards beginning with the bad leg. Practice lateral stepping, first to the healthy side and then to the bad side. Climbing steps is good exercise."

It is difficult to understand why the progressive ideas of Hirschberg did not take hold, or, for that matter, why it took almost a half-century to rediscover them.

Tertiary syphilis has become such a rarity among civilized peoples that it is difficult to imagine how common it had become toward the end of the century. Ataxia of luetic origin was one of the most frequently diagnosed diseases of the spinal cord. The first to prescribe exercises to overcome ataxia was Mortimer Granville, who wrote about them in 1881 (65). In 1889 H. S. Frenkel of Switzerland read a revolutionary paper at Bremen. It was difficult to believe that an ataxic gait resulting from nerve cell destruction could be improved merely by repetitive attempts at supervised ambulation; yet that is what Frenkel claimed and that is what he did. By 1897 he had

---

[44] Raymond (113) coined the phrase "motor re-education" in 1896. The phrase was made the title of a book (47) in which Faure mentioned that "already there is an intelligent understanding between workmen's compensation insurance companies and institutes of mechanotherapy in France."

convinced so many physicians of the utility of his method that more than two dozen confirmatory papers, in several languages, were published (49). Luetic ataxia is a thing of the past, but ataxia remains, as does Frenkel's approach to it.

Frenkel wrote, "Theoretically, the transformation of an ataxic movement into a normal movement takes place in tabetic subjects according to the same laws as the acquisition in healthy persons of a complicated movement which acquires the differentiation of tactile impressions of minute strength. A certain minimum of sensation, however, is absolutely necessary; complete anesthesia precludes this application of the treatment by exercise, but fortunately, such cases are very rarely, if at all met with." Although Frenkel did not rely on elaborate equipment, he did insist on floor markings for the successive placement of the feet in walking. He preferred long paths to tiresome turnings. He advocated group exercises and suggested groups of three to six patients with similar degrees of ataxic involvement. His great contribution was the insistence on repetition.

MEDICAL GYMNASTICS IN RUSSIA

The reason for including paragraphs devoted only to Russia is that (a) there is so little information on the subject in the English language about what happened there in this area and (b) Vinokurov (130) published a book on the subject in 1959 with a summary of the history of therapeutic exercise in that country. The following two paragraphs are based on that chapter.

The first record of therapeutic exercise in Russia dates to the beginning of the seventeenth century. Physicians to the second Romanoff czar, Alexei Michaelovich, prescribed horseback riding, walking, running and hunting for his obesity. In 1765, the first Russian anatomist, A. P. Protasov, lectured on "The Importance of Motion in the Maintenance of Health." Ten years later, S. G. Zybelin of Moscow University recommended special exercises for both healthy and sick children. In the first Russian text on surgery, Busch wrote in 1810 that special motions are necessary to loosen tight joints following injury. M. J. Mudrow was the first Russian physician to insist that "we must treat the patient not his illness." In 1820 he wrote about the necessity of rational exercise and rest during illness.

In his book, *A Course in Internal Medicine*, S. P. Botkin wrote, "A patient who suffers from a heart attack and who has wrong ideas about hygiene and stubbornly keeps his muscles inactive will have shortness of breath on the slightest exertion. On the other hand, a patient with similar complaints who has not neglected exercise of his respiratory organs will perform motions without dyspnea."

The Twentieth Century

The most prominent new feature in medical practice during the nineteenth century was the appearance of specialization. Early in that century, pathology lead the way to improved diagnosis, and this was augmented by the coming of bacteriology and other basic sciences. The scope and frequency of major surgery were greatly enhanced by the use of anesthesia and sterilization; experimental pharmacology, begun by Magendie, advanced therapeutics. The concentration of war casualties in military hospitals and the rapid increase in the number of civilian hospitals lead to the segregation of patients with allied diseases. These were the principal events which gave birth to organized specialties. As the twentieth century opened, specialists in physical therapy were primarily concerned with electrotherapy, and therapeutic exercise was the domain of the orthopedists, the neurologists and the physicians at the spas. It was not until the Second World War that therapeutic exercise became an important part of physical medicine.

The twentieth century began in a world with less than the usual amount of strife. A generation had passed without a large-scale war between major powers. The automobile was a curious novelty, which the horse could outrace in a hundred yards and outdo in the number of traffic casualties caused. Mechanization on the farm, in the factory and in transportation accounted for relatively little skeletal trauma and the need for postsurgical exercise. With the world once more at peace, men could concentrate on peacetime diseases. Once more, scoliosis commanded attention, and, in 1904, Klapp[45] introduced a fresh idea in its management.

Klapp (73) believed that, if he could "mobilize" the spine and develop the trunk muscles with the patient in the prone position, he could correct or at least halt the progress of spinal deformity. He suggested that during their formative years, children with scoliosis should creep or crawl on all fours (73), with special attention to the inclination of the trunk. The nearer the trunk is to the vertical position, the lower in the spine is the region of greatest mobility. He contended that 1 hour of crawling was made useless by 11 hours of bad posture. He steadily increased the duration of crawling, so that eventually his patients spent their entire time as quadrupeds, even during meals and school periods. In 1926, he opened his first "home" for scoliotic children in Potsdam. They spent all their hours on all fours. "Considerable commotion was created when on one fine summer afternoon, all the children in the home started crawling on all fours out of the garden, along the street to the swimming pool. A policeman on duty followed this procession, shaking his head in perplexity." Klapp had to abandon the home because of several difficulties, chiefly, because the knees of the

---

[45] Rudolph Klapp was born in Arolsen in 1873. He studied medicine at Würzburg and received his medical license in Kiel, where he met August Bier, a surgeon who made great contributions to physical therapy. The two became fast friends and died in the same year— 1949. Both went to Bonn in 1904, and it was during that year that Klapp first introduced his "creeping exercises." He later wrote that the idea of walking on all fours came to him as he watched the back of his dog in motion. His technqiue was further developed by two gymnasts, Gertrude Schulz and Marianne Arnold. The famous Klapp School established by him in Marburg in 1928 was taken over by the state in 1944. The method of Klapp was attacked for overmobilization of the spine and because the children were treated in groups instead of individually. Klapp replied that it was too uneconomical to treat most patients with his method except on a group basis.

children were traumatized, and it was economically impossible to keep the children in the home long enough for their spines to straighten out. Although the full program of Klapp was not continued, the principles evolved by his school were widely used for spinal curvature.

With the advent of the First World War there was a marked increase in the use of restorative exercises in the military hospitals of all the belligerents. Examples of the progress made may be found in the works of Kouindjy (75) in France, McKenzie (90) in the United States and Deane (41) in England. Deane called attention to the fact that exercises had been used too infrequently in those recovering from trauma. "Much valuable time is lost by not putting men on gymnastic treatment early enough." He believed in varying the monotony of exercise by maximum use of simple but interesting apparatus, especially the parallel bars, "adaptable to disabilities of the body from the neck to the toes." He felt strongly that the sound limb should be used to a maximum to assist the weakened limb in exercising. He prescribed quadriceps setting exercises in knee disabilities. He also prescribed games as a form of exercise for the disabled. Occupational therapy as a form of medical gymnastics dates from this period. It was first instituted in a French military convalescent center by Bergonie, and the idea soon spread to military hospitals on both sides of the firing line.

There is strong evidence that poliomyelitis existed in ancient times; yet it was not until 1789 that Underwood first described it and not until 1907 that it became a serious problem in America. Robert W. Lovett, a Boston orthopedist, was called to Vermont to assist in the first severe epidemic in the United States. He soon concluded (85) that "muscle training constitutes the most important of the early therapeutic measures" and turned the exercise program over to his senior assistant, Miss Wilhelmine G. Wright. She developed many techniques, but most notably, the training of paraplegics to ambulate on crutches with the use of upper extremity muscles (135). In our opinion, the ambulation of paraplegics is the greatest of all achievements in the history of therapeutic exercise.

In Sweden, with its tradition of gymnastics, interest in therapeutic exercise never lapsed. Arvedson (8) recognized the value of exercises in musculoskeletal disabilities, especially poliomyelitis. "We know that the nerve cells which have been destroyed cannot be replaced by the formation of new nerve cells. But if such a cell is not completely destroyed it may recover. In poliomyelitis it not infrequently happens that some nerve cells at the seat of disease are not completely destroyed and because of this, as a rule, improvement gradually takes place in addition to that which appears early as a result of the subsidence of swelling in the disease focus.

"By gymnastic treatment, we can certainly not directly influence the healing process in the cord, but we can and should work to keep the joints, muscles and nerves in fit condition until the process of repair in the spine has progressed so far that the nerve cells which are not destroyed begin to recover their functional power. This should then be exercised in the best possible way.

"Impending contractures should be prevented by strong and continuous stretching of the antagonists of the paralyzed or weakened muscles. We should endeavor to discover and exercise the slightest remnant of power in the paralyzed muscles. It often happens that there is such power, though it may only be discovered by careful examination . . . Finally, we should try to exercise to the utmost, the patient's power of allowing healthy muscles to act in place of those which are paralyzed . . . To train such vicarious motions (as the tensor fasciae latae for the knee extensors) we should ask the patient to carry out the movement previously done by the paralyzed muscle in any way he can without regard to form. Formerly, it was believed that paralysis which remained after 6 months, in spite of proper treatment, would be permanent, but according to the experience of recent years, even after this time good results have been obtained, especially if the patient had not previously received gymnastic therapy." Little else has been added to the gymnastic treatment of poliomyelitis since, except for hydrogymnastics.

Exercise under warm water was recommended for paralysis by Aurelianus (10), but, as used today, hydrogymnastics as a word[46] and method is an American offering. Charles L. Lowman of Los Angeles, during a visit to Chicago in 1924, saw some paralyzed patients exercising in a wooden tank at the Spaulding School for Crippled Children. On returning to California, he converted a lily pond into two treatment pools and described its use in the treatment of paralysis in the December 1924 issue (86) of *Nation's Health*.

It has always been costly to build an indoor swimming pool; it has always been costly to maintain its environmental temperature in cold climates. But a large pool was not necessary. In 1928, Henry Pope asked the Chicago engineer Hubbard to build an indoor tank large enough for a man to stretch in, with room enough for the free movement of all the parts, not possible in an ordinary bathtub. One of the first to use indoor hydrogymnastics for poliomyelitis was Hansson (63), who, more than any other physiatrist in the United States, emphasized the value of gymnastics for musculoskeletal disease, between the two world wars. During that period, one of the very few papers prepared by a physical therapist (as specialists were called then) on therapeutic exercise (46) was delivered by Elsom in 1926. He spoke of it as "a neglected method in physiotherapy," but himself

---

[46] The word "hydrogymnastics" was coined by Dr. Lowman in 1924. Carl Hubbard installed the first metal tank in a hospital at the request of Dr. W. P. Blount, an orthopedic surgeon. (*J. Bone Joint Surg., 10:* 506, 1928.) The first modern indoor use of underwater exercise occurred at the end of the last century in the Petersburger Klinik (v. Leyden, E. and Goldscheider, A.: Ueber kineto-therapeutische Bäder. *Zeit. Diät. Phys. Ther., 1:* 112, 1898.)

neglected all forms of exercise therapy except those used in obesity, neurosis, digestive and cardiac disorders.

Since hydrogymnastics in the cold of the winter can be expensive, a substitute for it was proposed by Olive Guthrie-Smith, along with Sir Arthur Porritt (108). She placed limbs to be moved in canvas slings suspended by springs from an overhead frame. She called spring-resistance exercises "eutonic." In spite of little encouragement Mrs. Guthrie-Smith continued to improve her apparatus and method until the Second World War at which time interest in them spread throughout England and, in a small way, through other lands where they were finally recognized as the nearest thing to dry hydrogymnastics.

Backache has been so common among so many people for so long that a vast literature has accumulated on the subject. Until the twentieth century the diagnosis was usually divided among a few causes: rheumatism, sciatica, kidney disease and gynecologic pathology. With the advent of the x-ray, it was possible to identify curvatures of the spine previously neglected on clinical examination, and the narrowing of intervertebral spaces. There were occasional diagnoses of vertebral pressure on spinal nerves.[47] Fielding Garrison labeled "remarkable" the orthopedic group in Boston of which Lovett was a leader. In that city in 1934 there appeared the book "Essentials of Body Mechanics" which helped support that designation. Goldthwait (59) and his colleagues taught that many previously undiagnosed backaches were due to faulty posture or habits. A few years later Dandy called attention to the role of a previously ignored anatomical structure—the intervertebral disc as a principal factor in the etiology of back pain. Surgical intervention helped many but there remained those who were not improved and those for whom surgery was not recommended. In 1953, Paul C. Williams applied the principles of vector analysis to the rhomboid of spine flexors and extensors which control the lumbosacral spine. He proposed a series of postural exercises to strengthen those muscles and relieve backache. These have come to be known as Williams' exercises and are described in his scholarly book (133) published in 1965.

Ernest A. Codman, a Boston surgeon had some positive, but at the time, unorthodox ideas about the causes and treatment of shoulder pain. He wrote a book on the subject for which he could find no publisher, so he published it himself (33). He pointed out that in the erect position, the little supraspinatus must pull on the tuberosity firmly to keep it from touching the acromion. If the patients abducts the arm in that position, the strain causes great pain in the diseased supraspinatus, but, if the shoulder is abducted in the stooping position, the arm moves under the influence of gravity and the supraspinatus relaxes, permitting shoulder motion without pain. It required only a simple step from this to the *pendulum* or *stooping* exercises which bear the name of Codman.

---

[47] P. C. Williams: Reduced lumbosacral joint space—its relation to sciatric irritation. *J.A.M.A., 99:* 1677, 1932.

Exercises had been recommended for cardiac diseases, but not until 1910 were they proposed for peripheral vascular disease. Leo Buerger (23) proposed a series system of positionings in vascular disease, in which the effect of gravity and posture was applied to the vascular musculature and the blood column. The exercises which bear his name have been used most in the vascular disease which was named after him.

Even the most optimistic of gymnastic enthusiasts would hardly have dared to suggest that a simple exercise could be limb or life saving, yet that suggestion was made and documented for vascular disease. In 1951, Veal (29) showed that active and passive exercises instituted at the earliest possible moment could save a limb involved with the relatively uncommon condition, acute massive venous occlusion.

Following the First World War, there was a change in attitude toward exercises in Germany (74), and relaxation was stressed increasingly, especially since it was believed that such an approach was best for the great number of neuroses caused by the war and its aftermath. August Bier insisted that relaxation exercises be included in remedial exercise. He believed that sports and games were more relaxing than conventional exercises and insisted that they be included in the gymnastic program for patients. Exercises and sports for psychotics had been recommended as far back as the beginning of the Christian Era by Celsus (29) and resurrected in the nineteenth century by all the humane psychiatrists who subscribed to Pinel's new "moral treatment."[48] The management of psychiatric patients has varied with the number, quality and supervision of aides those in charge were were willing to pay for. In the early part of this century interest had fallen markedly in most places. During the Second World War, psychiatry came into its own and money. Auxiliary personnel were hired by mental hospitals in increasing numbers; activity and exercise programs assumed a new importance and appreciation.

In 1920, Kohlrausch adopted the relaxation philosophy of Bier in the treatment of internal diseases where hypertonicity seemed to influence the pathology. This led to the development of "crouching gymnastics." While sitting on a small bench, movement of the vertebral column can be performed smoothly; so can movement of the abdominal muscles. Kohlrausch believed that with relaxed abdominal muscles, such conditions as peptic ulcer and other functional diseases of the gastrointestinal tract are benefited. He reasoned that, whereas resistance exercises help those with atonic conditions, relaxing exercises help diseases in which the tissues are hypertonic.

The crouching position, with the patient sitting on his heels, has become

---

[48] Soon after the French Revolution, Philippe Pinel helped revolutionize the treatment of the insane by treating victims with human dignity—*morally*. The new treatment included a supervised activity program. In 1840, F. Leuret wrote in *Du Traitement Moral de la Folie*, "Those patients who can walk but cannot or will not work are gathered in the hospital yard and given exercise in the form of military drill . . . It is the beginning of a methodic, regular and reasonable activity which can be a starting point for the other activities."

a favorite in Scandinavia for relaxing the abdomen in breathing exercises. As the second quarter of this century began, thoracic surgery for pulmonary lesions became increasingly more frequent, first for tuberculosis and then for tumor. T. Holmes Sellors (120), who established a program of breathing exercises at the Brompton Hospital in 1936, credits J. E. H. Roberts as having originated the idea with the help of a speech therapist, Courtland McMahon.[49] So-called segmental breathing exercises were introduced there about 1940. After the war breathing exercises were also introduced for other pulmonary diseases such as asthma and emphysema, but Sinclair (122) seriously questioned whether these had any lasting value. Similar criticism has been aimed at breathing exercises for cardiac disease.

Therapeutic exercise has always proven most useful in reversible muscle weakness, that is, following trauma to long bones and peripheral nerves. Although there are more traumatic casualties each year in peacetime than in war, peacetime casualties are scattered; the military are concentrated. Each war during the past century has seen increasingly greater use of restorative exercises, and World War II followed the pattern. In addition to exercise departments at hospitals, many convalescent centers were established by all the belligerents where "convalescent exercises" (123) were prescribed for many hours a day. Once more, exercises were given in groups according to disability. There were "ankle classes" and "shoulder classes." Calisthenics and other exercises were given to patients while still bedridden, and programs of "adapted sports" were introduced, such as "wheelchair basketball" for paraplegics. Renewed emphasis was placed on "reconditioning exercises" to counteract the deconditioning, and the "abuse of rest" was rediscovered. Special centers were activated for some of the major disabilities. At centers for the newly blind, orientation in walking was given along with instruction in games; at centers for amputees, stumps were moved early and through maximum range in preparation for the prosthesis, which would require still another set of exercises for best use.

But the greatest stimulus of all to therapeutic exercise came from a young Alabama physician who had just been awarded his medical degree in 1943. Thomas DeLorme was an amateur weight lifter who carried his hobby with him into the army. While assigned to a military hospital in Chicago he noted that, following knee surgery, the quadriceps which became so weak, so soon, in so many, could be restored to full strength rapidly by increasing the resistance applied to exercising muscles (43). The method, which he called Progressive Resistance Exercise (P.R.E.), was adopted more rapidly and widely than any other gymnastic proposal in this century,[50] except for *early ambulation*.

---

[49] The techniques were later developed by the Misses Linton and Reed of the Brompton Hospital.

[50] The idea of progressively increasing resistance in exercise programs was not new, as DeLorme himself was the first to state. In 1841, Bienaimé (13) wrote, "It is not enough to

The most revolutionary change in exercise connected with medical practice in the twentieth century is concerned with patient activity following major surgery. With very few exceptions, it had been customary, following any abdominal surgery, for patients to remain bedfast for at least a week. In 1938, Daniel J. Leithauser (78) performed an appendectomy on a 38-year-old man who defied the virtually sacred regime of bed rest and insisted on leaving his bed and the hospital on the first postoperative day. The patient returned rapidly to his routine of daily activities. He did so well that Leithauser prescribed early rising and physical activity for all postoperative appendectomies, and soon for almost all patients following abdominal surgery. In addition, he prescribed "bed exercises" to prevent deconditioning and to dissuade the patient from thinking in terms of invalidism. Although at least fifty surgeons had previously reported on the benefits of early rising following surgery, it was the careful and convincing work of Leithauser which soon made postoperative bed rest as uncommon as it had been common previously.

Early rising following childbirth was not a new idea; primitive peoples practiced it, but in modern times attempts to alter the "time honored custom to allow the puerperal woman to sit up on the tenth day" resulted only in a shortening of the "lying-in" period.[51] In 1909, G. Gellhorn of St. Louis advocated post-partum exercises to strengthen the abdominal wall.[52] He described a rotary motion of the abdominal wall "familiar to all of you from the exhibition of Egyptian dancers." It was not until about 10 years later that post-partum exercises became popular in England. Another form of post-partum exercise to strengthen perineal muscles was introduced by Kegel.[53] At about the same time, Harvey Billing[54] introduced postural exercises for the relief of dysmenorrhea.

When Andry tickled the toes of children to secure a degree of motion not otherwise possible, he did not call it reflex exercise therapy, for he died just 9 years before Robert Whytt described the reflex arc.[55] It took another

---

turn the exercise wheel handle. The patient must experience the resistance, for without resistance the exercise has no effect . . . we must turn the thumb screw a little tighter each day to increase the resistance gradually and with it the muscular effort to overcome it."

[51] According to Williams, White in England had recommended early rising in 1776, as did Küstner in Germany in 1899. Williams, J. W.: *Obstetrics*. New York, 1927.

[52] "A revolutionary idea at the time." Adair, F. L. and Stieglitz, E.: *J. Obstetric Medicine*. Philadelphia, 1934.

[53] A pneumatic rubber chamber is inserted into the vagina. The patient presses down on the bladder, which is connected to a mercury manometer. She can observe the development of progressive strengthening with the "perineometer." Kegel, A. H. Progressive resistance exercise in the functional restoration of the perineal muscles. *Am. J. Obstet. Gynecol.*, *56:* 238, 1948.

[54] According to Billig, dysmenorrhea is the result of a postural defect of contracted ligaments which compress nerves. The exercises are supposed to relieve nerve compression through postural correction. Golub, L. J. Billig exercises for dysmenorrhea. *Philadelphia Med.*, *45:* 303, 1949.

[55] In his treatise *On the Vita and Other Involuntary Motions of Animals* published in Edinburgh in 1751, he showed that the reflex arc was independent of higher nerve centers.

century and a half for another Briton to explore reflexes minutely. At the end of the nineteenth century, Charles Scott Sherrington, an experimental neurophysiologist, developed the concepts to reciprocal innervation and inhibition. Several physicians were instrumental in introducing normal and pathological reflexes into exercise therapy, but chief among these was another neurophysiologist, Herman Kabat, who left the laboratory in search of a medical degree to put his ideas into clinical practice. He used the stretch reflex of Sherrington, the flexion reflex of von Bechterew and the tonic neck reflex of Magnus (among others) and called his method *facilitation*. Facilitation is especially recommended in patients with paralysis because of the high synaptic resistance produced by disease and disuse. Pavlov had shown that repeated transmission of impulse across synapses decreased synaptic resistance and resulted in new functional pathways in the central nervous system. By empirically trying different approaches, Kabat arrived at more effective techniques.

Among other physicians who developed reflex techniques in exercise therapy were Temple Fay, who proposed the amphibian reflex to reduce spasticity in children with cerebral palsy, and Frances Hellebrandt, who showed that by means of the crossed reflex it was possible to exercise one muscle and strengthen its contralateral mate.

In addition to exteroceptive and proprioceptive stimulation, facilitation can also be achieved with voluntary reinforcement. There is a rare form of speech loss which follows spontaneous unilateral superior recurrent laryngeal nerve paralysis. There results a unilateral vocal cord atrophy which prevents approximation of the two cords and thus normal speech projection. Brodnitz (21) was successful in producing hypertrophy of the remaining good cord by reinforcing exercises. He reasoned that since the cords approximate during certain forms of stress, as in moving the bowels but also in forceful gestures as in pounding the table while arguing, that his patients should make plosive sounds while extending their upper limbs with clenched fists.

In the eighteenth century, Hoffman said that exercise improved the action of drugs, but the action of drugs to improve exercise is a twentieth century idea. It is difficult to name a starting point acceptable to all. We choose the case of Doctor Harriet Edgeworth, herself a victim of myasthenia gravis, who reported on her ability to delay fatigue on muscle exertion by taking ephedrine.[56] This was not only empiric but fortuitous for it was later shown that fewer than 20% of such patients benefit from the drug. Truly remarkable was the work 4 years later of another woman physician, M. B. Walker of England. She reasoned[57] that the muscular weakness of myasthenia gravis was clinically identical with curare poisoning and treated the patient with the antidote and later its analogue,

---

[56] A report of progress in the use of ephedrine in a case of myasthenia gravis. *J.A.M.A.,* *94:* 1136, 1930.

[57] Treatment of myasthenia gravis with physostigmine. *Lancet, 1:* 1200, 1934.

neostigmine. In 1947, Ransahoff[58] reversed the procedure; he administered curare to "spastic" poliomyelitis muscles so that he could passively exercise them and prevent deformity.

Two years later the world was electrified by the announcement of a new milestone in therapy — adrenocortical steroid[59] which, by reducing inflammation of rheumatoid joints rapidly, made motion possible in sufferers for the first time in a long time. Soon after, steroid preparations were injected into joints suffering from traumatic arthritis, or into inflamed bursae and again made motion possible much earlier than previously feasible.

The greatest deterrent to voluntary motion in an innervated muscle is spasticity. The long search for a spasmolytic drug that would not produce weakness or drowsiness was reviewed by Lensman (79) in 1970. A few years later, the vaunted drug diazepam was challenged by dantrolene sodium. Mayer et al. (93) found that dantrolene reduced clonus, spontaneous mass reflex responses and was beneficial in therapeutic exercise programs in mild spasticity. The search for antispastic drugs continues as "drug potentiated gymnastics" captures the imagination of pharmacologists and clinicians.

In 1953, Hettinger and Müller (64) compared the relative merits of isotonic and isometric exercises in healthy persons to determine the value of such parameters as duration, stress and frequency of exercise. There were a few clinical trials of brief isometric exercises with results so equivocal that the method has not survived in the therapeutic armamentarium.

The first use of electrotherapy was to contract impaired muscles. Since the middle of the eighteenth century, there have been waves of interest and neglect of the ability of electrical stimuli to produce a lasting therapeutic or desirable effect. In 1962, Liberson and his co-workers (82) resurrected the subject by programming impulses to lower limb muscles in hemiplegics learning to walk again. A considerable interest in the idea lead to trials in several countries but because of the limited number of suitable patients, the costs and the technological problems involved, its use is not spreading.

ISOKINETIC EXERCISE

Time and again there have been therapeutic proposals based on scientific (as opposed to intuitive or metaphysical) ideas which sound so attractive that their failure to survive taxes the loyalty of scientifically minded supporters. One of these concepts is that of isokinetic exercise. Hislop and Perrine (66) reasoned that since muscular performance can be reduced to the physical parameters of force, work, power and endurance, the specificity attainable should be determined by an exercise system designed to

---

[58] Curare and intensive physical therapy in the treatment of acute anterior poliomyelitis. *Bull N. Y. Acad. Med., 23:* 51, 1947. In the following year, Kottke and his associates showed that curare added nothing to the treatment of poliomyelitis except expense.

[59] Philip S. Hench and his associates first used the drug synthesized by Kendall in 1949. J.A.M.A., *139:* 1274, 1949.

control each training need. This was the first new approach to applied muscle contraction since muscle setting (isometric) was introduced during World War I, as a step beyond the traditional usual contraction of daily work (isotonic). Isokinetic contraction is the control of the speed of muscle performance under a constant load. Although this can be achieved partially under water, or with the use of springs, in order to fulfill the difficult demands of continuously uniform stress through the full range of motion of most body joints, an apparatus was built by a manufacturer whose costs were so great that he asked a price which few could afford or were willing to pay for a device which was theoretically attractive but practically no more beneficial than coventional methods.

BIOFEEDBACK

The principle of the triode (radio tube) is that electrons emitted by a filament will move to a nearby positively charged plate whence they can be returned to the circuit to an interposed grid which can then be charged and discharged in a manner which will control the flow of electrons. The return of the electrons in the closed circuit was labeled feedback. Psychologists used the same word to mean that knowledge of any behavior returns to the system to control further behavior. The prefix *bio-* was added to emphasize that the energy fed back was of animal (usually bioelectric) origin. The electric energy generated by muscle contraction can be converted into sound or sight (electromyography). Perhaps the first American physician to publicize clinical electromyography was A. A. Marinacci. In 1960, along with Horande (92) he published the first article on biofeedback which he called audio-neuromuscular reeducation. He recommended that patients with neurogenic muscle weakness listen to the electrical potentials generated by their contracting muscle to identify minimal contractions and voluntarily "to bring these contractions once more under useful voluntary control." He reported results obtained in five different patients suffering from a variety of upper and lower motor neuron lesions and demonstrated that he fully grasped the procedure which was not used by others for another decade. "A 64-year-old man suffered from thrombosis of the right middle cerebral artery resulting in hemiplegia . . . The needle was then placed in the normal right deltoid and the patient was instructed how to generate the motor units . . . Again the needle was inserted into the paralyzed left deltoid. At once the patient was able to generate 10 to 15% of the motor units in this location from which there had previously been no detectable activity. The same procedure was followed in the triceps, extensors and flexors and the muscles of the left hand. Within an hour, the patient was able to develop 20% function in the muscles of the left upper extremity . . . in cerebral arterial thrombosis a certain percentage of cells have survived and they can be reeducated to transmit muscular impulses."

In 1969, Booker and his co-workers (18) utilized the visual display of myoelectric responses to achieve improved voluntary contractions in weakened muscles and this was soon followed by a spreading interest in biofeedback, not only for muscle reeducation but to reduce spasticity. (5).

Beginning in 1972 there was a rapidly increasing number of reports in the American literature on biofeedback as an adjuvant to the strengthening of weakened muscle, particularly in hemiplegics. The evidence at the time of this writing indicates that in some patients myofeedback is useful in reactivating lapsed control of voluntary motion.[60]

OPERANT CONDITIONING

Most patients are willing to give prescribed exercises a fair trial. Motivation, enthusiastic encouragment and individual improvement lead to perseverance. There are some patients, who because of mental depression, brain damage or low interest need to be prodded. There are many approaches to this problem. One of the more publicized in recent years has been that of operant conditioning. Skinner proposed the word operant to mean a nonspecific stimulus which produces a specific effect. Conditioning is another word for learning. Fordyce, a clinical psychologist, introduced the concept of operant conditioning into rehabilitation (48). The operants he used could be described as "the carrot and the stick." The treatment staff is prepared in anticipation of the arrival of the patient at the therapeutic setting to respond effectively but not obviously to patient attitude and performance. Thus, if a patient exhibits punctuality, industry and other elements of cooperation in his treatment program, members of the staff show by their speech, gestures and attitude that they are pleased. If the patient is inactive beyond the probable dictates of his disability, staff members show their displeasure by an apparent disinterest in him. Although the method was originally designed to attack the problem of pain, it is also used as an adjunct to exercise therapy. It would be proper to label this method a form of feedback.

Rehabilitation is a twentieth-century word.[61] At first it meant restoration, then it was used synonymously with the practice of good medicine. In the field once called physical medicine, it has come to mean almost any physical therapy, but most of all, therapeutic exercise (and often, only therapeutic exercise). There is safety in vagueness and comfort in using a comprehensive word, but there is not the accuracy which commands respect. Since exercise can be a precise therapeutic tool, it behooves those who prescribe and supervise it to call it by its proper name to reflect the scientific attitude which health personnel should bring to it.

---

[60] S. Licht: Biofeedback: Retrospect and Prospect. A paper read at the annual meeting of the American Academy of Physical Medicine and Rehabilitation, Bal Harbour, Florida, November 3, 1976.

[61] Although the word was used on rare occasions earlier, its present meaning (or, unfortunately, meanings) is quite new. See the editorial, "The Word Rehabilitation," in *Occ. Ther. Rehab., 27:*,124, 1948.

REFERENCES

1. ADAMS, F. *Aretaeus, The Extant Works of.* London, 1856.
2. ADAMS, F. *Hippocrates, The Genuine Works of.* London, 1849.
3. ADAMS, F. *Paulus Aegineta, The Seven Books of.* London, 1844.
4. ALLBUTT, C. *Greek Medicine in Rome.* London, 1921.
5. AMATO, A., HERSMEYER, G. A., AND KLEINMAN, K. M. Use of electromyographic feedback to increase inhibitory control of spastic muscles. *Phys. Ther., 53*: 1063, 1973.
6. ANDRY, N. *L'Orthopédie.* Paris, 1741.
7. ARNALDUS OF VILLANOVA. *The Conservation of Youth.* Translation by J. Drummond. Woodstock, 1912.
8. ARVEDSON, J. *Diseases Treated by Medical Gymnastics.* Philadelphia, 1921.
9. *Asclepiades, His Life and Writing.* Translation by R. M. Green. New Haven, 1955.
10. AURELIANUS, C. *On Chronic Diseases.* Translation by I. E. Drabkin. Chicago, 1950.
11. BARTHEZ, P. J. *Nouvelle Méchanique des Mouvements de l'Homme et des Animaux.* Carcassonne, 1798.
12. BASEDOW, J. B. In (38).
13. BIENAIMÉ, L. *Examen Pratique des Différents Osseuses.* Paris, 1841.
14. BLUNDELL, J. W. F. *The Muscles and Their Story.* London, 1864.
15. BOERHAAVE, H. *Academical Lectures on the Theory of Physic.* London, 1746.
16. BOERNER, F. *De Arte Gymnastica.* Helmstadt, 1748, in (38).
17. BONNET, A. *Traité de Thérapeutique des Maladies Articulaires.* Paris, 1853.
18. BOOKER, H. E., RUBOW, R. T., AND COLEMAN, A. J. Simplified feedback in neuromuscular retraining. *Arch. Phys. Med. Rehabil., 50:* 621, 1969.
19. BORELLI, G. A. *De Motu Animalium.* Rome, 1680, in (11).
20. BRIGHT, T. *Hygieina.* London, 1583, in (35).
21. BRODNITZ, F. S. Rehabilitation of voice and speech in malignancies and other organic disorders. *Am. Acad. Ophthalmol. Otolaryngol.,* New York, 1959.
22. BUCHOLZ, C. H. *A Manual of Therapeutic Exercise and Massage.* Philadelphia, 1917.
23. BUERGER, L. *Circulatory Disorders.* Philadelphia, 1924.
24. BUSQUEY TORRO, S. *Gimnastica, Hygienica, Medica y Ortopedica.* Madrid, 1865.
25. BUZAGLO, A. *A Treatise on Gout.* London, 1778.
26. CAGNATUS, M. *De Sanitate Tuendae.* Rome, 1590, in (69).
27. CANAPE, J. *L'Anatomie du Mouvement et des Muscles de Galien.* Paris, 1541, in (62).
28. CARDANUS. H. *De Subtilitate Libri XXI.* Paris, 1551, in (69).
29. CELSUS, A. C. *De Medicina.* Translation by M. Ninnin. Paris, 1753.
30. CHANCEREL, F. *Historique de la Gymnastique Médicale.* (Thèse) Paris, 1864.
31. CHEYNE, G. *An Essay on Health and Long Life.* London, 1724.
32. CLIAS, P. *Cours Elémentaire de Gymnastique.* Paris, 1819.
33. CODMAN, E. A. *The Shoulder.* Boston, 1934.
34. CORNARO, L. *Discorsi Della Vita Sobria.* Padua, 1558.
35. COULTER, J. S. *Physical Therapy.* New York, 1932.
36. CULPEPER, N. *Galen's Art of Physick.* London, 1652.
37. CYRIAX, E. F. *Bibliographia Gymnastica Medica.* Wörishofen, 1909.
38. DALLY. N. *Cinésiologie ou Science du Mouvement.* Paris, 1857.
39. DAREMBERG, C. *Essai sur la Détermination des Périodes de l'Histoire de la Médecine.* Paris, 1850.
40. DAVID, J. *On the Effects of Motion and Rest.* London, 1790.
41. DEANE, H. E. *Gymnastic Treatment for Joint and Muscle Diseases.* London, 1918.
42. DECHAMBRE. A. *Dictionnaire Encyclopédique des Sciences Médicales.* Paris, 1856.
43. DeLEORME, T. L. Restoration of muscle power by heavy resistance exercises. *J. Bone Joint Surg., 27:* 645, 1945.
44. DELPECH, J. M. *L'Orthomorphie.* Paris, 1828.
45. DUCHESNE, J. *Le Pourtraict de la Santé.* Paris, 1606, in (38).
46. ELSOM, J. C. Therapeutic exercise. *Arch. Phys. Ther., 7:* 65, 1926.
47. FAURE, M. *La Rééducation Motrice.* Paris, 1902.
48. FORDYCE, W. E., FOWLER, R. S., JR., ET AL. Operant conditioning in the treatment of

chronic pain. *Arch. Phys. Med. Rehabil., 54:* 299, 1973.

49. FRENKEL, H. S. *The Treatment of Tabetic Ataxia by Means of Systematic Exercise.* London, 1902.
50. FUCHS, L. *De Motu et Quiete.* Tübingen, 1565, in (88).
51. FULLER, F. *Medicina Gymnastica.* London, 1705.
52. GALEN. *De Sanitate Tuendae.* Translation by R. M. Green. Springfield, 1951.
53. GALEN. *De Parva Pilu.* Translated by R. M. Green for the author.
54. GAZIUS, A. *Florida Corona.* Lyons, 1510.
55. GENTRY, M. Un ami de Pichegru. *Prog. Méd., 6:* 49, 1929.
56. GEORGII, A. *Kinésithérapie.* Paris, 1847.
57. GERIKE, F. *De Gymnasticae Medicae Veteris Inventoribus.* Helmstadt, 1748, in (38).
58. GOLDSCHEIDER, A., AND JACOB, P. *Handbuch der physikalischen Therapie.* Leipzig, 1901.
59. GOLDTHWAIT, J. E., BROWN, L. T., SWAIM, L. T., AND KUHNS, J. G. *Essentials of Body Mechanics.* Boston, 1934.
60. GRASSET, H. *La Médecine Naturiste.* Paris, 1911.
61. GUERMONPREZ, F. *La Gymnastique des Convalescents.* Paris, 1905.
62. GUTS MUTH, J. F. *Gymnastik für die Jugend.* Schnepfenthal, 1793.
63. HANSSON, K. G. Hydrogymnastics in infantile paralysis. *Arch. Phys. Ther., 12:* 589, 1931.
64. HETTINGER, T., AND MÜLLER, E. A. Muskelleistung und Muskeltraining. *Arbeitsphysiol., 15:* 111, 1953.
65. HIRSCHBERG, R. In, Durey, L. *Manuel Pratique de Kinésithérapie.* Paris, 1903.
66. HISLOP, H. J., AND PERRINE, J. A. The isokinetic concept of exercise. *Phys. Ther., 47:* 114, 1967.
67. HOFFMANN, F. *Dissertationes Physico-Medicae.* Hague, 1708, in (38).
68. HUNTER, J. *The Complete Works of.* Philadelphia, 1841.
69. JOSEPH, L. Gymnastics from the Middle Ages to the 18th century. *Ciba Symposium, 10:* 1030, 1949.
70. JOUBERT, L. *De Gymnasiis et Generibus Exercitationum.* Lyons, 1582, in (38).
71. KABAT, H. Personal communication.
72. KLAPP, B. *Das Klapp'sche Kriechverfahren.* Stuttgart, 1952.
73. KLAPP, R. *Funktionelle Behandlung der Skoliose.* Jena, 1910.
74. KOHLRAUSCH, O. Personal communication.
75. KOUINDJY, P. *La Kinésithérapie de Guerre.* Paris, 1916.
76. LAGRANGE, F. *La Médication par l'Exercice.* Paris, 1894.
77. LeCLERC, D. *Histoire de la Médecine.* Amsterdam, 1723.
78. LEITHAUSER, D. J. *Early Ambulation.* Springfield, 1946.
79. LENSMAN, J. A. R. The use of drugs in the treatment of spasticity. *Proc. Roy. Soc. Med., 63:* 935, 1970.
80. LEONARD, F. E. AND AFFLECK, G. B. *A Guide to the History of Physical Education.* Philadelphia, 1947.
81. LEVERTIN, A. *Dr. Gustav Zander's Medico-Mechanical Gymnastics.* Stockholm, 1893.
82. LIBERSON, W. T., HOLMQUEST, H. ET AL. The peroneal nerve synchronized with the swing phase of the gait of hemiplegic patients. *Arch. Phys. Med. Rehabil., 43:* 547, 1962.
83. LITTRÉ, E. *Oeuvres Complètes d'Hippocrate.* Paris, 1839–1861.
84. LONDE, C. *Gymnastique Médicale.* Paris, 1821.
85. LOVETT, R. W. *The Treatment of Infantile Paralysis.* Philadelphia, 1916.
86. LOWMAN, C. L. AND ROEN, S. G. *Therapeutic Use of Pools and Tanks.* Philadelphia, 1952.
87. LICAS-CHAMPIONNIÈRE, J. Le massage et la mobilisation dans le traitement des fractures. *J. Méd. Chir. Prat.,* 1889, in (95).
88. MACAULIFFE, L. *La Thérapeutique Physique d'Autrefois.* Paris, 1904.
89. MACKENZIE, J. *The History of Health and the Art of Preserving It.* Edinburgh, 1759.
90. MCKENZIE, R. T. *Exercise in Education and Medicine.* Philadelphia, 1900 and 1923.

91. Marfort, J. E. *Manuel Pratique de Gymnastique Médicale*. Paris, 1907.
92. Marinacci, A. A., and Horande, M. Electromyogram in neuromuscular reeducation. *Bull. Los Angeles Neurol. Soc., 25:* 57, 1960.
93. Mayer, N., Mecomber, S. A., and Herman, R. Treatment of spasticity with dantrolene sodium. *Am. J. Phys. Med., 52:* 18, 1973.
94. Mead, R. *Monita et Praecepta Medica*. London, 1751, in (88).
95. Mennell, J. B. *Treatment by Mobilisation and Massage*. London, 1911.
96. Mercurialis, H. *De Arte Gymnastica*. Venice, 1569.
97. Messerli, F. *Histoire Générale de Culture Physique*. Paris, 1916.
98. Montaigne, M. de. *Education des Enfants*. Paris, 1572, in (88).
99. Nágera, J. M. Personal communication.
100. Nenci, G. *Discorsi Sopra la Gimnastica nella Medicina Pratica*. Luca, 1766.
101. Oertel, O. In *Ziemmen's Handbuch der Speciellen Pathologie und Therapie*. Leipzig, 1885.
102. Oribase. Translation by C. Daremberg. Paris, 1851.
103. Pagel, J. In Durey, L. *Manuel Pratique de Kinésithérapie*. Paris, 1903.
104. Paré, A. *Oeuvres*. Paris, 1840.
105. Petrarca, F. *Opera*. Basle, 1554, in (69).
106. Philostratus, F. *Gymnasticon*. Translation by C. Daremberg. Paris, 1858.
107. Pichery, J. L. *Gymnastique de l'Opposant*. Paris, 1867.
108. Porritt, A. E., and Smith, O. F. G. Method of exciting incipient movement in weakened muscles. *Br. Med. J., 1:* 54, 1931.
109. Pravaz, C. G. *Méthode Nouvelle pour le Traitement des Déviations de la Colonne Vertébrale*. Paris, 1827.
110. Pugh, J. A. *Physiologic Treatise on the Science of Muscular Action*. London, 1794.
111. Puschmann, T. A. *History of Medical Education*. London, 1891.
112. Quelmalz, S. T. *Novum Sanitatis Praesidium ex Equitatione Machinae Beneficis Instituendi*. Leipzig, 1735, in (38).
113. Raymond, F. La rééducation des muscles. *Rev. Intern. Thér.*, 1896, in (88).
114. Rédard, P. *Gymnastique Orthopédique*. Paris, 1762.
115. Rousseau, J. J. *Emile, ou Traité de l'Education*. Paris, 1762.
116. Rowley, W. *An Essay on the Cure of Ulcerated Legs Without Rest*. London, 1770.
117. Sanctorius, S. *De Medicina Statio Aphorismi*. Venice, 1614, in (69).
118. Schott, T. *Physikalische Behandlung der Herzkrankheiten*. Berlin, 1916.
119. Schreiber, J. A. *Manual of Treatment by Massage and Exercise*. Philadelphia, 1887.
120. Sellors, T. H. Personal communication.
121. Shaw, J. *Curvature of the Spine*, London, 1825.
122. Sinclair, J. D. The effect of breathing exercises in pulmonary emphysema. *Thorax, 10:* 246, 1955.
123. Stafford, G. T. *Exercise During Convalescence*. New York, 1947.
124. Stahl, G. E. *De L'Equitation, Nouveau Spécifique Antiphthisique*. Halle, 1699, in (35).
125. Stahl, G. E. *De Motu Corporis Humani*. Erfurt, 1733, in (38).
126. Taylor, G. H. *The Swedish Movement Cure*. New York, 1860.
127. Thorne, B. *The Schott Method of the Treatment of Chronic Diseases of the Heart*, Philadelphia, 1899.
128. Tissot, C. J. *Gymnastique Médicinale et Chirurgicale*. Paris, 1781.
129. Veal, J. R., Dugan, T. J. et al. Acute massive venous occlusion of the lower extremities. *Surgery, 29:* 355, 1951.
130. Vinokurov, P. A. *Lechebnaya Fizicheskaya Kultura*. Moscow, 1959.
131. Westerblad, C. A. *Ling, the Founder of the Swedish Gymnastics*. London, 1909.
132. Wetterwald, F. In Durey, L. *Manuel Pratique de Kinésithérapie*. Paris, 1903.
133. Williams, P. C. *The Lumbosacral Spine*. New York, 1965.
134. Withington, E. T. *Hippocrates, with an English Translation*. New York, 1927.
135. Wright, W. Crutch walking as an art. *Am. J. Surg., 1:* 372, 1926.
136. Zander, G. *L'Etablissement de Gymnastique Médicale Méchanique*. Paris, 1879.

2

The Morphological and Functional Basis of Therapeutic Exercise

_____ STEVEN L. WOLF

Accompanying the growth and sophistication of physical rehabilitation techniques, the more slowly developing body of academic and scientific knowledge provides growing justifications for application of these technological advancements. An underlying tenet of physical restoration has remained unchanged during this period: facilitation of purposeful movement in patients with neuromuscular dysfunction requires the application of professional hands directed by minds abundant with relevant information. To render a successful therapeutic outcome requires a firm foundation in all elements of the neuromuscular system. Without such a basis the formulation of an exercise program and the evaluation of its outcome are impeded. This chapter, then, is devoted to a review of muscle structure and contractile properties. Considerable attention is given to many aspects of the basic motor unit – the essential building block for motion.

Several important components of exercise physiology extend beyond the scope of this chapter. The reader may gain considerable information from excellent texts which discuss: cardiovascular (3, 14, 125, 141, 144, 200, 203), metabolic (6, 91, 144, 145, 147, 182, 213), nutritional (6, 26, 215), climatic (6, 88, 121, 133, 172, 181), respiratory (5, 6, 59, 72, 144, 181, 200, 214), blood flow (5, 242) and heat regulatory (5, 74, 132) components of therapeutic exercise.

Muscles are mainly formed by the union of extrafusal contractile elements which receive their innervation from axons that emerge from ventral roots of the spinal cord. The cell body, or soma of the axon, resides in the ventral horn as an alpha (α) motoneuron. Each motor cell supplies varying numbers of muscle fibers by successive bifurcations of its axis cylinder. The motoneuron, its axon, and all the muscle fibers innervated by terminal aborizations of this nerve fiber are referred to as the _motor_ *unit.* The outflow from α motoneurons is what Sherrington (207) termed "the final common pathway"; for it is through the expression of motor unit activity that movement occurs. Since therapeutic exercise denotes a variety and orderly succession of procedures designed to restore functional movement, it would appear that an awareness of motor unit properties could serve well as a basis for appropriate treatment plans.

Microscopic Structure of Muscle Fibers

The muscle fiber is a large syncytial cell of variable width and length. Like other cells, it is formed by a protoplasm, the sarcoplasm, which contains sarcolemmal nuclei, and is limited by a cell membrane, the sarcolemma. The myofibrils are a cytoplasmic differentiation in relation to the contractile specialization of this cell (Fig. 2.1).

The sarcolemma is a thin continuous membrane which corresponds to the plasma membrane found in other cells (235), and can be vitally stained by janus green (62). Under the electron microscope it appears to be a true membrane 20–100Å in thickness (99, 142). Since the nuclei of the muscle fiber are beneath this membrane, they are called sarcolemmal or subsarcolemmal nuclei. These nuclei are elongated and parallel to the long axis of the fiber and always occupy a peripheral position.

Outside the cell membrane of the muscle fiber is another layer colored by stains selective for connective tissue and reticulum. It consists of a network containing fibroblastic nuclei, more plump than the sarcolemmal nuclei and not strictly parallel with the muscle fiber. This outer membrane must not be confused with sarcolemma, a term reserved for the inner cell membrane, the active interface between the intracellular and extracellular medium, where the ionic changes inducing the action potential take place. The outer layer, designated as a basal lamina by Fawcett (89) is thicker than the sarcolemma.

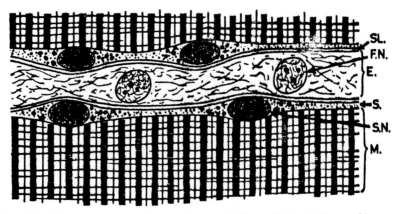

Fig. 2.1. Microscopic structure of muscle fiber. Abbreviations: *SL*, sarcolemma; *S*, sarcoplasm; *S.N.*, sarcolemmal nuclei; *M*, myofibrils; *E*, endomysium; *F.N.*, fibroblastic nuclei.

The sarcoplasm is the undifferentiated protoplasm in which the myofibrils are embedded. It surrounds the sarcolemmal and end-plate nuclei and varies in amount from muscle to muscle. As a rule, muscles in constant activity (ocular, respiratory) have the greatest amount of sarcoplasm, whereas muscles which contract quickly and fatigue readily contain the fewest (1). The sarcoplasm contains a diversity of granules of different sizes: mitochondria (sarcosomes), fat, and lipoprotein droplets.

The muscle fibers which contain much sarcoplasm or many fatty granules appear darker. There is some relationship between the general pigmentation or redness of a muscle and the proportion of dark to light fibers. For example, the red muscles usually have a contraction time two to three times slower than that of white muscles (60) (see p. 60).

This correlation between differences in granularity and abundance of sarcoplasm and differences in the physiology of muscle fibers has occasionally been erroneously interpreted as indicating a special contractile function of the sarcoplasm. Direct evidence of sarcoplasmal contractility in adult vertebrate striated muscles is entirely lacking, as Barer (15) has shown. The sarcoplasm must be considered as having mainly a metabolic function: storage of glycogen and specific enzymes used during contraction of the myofibrils. This role is sufficient to explain some variations in sarcoplasmic appearance in relation to differences in the muscle behavior.

The myofibrils are the only contractile elements of the muscle fiber. From Figure 2.2 we can see that the myofibril is but one component in a microscopic continuum ranging from the muscle fiber to its molecular constituents. Recalling that one micron (μ) is one thousandths of a millimeter and that one Ångstrom unit is one ten thousandths of a micron we can appreciate the size of the 0.5–1 μ wide and closely packed myofibrils. They are oriented in a longitudinal direction, parallel to one another, and run the entire length of the fiber (Fig. 2.2). In transverse sections, the myofibrils tend to be grouped into bundles known as Cohnheim's fields. In longitudinal sections, they have a periodic structure consisting of alternating bands of approximately equal length: dark (anisotropic "A" band) and light (isotropic "I" band). These bands are not homogeneous. Thus, "A" contains in its mid-part a clearer zone (H zone), in the middle of which we may find a dark line (M line). The "I" band is divided in two equal parts by the Z line (Fig. 2.3a). This line is probably a link between the myofibrils, whereas the other parts are independent. The dark band of each myofibril in a single muscle fiber is normally opposite the dark band of all other fibrils. This alignment is responsible for the cross-striation.

The contractile unit (sarcomere) is the portion of the myofibril included between two Z lines. It is 2.3 μ in length in the relaxed state. During passive stretching, we observe a lengthening of "I" and an enlargement of the H zone (Fig. 2.4a). During isometric contraction, "I" shortens and H disappears (Fig. 2.4b). At 60% shortening, "I" is replaced by a narrow band, the contraction "C" band. In this state, the length of the sarcomere is reduced to 1.4 μ. A slight shortening of "A" occurs only in full contraction.

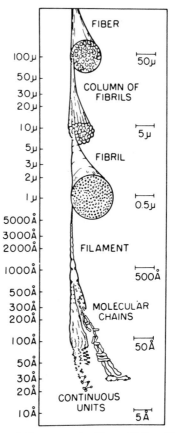

Fig. 2.2. Components of the muscle fiber. (After Buchthal and Kaiser as shown by Ricci (200).)

Electron microscopic investigations (131) and theoretical models (195) have revealed the complicated pattern of myofibrils and their modification during stretching and contraction (Fig. 2.3b). The "A" band is formed by protidic filaments of myosin 110 Å thick except at the level of the "M" line, where their diameter reaches 140 Å. They are parallel to each other and regularly arranged in hexagonal figures, as seen in transverse sections (Fig. 2.3c). The distance between two adjacent filaments is constant, from 200 to 300 Å. The "I" band is formed by filaments of actin 40 Å thick inserted between filaments of myosin so that each is surrounded by six filaments of actin. In a lateral view they are seen to overlap the "A" band up to the level of the H zone. Hanson and Huxley (116) believe that they are linked together at the Z band and the H zone by a thin elastic thread.

During passive stretching, actin filaments slide along myosin molecules. During contraction, they slide in the opposite direction and penetrate into the H zone until they meet at the level of M (Fig. 2.4). There is also shortening of actin filaments during this process. When contraction is complete, myosin filaments also shorten. Examinations of muscle with the electron microscope have shown that cross-bridges between the myosin and actin filaments extend across a gap of about 130 Å. Cross-bridges actually appear to be projections on the myosin filaments which may be the heavy meromyosin (HMM) end of the myosin molecule (156). The myosin molecules are arranged in bundles to make up the thick myosin filaments so that the heads (HMM end) of these molecules are always oriented in the same direction and always at the midpoint of the myosin filament. Thus in one half of the "A" band the myosin molecules are oriented in one direction and in the other half of the "A" band, they are pointing in the opposite direction. Therefore, during contraction, when actin filaments in each half of the sarcomere are drawn toward the center of the "A" band, they must be acted upon by "sliding" forces moving in opposite directions in either half of

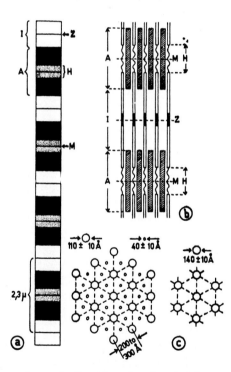

Fig. 2.3. Microscopic and ultramicroscopic structure of the myofibril. (a) Microscopic appearance of a myofibril in resting state. (b) Schematic representation of the ultrastructure of a myofibril in longitudinal section, showing the parallel arrangement of actin and myosin molecules. (c) Schematic representation of the arrangement of protidic molecules in transverse section at the level of the A band. At left, section outside the H zone; at right, section within H zone. Each molecule of myosin is surrounded by six molecules of actin. (After Hanson and Huxley (116).)

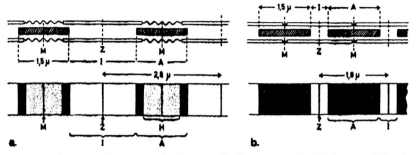

Fig. 2.4. Structural changes in the myofibril compared with the modifications of protein relationships: (a) during passive stretch; (b) during active contraction. (After Hanson and Huxley (116).)

the "A" band. The changes noted above for molecular arrangements are responsible for the sequence of events seen in light microscopy during stretching and contraction.

Orientation and Attachment of Muscle Fibers

There are several ways in which muscle fibers attach to tendons. In some flat muscles (e.g., sternomastoid, sartorius, gluteus maximus), fleshy fibers run *parallel* to the longitudinal axis and terminate in tendons or aponeuroses (Fig. 2.5a). *Fusiform* muscles, such as the biceps brachii, are considered to have a parallel array of fasciculi. Other muscles contain fasciculi converging upon one side of a tendon and run the entire muscle length. These muscles are referred to as *penniform* or *pennate* muscles (Fig. 2.5b) and may be *unipennate* (e.g., extensor digitorum longus), *bipennate* (e.g., peroneus longus), *multipennate* with fasciculi converging on several tendons (e.g., deltoideus), or *circumpennate* (e.g., tibialis anterior). The fibers of yet other muscles (e.g., adductor longus) may converge at a point after originating from a wide area (Fig. 2.5c). These muscles are termed *radial* or *triangular*.

The nature of the attachment of muscle fiber to tendon has long been controversial. Some authors believed that the myofibrils were attached to the inner surface of the sarcolemma at the end of the muscle fiber and were separated from the tendon fibrils which were attached to the outer surface (99). Others thought that the myofibrils were continuous with the tendon fibrils through the end of the fiber (49). Electron microscopic investigations have settled the question: at musculotendinous levels, the sarcolemma undergoes a profuse folding and the ends of the myofibrils are attached to the inner surfaces of the folded sarcolemma; the collagen fibrils of the tendon are attached to its outer surfaces (66, 99).

Histochemical studies have shown at the level of the musculotendinous junction an important accumulation of cholinesterasic activity (22, 65), which seems to be localized in the folded sarcolemma. These cholinesterasic cuffs are conical and form a cup underlining the end of each muscle fiber (Fig. 2.6). They have no synaptic function like the subneural apparatus of the motor end-plate. Whatever their significance, these cuffs have the practical interest of showing clearly where the muscle fibers end and thus allow some fundamental deductions concerning the anatomy of motor units.

Dimensions of Muscle Fibers

The diameter of muscle fibers can easily be measured on histological cross sections, in which they appear round or polygonal-shaped; their length can be estimated only by dissection of individual fibers or by indirect methods.

Diameter. The average diameter of fibers in most muscles is 40–50 μ (1), with each myofibril accounting for 1–3 μ of this diameter (92). There is a marked variation in estimated values from 20–80 μ, with a unimodal distribution curve (54, 160). For example the diameter of muscle fibers in the adult vastus medialis distribute about a measurement of 42 μ. There are also marked variations in mean diameter from one muscle to another. In the thigh and gluteal muscles, the average width is 87.5 μ; in ocular muscle, 17.5 μ (114). According to Feinstein et al. (90), the following differences in mean fiber diameters may be found: brachioradialis, 34.0 μ; first lumbrical, 18.7 μ; tibialis anterior, 56.7 μ; and medial head of gastrocnemius, 54.1 μ. Thus the average width of the muscle fibers is roughly proportional to the size of the muscle. In the same muscle, there are also marked differences in fiber diameter among people. For example, Coërs (54) has found in deltoideus 5 different mean values of 51.8, 46.7, 62.8, 62.9 and 48.5 μ. These values are considered to be high because of the frozen section technique of histology employed.

Length. It is generally believed that the fibers do not extend the whole length of the muscle, except in short muscles. This statement is based on the assumption that the length of muscle fibers seldom exceeds 5 cm (1) and usually ranges from a few to over 30 mm. However, a fiber 34 cm long was once isolated from a human sartorius (161), indicating the possibility

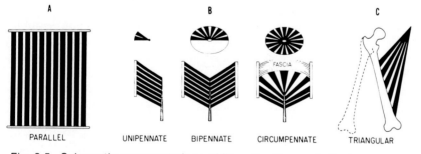

Fig. 2.5. Schematic representations of fiber direction and attachments which contribute to architectural nomenclature of muscles. (After Grant and Basmajian (102).)

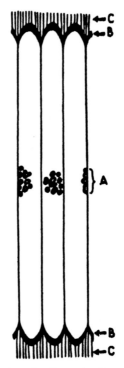

Fig. 2.6. Cholinesterase localizations in the muscle fibers. (A) Subneural apparatus, (B) cholinesterasic cuffs at musculotendinous level, (C) tendon.

that some fibers may extend almost the entire length of long muscles. Feinstein et al. (90) in a careful study were able to show that in some muscles with short fasciculi (interosseus, lumbrical, anterior tibial, medial head of gastrocnemius) all single fibers examined extended the length of the bundles. In one longer muscle (brachioradialis) a great number of fibers extending the entire length of the muscle bundles were also observed. On sections of this muscle, however, some fibers terminating in the middle of the muscle were observed.

As already noted, the end of each muscle fiber is outlined by a cholinesterasic cuff in histochemical preparations. The spatial distribution of these terminal cuffs shows clearly the mode of attachment of muscle fibers and indicates their length more precisely than the very difficult process of tracing an entire muscle fiber by microdissection or in serial sectioning.

The Koelle histochemical technique (149, 150) and its modifications (61, 134, 193, 231) enable investigators to localize cholinesterase in muscle. Coërs and Durand (56) were thus able to find enzymatic cuffs only in the vicinity of the region of tendinous or aponeurotic attachment of muscle (Fig. 2.12). Thus, it may be assumed that in these muscles most, if not all, of the fibers extend from one tendinous insertion to the other and in many cases are much longer than is usually believed, for instance, in some muscles formed by long parallel fasciculi, such as the biceps brachii or vastus medialis. Coërs and Woolf (57) have found only two limb muscles, the gracilis and sartorius, in which the cholinesterase cuffs were scattered along their entire length (Fig. 2.12d) thus providing evidence that these muscles are formed mainly by parallel bundles of short fibers which are intimately linked.

Innervation of Muscles

The muscular nerves contain a majority of myelinated fibers of various diameters ranging from 2 to 20 μ and distribute into two general groups (small: 2–8 μ; large: 9–20 μ). Among these fibers, approximately 40 per cent are sensory and come mainly from muscle spindles and Golgi tendon organs. These afferent fibers are in the large-sized group. The remaining 60% are the motor efferent fibers. About 30% of them fall in the small-sized group. This is the small nerve motor system (fibers) devoted to the motor innervation of muscle spindles (175). The remaining efferent axons (α fibers) supply the ordinary muscle fibers and fall in the large-sized group. They are 8–14 μ in diameter. Motor nerves also contain thin sympathetic fibers terminating in the walls of intramuscular blood vessels, which do not participate in the innervation of muscle fibers.

INNERVATION OF MOTOR UNITS

The ramification of the anterior horn cell axis cylinders begins only before the penetration of the nerve into the muscle. The greater part of the branching occurs after the penetration (77, 148) and continues up to the terminal nerve bundles, which spread in a bunch of nerve fibers, each of them forming a terminal arborization on a muscle fiber. The innervation ratio of the lower motor neuron (number of muscle fibers it innervates) measures the size of the motor unit. This innervation ratio may also be applied to the motor nerve fibers. It remains approximately constant in the proximal part of the nerves and begins to diminish when the nerve penetrates the muscle, each bifurcating fiber having a lower ratio than its parent fiber. The innervation ratio of the terminal axons coming from the last nerve bundles is of course very near unity. In fact, these terminal fibers are occasionally the site of a final branching, so that their average terminal innervation ratio is about 1.1:1 (54, 78) (Fig. 2.7).

Myoneural Junction

The motor axon produces a terminal arborization on the surface of the muscle fiber. The appearance of this branching is dependent upon the staining procedure employed. In methylene blue preparations many swellings are seen on the branches and on the extremities of the arborizations (57, 86) (Fig. 2.8). These neuroplasmic collateral and terminal dilatations are not stained by silver impregnation, which shows only neurofibrillar twigs, ending in tapered points.

As demonstrated by Couteaux (63, 64), the axoplasm does not penetrate

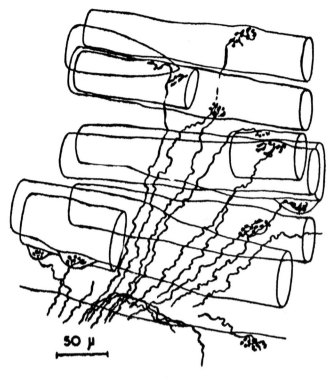

Fig. 2.7. Pattern of terminal motor innervation in human muscle. Only 1 out of the 10 terminal axons is the site of a bifurcation and innervates two muscle fibers, so that the terminal innervation ratio of this axonal grouping is 11:10. (Camera lucida drawing of a methylene blue preparation.)

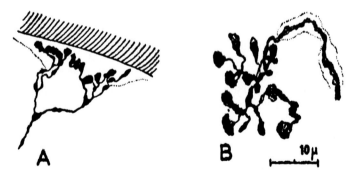

Fig. 2.8. Camera lucida drawing of human terminal arborizations vitally stained with methylene blue. (A) Lateral view; (B) frontal view.

into the sarcoplasm of the muscle fiber but lies in grooves on its surface. At these grooves, the sarcoplasm forms a structure with a spiny appearance, called by Couteaux the *subneural apparatus* (Fig. 2.9). This spiny or lamellar arrangement is due to a profuse folding of the sarcoplasmic membrane as shown by electron microscopy (84, 118, 201). These junctional folds, 500–700 Å thick, separate axoplasm from sarcoplasm at the ending (Fig. 2.10). Thus it is certain that there is a distinct barrier between the branches of the motor nerve endings and the sarcoplasm. The subneural apparatus can be considered as the postsynaptic part of the myoneural junction. It shows extremely high acetylcholinesterasic activity (64) and is very easily stained by histochemical methods for this enzyme, for example, Koelle's method.

In comparing histochemical to methylene blue vitally stained preparations, Coërs has noticed in human muscles that only the axoplasmic swellings of the terminal arborization come into contact with the sarcoplasmic membrane (58). Thus, in man, the subneural apparatus is formed by separate units having the shape of cuplets (Fig. 2.11) and does not consist of ramified gutters as seen in other animals.

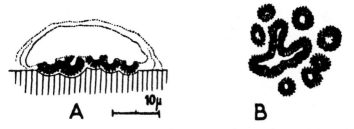

Fig. 2.9. Camera lucida drawing of human subneural apparatus stained by modified Koelle's histochemical method for cholinesterase. (A) Lateral view; (B) frontal view.

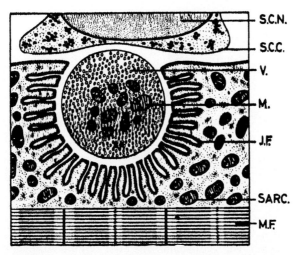

Fig. 2.10. Diagram of the myoneural junction from electron microscopic observations. Abbreviations: M.F., myofibrils; SARC., sarcosomes; J.F., junctional folds (subneural apparatus); AX., axoplasm; M, mitochondria; S.C.N., Schwann cell nucleus; S.C.C., Schwann cell cytoplasm; V, synaptic vesicles.

In a given species, the structure of the subneural apparatus is fairly constant, and variations consist mainly of differences in individual sizes in a given muscle and in average sizes in the different muscles. The average size of the subneural apparatuses in a variety of limb muscles in man is 32.2 μ. The extremes of normal variations are 10 μ and 80 μ. The distribution curve of individual values is unimodal like histograms of muscle fiber diameters (53). The variations in size of the subneural apparatuses seem to be parallel to the variations in diameter of the muscle fibers. In a given muscle, this correlation has been found statistically significant (53).

Thus, in human limb muscles the synaptic junction between terminal arborization and sarcoplasm is fairly uniform, and there is no morphological evidence that subneural apparatuses might be classified according to the possibility of two types of motor endings. The distinction between *terminaisons en plaques* and *terminaisons en grappes* established from observation of terminal arborizations only (78) has no value as far as the synaptic junction itself is concerned. This distinction has no functional significance and can no longer be considered as indicating a specialization of certain muscle fibers in relation to muscle tone.

TOPOGRAPHY OF TERMINAL MOTOR INNERVATION

The nerve endings are not scattered at random within the muscle but are concentrated in narrow zones. In most muscles, there is only one such area,

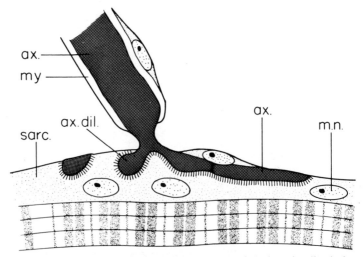

Fig. 2.11. Drawing of a motor end plate as seen in a longitudinal view of the muscle fiber. Terminal nerve branches lie in synaptic gutters and directly under the axoplasm-sarcoplasm interface, transverse sections of the subneural lamellae appear as rodlets. The axoplasmic dilatations of the terminal axonal arborization come into contact with the subneural apparatus. Abbreviations: *ax,* axoplasm with its mitochondria; *my,* myelin sheath; *sarc,* sarcoplasm and mitochondria; *mn,* muscle nuclei; *ax. dil.,* axonal dilatations. (After Couteaux (67).)

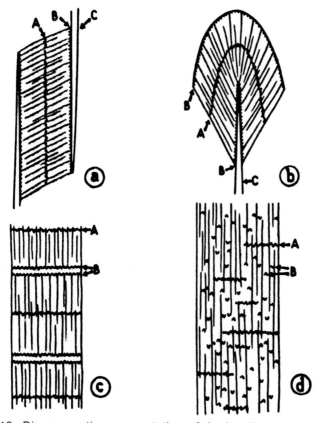

Fig. 2.12. Diagrammatic representation of the localization of subneural apparatuses and cholinesterasic cuffs in muscle fibers of various muscles. (a) Unipennate muscle, (b) circumpennate muscle, (c) metameric muscle (rectus abdominis), (d) gracilis or sartorius; (A) subneural apparatuses, (B) cholinesterasic cuffs, (C) tendon.

the shape of which depends upon the architecture of the muscle and the mode of insertion of its fibers (Fig. 2.12).

In unipennate muscles (soleus) and in most muscles composed of long parallel fibers (biceps brachii, vastus medialis), this area is straight and remains midway between the zone of origin and insertion of the muscle fibers. In bipennate or circumpennate muscles (palmaris longus, tibialis anterior), it occupies a curved surface, having in longitudinal section a more or less parabolic shape. These narrow bands are always midway between the zones of origin and insertion of the muscle fasciculi. In metameric muscles of the abdominal wall, such as the rectus abdominis, there is one zone of innervation in each metamere so that cholinesterasic activity is localized in equidistant bands containing in turn the subneural apparatuses and the enzymatic cuffs ending the muscle fibers (49, 55, 206).

In most muscles the fibers extend without interruption from one tendon to the other. Therefore, it should be concluded from the topography of the terminal innervation bands that each muscle fiber is supplied by only one motor end-plate, which is always situated at its midpoint. In the sartorius and gracilis, which are formed by parallel bundles of short fibers linked together, the distribution of motor endings does not follow this rule; they contain several bands of innervation scattered throughout their whole length (Fig. 2.12d). It seems likely that this disposition of end-plate does not necessarily indicate a multiple innervation of the muscle fibers as could be argued on physiological ground but, rather, mirrors the serial arrangement of the fibers and represents the usual simple innervation of these fibers at various levels in the muscle. However, since very long fibers have been isolated from a human sartorius (161), the possibility that a small proportion of these muscles could have a multiple innervation cannot be entirely excluded on morphological grounds.

Muscle Spindle

Structure. The muscle spindle is formed by a grouping of small striated muscle fibers enclosed in a collagenous sheath from which they are separated by a lymphatic space. This space is broader at the central, or equatorial, part of the organ and thus this muscle receptor appears fusiform, or spindle-like, in shape. The spindle length varies from 4 to 7 mm and its width can approach 200 μ. The grouping of striated muscle fiber is often called an *intrafusal bundle* which contains two types of fiber: *nuclear bag* and *nuclear chain*. Bag fibers are generally thicker and longer and have a group of nuclei near the equator lying in two or three rows (Fig. 2.13). Chain fibers usually display a single row of nuclei which are aligned down the center of the fiber. Beyond a 300 μ radius from the equator chain and bag fibers contain few nuclei.

Innervation: Sensory. The primary receptor ending or *annulospiral ending* is derived from large myelinated fibers and enwrap the central 300 μ of bag and chain fibers lying within a spindle. Smaller, less myelinated secondary receptor endings, or *flower-spray endings,* predominantly innervate chain fibers and usually are found beside the primary afferent ending. As noted by Matthews (176) the essential morphological differences between primary and secondary afferent endings rests in their location within the spindle and in their relationship to intrafusal fibers and not in their microscopic structure. Because of their larger size, primary spindle afferents are known to transmit sensory impulses at a greater speed than secondaries. While several essential differences exist between these two sensory muscle spindle components perhaps of greatest significance is the fact that primary receptor endings are extremely sensitive to dynamic (velocity-dependent) changes in extrafusal muscle length while both primary and secondary endings are almost equally capable of signaling changes in muscle length.

Innervation: Motor. Spindles receive their efferent supply from gamma (γ) motor axons, the activation of which produces contractions in the polar ends of intrafusal fibers. The resulting intrafusal contractions stretch the equatorial region of the spindle causing a deformation and subsequent depolarization of primary afferent terminals. Fusimotor terminations upon intrafusal fibers are called *plate endings* or *trail endings* (Fig. 2.13). Plate endings may be further subdivided into plate-1 (P_1) and plate-2 (P_2). Plate-1 endings terminate primarily upon the polar region of nuclear bag fibers and morphologically bear a strong resemblance to extrafusal end-plates (Fig. 2.13A). Plate 2 (P_2) endings (terminals for dynamic fusimotor fibers) are more diffuse and irregular than P_1 endings and appear predominantly upon nuclear bag fibers (Fig. 2.13A). Trail endings (terminals for static fusimotor fibers) are diffuse networks without specific termination loci and may extend over 80 μ along the intrafusal length of chain or static bag fibers (Fig. 2.13, *B* and *C*).

Spindle Response Characteristics. Stimulation of motor fibers produces no immediate visible extrafusal contraction; yet the involvement of the muscle proprioceptor efferent system is essential for maintenance of appropriate muscle tonus and for coordinated and integrated movement. The work of P. B. C. Matthews (173) became instrumental in delineating the behavior of fusimotor fibers. Both primary and secondary endings are capable of producing *static* muscle spindle responses which are simply the discharge rates at a specific muscle length. *Static fusimotor fibers* are known to decrease the velocity response of a spindle at the beginning or end of a dynamic stretch. They can also increase the static response of both primary and secondary spindle sensory fibers. The *dynamic response* of a muscle spindle afferent implies a discharge rate which can be measured during the course of a muscle stretch. The primary muscle spindle affer-

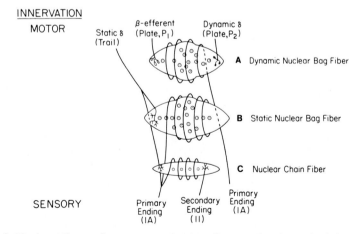

Fig. 2.13. Locations of sensory and motor innervation in typical dynamic (*A*) and static (*B*) nuclear bag and nuclear chain (*C*) intrafusal fibers. See text for details (After Eyzaguirre and Fidone (87) and Boyd et al. (28)).

ents are mainly responsible for this dynamic response. *Dynamic fusimotor fibers* are characterized by increasing the normal velocity response upon commencing or terminating the dynamic phase of a muscle stretch. Evidence accumulated thus far (83) seems to indicate the absence of any "intermediate" fusimotor fiber which would function somewhere between the range of static and dynamic γ axons.

Efferent fibers which end as P_1 plates have been identified as *skeletofusimotor* or *β axons*. These axons presumably innervate extrafusal fibers as well as striated spindle muscle fibers. The β axons have been shown to exert a dynamic action on the sensitivity of primary spindle endings during stretch (82). They can also activate the tension receptors, *Golgi tendon organs*, which lie in series with extrafusal muscle fibers. These receptors are simple in structure and are about 700 μ long and 180 μ wide. They reside at the musculo-tendinous junction or within the tendon itself (208, 209). Physiologically tendon organs signal small to large changes in muscle tension and provide an inhibitory reflex affect upon the muscles in which they reside.

There is very little question that the fusimotor system is a key component in a servomechanism which is constantly modified and influenced by segmental and supraspinal inputs. The activity in this complex system is important to the control of movement, posture and muscle tonus. Our comprehension of the muscle proprioceptor and its influence upon movement is still in its infancy. A more elaborate discussion of this essential component for integrative motor activity transcends the scope of this chapter. Several excellent texts (100, 152, 155, 157, 175, 187) and review articles (151, 174, 176, 221) should be consulted for details. In addition the work of Boyd (27, 29), Barker (16–18) and the French laboratories (24, 82) offer a contemporary appraisal of sensory and motor innervation of the mammalian muscle spindle.

Within recent years considerable attention has been given to microneurography, a technique wherein recordings can be made directly from afferent peripheral nerve fibers in conscious human subjects. From the studies on human muscle spindle afferent fibers performed primarily by Swedish (112, 113, 237–241) and German (44) investigators we have learned that for mild passive isotonic motions or in isometric contractions the human muscle spindle performs much like those in lower mammals. Clinical microneurography has revealed that the human muscle spindle primary afferent responds to stretch or vibratory stimuli; however, the sensitivity indices of both primary and secondary afferent endings in man appear somewhat lower than observations made from cat. Evaluation of microneurographic data also suggests that under conditions of moderate isometric contraction human fusimotor drive is intimately linked to activity within the alpha motor system, thus affirming the α-γ coactivation concept developed by Granit (101). A further comprehension of the human muscle spindle system may emerge as a result of future advancements in microneurography.

Composition of Motor Units

The motor unit is essentially a physiological concept even though it is a morphological entity. For the physiologist, a motor unit represents a group of muscle fibers whose function is indivisible in terms of the all-or-nothing law. From primarily indirect evidence, it has been estimated that a motor unit contains about 100–200 muscle fibers (50) and that the small muscles of the hand and eye concerned with finer movements have smaller motor units than large limb muscles performing coarser motions. Bors, for example, has determined that only 5 or 6 muscle fibers contribute to the extraocular motor unit in man (25), while Lindhard (159) has made theoretical calculations which suggest that in upper limb muscles the nerve-muscle ratio is 1:275; for biceps brachii this ratio changes to 1:1000 (40). It is usually stated that the fibers belonging to a motor unit are not anatomically grouped within the muscle but are separated into several bundles, each with its electromyographic expression in the "subunit" action potential of Buchthal (40), which now is conceded to lack significance.

The most valuable morphological study of this question has been performed by Feinstein et al. (90). They found in several muscles a great difference in the mean number of fibers per motor unit: platysma — 22, first dorsal interosseous — 305, first lumbrical — 96 to 97, tibialis anterior — 506 to 592, medial head of gastrocnemius — 1471 to 1742. These values confirm the assumption that muscles performing delicate movements (intrinsic muscles of the hand) have smaller motor units than muscles concerned with postural activity (gastrocnemius). These data have been confirmed by Christensen (49), who found the following values: rectus superior oculi, 23; opponens pollicis, 13; biceps brachii, 163; sartorius, 300; rectus femoris, 305; gracilis, 507; semitendinosus, 713; gastrocnemius, 2,037 muscle fibers per motor unit.

Muscle fibers are grouped into bundles surrounded by a connective tissue, the perimysium. In this way as many as several hundred muscle fibers are combined to form compact primary bundles. Several of these bundles merge to form secondary and even tertiary bundles. It seems unlikely that these bundle divisions might correspond to an anatomical separation of motor units. In motor neuron diseases producing a progressive muscular atrophy, the atrophied and normal fibers remain grouped into distinct bundles of 10–50 fibers. This pathological change implies that motor units are not anatomically separate but are formed by numerous bundles which are mixed together (245). The branching of nerve bundles in small muscles (lumbricales) also suggests overlapping of motor units and a considerable scattering of the individual muscle fibers of a single motor unit. This scattering has been confirmed by electromyographic recording (41).

Important questions emerge from these preliminary observations. If, in fact, the population of muscle fibers comprising a motor unit is scattered, what is the motor unit distribution within a muscle? How might these motor units be visualized? What are the functional characteristics of motor unit populations for a given muscle? It would appear that answers to these inquiries should provide information which is essential to the development of an appropriate therapeutic exercise regime. The histochemical and physiological advances of the past decade have produced significant information. In the sections which follow we examine ways which lend clarity to our comprehension of motor unit profiles.

Contractile Properties of the Motor Unit

There is very little question that movement induced in an intact muscle is, "a function both of the contractile machinery and of the passive elastic elements" (43). Contractile mechanisms may vary between muscles and are related to force-velocity relationships and tetanic tensions. Elastic or compilance elements are inherent to muscle by virtue of associated connective tissue and tendon. Through the detailed work of Hill (128, 129), we have come to better understand the time course of the "active" muscle. The rise time for a contraction occurs quickly, in the order of just a few milliseconds. The duration of a contraction is dependent upon the nature of contractile elements within the muscle and is modified by elastic elements. The unique contributions offered by each muscle are contingent upon the muscle's basic constituents. Thus, such factors as rate of rise, maximal tension output, and duration and frequency of contraction define the participation of each motor unit during volitional or reflexly induced movement.

Evidence (75, 109, 115, 130) accumulated thus far suggests that differentiation of muscle fiber types occurs at various times following birth. Muscles in many newborn mammals possess a large number of slow-twitch motor units compared to their adult forms. Differences in physiological behavior among motor units within a muscle are based upon several measurements which have been derived primarily from investigations in adult animals. Some of these measurements include:

1. *Motor unit size*: The number of muscle fibers in one motor unit.
2. *Conduction velocity*: The speed (usually expressed as meters per second) required for an impulse to travel a defined distance along the motor axon innervating a group of muscle fibers.
3. *Twitch tension*: The amount of force (usually expressed in grams) generated by the isometric contraction of a motor unit in response to electrical or volitional activation of its motor axon.
4. *Tetanic tension*: The amount of isometric force (usually expressed in grams) generated by a motor unit in response to a tetanizing stimulus of know parameters applied to its motor axon.
5. *Twitch:Tetanus ratio*: The proportion obtained by dividing the value of a twitch tension of a motor unit by its tetanus tension value.
6. *Resistance to fatigue*: The ability of a motor unit to maintain a given isometric force during repetitive activation at known stimulation parameters for a defined time interval.
7. *"Sag" property*: A motor unit's display of reducing tension output during repetitive activation of its motor axon at submaximal (unfused) stimulating parameters for a tetanic contraction.

8. *Time to peak*: The amount of time required to achieve maximal tension in a motor unit following activation of its motor axon.
9. *Half-relaxation time*: The amount of time between peak tension to half this value for a motor unit.
10. *Twitch contraction post-tetanic potentiation*: The increased tension from activation of a motor unit following a high frequency tetanic stimulation of its motor axon.

There are additional properties of both the motor unit and its innervating motor neuron which can be used to characterize a grouping of muscle fibers. A discussion of these factors may be found elsewhere (45, 53, 87).

A muscle is comprised of varying numbers of motor units (see p. 59) which individually contribute to its total contraction speed, power, and resistance to fatigue. Generally muscles have been described as *phasic* and *tonic*, or *white* and *red*, on the basis of several considerations including those discussed above for motor units. There is very little question that all the muscle fibers of a motor unit are similar in their histochemical, morphological and functional composition. Many of the properties ascribed to phasic and tonic motor units can be seen in Table 2.1, and some of the essential differences between the time course of a twitch contraction of phasic and tonic motor units are shown in Figure 2.14. It is difficult to cite one unique characteristic that clearly separates these two unit types. Histochemical (see below) and physiological data suggest that in man

TABLE 2.1. *Some Anatomical and Physiological Characteristics of Motor Units*

Property	Motor Unit Type		
	Slow (red)	Fast (white)	Medium
1. Motor unit size	Small	Large	Intermediate to large
2. Conduction velocity	Slow	Fast	Similar to fast
3. Twitch tension	Low	High	Intermediate
4. Tetanic tension	Low	High	Intermediate
5. Twitch:tetanus ratio	High	Low	Intermediate
6. Resistance to fatigue	High	Low	High
7. "Sag" property	Absent	Rapidly occurring	Present
8. Time to peak	Slow	Fast	Intermediate
9. Half-relaxation time	Longer	Shorter	Intermediate
10. Twitch contraction post-tetanic potentiation	Poor → good	Good	Intermediate

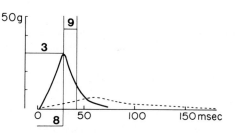

Fig. 2.14. Comparison of time course and magnitude of isometric twitch tension in a fast (heavy solid trace) and slow (dotted trace) motor unit. Numbers *3, 8,* and *9* refer to motor unit properties described in Table 2.1.

muscles which contain primarily tonic motor units are resistant to fatigue, adapted for prolonged contractions and participate in maintenance of posture (anti-gravity muscles). Most flexor muscles and many whose primary function is to extend a body segment contain predominantly phasic motor units. These muscles are capable of producing strong, rapid contractions which are essential for dynamic movements; but they are not fatigue-resistant. Several investigators (70, 146, 192) have attempted to describe the primary function of many human muscles.

As can be seen in Table 2.1, a third category of motor unit has been identified. The physiological properties of these motor units lie somewhere between those of the "fast-twitch" and "slow-twitch" variety. This third group is said to be *intermediate* in composition. It should be emphasized that intermediate motor units probably do not represent a specific class but possess characteristics which place them somewhere along a continuum which ranges from phasic to tonic. Whether intermediate fiber types are capable of changing to red or white fibers is uncertain but evidence to date argues against this possibility. A more plausible and teleological argument for the role of intermediate type motor units has been advanced by Stuart and colleagues (199, 225, 226) who feel that quantitative and qualitative differences for a muscle's intermediate units may be species dependent and determined by environmental and natural factors. These factors would probably include whether an animal was confined or free (i.e., domestic vs. wild), and whether powerful movements were required for survival.

SIZE PRINCIPLE AND THE RECRUITMENT OF MOTOR UNITS

From experiments in the decerebrate cat Henneman and co-workers (119, 120, 216) noted that smaller motoneurons, as determined from the relative amplitudes of ventral root filament recordings, usually were activated before larger motoneurons in response to controlled electrical stimulation. Since smaller motoneurons are known to be primarily "tonic" in function, it would follow that tonic motor units would be recruited before phasic units. The *size principle* which was hypothesized by Henneman would have obvious implications for therapeutic exercise. If correct, this theory would suggest that minimal contractions or forces which generate low muscle tension would preferentially activate tonic motor units. For example, knowing that this type of unit possesses a comparatively high resistance to fatigue would indicate that repeated mild contractions could be sustained for comparatively long periods as part of a training procedure. Grimby and colleagues (104) have demonstrated that during fatiguing exercise in spastic patients the recruitment order may reverse as fatigue is approached and ultimately become indefinite. The original tonic-to-phasic recruitment pattern may be restored, however, by rest or by tonic reflex support of voluntary muscle activation. To date, reflex testing experiments (230) in muscles of the human lower and upper limbs have provided evidence which supports the size principle as a basis for predicting motor unit recruitment. It should be noted that recruitment orders are not absolute (46) and may be altered by changes in the speed of movement, resistance to movement, co-contraction or by supraspinal influences (103, 179, 229).

Histochemical Properties of Motor Units

Because muscle fibers require energy to perform repeated contractions considerable research has been undertaken to determine metabolic pathways which may help to categorize motor unit behavior. Generally tonic muscle fibers have been shown to have a more plentiful capillary supply (202) thus providing these muscular elements with more oxygenated blood and contributing to their "red" appearance. By examining protein and enzymatic content in muscle fibers it has been concluded that red muscle fibers have a higher oxidative capacity and white fibers have a higher glycolytic activity per gram of muscle. Since phasic muscle units primarily utilize anaerobic metabolic pathways (glycogen metabolism) we can readily appreciate why lactate and pyruvate-related products accumulate with exercise and how these fibers can fatigue in comparatively short order. Conversely, the belief that tonic or slow-twitch fibers have a higher oxidative capacity is supported by the observation that red fibers are rich in mitochondria and mitochondrial protein and can utilize fat stores better than their white or fast-twitch counterparts.

From the volume of research concerning histochemical properties of muscle the novice may be easily confused about the diverse nomenclature which has developed within the literature (see, for example, reference 52). Generally type B or type I muscle fibers have become associated with red or slow muscle fibers (oxidative metabolism) while type A or type II muscle fibers are related to fast or white muscle fibers (glycolytic metabolism). Of course, as with physiological studies, so-called "intermediate" fiber types have been identified with histochemical techniques. These fibers are sometimes called type C or type III fibers, but because of their vast staining properties, they fit a wide range of categories. There are at least 36 histochemical assays for identifying enzymatic activity in muscle fibers. Information concerning histochemical stains of human muscle (76, 81, 85, 135, 146, 186, 197) and errors in staining procedures (31, 106–108) are readily available.

Histochemical analyses in human autopsy material (138) indicate that many human muscles contain both type I and II muscle fibers. Muscles which serve primarily a tonic function possess a preponderance of type I fibers, and those muscles which perform dynamic movements have more of the type II variety. Human muscles which fulfill both tonic and phasic functions (e.g., gastrocnemius, pectoralis major, deep portion of biceps brachii) do not show a significant difference in fiber type composition. Initial attempts to determine the spatial distribution of fiber types indicate that these are randomly dispersed in most muscles; however this method of exploration requires further systematic study utilizing biopsy techniques.

Examination of biopsied muscle samples taken from patients with various neuromuscular disorders has revealed interesting findings which may have physiological implications. For example several studies (13, 30, 42) have shown that in Duchenne muscular dystrophy type I fibers seem to predominate over type II fibers beyond control levels. Awareness of imbalances in muscle fiber types as a result of disease would be of value in dictating a therapeutic exercise regime. Histochemical profiles of muscles in patients with neuromuscular pathologies are being studied quite actively and should be assimilated as part of a basis for muscle training since these profiles may differ from those seen in healthy individuals (139, 243, 244).

Future Studies in Motor Unit Organization

It would appear that information concerning the physiological organization of motor units comprising human muscle would be of value to the clinician. Studies designed to obtain such data have already been explored in animal models (Fig. 2.15). By using microelectrode intracellular stimulation techniques, it is possible to repetitively activate an alpha motoneuron for a defined duration. Knowledge of which muscle this motoneuron innervates, recording the time course of the twitch tension, monitoring tension changes to tetanizing electrical stimuli delivered to the motoneuron and computing the motor axon conduction velocity enable us to determine the physiological properties of the motor unit. These data can then be supplemented with histological information obtained from the muscle. Figure 2.15 illustrates the results from employing such techniques. In this case physiological data reveal that this motoneuron to the medial gastrocnemius muscle of the cat innervated a fast-twitch motor unit (rapid axon conduction velocity, quickly fatiguing, and low twitch: tetanus ratio). The histological examination for glycogen depletion indicates that this unit (Fig. 2.15, white spots) represents widely dispersed muscle fibers which are confined to the dorsolateral aspect of the muscle.

Clinical research (21, 223, 224) has been modified from previous work (178) to reveal similar data. In these cases the minimal electrical stimulation necessary to cause the slightest contraction is provided cutaneously along the motor point and isometric tension is recorded about the joint activated by muscle stimulation. Following prolonged stimulation the muscle fibers which were observed to twitch in synchrony to the stimulation are biopsied and subjected to histochemical analyses. In this manner physiological and cytochemical data are obtained from one testing session.

This technique offers us the potential for learning the spatial distribution of motor unit types in man. Such information may be of significance since it will advance our knowledge concerning: 1) the relative quantity of fast- and slow-twitch units for any one muscle and 2) the distribution of unit types in two-joint muscles. As a result of such studies our enhanced awareness of muscle properties may enable us to train muscles or portions of muscle, i.e., two-joint muscles, in accordance with their precise properties.

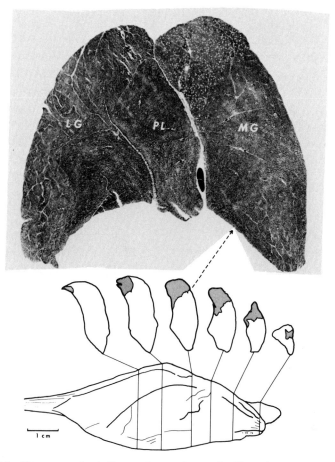

Fig. 2.15. Glycogen depletion pattern of muscle fibers in a single motor unit of cat medial gastrocnemius muscle. (Upper) Histological cross section of posterior leg showing glycogen depletion zone (light dots) in posterolateral area of medial gastrocnemius. (Lower) Entire medial gastrocnemius muscle with representative cross sections at different levels. Stippled area on each cross section shows longitudinal extent of the motor unit's glycogen-depleted fibers. Histological picture shown above is from center cross section (dashed line). Conduction velocity of motoneuron innervating these depleted fibers = 95.6 m/sec; twitch:tetanus ratio = 0.775. Abbreviations: LG, lateral gastrocnemius; PL, plantaris, MG, medial gastrocnemius. (Courtesy of Dr. W. D. Letbetter.)

During the past decade considerable attention has been drawn to the influence which peripheral nerves may exert upon muscle (neurotrophism) and the implication that this nerve-muscle relationship may have in the diagnosis of certain neuro- and myopathic conditions (for reviews see references 52, 105, 110, 111). Thus, for example, cross-innervation of a "fast" muscle nerve to a "slow" muscle, following removal of the latter's nerve supply, is capable of converting the "slow" muscle to a "fast" one.

The meaning of this work in terms of clinical implications is unclear at present.

Clinical Quantification of Motor Unit Populations

In recent years several groups of investigators have attempted to employ modern neurophysiological techniques to determine total numbers of motor units in specific muscles or muscle groups. This concept is indeed exciting. If valid and reliable motor unit determinations could be performed, then clinicians might be able to learn with more precision the mechanisms underlying specific myopathies and neuropathies. Furthermore, by noting changes in these quantitative values with serial examination in patients having specific diagnoses, decisions regarding such factors as physical and pharmacological therapy or vocational alternatives might be assessed more clearly.

Thus far motor unit determinations have been limited to a single muscle or muscle groups from which activity can be recorded in relative isolation with surface electrodes while incrementing stimulus intensities are presented to the appropriate peripheral nerve. These muscles include: extensor digitorum brevis, abductor hallucis, extensor hallucis brevis, thenar eminence group, hypothenar eminence group, and first dorsal interosseus.

Initial attempts to estimate motor unit populations in extensor digitorum brevis were undertaken by McComas and colleagues (162, 166, 168, 210) and subsequently repeated in hand muscles (212). Their quantification technique involves comparing the amplitude (69) of evoked motor unit potentials during incrementing stimulus strength with that potential evoked by a supramaximal nerve stimulus (Fig. 2.16A).

Assuming that each stimulus increment would excite an additional motor unit, calculations of the mean peak-to-peak amplitude of some 8–12 motor units can be made. Dividing this mean value into that obtained from the supramaximal stimulus would yield the motor unit estimate. These determinations have produced considerable normative data in various age groups (47, 169), and the technique has even been employed in animal models (158). McComas has presented data in a variety of pathologies. Motor unit populations appear to be reduced in muscles of hemiplegic patients (164, 170). Some functional motor unit compensation occurs in patients with partial nerve lesions (165). In patients with Duchenne muscular dystrophy (167) motor unit totals appear greatly reduced but potential sizes remain normal. A loss of motor units was also reported in patients with limb-girdle or facioscapulohumeral dystrophy (211) and surviving units appear to be larger in size, while in patients with thyrotoxicosis (171) a quantitative loss in motor unit numbers is reversible.

These observations have prompted McComas and colleagues to hypothesize a concept of "sick" motoneurons (163). Such cells are viewed as being unable to exert an excitatory or trophic influence on muscle fibers because of inherent properties of the acquired or inherited disease process. The

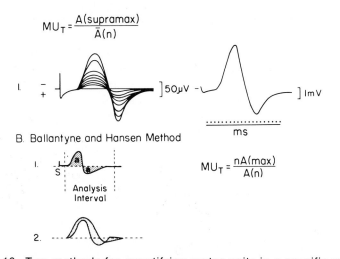

A. McComas Method

$$MU_T = \frac{A(supramax)}{\bar{A}(n)}$$

]50µV

]ImV

ms

B. Ballantyne and Hansen Method

$$MU_T = \frac{nA(max)}{A(n)}$$

Analysis Interval

Fig. 2.16. Two methods for quantifying motor units in a specific muscle or muscle group. (A) Amplitude method. 1. (left) superimposed responses to incrementing nerve stimuli and (right) response to supramaximal stimulation of nerve. Calibration: 1 msec between dots. (B) Calculation of the area of differences in potentials used to 1) derive absolute area, a, of a potential and 2) compare two potentials (shaded area). Abbreviations: MU , total number of motor units; (in A: A (supramax), amplitude of response to supramaximal nerve stimulation; Ā(n), mean amplitude of "n" incrementing nerve stimuli; in B: n, number of motor units in penultimate template; A(max), absolute area for supramaximally-evoked muscle action potential; A(n), absolute area of potential composed of n units.

duration of the dysfunctional stage in motoneurons is related to the pathology. Thus, in diseases of the motoneuron associated with possible improvement, only a few sick motor cells would exist, but in dystrophic patients, for example, motoneuron dysfunction could exist for several years before the cell would "die." The fact that increased motor unit counts can be obtained subsequently to a reduction in motor unit determination suggests that some sick motoneurons are capable of regaining function. A more plausible explanation for this observation and the occasional recording of large amplitude muscle potentials accompanying reduced total motor unit counts could be attributed to axonal sprouting from functional motoneurons (73).

Research undertaken by Panayiotopoulos and Scarpalezos (188–190, 204, 205) produced results on motor unit counts in patients with Duchenne muscular dystrophy, thyrotoxic myopathy, and limb-girdle dystrophy which were not in accord with McComas' findings. Significant differences in motor unit estimates between these patients and control subjects were not apparent. Although the amplitude method for determining motor unit population was used, Panayiotopoulos and Scarpalezos employed finer gradations in stimulus strength and examined amplitude differences following superimposition of several motor unit potential tracings at any one stimulus strength. Through these refinements in technique, it was deduced that the comparatively high noise level in the recording system of the McComas group would tend to obscure small units. This occurrence could lead to overestimations of total motor unit populations which, in turn, could result in interpretation errors. Additionally long latency unit response might be overlooked. It was argued that incremented responses used to calculate mean peak-to-peak amplitudes of motor units may not be representative of the entire population of abnormal units. The most important criticism put forth suggests that responses evoked by graded stimulation may not even correspond to the activation of single motor units in normal or dystrophic muscle. Recently clinical electrophysiological data (191) obtained from patients with dystrophia myotonia have yielded clues that this disease process may include myogenic and neural components.

Convincing information concerning motor unit estimates in normal (9) and dystrophic (11) individuals has recently been advanced by Ballantyne and Hansen. The method involves computer-based motor unit determinations which take into account not only amplitudes of electrically activated unit potentials but latency, duration, areas, and number of phases in peak-to-peak responses (Fig. 2.16 B). Units are stored as templates and each successively recruited unit is compared with respect to areas of difference between it and those already designated as templates. After 10–15 templates have been determined a supramaximally evoked muscle action potential is obtained and the total number of motor units is determined. By serial subtraction of templates the configuration of individual motor unit potentials can be visualized.

Based upon this method Ballantyne and Hansen were able to demonstrate that in the extensor digitorum brevis muscle a wide range of motor unit totals exist for all age groups and motor unit counts in normal subjects and myasthenic patients do not differ significantly. Furthermore while total motor unit estimates appear lower in patients with myotonic muscular dystrophy, patients with Duchenne, limb-girdle or facioscapulohumeral muscular dystrophies display motor unit totals are within a normal range.

W. F. Brown and his colleagues (33–36, 180) have devised yet another method of examining total motor unit populations and have concluded that any method which seeks to yield motor unit estimates should include a correction factor for variations in excitability and overlap in motor unit firing levels. Additionally larger recruited motor unit potentials should be incorporated in the estimate of a mean motor unit potential. Based upon these considerations Brown and Milner-Brown (37) have demonstrated that previous motor unit determinations result in overestimations in some patient groups.

ELECTROPHYSIOLOGICAL PARAMETERS IN MOTOR INNERVATION

In light of the continuing refinements in electrophysiological techniques and criticisms of existing measurements which have been developed to estimate total numbers of motor units the clinician may justifiably question the validity of such procedures. Of equal importance are two relevant questions which should emerge from the previous discussion—have the above methods generated any reliable information which may help the clinician to assess the status of his patient and, if so, might this information be applicable to the formulation and implementation of therapeutic exercise regimes? The answer on both counts is unquestionably affirmative.

It should be recalled, for example, that in computing motor unit estimates Ballantyne and Hansen evaluated all components (latency, amplitude, peak-to-peak area, duration and numbers of phase changes) comprising a muscle potential. An analysis of these characteristics (10) has revealed that reduced potential durations and increased latencies without changes in amplitude or area typify findings in myasthenia patients and are consistent with the notion that a terminal neuropathy is present in this disease. In most dystrophic patients a similar analysis (12) indicates that significant increases in both motor unit potential latencies and durations are common. Alternative methods of assessing neuromuscular pathologies by intramuscular needle electrode examinations to determine fiber densities within motor units have been developed by Swedish clinicians (219, 233). The technique offers considerable promise as a relatively uncomplicated method to observe serial changes in muscle potential characteristics.

It would appear that assessing all electrophysiological parameters which comprise the evoked muscle potential response might provide definite data to supplement clinical impressions. An evaluation of these data, obtained from any one patient over time, would have apparent implications with respect to neuromuscular status and fatiguability in the patient. Additionally, a new perspective regarding the duration and type of exercise may emerge from this analysis.

Training and Fatigue During Exercise

Musculoskeletal, circulatory and respiratory adaptations to increase strength and work capacity are an integral component of *training* or *conditioning*. The deconditioning effects of inactivity (and, in part, of illness) are the reverse of training effects (71, 231). Although the chronic effects of exercise in conditioning are bound to influence muscular strength and skill, the most striking effects are on the circulation.

The overall result of an exercise program is to enhance the metabolic capacity of working muscle. The general effects are most striking when the exercise involves multiple large muscle groups and is sufficiently prolonged and strenuous to induce metabolic and circulatory stress. Thus, the severity of the exercise must be continually adjusted to the training status of the subject and increased as training progresses.

The working metabolism of the muscles is conveniently divided into aerobic and anaerobic for this discussion. The aerobic metabolism in exercise is made possible by an increase in pulse rate, in stroke output of the heart and in arteriovenous oxygen difference. In training, the most dramatic change is in stroke output, which is probably achieved both by more effective venous return to the heart and by more forceful pump action of the heart. In strenuous exercise programs, the latter is accompanied by genuine moderate hypertrophy of the heart, which in normal hearts is physiologic, harmless and reversible. The result of increased stroke output in a fixed moderate task is that the pulse rate is less elevated than before training. However, if the work rate is increased, a higher ceiling of pulse rate may be attained after training. The net result of these circulatory changes is that the maximal O_2 consumption is genuinely increased and accumulation of lactic acid begins at a higher rate of work than before training. In older men the effects of training can be likewise demonstrated, but the achievable levels of O_2 consumption, pulse rate and stroke output decrease progressively with age.

Anaerobic capacity for work is similarly increased with training, but the mechanisms are less well understood. Tolerable levels of lactic acid and oxygen debt are raised. Presumably, the adaptive changes are at a cellular level and are not wholly in the muscles themselves.

Practical measurement of the state of training or conditioning has been a subject of considerable interest. From a theoretical point of view, any of the variables which change could be used as an index. Maximal O_2 consumption is a central value but is difficult to measure routinely. Lactic acid accumulation is also a valid index. Practical tests for mass use have usually utilized the pulse rate as an index (140), based on the evidence that efficient circulation of the trained individual is characterized by slow pulse (and high stroke volume) during exercise and by a prompt return toward resting conditions after exercise (Fig. 2.17). Since the resting pulse rate is affected by emotion and is a poor index and since pulse rate during exercise is difficult to measure, the pulse rate in recovery from nearly exhausting work has been the favored measurement. Pulse rates early in recovery are a rough measure of those in exercise; those later in recovery are an index of the speed of readaptation to rest. Pulse rate during severe exercise and the first five minutes afterward is relatively little affected by emotion. Tests of this or a more complex type have been named *tests of physical fitness*. Since physical fitness is not a single attribute, the term should be qualified to refer to "cardiovascular fitness" or "fitness for heavy unskilled muscular work."

Fatigue in relationship to the physiology of exercise has a much more definite meaning than is common in clinical usage. In a strict physiologic sense, fatigue is the falling off of response to a stimulus. The stimulus may be electric, reflex or a voluntary effort. When a local muscle group is continually exercised and its motion and strength are measured or ob-

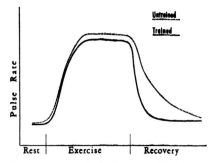

Fig. 2.17. Pulse rate responses in trained and untrained subjects to moderately severe unskilled work.

served, the response will begin to diminish and, if carried far enough, will fall to zero. That this is not fatigue of the local nerve or muscles is easily demonstrated by electrical stimulation of the nerves to the fatigued muscles, which respond well. Except in myasthenia gravis, curare poisoning and possibly in diseases of muscle, the peripheral neuromuscular apparatus has a high threshold to fatigue which is rarely reached in voluntary exercise but may be achieved under unique circumstances (222).

The fatigue met clinically or brought on by whole body exercises is more likely to be a symptom than a measurable decrement in performance. Of course, the body fatigue of very strenuous exercise, with its cardiovascular stress and lactic acid accumulation, is measurable physiologic fatigue, but it is rarely encountered except in athletics, the armed services and in a few strenuous occupations. The type of fatigue observed in most occupations and most individuals is a much subtler process (177). Studies of industrial production have shown that the emotional factors involved in interpersonal relationships with supervisors and fellow workers are usually the most significant. Factors of temperature, light and noise play a lesser role. In the more intellectual occupations, basic interests, diverting emotional factors and the whole gamut of motivational influences are probably involved. Whether fatigue in these conditions represents a block at higher synapses in the CNS requires further investigation.

While cardiovascular adjustments are important factors in appreciating conditioning and fatigue in muscle, it would appear that considerable information may be acquired by studying changes in motor unit and muscular properties during exercise. The recognition of such changes offers the potential for more clearly developing therapeutic exercise principles directed at specific muscles or groups of muscles.

Considerable information concerning the effects of training and fatiguing exercise on animal muscle at both the macro- and microscopic level are now available. Using the rat as an experimental model, it has been possible to demonstrate that isometric (184, 232), spring (126, 220) or endurance (8, 23, 183) exercise is capable of inducing quantitative histochemical or physiological changes in hind limb muscle composition. Chronic electrical stimulation of hindlimb muscle on a daily basis and for as little as 1 month is capable of minimizing fatigue and inducing changes toward increased oxidative muscle metabolism and tonic muscular contraction in the rabbit (32, 196) and cat (194). Studies (79, 153) have demonstrated that electrical stimulation to rat or guinea pig nerve fiber, nerve trunk or muscle can produce a preferential glycogen depletion in glycolytic, type A muscle fibers. Endurance training in the primate has been shown to induce increased oxidative metabolic capacities without significantly altering physiological properties in the plantaris muscle (80). Using the mouse soleus muscle as a model Spande and Schottelius (217) have been able to implicate phosphocreatinine depletion as a primary factor in causing fatigue. Conversely, the effect of tenotomy or immobilization has been shown to cause physiological and structural muscular changes in a variety of animals (68, 127, 198, 227, 234).

Recent work by Herbison and colleagues (122, 123) has added a temporal element to considerations of exercise effects upon striated muscle. From experiments on rats with induced peripheral nerve lesions these investigators have demonstrated that strenuous exercise soon after nerve trauma may actually cause excessive protein breakdown in denervated muscle and retard return of functional muscle activity.

Research designed to evaluate the effects of exercise and training on properties of human muscle is still in its infancy. Significant contributions toward our understanding of muscle fiber composition following exercise have been provided by Gollnick and his colleagues (93–97, 197) as well as by Swedish investigators (124, 143). Muscle biopsy samples have been taken from primarily the deltoid and vastus lateralis muscles during varying exercise loads and conditions. Slow-twitch muscle fiber types appear to predominate in trained subjects compared to the wide variety of fiber types existing in these two muscles in untrained men (93). Endurance training has been shown to increase muscle glycogen storage and oxidative capacity following exercise. Prolonged training over a 5-month period is capable of increasing oxidative capacities of both slow- and fast-twitch muscle fibers while preferentially augmenting glycolytic capacities in fast-twitch units. This type of exercise regime does not result in a relative percentage change of fiber types but slow-twitch muscle fibers appear larger and occupy a greater muscle area. Muscle glycogen storage may be increased by a factor of 2.5 over control conditions after several months of exercise. No differences in the rate of glycogen resynthesis following exercise has been demonstrated in trained versus non-trained subjects (197).

Glycogen depletion patterns in human vastus lateralis muscle can be differentiated by the type of exercise program. Short duration, high intensity work first depletes low-oxidative, high-glycolytic fast-twitch fibers of glycogen. This finding is in contrast to metabolic events seen in moderate-intense exercise where high-oxidative slow-twitch fibers are the first to lose glycogen reserves (95, 97).

Diet has been shown to affect muscle metabolism during exercise (94). High fat and protein diets during exercise can result in elevated glycogen storage in fast-twitch fibers and reduced glycogen metabolism during performance. Total glycogen depletion while exercising appears to be less in fast- than slow-twitch fibers after controlled or high carbohydrate diets but greater after high fat and protein meals.

While the above work has been directed toward examining muscle activity during training, it must be pointed out that clinical studies designed to evaluate quantitative or qualitative changes in muscle structure or function during *therapeutic* exercise regimes have been extremely limited. It would appear that for the clinician to derive maximal value from studies on muscle fiber composition during exercise, testing regimes analogues to those employed in the treatment of musculoskeletal disorders should be incorporated into future studies. Recent data (136) have suggested that equal gains in muscle strength can be obtained through either eccentric or concentric exercise though the former may be more beneficial for patients with joint mobility limitations due to pain.

Additional Physiological Cues for Therapeutic Exercise: Biofeedback

The information presented in this chapter has dealt primarily with subunits of muscle and with muscle groups in total. In most therapeutic exercise procedures the individual patient can make accurate motor responses to sensory cues by successfully processing kinesthetic and proprioceptive input. These inputs are provided through volitional effort or by assistive procedures such as resistance to movement or passive stretch. For several years Basmajian and his colleagues (19) have demonstrated that through the use of audio and visual feedback from muscle contractions man is capable of isolating and controlling single motor units. Such precise neuromuscular control may occur without visualization of muscle activity. As a result of these findings the concept of electromyographic feedback for assisting patients with musculoskeletal or neurological impairments to regain functional motor control has emerged.

Like other forms of information feedback, muscle biofeedback enables the patient to use visual and auditory representations of physiological events which are not normally perceived. In this situation visual or auditory signals are true indications of electromyographic activity. Through adequate training, a patient can learn to initiate and control appropriate muscle responses. While many other forms of exercise rely most heavily upon proprioceptive cues, effector responses using muscle biofeedback must, to a large extent, depend upon signal processing through vision or audition. This form of sensory-motor integration can, of course, be supplemented and "shaped" by the addition of proprioceptive inputs resulting from any combination of muscle stretch, resistance, vibration, or cuta-

THERAPEUTIC EXERCISE

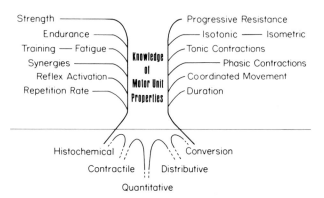

Strength —————————— Progressive Resistance
Endurance ———— Isotonic —— Isometric
Training — Fatigue —— Knowledge Tonic Contractions
Synergies ———— ol Phasic Contractions
Reflex Activation— Motor Unit Coordinated Movement
Repetition Rate —— Properties Duration

Histochemical Conversion
Contractile Distributive
Quantitative

Fig. 2.18. Neuromuscular component of a hypothetical therapeutic exercise "tree" using the motor unit as the basic element.

neous stimulation. Indeed significant clinical gains have already been achieved using biofeedback in stroke patients (2, 4, 7, 20, 38, 137, 185, 228), patients with cerebral palsy (117, 218, 246) or torticollis (39, 51) and in patients with joint motion restriction (155). To date little information is available concerning muscle feedback application in traumatic musculo-skeletal disorders.

Despite these recent advances EMG biofeedback is still in its infancy as a therapeutic modality. Factors such as patient strategies, physiological processing mechanisms and behavior "shaping" require concentrated explorations. By implementing many of the physiological and anatomical correlates of muscle activity a more precise plan of action may be administered in using this modality. Awareness of the primary physiological and histochemical constituents (see pp. 00–00) of the muscle being explored will inevitably lead to a rationale for the training procedure. For example, knowing that a muscle contains primarily slow-twitch units with high oxidative metabolic activity will dictate that static contraction rather than dynamic movements should be undertaken employing visual or auditory feedback. Even more precise strategies can be developed in patients who are able to initiate localized contractions in a confined portion of a muscle mass if the physiological characteristics of the motor units within that muscle area are known.

Conclusions

An understanding of muscle morphology, composition and innervation facilitates our ability to establish a basis for therapeutic exercise. Within the past decade considerable research has been devoted to muscle fiber groupings (motor units) whose activity not only produces the phenomenon of movement but also expresses a definitive output derived from the highly complex and integrative action of the central nervous system.

In this chapter we have reviewed the basic structure of muscle and have approached the neuromuscular component of therapeutic exercise through an examination of motor unit properties. While significant advancements have been made toward comprehending muscle activity, it should be apparent to the reader that the clinical implication of these findings will require further investigation. We now have some appreciation of muscle fiber composition in man. This lesson has been learned through arduous research which has employed anatomical, histochemical and physiological techniques under clinical and animal laboratory conditions.

We can view the muscle component of the neuromuscular basis for exercise techniques as a developing tree (Fig. 2.18). These techniques stem from an appreciation of motor unit properties which are rooted in essential scientific considerations. As these roots become well implanted, our awareness of such factors as: the spatial distribution of motor unit types within a muscle, the changes in muscle composition resulting from exercise, reinnervation (or nerve transplantation), the meaning and significance of abnormal electrophysiological measurements in nerve or muscle disease and the importance of nutrition or accessory modalities in muscle function, to name but a few, will be enhanced. The results of this scientific enlightenment should enable us to apply therapeutic techniques more appropriately and meaningfully.

REFERENCES

1. ADAMS, R. D., DENNY-BROWN, D., AND PEARSON, C. M. *Diseases of Muscle*. New York, 1953.
2. AMATO, A., HERMSMEYER, C. A., AND KLEINMAN, K. M. Use of EMG feedback to increase inhibitory control in spastic muscles. *Phys. Ther., 53*: 1063, 1973.
3. ANDERSEN, K. L. The Cardiovascular System in Exercise. In *Exercise Physiology*, edited by H. B. Falls. Academic Press, New York, 1968.
4. ANDREWS, J. M. Neuromuscular re-education of the hemiplegic with the aid of the electromyograph. *Arch. Phys. Med. Rehabil., 45*: 530, 1964.
5. ASMUSSEN, E. Muscular Exercise. In *Handbook of Physiology*, Section 3, Respiration, Volume 2, edited by W. O. Fenn and H. Rahn. American Physiological Society, Washington, D.C., 1964.
6. ÅSTRAND, P. O., AND RODAHL, K. *Textbook of Work Physiology*. McGraw-Hill, New York, 1970.
7. BAKER, M., REGNEOS, E., WOLF, S. L., AND BASMAJIAN, J. V. Developing strategies for biofeedback applications in neurologically handicapped patients. *Phys. Ther.* (in press).
8. BALDWIN K. M. WINDER, W. W., AND HOLLOSZY, J. O. Adaptation of actomyosin ATPase in different types of muscle to endurance exercise. *Am. J. Physiol., 229*: 422, 1975.
9. BALLANTYNE, J. P., AND HANSEN, S. A new method for the estimation of the number of motor units in a muscle. *J. Neurol. Neurosurg. Psychiatry, 37*: 907, 1974.
10. BALLANTYNE, J. P., AND HANSEN, S. Computer method for the analysis of evoked motor unit potentials. 1. Control subjects and patients with myasthenia gravis. *J. Neurol. Neurosurg. Psychiatry 37*: 1187, 1974.
11. BALLANTYNE, J. P., AND HANSEN, S. New method for the estimation of the number of motor units in a muscle. 2. Duchenne, limb-girdle and facioscapulohumeral, and myotonic muscular dystrophies. *J. Neurol. Neurosurg. Psychiatry 37*: 1195, 1974c.

12. BALLANTYNE, J. P., AND HANSEN, S. Computer method for the analysis of evoked motor unit potentials. 2. Duchenne, limb-girdle, facioscapulohumeral and myotonic muscular dystrophies. *J. Neurol. Neurosurg. Psychiatry 38:* 417, 1975.

13. BALOH, R., AND CANCILLA, P. A. An appraisal of histochemical fiber types in Duchenne muscular dystrophy. *Neurology, 22:* 1243, 1972.

14. BARCROFT, H. Circulation in Skeletal Muscle. In *Handbook of Physiology*, Section 2: Circulation. Volume II. American Physiological Society, Washington, 1963.

15. BARER, R. The structure of the striated muscle fiber. *Biol. Rev., 23:* 159, 1948.

16. BARKER, D., EMONET-DÉNAND, F., LAPORTE, Y., PROSKE, U., AND STACEY, M. J. Morphological identification and intrafusal distribution of the endings of static fusimotor axons in the cat. *J. Physiol. (Lond.), 230:* 405, 1973.

17. BARKER, D. The Morphology of Muscle Receptors. In *Handbook of Sensory Physiology*, Volume 3, edited by C. C. Hunt. Springer-Verlag, Heidelberg, 1974.

18. BARKER, D., EMONET-DÉNAND, F., HARKER, D. W., JAMI, L., AND LAPORTE, Y. Distribution of fusimotor axons to intrafusal muscle fibres in cat tenuissimus spindles as determined by the glycogen-depletion method. *J. Physiol. (Lond.), 261:* 49, 1976.

19. BASMAJIAN, J. V. *Muscles Alive: Their Functions Revealed by Electromyography*, Ed. 3, Williams & Wilkins Co., Baltimore, 1974.

20. BASMAJIAN, J. V., KUKULKA, C. G., NARAYAN, M. G., AND TAKEBE, K. Biofeedback treatment of foot-drop after stroke compared with standard rehabilitation technique: effects on voluntary control and strength. *Arch. Phys. Med. Rehabil., 56:* 231, 1975.

21. BEASLEY, M. A., O'DONOVAN, M. J., STEPHENS, J. A., TAYLOR, A., AND USHERWOOD, T. P. Unit studies in normal human gastrocnemius by microstimulation, glycogen depletion and needle biopsy. *J. Physiol. (Lond.), 260:* 11P, 1976.

22. BECKETT, E. B., AND BOURNE, G. H. The histochemistry of normal and abnormal human muscle. *Proc. Roy. Soc. Med., 50:* 18, 1957.

23. BENZI, G. PANCERI, P., DE BERNARDI, M., VILLA, R., ARCELLI, E., D'ANGELO, L., ARRIGONE, E., AND BERTÈ, F. Mitochondrial enzymatic adaptation of skeletal muscle to endurance training. *J. Appl. Physiol, 38:* 565, 1975.

24. BESSOU, P., AND PAGÈS, B. Cinematographic analysis of contractile events produced in intrafusal muscle fibres by stimulation of static and dynamic fusimotor axons. *J. Physiol. (Lond.), 252:* 397, 1975.

25. BORS, E. Ueber das Zahlenverhatnis Zwischen Nerven- und Muskelfasern. *Anat. Anz. 60:* 444, 1926.

26. BOURNE, G. H. Nutrition and Exercise. In *Exercise Physiology*, edited by H. B. Falls. Academic Press, New York, 1968.

27. BOYD, I. A., AND WARD, J. Motor control of nuclear bag and nuclear chain intrafusal fibres in isolated living muscle spindles of the cat. *J. Physiol. (Lond.), 244:* 83, 1975.

28. BOYD, I. A., GLADDEN, M. H., McWILLIAM, P. N. AND WARD, J. 'Static' and 'dynamic' nuclear bag fibres in isolated cat muscle spindles. *J. Physiol. (Lond.), 250:* 11P, 1975.

29. BOYD, I. A. The response of fast and slow nuclear bag fibres and nuclear chain fibres in isolated cat muscle spindles to fusimotor stimulation, and the effect of intrafusal contraction on the sensory endings. *Q. J. Exp. Physiol., 61:* 203, 1976.

30. BROOKE, M. H., AND ENGEL, W. K. The histologic diagnosis of neuromuscular diseases: a review of 79 biopsies. *Arch. Phys. Med. Rehabil., 47:* 99, 1966.

31. BROOKE, M. H., AND KAISER, K. K. Muscle fiber types: how many and what kind? *Arch. Neurol., 23:* 369, 1970.

32. BROWN, M. D., COTTER, M. HUDLICKA, O., SMITH, M. E., AND VRBOVÁ, G. The effect of long-term stimulation of fast muscles on their ability to withstand fatigue. *J. Physiol. (Lond.), 238:* 47P, 1973.

33. BROWN, W. F. A method for estimating the number of motor units in thenar muscles and the changes in motor unit count with ageing. *J. Neurol. Neurosurg. Psychiatry 35:* 845, 1972.

34. BROWN, W. F., AND FEASBY, T. Estimates of motor axon loss in diabetics. *J. Neurol. Sci., 23:* 275, 1974.

35. BROWN, W. F., AND JAATOUL, N. Amyotrophic lateral sclerosis; electrophysiological study (number of motor units and rate of decay of motor units). *Arch. Neurol., 30:* 242, 1974.
36. BROWN, W. F., MILNER-BROWN, H. S., AND DEAKE, J. Errors in Motor Unit Estimates. In *Abstracts of the 3rd International Congress on Muscle Disease,* edited by W. G. Bradley. Excerpta Medica, Amsterdam, 1974.
37. BROWN, W. F., AND MILNER-BROWN, H. S. Some electrical properties of motor units and their effects on the methods of estimating motor unit numbers. *J. Neurol. Neurosurg. Psychiatry 39:* 249, 1976.
38. BRUDNY, J. Sensory feedback therapy as a modality of treatment in CNS disorders of voluntary movement. *Neurology, 24:* 925, 1974.
39. BRUDNY, J., GRYNBAUM, B. L. AND KOREIN, J. Spasmodic torticollis: treatment by feedback display of EMG. *Arch. Phys. Med. Rehabil., 55:* 403, 1974.
40. BUCHTAHL, F., AND MADSEN, A. Synchronous activity in normal and atrophic muscles. *Electroencephalogr. Clin. Neurophysiol., 2:* 425, 1950.
41. BUCHTAL, F. The functional organization of the motor unit. *Proc. First Int. Cong. Neurol. Sci.,* 1957.
42. BUCHTAL, F., SCHMALBRUCH, H., AND KAMIENIECKA, Z. Contraction times and fiber types in patients with progressive muscular dystrophy. *Neurology, 21:* 131, 1971.
43. BULLER, A. J. The Physiology of the Motor Unit. In *Disorders of Voluntary Muscle,* Ed. 3, edited by J. N. Walton. Churchill Livingstone, London, 1974.
44. BURG, D., SZUMSKI, A. J., STRUPPLER, A., AND VELHO, F. Afferent and efferent activation of human muscle receptors involved in reflex and voluntary contraction. *Exp. Neurol., 41:* 754, 1973.
45. BURKE, R. E. On the Central Nervous System Control of Fast and Slow Twitch Motor Units. In *New Developments in Electromyography and Clinical Neurophysiology,* Vol. 3, edited by J. E. Desmedt. Karger, Basel, 1973.
46. BÜDINGEN, H. J., AND FREUND, H.-J. The relationship between the rate of rise of isometric tension and motor unit recruitment in human forearm muscle. *Pflügers Arch., 362:* 61, 1976.
47. CAMPBELL, M. J., McCOMAS, A. J., AND PETITO, F. Physiological changes in ageing muscles. *J. Neurol. Neurosurg. Psychiatry 36:* 174, 1973.
48. CARR, R. W. Muscle-tendon attachment in the striated muscle of fetal pig. Demonstration of the sarcolemma by electric stimulation. *Am. J. Anat., 49:* 1, 1931.
49. CHRISTENSEN, E. Topography of terminal motor innervation in striated muscles from stillborn infants. *Am. J. Phys. Med., 38:* 65, 1959.
50. CLARK, D. A. Muscle counts of motor units. A study in innervation ratio. *Am. J. Physiol., 96:* 296, 1931.
51. CLEELAND, C. S. Behavioral techniques in the modification of spasmodic torticollis. *Neurology, 23:* 1241, 1973.
52. CLOSE, R. I. Dynamic properties of mammalian skeletal muscles. *Physiol. Rev., 52:* 129, 1972.
53. COËRS, C. Contribution a l'étude de la jonction neuromusculaire. II. Topographie zonale de l'innervation motrice terminale dans les muscles striés. *Arch. Biol., 64:* 495, 1953.
54. COËRS, C. Les variations structurelles normales et pathologiques de la jonction neuromusculaires. *Acta Neurol. Psychiatr. Belg., 55:* 742, 1955.
55. COËRS, C. AND DURAND, J. Donneés morphologiques nouvelles sur l'innervation des fuseaux neuromusculaires. *Arch. Biol., 67:* 685, 1956.
56. COËRS, C. AND DURAND, J. La répartition des appareils cholinestérasiques en cupule dans divers muscles striés. *Arch. Biol., 68:* 209, 1957.
57. COËRS, C., AND WOOLF, A. L. *The Innervation of Muscle. A Biopsy Study.* Oxford, 1959.
58. COËRS, C. Structure and organization of the myoneural junction. *Int. Rev. Cytol., 22:* 239, 1967.
59. CONSOLAZIO, C. F., JOHNSON, R. E., AND PECORA, L. J. *Physiological Measurements of*

Metabolic Functions in Man. McGraw-Hill, New York, 1963.

60. COOPER, S., AND ECCLES, J. C. The isometric response of mammalian muscles. *J. Physiol., 69:* 377, 1930.

61. COUPLAND, R. E., AND HOLMES, R. L. The use of cholinesterase techniques for the demonstration of peripheral nerve structures. *Q. J. Microsc. Sci., 98:* 327, 1957.

62. COUTEAUX, R. Contribution a l'étude de la synapse myoneurale; Buisson de Kuhne et plaque motrice. *Rev. Can. Biol., 6:* 563, 1947.

63. COUTEAUX, R. *Contribution a l'etude de la synapse myoneurale.* Montreal, 1947.

64. COUTEAUX, R. Recherches histochimiques sur la distribution des activities cholinestérasiques au niveau de la synapse myoneurale. *Arch. Anat. Microsc. Morphol. Exp., 41:* 352, 1952.

65. COUTEAUX, R. Particularités histochimiques des zones d'insertion du muscle strié. *C. R. Soc. Biol., 147:* 1974, 1953.

66. COUTEAUX, R. Sur le mode de terminaison des myofibrilles et leurs connexions avec la membrane sarcoplasmique. *C. R. Acad. Sci., 246:* 307, 1958.

67. COUTEAUX, R. Motor End Plate Structure. In *The Structure and Function of Muscle,* Ed. 2, Volume 2, edited by G. H. Bourne. Academic Press, New York, 1973.

68. CROCKETT, J. L., AND EDGERTON, V. R. Exercise and restricted activity effects on reinnervated and cross-innervated skeletal muscles. *J. Neurol. Sci., 25:* 1, 1975.

69. CURRIER, D. P. Value of the magnitude of muscle action potentials. *Phys. Ther., 51:* 1000, 1971.

70. DAWSON, D. M., AND KAPLAN, N. O. Factors influencing the concentration of enzymes in various muscles. *J. Biol. Chem., 240:* 3215, 1965.

71. DEITRICK, J. E., WHEDON, G. D., AND SHORR, E. Effects of immobilization upon various metabolic and physiologic functions in normal man. *Am. J. Med., 4:* 3, 1948.

72. DEJOURS, P. Control of Respiration in Muscular Exercise. In *Handbook of Physiology,* Section 3, Respiration, Volume 1, edited by W. O. Fenn and H. Rahn. American Physiological Society, Washington, D.C., 1964.

73. DESMEDT, J. E., AND BORENSTEIN, S. Collateral innervation of muscle fibres by motor axons of dystrophic motor units. *Nature New Biol., 246:* 500, 1973.

74. DILL, D. B. *Life, Heat, and Altitude.* Harvard University Press, Cambridge, 1938.

75. DRACHMAN, D. B., AND JOHNSTON, D. M. Development of a mammalian fast muscle; dynamic and biochemical properties correlated. *J. Physiol. (Lond.), 234:* 29, 1973.

76. DUBOWITZ, V. Histochemical Techniques in the Analysis of Neuromuscular Disease. In *Studies on Neuromuscular Disease,* edited by K. Kunze and J. E. Desmedt. Karger, Basel, 1975.

77. ECCLES, J. C., AND SHERRINGTON, C. S. Numbers and contraction values of individual motor units examined in some muscles of the limbs. *Proc. R. Soc., 106B:* 326, 1930.

78. EDDS, M. JR. Collateral regeneration of residual motor axones in partially denervated muscles. *J. Exp. Zool., 113:* 517, 1950.

79. EDGERTON, V. R., BARNARD, R. S., PETER, J. B., SIMPSON, D. R., AND GILLESPIE, C. A. Responses of muscle glycogen and phosphorylase to electrical stimulation in trained and non-trained guinea pigs. *Exp. Neurol., 27:* 46, 1970.

80. EDGERTON, V. R., BARNARD, R. S., PETER, J. B., GILLESPIE, C. A., AND SIMPSON, D. R. Overloaded skeletal muscles of a non-human primate *(Galago senegalensis). Exp. Neurol., 37:* 322, 1972.

81. EDSTRÖM, L., AND NYSTRÖM, B. Histochemical types and sizes of fibres in normal human muscles. *Acta Neurol. Scand., 45:* 257, 1969.

82. EMONET-DÉNAND, F., JAMI, L., AND LAPORTE, Y. Skeleto-fusimotor axons in hindlimb muscles of the cat. *J. Physiol. (Lond.), 249:* 153, 1975.

83. EMONET-DÉNAND, F., LAPORTE, Y., MATTHEWS, P. B. C., AND PETIT, J. Experimental observations on the sharpness of classification of fusimotor fibres into static and dynamic types. *J. Physiol. (Lond.), 260:* 68P, 1976.

84. ENGEL, A. G. Locating motor end plates for electron microscopy. *Mayo Clin. Proc., 45:* 450, 1970.

85. ENGEL, W. K. The essentiality of histo- and cytochemical studies of skeletal muscle in investigation of neuromuscular disease. *Neurology, 12:* 778, 1962.
86. EVANS, R. H., HAYNES, J., MORRIS, C. J., AND WOOLF, A. L. *In vitro* staining of intramuscular nerve endings. *J. Neurol. Neurosurg. Psychiatry, 33:* 783, 1970.
87. EYZAGUIRRE, C., AND FIDONE, S. J. *Physiology of the Nervous System,* Ed. 2. Year Book Medical Publishers, Chicago, 1975.
88. FAULKNER, J. A. Maximum Exercise at Medium Altitude. In *Frontiers of Fitness,* edited by R. J. Shephard. Charles C Thomas, Springfield, Ill., 1971.
89. FAWCETT, D. W. *The Cell: An Atlas of Fine Structure.* W. B. Saunders Co., Philadelphia, 1966.
90. FEINSTEIN, B., LINDEGÅRD, B., NYMAN, E., AND WOHLFART, G. Morphologic studies of motor units in normal human muscles. *Acta Anat., 23:* 127, 1955.
91. FRÖBERG, S. O. Metabolism of Lipids in Blood and Tissues During Exercise. In *Biochemistry of Exercise,* edited by J. R. Poortmans. University Park Press, Baltimore, 1968.
92. GARAMVÖLGYI, N. The Functional Morphology of Muscle. In *Contractile Proteins and Muscle,* edited by K. Laki. Marcel Dekker, Inc., New York, 1971.
93. GOLLNICK, P. D., ARMSTRONG, R. B., SAUBERT, C. W., IV, PIEHL, K., AND SALTIN, B. Enzyme activity and fiber composition in skeletal muscle of untrained and trained men. *J. Appl. Physiol., 33:* 312, 1972.
94. GOLLNICK, P. D., PIEHL, K., SAUBERT, C. W., IV, ARMSTRONG, R. B., AND SALTIN, B. Diet, exercise and glycogen changes in human muscle fibers. *J. Appl. Physiol., 33:* 421, 1972.
95. GOLLNICK, P. D., ARMSTRONG, R. B., SAUBERT, C. W., IV, SEMBROWICH, W. L., SHEPHERD, R. E., AND SALTIN, B. Glycogen depletion patterns in human skeletal muscle fibers during prolonged work. *Pflügers Arch., 344:* 1, 1973.
96. GOLLNICK, P. D., ARMSTRONG, R. B., SALTIN, B., SAUBERT, C. W., IV, SEMBROWICH, W. L., AND SHEPHERD, R. E. Effect of training on enzyme activity and fiber composition of human skeletal muscle. *J. Appl. Physiol., 34:* 107, 1973b.
97. GOLLNICK, P. D., ARMSTRONG, R. B., SEMBROWICH, W. L., SHEPHERD, R. E., AND SALTIN, B. Glycogen depletion pattern in human skeletal muscle fibers after heavy exercise. *J. Appl. Physiol., 34:* 615, 1973.
98. GOSS, C. M. The attachment of skeletal muscle fibers. *Am. J. Anat., 74:* 259, 1944.
99. GOULD, R. P. The microanatomy of Muscle. In *The Structure and Function of Muscle,* Ed. 2, Volume 2, edited by G. H. Bourne. Academic Press, New York, 1973.
100. GRANIT, R. *Receptors and Sensory Perception,* Ed. 3. Yale University Press, New Haven, 1967.
101. GRANIT, R. *The Basis of Motor Control,* Academic Press, New York, 1970.
102. GRANT, J. C. B., AND BASMAJIAN, J. V. *Grant's Method of Anatomy,* Ed. 7, Williams & Wilkins Co., Baltimore, 1965.
103. GRIMBY, L., AND HANNERZ, J. Recruitment order of motor units on voluntary contraction; changes induced by proprioceptive afferent activity. *J. Neurol. Neurosurg. Psychiatry, 31:* 565, 1968.
104. GRIMBY, L., HANNERZ, J., AND RÅNLUND, T. Disturbances in the voluntary recruitment order of anterior tibial motor units in spastic paraparesis upon fatigue. *J. Neurol. Neurosurg. Psychiatry 37:* 40, 1974.
105. GUTH, L. Trophic influence of nerve on muscle. *Physiol. Rev., 48:* 645, 1968.
106. GUTH, L., AND YELLIN, H. The dynamic nature of so-called "fiber types" of mammalian skeletal muscle. *Exp. Neurol., 31:* 277, 1971.
107. GUTH, L., AND SAMAHA, F. J. Erroneous interpretations which may result from application of the "myofibrillar ATPase" histochemical procedure to developing muscle. *Exp. Neurol., 34:* 465, 1972.
108. GUTH, L. Fact and artifact in the histochemical procedure for myofibrillar ATPase. *Exp. Neurol., 41:* 440, 1973.
109. GUTMANN, E., MELICHNA, J., AND SYROVÝ, I. Developmental changes in contraction

time, myosin properties and fibre pattern of fast and slow skeletal muscles. *Physiol. Bohemoslov., 23:* 19, 1974.

110. GUTMANN, E. Neurotrophic relations. *Ann. Rev. Physiol., 38:* 177, 1976.

111. GUTMANN, E., AND HANZLÍNKOVÁ, V. Fast and slow motor units in ageing. *Gerontology, 22:* 280, 1976.

112. HAGBARTH, K. -E., AND VALLBO, A. B. Discharge characteristics of human muscle afferents during stretch and contraction. *Exp. Neurol., 22:* 674, 1968.

113. HAGBARTH, K. -E., AND VALLBO, A. B. Single unit recordings from muscle nerves in human subjects. *Acta Physiol. Scand., 76:* 321, 1969.

114. HALBAN, J. Die Dicke der Quergestreifen Muskelfasern und ihre Bedeuntung. *Anat., 3:* 267, 1894.

115. HAMMARBERG, C., AND Kellerth, J. -O. The postnatal development of some twitch and fatigue properties of the ankle flexor and extensor muscles of the cat. *Acta Physiol. Scand., 95:* 166, 1975.

116. HANSON, J., AND HUXLEY, H. The structural basis of contraction in striated muscles. *Symp. Soc. Exp. Biol., 9:* 228, 1955.

117. HARRIS, F. A., SPELMAN, F. A., AND HYMER, J. W. Electronic sensory aids as treatment for cerebral-palsied children. In Approprioception, Part II. *Phys. Ther., 54:* 354, 1974.

118. HARVEN, E., DE, AND COËRS, C. Electron microscope study of the human neuromuscular junction. *J. Biophys. Biochem. Cytol., 6:* 7, 1959.

119. HENNEMAN, E. Relation between size of neurons and their susceptibility to discharge. *Science, 126:* 1345, 1957.

120. HENNEMAN, E., SOMJEN, G., AND CARPENTER, D. O. Functional significance of cell size in spinal motoneurons. *J. Neurophysiol. 28:* 560, 1965.

121. HENSCHEL, A. The Environment and Performance. In *Physiology of Work Capacity and Fatigue,* edited by E. Simonson. Charles C Thomas, Springfield, Ill., 1971.

122. HERBISON, G. J., JAWEED, M. M., DITUNNO, J. F., AND SCOTT, C. M. Effect of overwork during reinnervation of rat muscle. *Exp. Neurol., 41:* 1, 1973.

123. HERBISON, G. J., JAWEED, M. M., AND DITUNNO, J. F. Effect of swimming on reinnervation of rat skeletal muscle. *J. Neurol. Neurosurg. Psychiatry 37:* 1247, 1974.

124. HERMANSEN, L., HULTMAN, E., AND SALTIN, B. Muscle glycogen during prolonged severe exercise. *Acta Physiol. Scand., 71:* 129, 1967.

125. HEYMANS, C., AND NEIL, E. *Reflexogenic Areas of the Cardiovascular System.* Little, Brown & Co., Boston, 1958.

126. HICKSON, R. C., HEUSNER, W. W., AND VAN HUSS, W. D. Skeletal muscle enzyme alterations after spring and endurance training. *J. Appl. Physiol., 40:* 868, 1975.

127. HIKIDA, R. S. Morphological transformation of slow to fast muscle fibers after tenotomy. *Exp. Neurol., 35:* 265, 1972.

128. HILL, A. V. The abrupt transition from rest to activity in muscle. *Proc. R. Soc. (Lond.), Ser. B, 136:* 399, 1949.

129. HILL, A. V. The series elastic component of muscle. *Proc. R. Soc. (Lond.), Ser. B, 137:* 273, 1950.

130. HUDLICKÁ, O., PETTE, D., AND STAUDTE, H. The relation between blood flow and enzymatic activities in slow and fast muscles during development. *Pflügers Arch., 343:* 341, 1973.

131. HUXLEY, H. E. Molecular basis of contraction. In *The Structure and Function of Muscle,* Ed. 2, Volume 1, edited by G. H. Bourne, Academic Press, New York, 1973.

132. IAMPIETRO, P. F., AND ADAMS, T. Thermal balance during exercise and environmental stress. In *Exercise Physiology,* edited by H. B. Falls, Academic Press, New York, 1968.

133. IAMPIERTRO, P. F. Exercise in hot environments. In *Frontiers of Fitness,* edited by R. J. Shephard. Charles C Thomas, Springfield, Ill., 1971.

134. IP, M. C. Some morphological features of the myoneural junctions in certain normal muscles of the rat. *Anat. Rec., 180:* 605, 1974.

135. JAMES, N. T. Histochemical demonstration of myoglobin in skeletal muscle fibres and muscle spindles. *Nature, 219:* 1174, 1968.

136. JOHNSON, B. L. Eccentric vs. concentric muscle training for strength development. *Med. Sci. Sports, 4:* 111, 1972.

137. JOHNSON, H. E., AND GARTON, W. H. Muscle re-education in hemiplegia by use of an electromyographic device. *Arch. Phys. Med. Rehabil., 54:* 320, 1973.

138. JOHNSON, M. A., POLGAR, J., WEIGHTMAN, D., AND APPLETON, D. Data on the distribution of fiber types in thirty-six human muscles. An autopsy study. *J. Neurol. Sci., 18:* 111, 1973a.

139. JOHNSON, M. A., SIDERI, G., WEIGHTMAN, D., AND APPLETON, D. A comparison of fibre size, fibre type constitution and spatial fibre type distribution in normal human muscle and in muscle from cases of spinal muscular atrophy and from other neuromuscular disorders. *J. Neurol. Sci., 20:* 345, 1973b.

140. JOHNSON, R. E., BROUHA, L., AND DARLING, R. C. Test of physical fitness for strenuous exertion. *Rev. Can. Biol., 1:* 491, 1942.

141. JOKL, E. *The Scope of Exercise in Rehabilitation.* Charles C Thomas, Springfield, Ill., 1964.

142. JONES, W. M., AND BARER, R. Electron microscopy of the sarcolemma. *Nature, 161:* 1012, 1947.

143. KARLSSON, J. Lactate and phosphagen concentrations in working muscles of man. *Acta Physiol. Scand., 80:* Suppl. 358, 1971.

144. KARPOVICK, P. V. *Physiology of Muscular Activity,* Ed. 6. W. B. Saunders Co., Philadelphia, 1965.

145. KEUL, J., AND DOLL, E. The Influence of Exercise and Hypoxia on the Substrate Uptake of Human Heart and Human Skeletal Muscles. In *Biochemistry of Exercise,* edited by J. R. Poortmans. University Park Press, Baltimore, 1968.

146. KEUL, J., DOLL, E., AND KEPPLER, D. Characteristics of "White" and "Red" Muscles. In *Energy Metabolism of Human Muscle.* Karger, Basel, 1972.

147. KLEIBER, M. Respiratory Exchange and Metabolic Rate. In *Handbook of Physiology,* Section 3, Respiration, Volume 2, edited by W. O. Fenn and H. Rahn. American Physiological Society, Washington, D.C., 1964.

148. KOBAYASHI, Y., OSHIMA, K., AND TASAKI, I. Analysis of afferent and efferent systems in the muscle nerve of the toad and cat. *J. Physiol. (Lond.), 117:* 152, 1952.

149. KOELLE, G. B. The histochemical differentiation of type of cholinesterases and their localization in tissues of the cat. *J. Pharmacol. Exp. Ther., 100:* 158, 1950.

150. KOELLE, G. B., AND FRIEDENWALD, J. S. A histological method for localizing cholinesterase activity. *Proc. Soc. Exp. Biol. Med., 70:* 617, 1949.

151. KOEZE, T. H. Muscle spindle afferent studies in the baboon. *J. Physiol. (Lond.), 229:* 297, 1973.

152. KONORSKI, J. *Integrative Activity of the Brain: An Interdisciplinary Approach.* University of Chicago Press, Chicago, 1967.

153. KUGELBERG, E., AND EDSTRÖM, L. Differential histochemical effects of muscle contractions on phosphorylase and glycogen in various types of fibres; relation to fatigue. *J. Neurol. Neurosurg. Psychiatry 31:* 415, 1968.

154. KUKULKA, C. G., BROWN, D. M., AND BASMAJIAN, J. V. Biofeedback training for early finger joint mobilization. *Am. J. Occup. Ther., 29:* 469, 1975.

155. KUNZE, K., AND DESMEDT, J. E. *Studies on Neuromuscular Diseases.* S. Karger, Basel, 1975.

156. LAKI, K. Size and Shape of the Myosin Molecule. In *Contractile Proteins and Muscle,* edited by K. Laki. Marcel Dekker, Inc., New York, 1971.

157. LANGWORTHY, O. R. *The Sensory Control of Posture and Movement.* Williams & Wilkins, Baltimore, 1970.

158. LAW, P. K., AND CACCIA, M. R. Physiological estimates of the sizes and the numbers of motor units in soleus muscles of dystrophic mice. *J. Neurol. Sci., 24:* 251, 1975.

159. LINDHARD, J. *Ergebn. Physiol., 33:* 337, 1931 (quoted in Feinstein et al. [90]).

160. LOCKHART, R. D. Anatomy of Muscles and Their Relation to Movement and Posture. In *The Structure and Function of Muscles,* Ed. 2, Volume 1, edited by G. H. Bourne.

Academic Press, New York, 1973.

161. LONG, M. E. Development of the muscle-tendon attachment in the rat. *Am. J. Anat., 81:* 159, 1947.

162. McComas, A. J., SICA, R. E. P., AND CURRIE, S. Evidence for a neural factor in muscular dystrophy. *Nature New Biol., 20:* 1263, 1970.

163. McComas, A. J., SICA, R. E. P., AND CAMPBELL, M. J. "Sick" motoneurones; a unifying concept of muscle disease. *Lancet, 1:* 321, 1971.

164. McComas, A. J., SICA, R. E. P., UPTON, A. R. M., AGUILERA, N., AND CURRIE, S. Motoneurone dysfunction in patients with hemiplegic atrophy. *Nature New Biol., 233:* 21, 1971.

165. McComas, A. J., SICA, R. E. P., CAMPBELL, M. J., AND UPTON, A. R. M. Functional compensation in partially denervated muscles. *J. Neurol. Neurosurg. Psychiatry, 34:* 453, 1971.

166. McComas, A. J., AND SICA, R. E. P. Properties of motor units in normal and partly denervated human muscles. *J. Physiol. (Lond.), 212:* 28P, 1971.

167. McComas, A. J., SICA, R. E. P., AND CURRIE, S. An electrophysiological study of Duchenne dystrophy. *J. Neurol. Neurosurg. Psychiatry 34:* 461, 1971.

168. McComas, A. J., FAWCETT, P. R. W., CAMPBELL, M. J., AND SICA, R. E. P. Electrophysiological estimation of the number of motor units within a human muscle. *J. Neurol. Neurosurg. Psychiatry, 34:* 121, 1971.

169. McComas, A. J., SICA, R. E. P., AND PETITO, F. Muscle strength in boys of different ages. *J. Neurol. Neurosurg. Psychiatry, 36:* 171, 1973.

170. McComas, A. J., SICA, R. E. P., UPTON, A. R. M., AND AGUILERA, N. Functional changes in motoneurones of hemiparetic patients. *J. Neurol. Neurosurg. Psychiatry, 36:* 183, 1973.

171. McComas, A. J., SICA, R. E. P., McNABB, A. R., GOLDBERG, W. M., AND UPTON, A. R. M. Evidence for reversible motoneurone dysfunction in thyrotoxicosis. *J. Neurol. Neurosurg. Psychiatry, 37:* 548, 1974.

172. MARGARIA, R., AND CERRETELLI, P. The Respiratory System and Exercise. In *Exercise Physiology,* edited by H. B. Falls. Academic Press, New York, 1968.

173. MATTHEWS, P. B. C. The differentiation of two types of fusimotor fibre by their effects on the dynamic response of muscle spindle primary endings. *J. Exp. Physiol., 47:* 324, 1962.

174. MATTHEWS, P. B. C. Muscle spindles and their motor control. *Physiol. Rev., 44:* 219, 1964.

175. MATTHEWS, P. B. C. *Mammalian Muscle Receptors and Their Central Actions.* Williams & Wilkins Co., Baltimore, 1972.

176. MATTHEWS, P. B. C. Receptors in Muscles and Joints. In *The Peripheral Nervous System,* edited by J. I. Hubbard. Plenum Press, New York, 1974.

177. MAYO, E. *Human Problems of an Industrial Civilization.* Cambridge, 1946.

178. MILNER-BROWN, H. S., STEIN, R. B., AND YEMM, R. The contractile properties of human motor units during voluntary isometric contraction. *J. Physiol. (Lond.), 228:* 285, 1973.

179. MILNER-BROWN, H. S., STEIN, R. B., AND LEE, R. G. Synchronization of human motor units; possible roles of exercise and supraspinal reflexes. *Electroencephalogr. Clin. Neurophysiol., 38:* 245, 1975.

180. MILNER-BROWN, H. S., AND BROWN, W. F. New method of estimating the number of motor units in a muscle. *J. Neurol. Neurosurg. Psychiatry, 39:* 258, 1976.

181. MOREHOUSE, L. E., AND MILLER, A. T., JR. *Physiology of Exercise,* Ed. 5. C. V. Mosby Co., St. Louis, 1971.

182. MOTTRAM, R. F. Metabolism of Exercising Muscle. In *Frontiers of Fitness,* edited by R. J. Shepherd. Charles C Thomas, Springfield, Ill., 1971.

183. MÜLLER, W., AND VOGELL, L. Temporal progress of muscle adaptation to endurance training in hindlimb muscles of young rats. *Cell Tissue Res., 156:* 61, 1974.

184. MÜLLER, W. Isometric training of young rats—effects upon hindlimb muscles. *Cell Tissue Res., 161:* 225, 1975.
185. NAFPLIOTIS, H. Electromyographic feedback to improve ankle dorsiflexion, wrist extension, and hand grasp. *Phys. Ther., 56:* 821, 1976.
186. OGATA, T., AND MURATA, F. Cytological features of three fiber types in human striated muscle. *Tohoku J. Exp. Med., 99:* 225, 1969.
187. OLKOWKSI, Z., AND MANOCHA, S. L. Muscle Spindle. In *The Structure and Function of Muscle,* Ed. 2, Volume 2, edited by G. H. Bourne. Academic Press, New York, 1973.
188. PANAYIOTOPOULOS, C. P., AND SCARPALEZOS, S. Hypertrophy of extensor digitorum brevis in limb-girdle muscular dystrophy. *Lancet, 2:* 230, 1974.
189. PANAYIOTOPOULOS, C. P., AND SCARPALEZOS, S. Electrophysiological estimation of motor units in Duchenne muscular dystrophy. *J. Neurol. Sci., 23:* 89, 1974.
190. PANAYIOTOPOULOS, C. P., SCARPALEZOS, S., AND PAPAPETROPOULOS, TH. Electrophysiological Estimation of Motor Units in Neuromuscular Diseases. In *Abstracts of the 3rd International Congress on Muscle Diseases,* edited by W. G. Bradley, Excerpta Medica, Amsterdam, 1974.
191. PANAYIOTOPOULOS, C. P., AND SCARPALEZOS, S. Dystrophia myotonica. *J. Neurol. Sci., 27:* 1, 1976.
192. PARTHENIU, A. L'intervalle phasico-tonique de l'excitabilité neuromusculaire. *Int. Z. Angew. Physiol., 24:* 333, 1967.
193. PEARSE, A. G. E. *Histochemistry, Theoretical and Applied,* Ed. 2. Churchill Ltd., London, 1960.
194. PECKHAM, P. H., MORTIMER, J. T., AND VAN DER MEULEN, J. P. Physiologic and metabolic changes in white muscle of cat following induced exercise. *Brain Res., 50:* 424, 1973.
195. PELL, K. M., AND STANFIELD, J. W., Jr. Mechanical model of skeletal muscle. *Am. J. Phys. Med., 51:* 23, 1972.
196. PETTE, D., MÜLLER, W., LEISNER, E., AND VRBOVÁ, G. Time dependent effects of contractile properties, fibre population, myosin light chains and enzymes of energy metabolism in intermittently and continuously stimulated fast twitch muscles of the rabbit. *Pflügers Arch., 364:* 103, 1976.
197. PIEHL, K. Glycogen storage and depletion in human skeletal muscle fibres. *Acta Physiol. Scand., 90:* Suppl. 402, 1974.
198. RATLIFF, R. A., AND LAMB, D. R. Glycogen replenishment following exercise: effects of denervation and tenotomy. *J. Appl. Physiol., 38:* 961, 1975.
199. REINKING, R. M., STEPHENS, J. A., AND STUART, D. G. The motor units of cat medial gastrocnemius; problem of their categorisation on the basis of mechanical properties. *Exp. Brain Res., 23:* 301, 1975.
200. RICCI, B. *Physiological Basis of Human Performance.* Lea & Febiger, Philadelphia, 1967.
201. ROBERTSON, J. D. The ultra structure of a reptilian myoneural junction. *J. Biophys. Biochem. Cytol., 2:* 381, 1956.
202. ROMANUL, F. C. A. Capillary supply and metabolism of muscle fibers. *Arch. Neurol., 12:* 497, 1965.
203. ROWELL, L. B. Cardiovascular Limitations to Work Capacity. In *Physiology of Work Capacity and Fatigue,* edited by E. Simonson. Charles C Thomas, Springfield, Ill., 1971.
204. SCARPALEZOS, S., AND PANAYIOTOPOULOS, C. P. Duchenne muscular dystrophy—reservations to the neurogenic hypothesis. *Lancet, 2:* 458, 1973a.
205. SCARPALEZOS, S., AND PANAYIOTOPOULOS, C. P. Myopathy or neuropathy in thyrotoxicosis? *N. Engl. J. Med., 289:* 918, 1973b.
206. SCHWARZACHER, H. G. Zur lage der motorischen endplatten in der Skeletmuskeln. *Acta Anat., 30:* 758, 1957.
207. SHERRINGTON, C. S. The Integrative Action of the Nervous System. *Silliman Memorial*

Lectures. Yale University Press, New Haven, 1906.

208. SHOULTZ, T. W., AND SWEET, J. R. Ultrastructural organization of the sensory fibers innervating the Golgi tendon organ. *Anat. Rec., 179:* 147, 1974.

209. SHOULTZ, T. W., AND SWEET, J. R. The fine structure of Golgi tendon organs. *J. Neurocytol., 1:* 1, 1972.

210. SICA, R. E. P., AND McCOMAS, A. J. Fast and slow twitch units in a human muscle. *J. Neurol. Neurosurg. Psychiatry, 34:* 117, 1971.

211. SICA, R. E. P., AND McCOMAS, A. J. An electrophysiological investigation of limb-girdle and facioscapulohumeral dystrophy. *J. Neurol. Neurosurg. Psychiatry, 34:* 469, 1971.

212. SICA, R. E. P., McCOMAS, A. J., UPTON, A. R. M., AND LONGMIRE, D. Motor unit estimations in small muscles of the hand. *J. Neurol. Neurosurg. Psychiatry, 37:* 55, 1974.

213. SIMONSON, E. Accumulation of Metabolites. In *Physiology of Work Capacity and Fatigue,* edited by E. Simonson. Charles C Thomas, Springfield, Ill., 1971.

214. SIMONSON, E. Regulation of Respiration in Work and Fatigue. In *Physiology of Work Capacity and Fatigue,* edited by E. Simonson. Charles C Thomas, Springfield, Ill., 1971.

215. SIMONSON, E. Nutrition and Work Performance. In *Physiology of Work Capacity and Fatigue,* edited by E. Simonson, Charles C Thomas. Springfield, Ill., 1971.

216. SOMJEN, G., CARPENTER, D. O., AND HENNEMAN, E. Responses of motoneurons of different sizes to graded stimulation of supraspinal centers of the brain. *J. Neurophysiol., 28:* 958, 1965.

217. SPANDE, J. I., AND SCHOTTLIUS, B. A. Chemical basis of fatigue in isolated mouse soleus muscle. *Am. J. Physiol., 219:* 1490, 1970.

218. SPEARING, D. L., AND POPPEN, R. The use of feedback in the reduction of foot dragging in a cerebral palsied client. *J. Nerv. Ment. Dis., 159:* 148, 1974.

219. STÅLBERG, E., AND THIELE, B. Motor unit fibre density in the extnesor digitorum communis muscle. *J. Neurol. Neurosurg. Psychiatry, 38:* 874, 1975.

220. STAUDTE, H. W., EXNER, G. U., AND PETTE, D. Effects of short-term, high intensity (sprint) training on some contractile and metabolic characteristics of fast and slow muscle of the rat. *Pflügers Arch., 344:* 159, 1973.

221. STEIN, R. B. Peripheral control of movement. *Physiol. Rev., 54:* 215, 1974.

222. STEPHENS, J. A., AND TAYLOR, A. Fatigue of maintained voluntary muscle contraction in man. *J. Physiol. (Lond.), 220:* 1, 1972.

223. STEPHENS, J. A., AND TAYLOR, A. Human motor unit contractions studied by controlled intramuscular microstimulation. *J. Physiol. (Lond.), 252:* 8P, 1975.

224. STEPHENS, J. A., AND USHERWOOD, T. P. The fatigability of human motor units. *J. Physiol. (Lond.) 250:* 27P, 1975.

225. STEPHENS, J. A., AND STUART, D. G. The motor units of cat medial gastrocnemius. *Pflügers Arch., 356:* 359, 1975.

226. STEPHENS, J. A., AND STUART, D. G. The motor units of cat medial gastrocnemius; speed-size relations and their significance for the recruitment order of motor units. *Brain Res., 91:* 177, 1975.

227. TABARY, J. C., TABARY, C., TARDIEU, C., TARDIEU, G., AND GOLDSPINK, G. Physiological and structural changes in the cat's soleus muscle due to immobilization at different lengths by plaster casts. *J. Physiol. (Lond.), 224:* 231, 1972.

228. TAKEBE, K., KUKULKA, C. G., NARAYAN, M. G., AND BASMAJIAN, J. V. Biofeedback treatment of foot drop after stroke compared with standard rehabilitation technique (Part 2); effects on nerve conduction velocity and spasticity. *Arch. Phys. Med. Rehabil., 57:* 9, 1976.

229. TANJI, J., AND KATO, M. Discharges of single motor units at voluntary contraction of abductor digiti minimi muscle in man. *Brain Res., 45:* 590, 1972.

230. TANJI, J., AND KATO, M. Recruitment of motor units in voluntary contraction of a finger muscle in man. *Exp. Neurol., 40:* 759, 1973.

231. TAYLOR, H. L., HENSCHEL, A., BROZEK, J., AND KEYS, A. Effects of bed rest on cardiovascular function and work performance. *J. Appl. Physiol., 2:* 223, 1949.

232. TERJUNG, R. L. Muscle fiber involvement during training of different intensities and durations. *Am. J. Physiol., 230:* 946, 1976.

233. THIELE, B., AND STÅLBERG, E. Single fibre EMG findings in polyneuropathies of different aetiology. *J. Neurol. Neurosurg. Psychiatry, 38:* 881, 1975.

234. TOMANEK, R. J., AND COOPER, R. R. Ultrastructural changes in tenotomized fast- and slow-twitch muscle fibres. *J. Anat., 113:* 409, 1972.

235. TONOMURA, Y. *Muscle Proteins, Muscle Contraction and Cation Transport.* University Park Press, Baltimore, 1973.

236. TSUJI, S. On the chemical basis of thiocholine methods for demonstration of acetylcholinesterase activities. *Histochemistry, 42:* 99, 1974.

237. VALLBO, Å. B. Muscle spindle response at the onset of isometric voluntary contractions in man. Time difference between fusimotor and skeletomotor effects. *J. Physiol. (Lond.), 218:* 405, 1971.

238. VALLBO, Å. B. The Significance of Intramuscular Receptors in Load Compensation during Voluntary Contractions in Man. In *Control of Posture and Locomotion,* edited by R. B. Stein, K. B. Pearson, R. S. Smith, and J. B. Redford. Plenum Press, New York, 1973.

239. VALLBO, Å. B. Muscle Spindle Afferent Discharge from Resting and Contracting Muscles in Normal Human Subjects. In *New Developments in Electromyography and Clinical Neurophysiology,* Volume 3, edited by J. E. Desmedt. Karger, Basel, 1973.

240. VALLBO, Å. B. Afferent discharge from human muscle spindles in non-contracting muscles. Steady state impulse frequency as a function of joint angle. *Acta Physiol. Scand., 90:* 303, 1974.

241. VALLBO, Å. B. Human muscle spindle discharge during isometric voluntary contractions. Amplitude relations between spindle frequency and torque. *Acta Physiol. Scand., 90:* 319, 1974.

242. WADE, O. L., AND BISHOP, J. M. *Cardiac Output and Regional Blood Flow.* Blackwell Scientific Publications, Oxford, 1962.

243. WARMOLTS, J. R., AND ENGEL, W. K. Open-biopsy electromyography. I. Correlation of motor unit behavior with histochemical muscle fiber type in human limb muscle. *Arch. Neurol., 27:* 512, 1972.

244. WARMOLTS, J. R., AND ENGEL, W. K. Correlation of Motor Unit Behavior with Histochemical Myofiber Type in Humans by Open-Biopsy Electromyography. In *New Developments in Electromyography and Clinical Neurophysiology,* Vol. 1, edited by J. E. Desmedt. Karger, Basel, 1973.

245. WOHLFART, G. Muscular atrophy in diseases of the lower motor neuron; contribution to the anatomy of the motor unit. *Arch. Neurol. Psychiatry, 61:* 599, 1949.

246. WOLPERT, R. AND WOOLRIDGE, C. P. The use of electromyography as a biofeedback therapy in the management of cerebral palsy. *Physiotherapy (Canada), 27:* 5, 1975.

3

Exercise for Strength and Endurance*

_____ BARBARA J. DE LATEUR

Theoretical Considerations

STRENGTH

Strength can be defined as the maximum force which can be exerted against an immovable object (static or isometric strength); the heaviest weight which can be lifted or lowered against gravity (dynamic or isotonic strength); or the maximal torque which can be developed against a pre-set rate-limiting device (isokinetic). The dynamic contractions can be subdivided into lengthening (eccentric) and shortening (concentric) contractions of varying velocities. These types of strength are not identical, but bear a definite relationship to each other. As velocity of shortening increases, the maximal tension which can be developed by the muscle decreases (1–3). The shape of the curve (which was measured for isometric and shortening contractions, and was calculated for lengthening contractions) is sigmoidal, with isometric tension occurring at the inflection point (4, 5). That is, the order of decreasing tension is as follows: fast lengthening, slow lengthening, isometric, slow shortening, and fast shortening contractions. An inverse relationship between velocity of (shortening) contraction and maximal torque has also been found on the isokinetic rate-limiting device (6).

The absolute muscle strength is a term used to indicate the maximum tension developed by muscle per unit of physiological cross section area (one or more sections taken at right angles to the muscle fibers so that all fibers are included). The figures generally given for the absolute muscle strength range from 3 to 4 kg per sq cm of physiologic cross section area (7–

---

* This chapter also forms part of the _Syllabus on Self-Study_, published by the American Academy of Physical Medicine and Rehabilitation. The Academy retains the right to publish this material without restriction.

9). Later work, in rats, suggested that performance of high force tasks may be improved without gross hypertrophy (10).

The ability to exert large, brief forces relates not only to muscle cross-sectional area, but also to motor-unit recruitment patterns. Utilizing bipolar needle electrodes and signal averaging techniques, Milner-Brown and co-workers found elevated synchronization ratios in weight lifters, compared with controls. The synchronization ratios of control subjects could then be increased by a 6-week weight-training program. A 20% increase in maximal isometric force was associated with a doubling of the synchronization ratio (11).

ENDURANCE AND ITS RELATIONSHIP TO STRENGTH

The endurance of a muscle may be defined as the ability of that muscle to continue a particular static or dynamic task. Although individual muscle endurance may be related to the endurance of the total individual, a distinction should be made between the two, because of the overwhelming importance of cardiovascular endurance (aerobic capacity) in the latter. The aerobic capacity of the individual will be covered in the chapters dealing with cardiovascular-pulmonary disease.

The extent to which muscle endurance is related to muscle strength, and the specificity of exercise programs designed to improve one or the other are subjects of considerable controversy. Some of the controversy may be resolved by defining a given test or training task in terms of percent maximal, rather than using the qualitative description of high-force, low-force, high-intensity, or low-intensity. Utilizing a constant load on the arm-ergograph, Monod and Scherrer (12) related movements per minute to the duration of work. The rate of movement ranged from 40% to near 100% of maximal. For an entirely different type of task, Rohmert (13) plotted a curve, based on 6,000 observations, of maximum holding time as a function of force, expressed as fractions of maximal. The range of fractions of force studied was 0.2 to 1.0. In both studies, the resultant curves were remarkably similar: hyperbolic curves with ends approaching the ordinate and abscissa asymptotically. The studies were carried out to more than 70 min in the former study (dynamic) and 11 min in the latter (static). This indicates that within limits, endurance at a given load may be increased by increasing the strength of a muscle. For example, if 20 lb is the maximum force which can be exerted (fraction = 1.0), the subject will be able to hold it only a few seconds (13, 14). An exercise program which doubles the maximum force to 40 lb shifts 20 lb to the left (fraction = 0.5) on the curve so that 20 lb may now be held approximately 1 min (13). It should be apparent that the new maximal force, 40 lb (fraction = 1.0) can only be held a few seconds.

Some experimental support for the notion of the interchangeability of relatively "high" and "low" weights was provided in the study, "A Test of the DeLorme Axiom" (15). Depending upon the strength of the individual subjects, the "high" weight of 55 lb represented about 85–100% maximal, and the "low" weight of 26 lb represented about 40–47% maximal. Training and test tasks were carried out to the point of fatigue. At the end of the series of training sessions, half of the low-weight group shifted to the high-weight task, half of the high-weight group shifted to the low-weight task, and all subjects then continued for four further (test) sessions. The performance curves in the test period did not differ significantly. Within the limits of the study (40–100% maximal), the results indicate that for otherwise identical tasks, "low" and "high" weights can be used interchangeably in training, as long as the task is continued to the point of fatigue. (Note that it took up to 15 times as long to fatigue with the low weight as with the high.) Two concepts elucidated in this study are those of biologic equivalence of a task (using fatigue as a biologic end-point) and the transfer of training acquired under one set of circumstances to performance under another set of circumstances.

Some cautions regarding generalization are in order, however. First, the similarity of the curves resulting from the Monod (12) and the Rohmert (13) studies does not permit the conclusion that isometric training will transfer fully to isotonic performance or vice versa. In cross testing (using a type of transfer-of-training design which showed initial transference only), Liberson and Asa (16) compared the results of an isotonic and an isometric training program. The isometric-trained group showed not only more improvement on the strain gage test (static), but also showed more improvement on the one-repetition maximum (dynamic) test. In contrast, utilizing a double-shift, transfer-of-training design with four test sessions (allowing study of delayed transference), deLateur et al. (17) found that subjects always did better on the type of task on which they had trained, i.e., isometric-trained did better on isometric tests; isotonic trained did better on isotonic tests. Thus, for qualitatively dissimilar tasks, the best training is that task itself.

A second caution regarding generalization is in order: the limits of interchangeability of "low" and "high" force exercise have not been established, but it seems clear that there must be some limit. It has been shown that there is an orderly sequence of recruitment of motor units. Milner-Brown et al. (18) found that the twitch tension of a motor unit varied nearly linearly as a function of the level of voluntary force at which it was recruited. The low-tension, low-threshold units show considerable fatigue resistance (19). Thus, below a certain limit (the exact value of which is not yet determined) genuine fatigue may not occur, and low-force training may have results which differ widely from higher force training.

There is, in fact, chemical and histochemical evidence that extremely different types of training have very different results. Studies in rats have shown a differential increase in myofibrillar proteins, reflecting an increase in strength, in weighted rats made to climb a pole (weight-lifting rats), whereas running rats had a selective increase in sarcoplasmic proteins, reflecting enhanced capacity for energy metabolism and local muscle endurance (20–23).

Running and weight lifting also produced quantitatively different regional changes in succinic dehydrogenase and phosphorylase enzyme activities (23). There is some species-specificity in these results, since they could not be duplicated in guinea pigs; in the latter animal, Helander (24) found an increase in actomysin (reflecting strength) in running animals. Thus, caution should be exercised in generalizing animal results to humans. However, human studies are proceeding. Gollnick and co-workers have used biopsy techniques to study effects of exercise in adults and children (25–29). They studied enzyme activities in the muscles of untrained individuals and of subjects trained in various types of athletics. Succinate dehydrogenase (SDH) activity, reflecting oxidative capacity, was much higher in the muscles of such athletes as bicyclists (legs higher than arms) canoeists (arms higher than legs), runners, and swimmers, than in the muscles of weight lifters, whose SDH activity was no higher than the untrained individuals. Gollnick subsequently studied the effects of a 5-month training program consisting of pedalling a bicycle ergometer 1 hour per day, 4 days per week, at a load requiring 75–90% of maximal aerobic power. He found that, although there was no alteration in the percentage number of the slow twitch (ST) (low-tension, early-recruited, fatigue-resistant) fibers, the ratio of the ST to fast twitch (FT) fiber areas increased from 0.82 to 1.11 ($P < 0.01$) after training. Oxidative capacity increased in both fiber types, whereas anaerobic capacity increased only in the FT fibers. Of particular interest on the low-force high-force specificity question are Gollnick's glycogen depletion studies after acute bouts of varying intensities of dynamic work or static contractions. Work intensities in bicycle exercise varied from 30 to 150% of $\dot{V}_{O_2}$ max. At all workloads below $\dot{V}_{O_2}$ max, slow twitch, high oxidative (ST) fibers were the first to lose glycogen, but progressive glycogen depletion occurred in FT fibers as work continued. These results indicated primary reliance upon ST fibers during submaximal endurance exercise with recruitment of FT fibers after the ST fibers were depleted of glycogen. This would tend to support the notion that FT fibers can be recruited with submaximal exercise if the exercise is continued long enough. In the studies of static (isometric) contractions, subjects performed repeated contractions, sustained until exhaustion, at 10, 15, 20, 25, 30, 35, 40, or 50% of maximal voluntary contractions force (MVC). From the selective glycogen depletion it was concluded that at sustained contractions below 20% MVC there is a major reliance upon ST fibers and above that level a primary reliance upon FT fibers.

It seems reasonable to summarize all these data by saying that for qualitatively identical exercise, there is *relative* interchangeability of loads between 30 and 100% of maximal, as long as the task is carried to the point of muscle fatigue. For extreme quantitative differences, or for qualitatively different tasks, the best training for a given task is that task itself.

Practical Programs

With some of these theoretical considerations in mind, one may then approach a number of practical exercise programs which have been developed.

One of the first systematic programs was described by DeLorme (30) and DeLorme and Watkins (31) who emphasized the rebuilding of strength by heavy-resistance, dynamic (isotonic) exercises. This program, widely used and known as progressive resistive exercise (PRE) has gone through a number of modifications, but commonly employs a series of 10 contractions at 25% maximal, and 10 each at 50, 75, and 100% maximal. Once a week a determination is made of the 10-RM, which is the maximal weight which can be lifted through the range of motion 10 times. As the name (PRE) suggests, this results in a progressive increase in load as the strength increases.

A modification of the DeLorme technique, in which the weight is taken off rather than added (10 repetitions each at 100, 75, 50, and 25%) is known as the Oxford technique (32). It was found that subjects could complete each training session with less fatigue with the Oxford than with the DeLorme technique, but the previous theoretical considerations and a recent study on training effects of fatigue (33) suggest that for that very reason the Oxford technique may be somewhat less effective than the DeLorme technique.

Hellebrandt (34) and Hellebrandt and Houtz (35, 36) have demonstrated that the work capacity of muscle can be improved, not only by progressive increase in load, but also by progressive increase in rate of repetition with a constant load. This requires use of a metronome and does not seem to be a widely used approach, but it is one of the options available.

The isokinetic exercise device (37–39) accommodates any torque developed throughout the range of motion. A study (40) comparing the results of a training program with this device with a comparable dynamic weight program showed no significant training results. However, in the study, performance of both groups was assured by monetary compensation. In the clinic the isokinetic exerciser offers the advantage that the patient can see an immediate printout of his progress, which has reinforcing (reward) value in itself.

Brief isometric exercise programs have been described by Hettinger and Müller (14), Liberson and Asa (16), and Rose et al. (41). These require a strain gage, so that information feedback about the force exerted and the progress made can be obtained. Their brevity and effectiveness in increasing isometric strength are advantages. However, since most ambulation and self-care tasks include some dynamic requirements, one should not rely entirely upon isometric exercise to train for these tasks.

The techniques described above are usually carried out in physical therapy departments. They can be duplicated, to a large extent, in the occupational therapy setting, which has the advantage of providing activities which many (but not all) patients find more interesting. Details and illustrations of such applications are to be found in the chapter on therapeutic exercise by Kottke in the *Handbook of Physical Medicine and Rehabilitation* (42).

REFERENCES

1. HILL, A. V. The maximum work and mechanical efficiency of human muscles and their most economical speed. *J. Physiol., 56:* 19-41, 1922.
2. FENN, W. O., BRODY, H., AND PETRILLI, A. The tension development by human muscle at different velocities of shortening. *Am. J. Physiol., 97:* 1-14, 1931.
3. FENN, W. O., AND MARSH, B. S. Muscular force at different speeds of shortening. *J. Physiol., 85:* 277-297, 1935.
4. WILKIE, D. V. The relation between force and velocity in human muscle. *J. Physiol., 110:* 249-280, 1950.
5. ABBOTT, B. C., BIGLAND, B., AND RITCHIE, J. M. The physiological cost of negative work. *J. Physiol., 117:* 380-390, 1952.
6. SCUDDER, G. N. A study of torque produced at controlled speeds of voluntary motion. MS thesis, University of Minnesota, 1969, quoted in *Handbook of Physical Medicine and Rehabilitation,* Ed. 2, Ch. 16, edited by F. H. Krusen, F. J. Kottke, and P. M. Ellwood, Jr. Philadelphia, 1971.
7. VON RECKLINGHAUSEN, H. *Gliedermechanik und Lähmungsprothesen.* J. Springer, Berlin, 1920.
8. HAXTON, H. A. Absolute muscle force in ankle flexors of man. *J. Physiol., 103:* 267-273, 1944.
9. RAMSEY, R. W., AND STREET, S. F. Isometric length-tension diagram of isolated skeletal muscle fibers in frog. *J. Cell. Comp. Physiol., 15:* 11-34, 1940.
10. GORDON, E. E., KOWALSKI, K., AND FRITTS, B. S. Changes in rat muscle fiber with forceful exercises. *Arch. Phys. Med., 48:* 577-582, 1967.
11. MILNER-BROWN, H. S., STEIN, R. B., AND LEE, R. G. Synchronization of human motor units; possible rôles of exercise and supraspinal reflexes. *Electroencephalogr. Clin. Neurophys., 38:* 245-254, 1975.
12. MONOD, H., AND SCHERRER, J. Capacité de travail statique d'un group musculaire synergique chez l'Homme. *C. R. Soc. Biol.* 151: 1358-1362, 1957. Cited in *Physiology of Work Capacity and Fatigue,* pp. 440-442, edited by E. Simonson. Charles C Thomas, Springfield, Ill., 1971.
13. ROHMERT, W. Ermittlung von Erholungspausen für statische Arbeit des Menschen. *Int. Z. Angew. Physiol. 18:* 123-164, 1960. Cited in Müller, E. A. Influence of training and of inactivity on muscle strength. *Arch. Phys. Med., 51:* 449-462, 1970.
14. HETTINGER, T., AND MÜLLER, E. A. Muskelleistung und Muskeltraining. *Arbeitsphysiol., 15:* 111-126, 1953. Cited in Müller, E. A. Influence of training and of inactivity on muscle strength. *Arch. Phys. Med., 51:* 449-462, 1970.
15. DELATEUR B. J., LEHMANN, J. F., AND FORDYCE, W. E. A test of the DeLorme axiom. *Arch. Phys. Med., 49:* 245-248, 1968.
16. LIBERSON, W. T., AND ASA, M. M. Further studies of brief isometric exercises. *Arch. Phys. Med., 40:* 330, 1959.
17. DELATEUR, B., LEHMANN, J., STONEBRIDGE, J., AND WARREN, C. G. Isotonic versus isometric exercise; a double-shift, transfer-of-training study. *Arch. Phys. Med., 53:* 212-217, 1972.
18. MILNER-BROWN, H. S., STEIN, R. B., AND YEMM, R. The orderly recruitment of human motor units during voluntary isometric contractions. *J. Physiol., 230:* 359-370, 1973.
19. FAULKNER, J. A. Muscle Fatigue. In *The Physiology and Biochemistry of Muscle as a Food,* pp. 555-575, edited by E. J. Briskey, R. G. Cassens, and B. B. Marsh, University of Wisconsin Press, Madison, 1970.
20. GORDON, E. E., KOWALSKI, K., AND FRITTS, M. Changes in rat muscle fiber with forceful exercises. *Arch. Phys. Med., 48:* 577-82, 1967.

21. GORDON, E. E., KOWALSKI, K., AND FRITTS, M. Protein changes in quadriceps muscle of rat with repetitive exercises. *Arch. Phys. Med., 48:* 296–303, 1967.
22. JAWEED, M. M., GORDON, E. E., HERBISON, G. J., AND KOWALSKI, K. Endurance and strengthening exercise adaptations; I. Protein changes in skeletal muscles. *Arch. Phys. Med., 55:* 513–517, 1974.
23. KOWALSKI, K., GORDON, E. E., MARTINEZ, A., AND ADAMEK, J. Changes in enzyme activities of various muscle fiber types in rat induced by different exercises. *J. Histochem. Cytochem., 17:* 601–607, 1969.
24. HELANDER, E. A. Influence of exercise and restricted activity on the protein composition of skeletal muscle. *Biochem. J., 78:* 478–482, 1961.
25. GOLLNICK, P. D., ARMSTRONG, R. B., SAUBERT, C. W., PIEHL, K., AND SALTIN, B. Enzyme activity and fiber composition in skeletal muscle of untrained and trained men. *J. Appl. Physiol., 33:* 312–319, 1972.
26. GOLLNICK, P. D., ARMSTRONG, R. B., SALTIN, B., SAUBERT, C. W., SEMBROWICH, W. L., AND SHEPHERD, R. E. Effect of training on enzyme activity and fiber composition of human skeletal muscle. *J. Appl. Physiol. 34:* 107–111, 1973.
27. ERIKSSON, B. O., GOLLNICK, P. D., AND SALTIN, B. The effect of physical training on muscle enzyme activities and fiber composition in 11-year-old boys. *Acta Paediatr. Belg., 28* (Suppl.): 245–252, 1974.
28. GOLLNICK, P. D., PIEHL, K., AND SALTIN, B. Selective glycogen depletion pattern in human muscle fibers after exercise of varying intensity and at varying pedalling rates. *J. Physiol., 241:* 45–57, 1974.
29. GOLLNICK, P. D., KARLSSON, J., PIEHL, K., AND SALTIN, B. Selective glycogen depletion in skeletal muscle fibers of man following sustained contractions. *J. Physiol., 241:* 59–67, 1974.
30. DELORME, T. L. Restoration of muscle power by heavy-resistance exercises. *J. Bone Joint Surg., 27:* 645–667, 1945.
31. DELORME, T. L., AND WATKINS, A. L. Technics of progressive resistance exercise. *Arch. Phys. Med., 29:* 263–273, 1948.
32. ZINOVIEFF, A. N. Heavy-resistance exercises; the "Oxford technique." *Br. J. Phys. Med., 14:* 129–132, 1951.
33. DELATEUR, B. J., LEHMANN, J. F., AND GIACONI, R. Mechanical work and fatigue; their roles in the development of muscle work capacity. *Arch. Phys. Med., 57:* 319–324, 1976.
34. HELLEBRANDT, F. A. Application of the overload principle to muscle training in man. *Am. J. Phys. Med., 37:* 278–283, 1958.
35. HELLEBRANDT, F. A., AND HOUTZ, S. J. Mechanisms of muscle training in man; experimental demonstration of the overload principle. *Phys. Ther. Rev., 36:* 371–383, 1956.
36. HELLEBRANDT, F. A., AND HOUTZ, S. J. Methods of muscle training; the influence of pacing. *Phys. Ther. Rev., 38:* 319–322, 1958.
37. MOFFROID, M., WHIPPLE, R., HOFKOSH, J., LOWMAN, E., AND THISTLE, H. Guidelines for Clinical Use of Isokinetic Exercise. *Rehabilitation Monograph XL.* Institute of Rehabilitation Medicine, New York University Medical Center, 1969.
38. THISTLE, H. G., HISLOP, H. J., MOFFROID, M., AND LOWMAN, E. Isokinetic contraction; new concept of resistive exercise. *Arch. Phys. Med., 48:* 279–282, 1967.
39. MOFFROID, M., WHIPPLE, R., HOFKOSH, J., LOWMAN, E., AND THISTLE, H. Study of isokinetic exercise. *Phys. Ther. 49:* 735–746, 1969.
40. DELATEUR, B., LEHMANN, J. F., WARREN, C. G., STONEBRIDGE, J., FUNITA, G., COKELET, K., AND EGBERT, H. Comparison of effectiveness of isokinetic and isotonic exercise in quadriceps strengthening. *Arch. Phys. Med., 53:* 60–64, 1972.
41. ROSE, D. L., RADZYMINSKI, S. J., AND BEATTY, R. R. Effect of brief maximal exercise on the strength of the quadriceps femoris. *Arch. Phys. Med., 38:* 157–164, 1957.
42. KOTTKE, F. J. Therapeutic Exercise. In *Handbook of Physical Medicine and Rehabilitation,* Ed. 2, Ch. 16, pp. 385–428, edited by F. H. Krusen, F. J. Kottke, and P. M. Ellwood, Jr. Philadelphia, 1971.

4

Facilitation Techniques in Therapeutic Exercise

_____ F. A. HARRIS

Introduction

While we will ultimately focus attention on the procedures utilized by the expositors of the major therapeutic exercise techniques,[1] this chapter begins with a discussion of the neurophysiological mechanisms upon which the effectiveness of these methods depends. During the years that therapeutic exercise procedures primarily relied on simple spinal reflex mechanisms, it was possible for therapists to function with minimal attention to neurophysiological principles, or even entirely on an empirical basis. Contemporary techniques are based on more complex sensorimotor mechanisms involving all levels of the neuraxis, however, and an increasing demand is placed on therapists for working knowledge of pathways and processing centers for cutaneous and even exteroceptive senses, as well as muscle input. Familiarity with the gamma (γ) efferent system is required, including its modulation from extrapyramidal motor areas in cerebral cortex (65), cerebellum and brainstem, in addition to knowledge concerning the classical corticospinal pathway consisting of upper and lower

---

[1] In the introductory sections of this chapter _therapeutic exercise_ is used to refer to any repetitive motor activities which a patient performs with the assistance of or under the supervision of a therapist, for the purpose of modifying muscle tone and/or increasing the strength and degree of control of voluntary movements. For the sake of brevity, the phrase _facilitation techniques_ will be used to refer to both facilitation and inhibition procedures. The phrase _proprioceptive neuromuscular facilitation_ (PNF) will be used in a general sense, to refer to any procedure where peripheral input via muscle, tendon and joint receptors is used for facilitation, rather than in specific reference to the PNF technique of Knott and Voss. Finally, in recognition of the predominance of women among therapists, the feminine gender has been used in references to therapist.

motoneurons. Responding to this challenge does bring benefits; rather than remaining duly-bound to any one method out of experience restricted to it or sheer faith in its expositor, therapists now have the opportunity to become ecclectic in practice. It is possible to select among a wide variety of techniques based on theoretical and practical considerations, and to employ them in concert or in sequence rather than in a mutually exclusive fashion, thus bringing greater benefits to the patient.

The theoretical discussion begins with a review of findings from classical research concerning spinal reflexes, which provide the basis for "traditional" PNF techniques. In the following section, we consider modifications in the view of motor mechanisms which occurred after investigation of the γ efferent system in the early 1950s, leading to development of Rood's cutaneous stimulation methods. Next, techniques involving head (i.e., vestibular) and neck reflexes and equilibrium reactions are examined, shading over into those procedures based on "central facilitation"—i.e., utilizing synergistic patterns and associated reactions. Finally, emerging sensory feedback and reinforcement concepts from contemporary behavioral psychology are examined in relation to traditional contemporary facilitation methods in order to arrive at the broadest possible view of the accomplishments to date and the potential for future development of therapeutic exercise as an extension of human motor learning.

Following the theoretical discussion, the major therapeutic exercise methods are compared in terms of their involvement or utilization of the above mentioned neural mechanisms, and a summary is drawn of the procedures which the present day therapist has at his or her disposal, to show the powerful armament which can be brought to bear on the patient's neurological problems with muscle tone, postural stability, range of motion, control of voluntary movement, strength and endurance (23).

The purpose for taking the therapist on a tour through the annals of traditional and contemporary neurobiology is to bring into clear focus and put into historical perspective those discoveries that provide the rationale for therapeutic exercise. One must be willing to make only one assumption: that neural mechanisms elucidated through studies of laboratory animals such as cats, monkeys, and baboons are operative in the human as well as in these animals—in order to relate the realms of basic science and clinical practice in physical therapy. This is not an unreasonable assumption; and, once the therapist makes it, he or she is equipped with at least one yardstick by which any therapeutic technique can be gauged. If the technique takes into consideration the anatomical organization and functional principles of the nervous system, it ought to work if properly applied.[2] The corollary to this statement is that if a new technique is

---

[2] While each technique is based on a broad principle, such as the use of muscle stretch for facilitation, there are many subtle aspects of the procedures which must be taken into consideration. These include the topographical relation between the area of the periphery stimulated and the weak muscle(s), the rate of stimulus application, the interval between

empirically discovered, the expositor(s) should endeavor to discover and understand the neural mechanisms upon which it depends. Thus, therapists should not be constrained from using techniques which are not presently explainable, but rather should be urged to seek comprehension of the neural mechanisms involved all the while new techniques are being used. In physical therapy, explanation of the basis for the method typically has followed the practical demonstration of its efficacy. (It is possible, however, to theoretically derive new concepts and procedures and then to test them in practice.)

Our present day review of theories and findings in the neurosciences also reveals the *incorrectness* of certain older views which were once put forth as fundamental "laws" and "axioms" concerning neural function. Since a number of approaches to therapeutic exercise rest heavily upon these presumed laws, these approaches should be revised in the light of contemporary knowledge. In the author's opinion, doing so broadens the scope of therapeutic exercise and leads to more effective techniques.

The effectiveness of therapeutic exercise for neuromuscular education, at least in terms of production of short-term changes in muscle tone and power of voluntary movements in both adult and pediatric patients, is indisputable. Since these techniques rely for their effectiveness on the manifestations of fundamental neuroanatomical structures and neurophysiological function, this is not very surprising. Debating the effectiveness of muscle stretch as a facilitatory stimulus, for example, amounts to challenging the existence of the stretch reflex. In the past, serious critics of facilitation techniques launched a more penetrating attack from the standpoint of questioning whether they have any lasting effects — whether any "carry-over" into improvement of everyday functional skills occurs as the result of daily repetition of short-term facilitatory effects during therapy. Even here, neuroscientists are beginning to fill in the theoretical edifice upon which facilitation techniques rest. Highly reputable neurobiologists have shown that the central nervous system (CNS) is capable of structural repair after injury. As will be discussed near the end of the chapter, CNS neurons spontaneously grow new processes and tend to re-establish connections even without any deliberate therapy going on (79) How much more likely it is, then, that with proper therapy, such inherent "plastic"

---

peripheral stimulation and the call for voluntary movement, and the intensity and duration of the facilitatory or inhibitory effect obtained in relation to the timing of voluntary movement. Thus the therapist might apply the "correct" stimulus in the broadest sense, and yet fail to achieve the desired effect due to lack of attention to these and other details. The classical "conditioning-testing interaction" used by neurophysiologists to assess excitatory and inhibitory influences, discussed in the context of Lloyd's studies of spinal reflexes (59, 60), in later paragraphs, provides an explicit model for the therapist to keep in mind while attempting to modify muscle tone or strength of voluntary contractions. This model focuses attention on all of the parameters which must be considered in evaluating the impact to any given stimulus on the excitability of CNS centers, including the spinal nuclei of alpha (α) motoneurons innervating voluntary musculature.

anatomical recovery processes may be guided toward an optimal functional outcome.

Theory

GENERAL CONSIDERATIONS — THE NEURAL BASIS FOR FACILITATION TECHNIQUES

The theoretical basis for certain facilitation and inhibition techniques used widely in both traditional and modern therapeutic exercise methods can be traced to Sherrington's time-honored findings from his investigations pertaining to spinal reflex physiology (84, 85). In fact, the target of Sherrington's investigations is identical to what should be the therapist's focus of attention, namely, the delineation of modulating influences upon the activity of spinal α motoneurons (also referred to as ventral horn cells) that innervate the voluntary musculature. Sherrington defined the concept of facilitation (Fig. 4.1) and inhibition in terms of how experimentally induced and naturally occurring inputs from peripheral nerves and receptors affected the excitability (i.e., tendency to discharge impulses) of these particular neural elements (59). For each stimulus affecting motoneurons at the spinal level — whether by way of central pathways conveying descending impulses of cortical, cerebellar, or brainstem origin, or by way of peripherally originating pathways conveying afferent impulses of cutaneous or muscle origin — the resulting impulse volley was shown to cause outright impulse discharge in a limited number of target motoneurons (i.e., those in the discharge zone) and to subliminally excite others in anatomical proximity (i.e., those in the subliminal fringe). Any superimposed or supplementary stimulus that could be shown to cause the recruitment of additional neurons from the subliminal fringe into the discharge zone was considered *facilitatory* (i.e., increased excitability); any stimulus that caused neurons to drop out of the discharge zone and fall back into the subliminal fringe was considered *inhibitory* (i.e., decreased excitability). Thus, in the process of carrying out his physiological studies of spinal reflex mechanisms, Sherrington also surveyed territory of great interest to the early therapists. The influences of peripheral origin — those carried via afferent fibers from muscle and tendon receptors, and from pain receptors in the skin — which he identified as most strongly and predictably influencing the excitability of alpha motoneurons are precisely the ones that came to be utilized in traditional facilitation techniques.

Thus, while viewing the patient as an intact human being, in all the complexity that implies, is a fundamental tenet of modern rehabilitation management, the therapist may nevertheless find it advantageous in planning and evaluating treatment to focus attention specifically on the patient's difficulties with bringing about and controlling alpha motoneuron discharge. The goal of evaluation is to determine 1) the distribution of abnormal muscle tone throughout the body, 2) the strength behind voluntary movements, and 3) the quality of coordination of voluntary move-

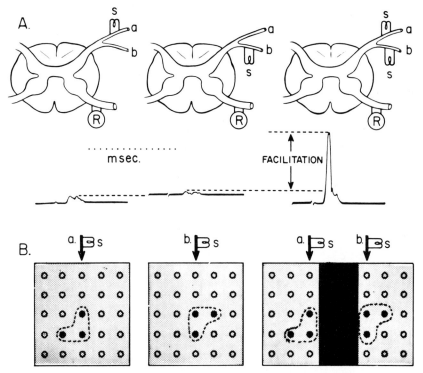

Fig. 4.1. (A) Demonstration of facilitation. Weak stimulation of each of two dorsal root strands, a and b, produces low-amplitude reflex responses shown in left and middle traces, respectively. Simultaneous stimulation of a and b elicited facilitated reflex discharge on the right, greater than the sum of the individual responses. (B) Mechanism of facilitation. On the left and in the middle are represented the motoneuron pools served by afferent sources, a and b. Input from each source discharges three motoneurons, and subliminally excites the remainder of the pool. The subliminal fringes of a and b partially overlap. Thus, when inputs a and b are provided simultaneously, additional neurons in the zone of overlap are brought to threshold, and eleven rather than six neurons fire. (From H. D. Patton, *Physiology and Biophysics*, 19th ed., W. B. Saunders Co., Philadelphia 1965 (71).)

ments that prevail at the time the patient presents for treatment. Once this has been accomplished, certain muscles or muscle groups can be selected as having the highest priority for attention, in terms of their functional importance for self-care activities, ambulation, and manipulation. The activity of weak muscles will require facilitation; that of spastic muscles will require inhibition. Muscles that contract in a tremorous or apparently erratic fashion will have to be brought under smooth volitional control.

In each instance, the problem can be conceptually reduced to that of regulation of α motoneuron discharge. In the case of weak muscles, the discharge of spinal motoneurons innervating those muscles must somehow be increased (i.e., their excitability level must be raised). In the case of spastic muscles, the "tonic" or "resting" level of discharge of spinal motoneurons innervating those muscles must somehow be decreased (i.e., their excitability must be diminished). In the case of tremorous or erratic muscle activity—such as in Parkinson's syndrome, ataxia, or athetoid cerebral palsy—the discharge rate of motoneurons innervating the affected muscles must be brought under reliable volitional control and "smoothed out," so that a given rate of discharge can be maintained for periods of time sufficient for postural stability, and transitions from one rate of firing to another may occur without under- or overshoot.

Having taken these initial conceptual steps in reducing the problem from consideration of overt movement, through 1) assessment of the tone and strength of synergistically and antagonistically operating muscles, and from there to 2) inference about the rate of discharge of spinal motoneurons innervating those muscles, the therapist is in a position to put both knowledge of the neurosciences and creativity into play in order to proceed with sound treatment. The therapist must then decide which neural influences, of peripheral and/or central origin, can be brought to bear on the rate of α motoneuron discharge to certain target muscles for the purpose of beneficially modifying muscle tone and strength of voluntary contraction—also taking into consideration the patient's individual motivational profile and capacity for motor learning, and the particular circumstances under which treatment will be carried out.

The following discussion provides an historical perspective on the methods devised as solutions for this problem—solutions which were understandably related to the state of knowledge about CNS and neuromuscular function which prevailed at each step during the evolution of physical therapy. In this evolution, five major approaches to facilitation can be recognized. These are:

1. Traditional PNF procedures
2. Cutaneous stimulation
3. Head and neck on body reflexes and equilibrium reactions
4. "Central" facilitation (i.e., synergies and associated reactions)
5. Motor learning (including EMG feedback, enhanced sensory feedback and contingent reinforcement).

TRADITIONAL PNF TECHNIQUES

We have indicated that the therapist may utilize mechanisms of peripheral or central origin to increase or decrease the probability of motoneuron discharge, thereby increasing muscle tone or voluntary motor output, or decreasing tone (i.e., promoting relaxation from a baseline state of hypertonicity or spasticity). That is, parts of the body and specific tissues comprising each part can be manipulated in such a fashion that sensory inputs having reflexly mediated synaptic excitatory or inhibitory effects on α motoneurons are produced; or, activity in cortically originating, descending pathways can be elicited through motivational and/or emotional stimulation, thereby modifying the degree of α motoneuronal discharge produced via the residual voluntary motor mechanism (e.g., those parts of the corticospinal and extrapyramidal pathway unaffected by the lesion).

Peripherally originating mechanisms are simplest and thus the best understood of neural mechanisms. Sherrington's comprehension of *spatiotemporal summation* of input from various sources affecting common α motoneurons, which gives these neurons an integrative ability, provided an explicit theoretical basis for the first proprioceptive facilitation techniques, in the strictest sense of this terminology. The occurrence of such summation or superimposition of diverse inputs has an obvious anatomical basis in synaptic convergence of peripheral and central input onto common motoneurons or onto common interneurons which in turn excite motoneurons. The functional correlate of this convergence has been documented through the use of neurophysiology's most refined technique—recording intracellularly from single α motoneurons (18, 64) or spinal cord interneurons (29) and showing that they are affected by stimulation of both central (e.g., motor cortex) and peripheral (e.g., muscle or cutaneous nerve branches) structures. In a comparable study performed on human subjects, with intramuscular electromyograph (EMG) recording from single motor units, it was shown that the same motor units could be activated by volitional input (i.e., through descending CNS pathways) and by both stretch reflex and nociceptive reflex inputs (3).

Thus it is a theoretically sound expectation that the therapist can modify the excitability of α motoneurons to descending volleys of central origin by "putting in" activity of peripheral origin which also impinges on these same motoneurons. The discharge of particular motoneurons can be facilitated (thus increasing muscle tone or strength of voluntary contraction) by using peripheral stimulation which sets up impulses in afferent fibers making excitatory connections with those "target" motoneurons (Fig. 4.2), or inhibited (thus bringing about muscle relaxation) by setting up activity in afferent fibers making inhibitory connections with them. The strength of the modulatory influence which the therapist is able to exert will reflect the type of stimulus applied, the anatomical relation between the part stimulated and the muscle or muscle group to be influenced, and certain details concerning the stimulus itself (e.g., rate of stimulus application). Thus the therapist can control or grade the modulatory effect, exerting a stronger influence initially and progressively "tapering off" her contribution as the patient improves in ability to independently mobilize the target motoneurons under centrally originating volitional drive.

Note that it is not necessary for a facilitatory stimulus to be independently capable of causing motoneuronal discharge; subthreshold synaptic effects are sufficient for facilitatory or inhibitory interactions between peripheral and central input to occur, since neurons can be shifted into or out of the discharge zone without actually causing them to fire impulses. As mentioned previously, the conditioning-testing interaction technique which the neurophysiologist uses to study neural pathways and synaptic

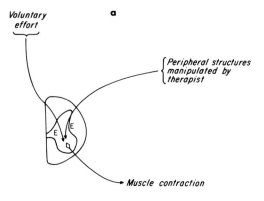

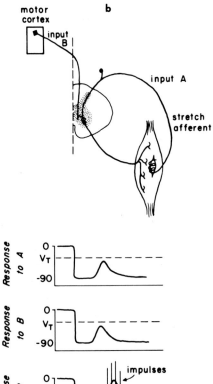

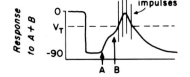

Fig. 4.2. (a) Diagrammatic representation of *spatiotemporal summation*, which provides the basis for facilitation of voluntary activation of muscles. Convergence of peripheral and central excitatory influences on α motoneurons

connections provides an excellent model for the therapist to employ in attempting to facilitate or inhibit the patient's efforts during therapeutic exercise activities. The physiologist interacts a conditioning stimulus from one source with a test stimulus from another in order to study synaptic interactions. Among the parameters varied are the relative strengths of the conditioning and test stimuli and the time interval between them. Using this procedure, Lloyd was able to establish a definite time course for both excitatory and inhibitory synaptic influences on spinal motoneurons. As Figures 4.3 and 4.4 indicate, a given conditioning input exerts a modulating influence on the test response which reaches a maximum after a brief delay and lasts a relatively short period of time. The therapist *must* keep these temporal factors in mind when using peripheral stimuli to modify the patient's spinal motoneuron output under volitional drive. The timing of the interval between the "conditioning" peripheral stimulus and the call for the "test" volitional effort from the patient is critical if the desired effect is to be obtained.

Obviously, the therapist's efforts at facilitation have a greater likelihood of success if the peripheral input can be *sustained* — which led first to the use of repetitive stimulation (i.e., "tapping" over the muscle belly rather than applying a single quick stretch) in the evolution of facilitation techniques, and eventually to the use of a mechanical vibrator (76), applied directly over the muscle belly or gripped by both the therapist and the patient, in contemporary variations on the traditional PNF techniques. In the following section, the use of muscle stretch as a facilitatory input will be examined in detail.

Reasons are immediately evident as to why the simplest and best understood of all peripheral mechanisms, the stretch reflex initiated through mechanical distortion of receptors within the muscles themselves, is the most powerful and most universally applicable of all facilitatory mechanisms. The large-diameter, rapidly conducting afferent fibers arising from stretch receptors within the muscle spindles make powerful monosynaptic

---

is the basis for facilitating discharge of the α motoneurons under volitional drive by "putting in" peripheral input such as muscle stretch. (b) A more detailed representation of the anatomical-physiological basis for facilitation techniques. Input A represents peripheral input to α motoneurons from stretch receptors; B represents descending input via the corticospinal tract and extrapyramidal routes. Both inputs converge upon common motoneurons. Intracellularly recorded responses of a single motoneuron to A or B alone are subthreshold; no impulse discharge results from either input in isolation. When B (representing volitional activation) follows closely after A (representing peripheral input which the therapist sets up by quick stretch of the muscle to be facilitated), the two inputs summate to produce a suprathreshold depolarization leading to impulse discharge. The two imputs come from different regions and must occur more or less simultaneously in order for the depolarizations they produce to add and thus exceed threshold; hence this process is referred to as *spatiotemporal summation*. (From F. A. Harris, *American Journal of Occupational Therapy, 23:* 397, 1969 (39), and F. A. Harris, *Physical Therapy, 51:* 391, 1971 (41).)

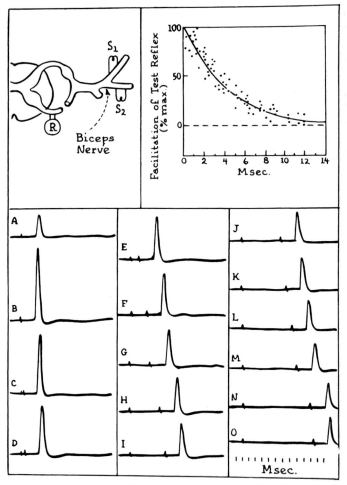

Fig. 4.3. Time course of facilitatory process. A conditioning stimulus applied to one branch of biceps nerve, activating Group I afferent fibers, elicited no reflex discharge. Test stimulus applied to the other branch elicited low-amplitude reflex discharge seen in A and O. Traces B through N show the reflex discharges elicited by combining the conditioning and test stimuli, separated by increasing intervals. The duration of the interval is indicated by the separation between the two small "blips" on the trace baseline, which represent the times at which the two stimuli were applied. The accompanying graph shows the relation between the increase in size of the test reflex (expressed as percentage of maximal) and the C-T interval. The greatest facilitation was obtained with near-simultaneous inputs from the two nerve branches; after a separation of only 10 msec, the facilitatory effect is entirely lost. (From D. Lloyd, *Journal of Neurophysiology, 9:* 421, 1946 (59).)

excitatory connections with α motoneurons innervating the muscle from which the afferent fibers arise. They also make polysynaptic inhibitory connections with motoneurons innervating the antagonist muscles, providing the physiological basis for Sherrington's *reciprocal innervation* principle. Thus the therapist may use muscle stretch for facilitation of the muscle stretched, or for relaxation of its antagonist(s).

While the "sign" (i.e., excitatory or facilitatory) of modulatory effects produced through proprioceptive stimuli is readily deduced from a knowledge of spinal reflex connections, there are additional, more subtle factors which also must be taken into account when using muscle stretch (which in fact is used in virtually every popular facilitation technique). One of these is the rate of stimulus application. Muscle stretch receptors produce a continuing "train" of impulses rather than a single impulse for a given stretch stimulus (Fig. 4.5), with frequency of impulses in the train depending both on the magnitude and the rate of applied stretch (49); therefore it is obvious that for a given magnitude of muscle stretch (i.e., amplitude of

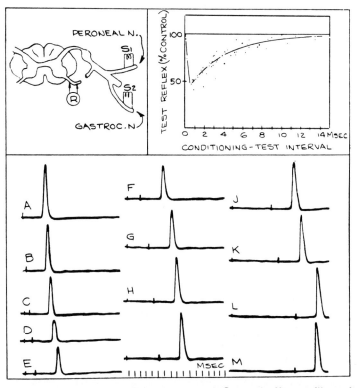

Fig. 4.4. Time course of inhibitory process. Group I afferent fibers from twc antagonistic muscles were used as input routes. Weak stimulus via peroneal n. elicited no reflex discharge. Stimulus to gastrocnemius n. elicited monosynaptic reflex seen in A and M. Traces B through L show discharges when two stimuli were combined, separated by increasing intervals. Accompanying graph shows relation between gastroc. n. test reflex response and input via peroneal n. preceding by various intervals. Maximal inhibition is obtained with C-T interval of about 1 msec, and the inhibitory effect is lost entirely with a separation of more than 14 msec. (From D. Lloyd, *Journal of Neurophysiology, 9:* 421, 1946 (59).)

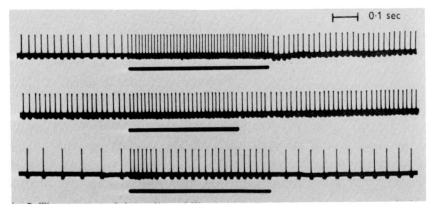

Fig. 4.5. Responses of a muscle stretch receptor to three different short stretches under varying physiological conditions. In each instance there is a resting or baseline "tonic" level of discharge that corresponds to the initial length of the muscle before it is stretched; the rate of discharge represents the length of the muscle. When the muscle is stretched, the rate of impulse discharge increases proportionately to the amount of elongation. As seen clearly in the bottom trace, there is usually a dynamic component of the response in which impulse frequency is proportional to rate of stretch, followed by a static component in which frequency is proportional to the length attained after stretch. When stretch is released, the impulse frequency returns to the baseline level as the muscle returns to its resting length. (From K. S. Janssen and P. B. C. Matthews, *Journal of Physiology (London), 161:* 357, 1962 (49)).

passive movement) a more powerful effect can be gotten the faster the stretch is applied. Thus, the greater the facilitatory effect sought, the brisker should be the movement producing muscle stretch. This is the reason for the effectiveness of applying "quick stretch" to a given muscle just before calling for its voluntary activation; it also explains the effectiveness of "tapping," which amounts to the application of a series of sudden muscle stretches, and also of the interposition of vibratory stimulators between the therapist and the patient, since muscle vibration is also the equivalent of a series of very quick stretches in its effect on the stretch receptors.

Rate of stretch is also important because relaxation of a given muscle — just the opposite effect from facilitation — can be obtained by stretching the muscle very slowly and maintaining stretch over a prolonged period of time. In this case, the stretch receptors are progressively "desensitized" (a process somewhat similar to anesthetization) because the excitatory process they set up adapts out under conditions of prolonged slow stretch (14). That is, the initial stretch stimulus "sneaks by" the stretch receptors without significantly increasing discharge rate if it is slowly enough applied, subsequently leaving them mechanically fatigued and unresponsive. As the normal "background" level of excitation of motoneurons via stretch afferent fibers is thus minimized or withdrawn during this process, a muscle after slow stretch will manifest lower tone compared to its status before slow stretch was applied. Thus, the therapist can obtain either facilitation or relaxation from a given muscle, utilizing the same stimulus of muscle stretch, depending on the rate at which the stimulus is applied and the duration of the interval over which it is maintained.

Since the mechanism underlying the relaxing effect of slow stretch is subtle and not readily appreciated by those who have not had direct experience with the physiological properties of receptors and afferent fibers, therapists seem to prefer more complex forms of stimulation (e.g., placing the patient in reflex-inhibiting positions) (6, 8, 9) to achieve the same effect. The fact remains that slow stretch is the best stimulus for obtaining relaxation of a given muscle or muscle group, just as quick stretch is the best facilitatory stimulus.

A phenomenon closely related to the above effect is involved in the use of prolonged cold application to obtain muscle relaxation (63). Cold application takes various forms; we must make a distinction between the use of deep, prolonged and penetrating cold to obtain relaxation and "superficial" cold stimulation as used by Rood to obtain facilitation. (The latter effect, which is based on γ efferent physiology, will be discussed in the section devoted to Rood's technique.) The relaxing effect of deep cold may be based on the same phenomenon as relaxation obtained through slow stretch, with the difference that slow stretch physiologically desensitizes the stretch receptors, thereby lowering the background level of stretch afferent input, while deep cold (penetrating the muscle mass) produces "cold block" of the receptor excitatory process or of the afferent fibers themselves. The latter is a state resembling blockage of impulse conduction which can be achieved by applying a local anesthetic to the nerve fibers. Just as a muscle can be reduced to a state of complete flaccidity by interrupting all dorsal root fibers carrying stretch afferent input to it, muscle tone can be diminished by cold block of conduction in the stretch afferents, which temporarily prevents impulse conduction while leaving the fibers themselves intact. Since the latter procedure is reversible upon warming, and since intact muscle afferent input is necessary for control of voluntary motor activities (35), it is clearly desirable to diminish tone functionally for a brief period through cold blockage and work toward neuromuscular re-education, rather than to lower tone permanently by deafferentation. (Partial deafferentation has been used in surgical approaches to diminish spasticity, but the degree of deafferentation is difficult to control and the resulting residual level of muscle tone is not predictable with any degree of accuracy (54, 94).)

Another relatively simple reflex mechanism studied by Sherrington, which has been utilized for both facilitation and inhibition, is the withdrawal reflex to noxious stimulation (i.e., stimulation that is painful or destructive of tissue) (84). Since the withdrawal reflex commonly manifests itself in the form of a flexion synergy for both upper and lower extremity, application of a mildly noxious stimulus (i.e., mechanical irritation at an intensity short of tissue injury) can be used to facilitate voluntary flexion patterns. Fortunately, "tickling" is also useful for this purpose in most individuals. Noxious stimulation elicits a multijoint, synergistic movement pattern in contrast to the selective contraction of a single flexor muscle produced by isolated stretch of that muscle. On the other hand, this gives us the first example of a situation where two facilitatory influences — one specific, through isolated muscle stretch, and the other generalized, through initiation of a withdrawal reflex — can be profitably superimposed in order to obtain an additive effect. Particularly in the case of a muscle developing almost zero contractile tension, facilitation through simultaneous elicitation of both stretch and withdrawal reflex response should produce sufficient increase in tone — perhaps even overt movement — to convince the patient that the supposedly paralyzed muscle has latent potential for recovery of voluntary contraction.

Noxious stimulation also can be used to obtain relaxation of extensors as well as facilitation of flexors. In the case of a patient with persisting lower extremity hypertonicity or spasticity, for example, noxious stimulation applied to the sole of the foot will tend to produce activation of flexors throughout the extremity and simultaneous reciprocal relaxation of all extensors. Here again, if a multijoint synergistic pattern is undesirable, production of a withdrawal reflex might be used to initiate generalized extensor relaxation, and then a specific extensor muscle selected for prolonged slow stretch to continue the relaxation process. Thus simultaneous or sequential application of the same or of different peripheral stimuli to one or more regions or tissues of the body, "heaping one facilitatory or inhibitory effect upon another," is a technique which the sophisticated therapist should be capable of using in order to obtain the maximal effect from facilitation methods.

MODERN TECHNIQUES BASED ON CUTANEOUS STIMULATION

In the 1960s, Margaret Rood introduced a new therapeutic procedure which extended the repertoire of the therapist beyond the scope of traditional methods involving muscle stretch, deep cold application, and elicitation of withdrawal reflexes. Her contribution is based on the use of gentle mechanical or superficial thermal stimulation of specific areas of the skin, affecting cutaneous receptors, in order to obtain localized facilitatory effects (77, 78). To some dubious observers the effects she is able to elicit by "brushing" against the direction of hair growth in the skin area overlying a given muscle appear so mysterious as to be highly suspect. Yet Rood's method is in fact firmly based on the physiology of the γ efferent system — which compared to those mechanisms studied by Sherrington is a "newcomer" to the neurophysiological scene (i.e., we have had detailed knowledge about it for only the last 15 years).

At the time when Rood introduced this technique, some therapists were prevented from using this approach because its purported neurophysiological basis was incomprehensible to physicians whose medical training had been completed prior to the discovery of the γ efferent system. However, Rood had simply succeeded in demonstrating that a neural mechanism that is clearly present in animals such as the cat and monkey (and which has definite adaptive or survival value) is also operative in the human. Hunt, Hagbarth and Megirian showed in basic neurophysiological studies that stimulation within the skin area overlying a given muscle (stroking against the direction of hair growth being a particularly potent stimulus) led to activation of the γ efferents innervating stretch receptors in that muscle, which in turn sensitized these receptors, i.e., made them more responsive to physiological muscle stretch (26, 38, 46, 47, 61). Rood simply applied the functional scheme elucidated in animals to the neurological patient; if the same mechanism were operative in humans, it is obvious that stimulation of the skin overlying a given muscle should increase the stretch afferent input from that muscle due to stretch under gravitational pull; and this in turn should reflexly increase the muscle's tone. What Rood accomplishes with "brushing and icing" (in the latter case, superficial, brief cold application) is bringing muscle stretch receptors to a heightened state of excitability, via γ efferent activation; now muscle stretch under gravitational force or deliberately applied by a therapist leads to an exaggerated afferent barrage (Figs. 4.6 and 4.7). Hence there is a more powerful facilitatory action for a given amount of muscle stretch.

Here again, we have a situation where the effectiveness of two approaches can be compounded by superimposition. Skin stimulation may be applied to heighten the excitability of stretch receptors in a given muscle, and then traditional quick stretch used as the ultimate facilitatory input to increase tone or even obtain observable muscle contraction and resulting limb movement.

While the results of basic neurophysiological investigations thus provide a clear-cut explanation for the Rood effect in terms of spinal cord mechanisms, further animal studies by Asanuma and his associates have revealed the existence of a complex cortically originating system which should provide a similar effect in parallel with that mediated by the γ efferent system (2, 80). These workers showed that stimulation of the skin overlying a given muscle tends to excite cortical motoneurons (pyramidal tract cells) whose axons descending via the corticospinal tract to make synaptic contact with alpha motoneurons innervating that muscle (Figs. 4.8 and 4.9). Again, stroking against the direction of hair growth is a particularly powerful stimulus. Evolution seems to have provided multiple sensorimotor networks, involving several levels of the CNS, to ensure that contact with an object increases mobility and results in a specific motor response increasing the likelihood of apprehending and manipulating it. The Rood technique is soundly based on the operation of these mechanisms which have obvious survival value.

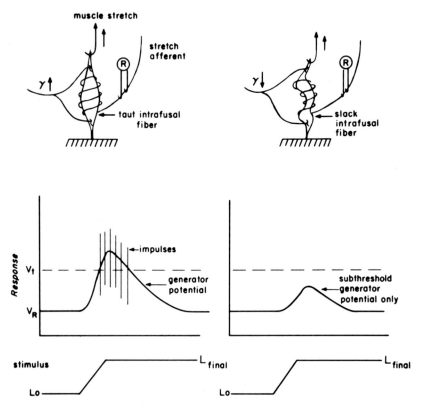

Fig. 4.6. Mechanical factors involved in control of stretch receptor sensitivity by gamma (γ) efferents. If the level of γ firing increases (*A*), the intrafusal fibers (IF) contract and become taut. This sensitizes the stretch receptors, wrapped around the IF fibers, by causing a partial distortion of the receptor membrane. If the muscle is subsequently stretched, externally and internally generated tensions will summate to cause suprathreshold membrane depolarization and impulse initiation. If the level of gamma firing decreases (*B*), the IF fibers will relax and go slack. Internal tension will be withdrawn, so the external stimulus must supply all of the force necessary to distort the receptor membrane. The same amount of stretch causing impulse discharge in *A* will fail to do so in *B*, because the amount of depolarization it produces in isolation is below the threshold for impulse initiation in the stretch afferent fibers. (From F. A. Harris, *Physical Therapy, 51:* 761, 1971 (42).)

REFLEXES AND EQUILIBRIUM REACTIONS ELICITED THROUGH VESTIBULAR AND NECK MUSCLE PROPRIOCEPTIVE STIMULATION

The application of peripheral stimuli through manipulation of the head, widely incorporated into traditional techniques, deserves special attention. Obviously, passive head movement within the physiological range produces sensory input via stretch afferents from receptors in the neck musculature as well as via vestibular afferents from receptors in the semicircular canals. Response to such stimulation includes: 1) simple stretch reflex-induced increase in tone of the muscles stretched, 2) more complex but predictably patterned symmetrical and asymmetrical reflexes to head rotation or tilt, and 3) exceedingly complex and variable equilibrium responses to changes in position of the head and body in space (7, 11, 87).

While the Bobath method in particular relies heavily on head manipulation for bringing about patterned facilitation effects, the fact remains that the above mentioned influences are relatively weak compared to the localized effects obtainable through selective techniques, such as quick stretch. While the classic example of the fencer's pose serves as an excellent mnemonic device for remembering the pattern of reflex response to

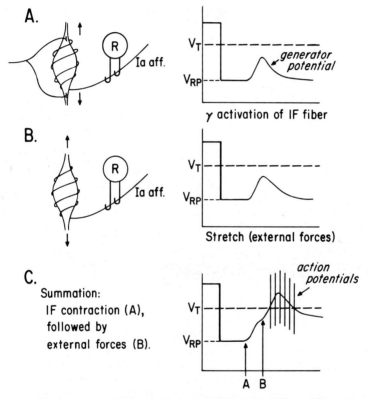

Fig. 4.7. Equivalence of external forces and intrafusal fiber (IF) contraction in producing receptor depolarization. (A) Generator potential (excitatory depolarizing change in membrane potential) produced by γ activation of intrafusal fiber. (B) Generator potential produced by muscle stretch under influence of external forces only. (C) Summation of subthreshold effects when IF fiber contraction is followed by muscle stretch. Here the generator potential exceeds the threshold for impulse initiation, and impulses headed for the CNS are set up in the stretch afferent fiber. Taut IF has "biased" or sensitized the receptor to stretch, so that amount of stretch that, in B, was insufficient to cause impulse discharge can now do so. (From F. A. Harris, *American Journal of Occupational Therapy*, 23: 397, 1969 (39).)

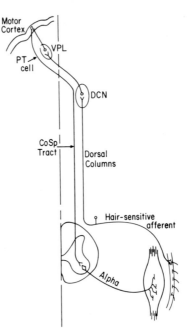

Fig. 4.8. Pyramidal (corticospinal) tract mechanism which parallels the γ system in mediating effects of cutaneous stimulation on underlying muscle. Hair receptors send projections to motor cortex by way of dorsal column-medial lemniscal pathway, exciting cells of origin of the pyramidal tract (PT). The mechanism operates selectively, so that the PT neurons excited by stimulating a particular area of skin are those which innervate the alpha motoneurons supplying the muscle underlying that area of skin. This mechanism, not involving γ efferents, may also be involved in production of specific muscle activation by means of skin stimulation. (From F. A. Harris, *American Journal of Occupational Therapy, 23:* 397, 1969 (39).)

head-turning in the spinal cat, it should be kept in mind that the human fencer does not assume his asymmetrical limb position by virtue of turning his head to one side (i.e., moving the head does not make the arms move into their characteristic position). Similarly in the example of the weight-lifter, who supposedly boosts his biceps output via the asymmetrical tonic reflex, the more likely explanation for the effectiveness of turning the head away from the flexed arm is that this puts the neck muscles on the side of the flexed arm under stretch and thus facilitates stabilization of the shoulder girdle as a suspension platform from which the biceps can exert stronger pull.

In the author's experience, attempts to facilitate or inhibit muscle activity in the upper extremities by turning the head are minimally, if at all, successful. We have here an example of a reflex mechanism which is moderately strong in a spinal animal, after other of the "multiple loops" mediating the animal's response to sensory input have been eliminated by low transection of the neuraxis; it has quite minimal strength in the intact human or neurologically impaired patient. In the author's opinion, facilitation of rolling from supine to prone or vice versa through passive head-turning is more likely based on avoidance of pain by the patient rather than on the initiation of vestibular or stretch reflex-induced responses of limbs, shoulder girdle and trunk to head-turning. That is, once the head has been passively turned past the limits to which the patient is accustomed, he begins to experience discomfort. He will allow himself to experience just so much discomfort before he finally responds by voluntarily moving his limbs, turning the shoulder girdle, and finally rotating his trunk in order to follow along with the head, thus completing the roll in order to eliminate the painful sensations experienced during the initial phase of passive head-turning.

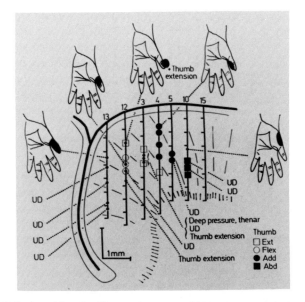

Fig. 4.9. Relationship of afferent input to efferent output in monkey motor cortex. *Vertical solid lines* indicate penetration tracks of microelectrodes inserted into the cerebral cortex for purposes of recording from single cells and passing stimulating current. The areas of skin that contained receptors giving rise to afferent projections to individual cells encountered along each track are indicated in the drawings of hand; the *dotted lines* interconnecting the two indicate which cells had excitatory skin areas corresponding to each patch of skin shaded in black. The motor effects produced by passing minute amounts of current directly in the vicinity of these cells are coded in terms of the superimposition of white or black circles and squares on the positions of particular cells along the penetration tracks. For a large proportion of the neurons thus studied, the cortical motor cells that received sensory input from a given patch of skin on the thumb led to activation of the muscle underlying that patch of skin when stimulated electrically. (From H. Asanuma et al., *Journal of Neurophysiology, 31:* 670, 1968 (2).)

Unfortunately, strong subjective belief in a method may preclude objectively monitoring the outcome of its application. The therapist must be particularly perceptive in cases such as this, so as to make a distinction between what expositors of various methods claim happens in response to certain stimuli and what may actually take place during treatment. Belief in the efficacy of head- and neck-on-body reflexes is so pervasive that the author has watched professional training films in which therapists describe a patient turning his own head to facilitate extension of one arm through the asymmetrical tonic neck reflexes (TNR), for example, while objective measurements indicate that no change in the position of either extremity took place during the voluntary head movement.

Although the tonic head and neck reflexes are weak, they can be used in combination with other forms of stimulation to cascade facilitatory effects toward a common goal. If the desire is to facilitate elbow extension, for example, greater success will be obtained if work begins with the patient in the supine position; placing him in prone will bias him toward flexion of all extremities, while placing him in supine will bias him toward extension (both effects mediated via γ efferent-induced changes in muscle tone distribution according to the prevailing pattern of vestibular stimulation) (24). Then, specific techniques such as quick stretch and brushing can be used to provide increasing amounts of facilitation to the triceps.

CENTRAL FACILITATION TECHNIQUES

"Central" facilitation should also be considered as an alternative or adjunct to peripheral stimulation. Methods utilizing irradiation, associated reactions, synergies and other mass action effects resulting from maximal effort exerted through residually functioning musculature, either with or without resistance, may be referred to as "central" facilitation because the synaptic connections at which supplementary excitation or inhibition occurs are exclusively between central nervous system elements, rather than between peripherally originating afferent fibers and spinal α motoneurons of other CNS elements. These methods do not rely upon peripheral input for facilitation, but rather on the recruitment of motoneurons supplying weak muscles into action patterns correlated with voluntary contraction of strong muscles. The author ascribes the effectiveness of such techniques to the existence of neural "circuits" at cortical, brainstem, cerebellar and spinal levels, all of which have been "programmed" in such a fashion that particular muscles tend to become active simultaneously or in a stereotyped temporal sequence (and, their antagonists reciprocally relax) while various movements are "played out" by the CNS. Some of these circuits, through genetic designation, are more or less uniform among all persons (i.e., "hard-wired"). Others, unique to the individual by virtue of his own personal motor learning experiences, are highly variable (i.e., "soft-wired") (5, 25).

A mechanism of this sort has been documented by Salmoiraghi (81) for the brainstem respiratory center, in which neurons driving expiratory effort mutually excite each other and reciprocally inhibit neurons whose activity produces inspiration; and, those driving inspiratory effort excite each other and inhibit the expiratory neurons. This simple programming of connections between respiratory neurons results in an oscillatory action, in which inspiratory neurons recruit others of their own kind into activity and inhibit their antagonists as inspiratory effort builds up. The inspiratory pool then fatigues near peak inspiration, and expiratory neurons are released from inhibition. The latter excite others of their own kind and their discharge rate spirals upward, with simultaneous inhibition of inspiratory neurons, until maximal expiration is reached. Finally, the expiratory neurons fatigue and the cycle repeats itself.

Sophisticated studies involving electrical stimulation of discrete areas within the motor cortex of the monkey have revealed a similar organization upon which all voluntary somatic muscle activity depends. The outcome of these experiments demands our rejection of "Beevor's hypothesis," often quoted by expositors of therapeutic exercise techniques, according to which the brain "knows nothing of muscles, but only of movements" (27, 28). The work of Chang and Ruch shows clearly that the brain does "know" of the individual muscles under its control; upper motoneurons representing individual muscles are grouped together in distinct areas of the motor cortex, so that these muscles are represented almost as if laid out on a piano keyboard (16). By selectively "depressing each key" (i.e., locally stimulating each cortical site) these workers produced isolated contractions of single muscles, one muscle corresponding to each stimulation site (Fig. 4.10). As stimulus intensity was increased, however, and more motoneurons were caused to fire, muscles began to contract in functionally related groups (i.e., in synergistic patterns) (Fig. 4.11). The most likely explanation for this is through programming in the motor cortex analogous to that observed in the respiratory center — with excitatory interconnections between neighboring cortical motoneurons so that strong activity in one pool of neurons begins to irradiate or "spill over" into activity of adjacent pools which innervate functionally related muscles. And, perhaps there are also inhibitory interconnections to "turn off" motoneurons innervating antagonists (58).

Much of the normal human motor repertoire probably depends on genetically determined or hard-wired circuits of this type. More complex associated activity patterns for lower and upper extremities, or sequential patterns chaining proximal and distal muscular activity (such as in throwing a ball) are built in through individualized motor learning, and thus depend on experience for their acquisition. According to this view, each identifiable motor action in the human repertoire would be represented by a "cell assembly" or synaptically interconnected group of motor neurons which tends to fire in the same sequence no matter how the activity is initiated, thus producing the same overt movement each time the pattern "plays through" the network (45).

If such neural organization is a prevailing feature at cortical, brain

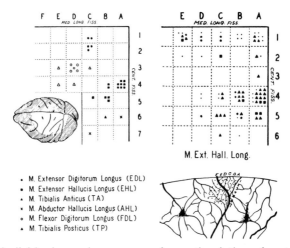

Fig. 4.10. Individual muscle responses from stimulation of motor cortex. The grid at the top shows isolated muscle contractions elicited from stimulation points that correspond to the smaller size grid superimposed on the leg area of the precentral cerebral cortex in the picture at the lower right. The large grid shows points from which response was obtained in a single foot or ankle muscle, with the particular muscle contracting coded in terms of symbols having various shapes and shadings according to the key provided. Grid points are 1 mm apart. (From H. T. Chang et al., *Journal of Neurophysiology, 10:* 39, 1947 (16).)

stem, cerebellar, and/or spinal levels of the CNS, it is not surprising that strong effort exerted with an extremity on the unaffected side in a hemiplegic can facilitate the same movement attempted with the weak side (37), or that a muscle which contracts weakly in isolation may come in quite strongly when involved in a synergistic pattern (e.g., contrast weak ankle dorsiflexion in supine, with the leg extended at the knee, to the strength of that obtainable in prone position with the knee flexed).

Therapists have engaged in controversy over whether or not associated reactions and other irradiated activity or mass patterns should be used in facilitation, above and beyond the question of whether or not they are effective over the short term. Some, fearing that the patient will learn to use these patterns for "trick movements," to the exclusion of being able to produce discrete muscle contraction for other functional movements, insist that all facilitation should be specific to one muscle at a time. Again, we must ask whether these options really are mutually exclusive. Why be limited to only one or the other approach? Where diffuse weakness is present, mass patterns can be used to produce some overt response, if for no other purpose than to motivate the patient through his observing that motor output is still possible. Then, local stimulation can be superimposed to selectively facilitate the contraction of particular muscles within the mass pattern that has emerged. Again, the therapist who adheres to only one method cannot hope to derive as much benefit as is possible from the compounding, superimposition, or sequential application of peripheral and central facilitation procedures.

BIOFEEDBACK THERAPY

To the extent that both neurophysiological and modern behavioral research have recently focused attention on the importance of sensory feedback for both the initial learning and the subsequent performance of skill motor acts (21, 33, 42, 51, 53, 55, 56, 67, 73, 90), so must this factor be taken into account in the development of new therapeutic techniques. The classical limb denervation experiments by Mott and Sherrington (66), later extended by Gilman and others (13, 33, 56, 57, 67, 92), provide ample documentation that motor outflow depends upon sensory inflow. These workers showed that monkeys, on which dorsal root sections had been performed so as to cut off afferent signals from one upper extremity, behaved as if that extremity were competely paralyzed. In fact, the impairment in function from sensory denervation far exceeded that usually

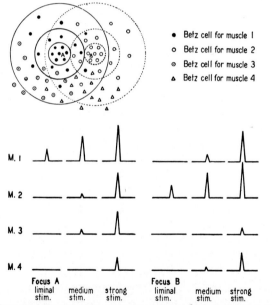

Fig. 4.11. Diagrammatic representation of hypothetical distribution of cortical Betz cells (pyramidal tract neurons) for individual muscles, showing how synergies might be produced. The cell group for each muscle has a focal distribution and a concentric fringe that overlaps those of other muscles. Each symbol stands for a Betz cell; the circles are spheres of excitation. The expected contraction of muscles to cortical stimulation at different strengths, recruiting more Betz cells as stimulus intensity is increased, is shown by myograms drawn in lower part of figure, in which magnitude of contraction corresponds to the numbers of Betz cells included in the sphere of excitation. Zones A and B represent about 4–8 sq mm of cortical tissue. (From H. T. Chang et al., *Journal of Neurophysiology, 10:* 39, 1947 (16).)

resulting from a lesion in the cortical motor area. There are two possible explanations for the fact that even though the outflow pathway to muscles in the affected extremity was intact and theoretically still normally operative, the limb was flail and could not be used for any functional activity by the animal: 1) the dorsal root section in effect produced a massive "disfacilitation"; that is, in the absence of background stretch receptor input from muscles in the affected limb, the motoneurons innervating those muscles were so depressed in excitability that they became unresponsive to descending volleys of impulses via central motor pathways; or 2) because the animal was deprived of accurate kinesthetic appreciation of the position of the affected limb in space, it had no basis for generating appropriate descending volleys to either stabilize the limb in fixed attitudes or to make phasic movements.

We are not yet in a position to determine which of these explanations is correct. Most likely, both factors have something to do with production of the observed symptoms. The inescapable conclusion, however, is that tonic postural and phasic motor outflow are both defective in the absence of sensory input.

Tabes dorsalis is one of several clinical conditions that particularly support interpretation of the defective movement problem in terms of faulty kinesthetic feedback. In this disease, as the result of lesions affecting conduction in the dorsal column pathway (which carries information important for appreciation of limb position), the patient has impaired coordination of movements of the extremities. In fact, a variety of clinical observations lead to the conclusion that lesions at any point along the sensory pathways carrying tactile and kinesthetic information can produce symptoms of impaired coordination or ataxia. A condition has been described, referred to as "pseudo-athetosis," in which there are continual involuntary movements of the extremities or other body parts affected, due to purely sensory lesions in peripheral nerve, spinal pathways, brain stem and thalamic relay nuclei, or somatosensory cortex (22, 44, 62). Thus, even if the extreme theoretical position that sensory feedback is necessary for any movement to occur at all proves untenable, it seems quite conservative to assert that postural stability and voluntary movements of normal quality depend on accurate kinesthetic feedback (which may include information from tactile as well as stretch receptors, since it is possible to monitor limb position strictly on the basis of tactile sensations).

Even a neurologically intact individual may gain insight into pathological movement phenomena through introspection—e.g., recalling occasions when he "pushed himself" to extremes in some athletic endeavor or physical work, resulting in excessive muscle fatigue. We interpret certain feelings coming from the extremities (i.e., the leaden, paresthetic quality of sensations, which are worsened by additional effort) as fatigue; these distorted feelings may also be responsible for the lack of coordination (i.e., shakiness or tremor, inability to hold a fixed position for very long or to move smoothly between the endpoints of any defined range of motion) which is a frequent accompaniment. In view of the similarities between these conditions and the symptoms of certain neuromuscular disorders, we must entertain the proposition that at least some, if not all, of the neurologically impaired individual's problems with postural stability and voluntary movement may result from distorted kinesthetic feedback. This distortion in turn could result from CNS lesions affecting areas which are primarily receptive or input-oriented rather than output-oriented (Figs. 4.12 and 4.13), or affecting mechanisms that control the sensitivity of kinesthetic receptors (e.g., the γ efferent system), thus deranging control mechanisms dependent upon information from these receptors (39, 42, 51, 56, 83, 86, 93, 94).

In this context, it is possible that the beneficial effects of peripheral stimulation may in part be the result of facilitating sensory rather than motor mechanisms—that is, of improving or restoring sensory capacity, or recalibrating the sensorimotor apparatus (i.e., establishing a new relationship between limb position and the afferent impulse pattern that represents it, via improved interrelated function of the residual sensory and motor elements) (Fig. 4.14).

Thus massage and passive manipulation may be efficacious by virtue of increasing the patient's awareness of the affected limb(s). The provision of additional input from skin, muscle and other kinesthetic receptors may simply increase the probability that he will attempt to use the affected limb through heightened awareness of it. Passive range of motion exercises may also help maintain normal stretch receptor sensitivity (e.g., by preserving normal elasticity of the intrafusal muscle fibers on which the stretch receptors are mounted) and/or assist the patient in establishing a new transmodality correlation between patterns of tactile sensation (resulting from both mechanical contact and thermal stimuli) and various limb positions. If this type of effect is to be maximized, however, the therapist must keep the patient "tuned in" to his movements through insistence on visual monitoring of the moving limb and concentration on any residual sensory impressions which may be related to limb position and movement. Neuromuscular re-education may be accomplished in a quite literal sense by helping the patient establish a new relationship between position and/or movement and the residual sensations derived via tactile and kinesthetic mechanisms (Fig. 4.15). (For example, elbow joint position can be monitored strictly in terms of tactile contact and thermal sensations that come from the areas of skin overlying the distal portion of the biceps and the proximal portion of the forearm flexors, as these areas are approximated during flexion and separated during extension.) A good deal of motor relearning may depend on the patient's attending to such sensations as a basis for position and movement feedback in place of the sensations normally derived from muscle and joint receptors.

Feedback of EMG signals via visual monitoring of an oscilloscope screen

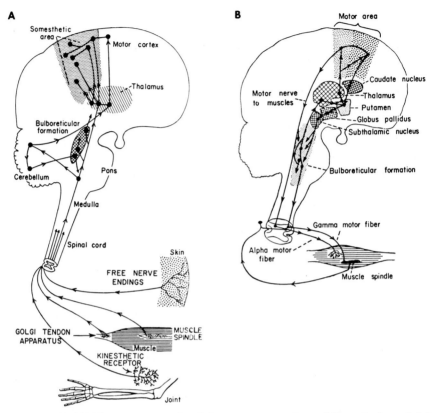

Fig. 4.12. (A) The sensory axis of the nervous system. Afferents from joint, muscle, tendon, and cutaneous receptors feed information comprising a multi-modality indication of limb position and movement to CNS. This information is processed at the spinal level for reflex modulation of tone, fed to the cerebellum for integration with vestibular input so as to allow control of equilibrium reactions, fed to the reticular formation to permit generalized regulation of γ efferent activity and muscle tone in accord with the degree of bodily activity, and distributed to the motor cortex from the thalamus both directly and via relay through the somesthetic area. (B) The motor axis. Information concerned with regulation of posture and movement is sent via the corticospinal pathway directly to α motoneurons at the spinal level, and indirectly via the extrapyramidal system to the γ efferents. Caudate nucleus, putamen, globus pallidus and other subcortical structures are included in the extrapyramidal pathway. The reticular formation serves as the main "funnel" for descending extrapyramidal signals, which influence the α motoneurons indirectly through the γ loop and generate a background level of tonic postural activity on which signals for phasic voluntary movements are superimposed. (From A. C. Guyton, *Textbook of Medical Physiology,* Ed. 4, W. B. Saunders Co., 1971 (36).)

or broadcast over a loudspeaker also can be used to teach the patient voluntary control down to the ultrafine level of individual motor units (4, 72); thus a correlate of contractile activity can be sensed, displayed for self-monitoring by the patient, and even reinforced automatically by reward dispensers set to be triggered when particular voltage levels have been reached. And, the technique which the author introduced, utilizing artificial sense organs to convert head and limb movements into proportional electrical variations that are then fed back to the patient in the form of exteroceptive (visual or auditory) signals (43, 53), carries the education process a step further in the direction of modern motor learning paradigms. That is, motivational aspects, the importance of which are becoming widely appreciated (82), can be explicitly incorporated into the therapeutic exercise regimen. Rather than relying on verbal behavior modification, requiring continual interaction between the therapist on a one-to-one basis (in which the therapist is overly burdened with providing verbal reinforcement to the patient in addition to guiding the exercise activities, supplying maximal resistance to movement, etc.), electronic devices can monitor the signals being fed back to the patient and automatically dis-

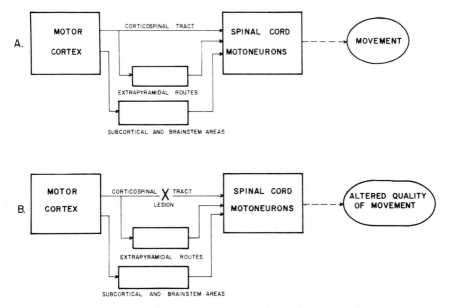

Fig. 4.13. Model of cerebral organization illustrating redundant representation of motor function. (A) Subcortical and brainstem areas (basal ganglia, red nucleus, reticular formation, etc.) are involved in motor outflow as well as cerebral cortical motor area, and these structures influence alpha motoneurons via extrapyramidal routes (rubrospinal, reticulospinal, etc.) paralleling the corticospinal tract. (B) Compensation for motor deficits caused by lesions interrupting the corticospinal tract is possible through circumventing the lesions (sending signals to the spinal motor nuclei via the alternate pathways mentioned above). The quality of movement thereby produced is different from normal in certain respects (particularly with regard to speed of execution and endurance), but functional voluntary movement even of the fingers is possible after interruption of the corticospinal tract at the level of the medullary pyramids. (From F. A. Harris, *American Journal of Occupational Therapy, 24:* 264, 1970 (40).)

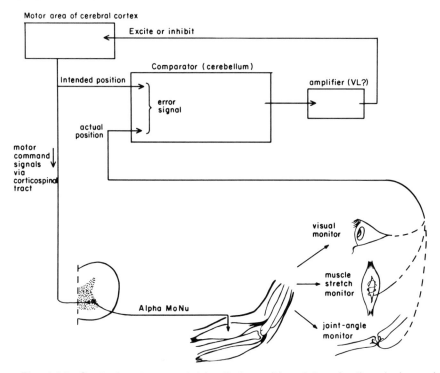

Fig. 4.14. Control system model for limb position determination during voluntary movement. A signal representing the intended position is fed into the cerebellum via collateral branches of the corticospinal tract fibers which excite α motoneurons at the spinal cord level to bring about muscle contraction. Information representing the actual limb position at any instant in time reaches the cerebellum via sensory projections from visual, muscle, joint, and perhaps even cutaneous receptors. The cerebellum derives a difference or error signal by subtracting the "feedback" signal from that representing intended movement and plays back upon the motor cortex to either increase (by excitation) or decrease (by inhibition) output to the muscles. Corrections cease when the error signal is zero—i.e., when intended and actual positions are identical. (From F. A. Harris, *Physical Therapy, 51:* 761, 1971 (42).)

pense rewards for success (i.e., turn on appliances or dispense tokens to be exchanged later for concrete reinforcers) or apply mild negative reinforcement for failure. Moreover, the threshold for success can be continually adjusted by the therapist to promote progressive improvement. As soon as the patient reaches a particular criterion, his goal can be shifted upward so that performance of the activity in which he has been involved continues to remain a challenge.

Using such devices as adjuncts to conventional therapy, a single therapist can work with several patients simultaneously, setting each a task consistent with his own interests and providing each with criteria for obtaining reinforcement consistent with his own changing ability. Finally, the electrical signals from movement transducers can be recorded to provide objective documentation of improvement in the patient's motor skills resulting from this form of therapeutic exercise. By changing reinforcement threshold levels at a reasonable pace, the therapist can use such devices to maintain a constant challenge and thus sustain the patient's interest in performing the desired activities (stabilizing particular joints, or moving an individual joint through a particular range, or moving a combination of joints in a synergistic pattern, etc.) over a considerable period of time. This is particularly advantageous, since in therapeutic

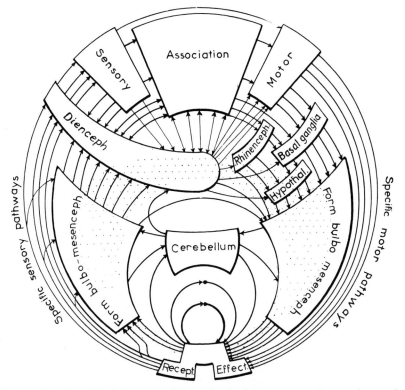

Fig. 4.15. Simplified diagram of the principal sensory, motor, and associative paths throughout the nervous system, illustrating the "multiple loop" organization of the sensorimotor system. Receptors feed information to all "levels" simultaneously, and input reaches the cortical motor area through routes of varying degrees of complexity—some direct, and others involving relay in subcortical structures and/or sensory and association cortex. Motor output is directed toward the effectors over parallel corticospinal and extrapyramidal routes, the former going directly to alpha motoneurons while the latter influence muscle tone and phasic contraction indirectly through gamma efferent regulation of stretch receptor sensitivity. The loops are all "closed" since muscle output invariably stimulates receptors which, by re-afferentation, signal any change in status to the CNS. (From J. Paillard, *Handbook of Physiology*, American Physiological Society, Washington, D.C., 1960 (70).)

exercise as well as in conditioning or body-building exercise, the greater the number of repetitions performed (within the limits of fatigue), the greater the gains in strength and control of voluntary movement. Note that in the above discussion the author construes therapeutic exercise quite broadly, as the performance of specifically prescribed activities under the supervision of a therapist, involving direct interaction with the thera- pist (as in resistive exercise) – while electronic devices may be used to monitor the patient's movements, record them objectively, and automati- cally reinforce successful efforts so as to sustain motivation and interest in the exercise activity.

CNS PLASTICITY AS THE BASIS FOR "CARRY-OVER"

According to traditional clinical neurological concepts, the circuitry of the CNS is comparable to the "hard-wired" electrical networks used in telephone or telegraph communications. The connections between various CNS centers are viewed as genetically predetermined and fixed after development, and if these centers or their interconnections are damaged, the resulting functional impairment is thought to be irreversible since the messages supposedly can no longer be processed in the normal manner. Thus, the patient's capacity for voluntary movement would be irreversibly lost if his "motor pathways" were interrupted, his expressive language function would be lost if his "speech center" were damaged, and so on (23).

Contemporary computer specialists hold a rather different view concern- ing the functional organization of the brain, however, and they readily envision the CNS as having the capacity to reorganize itself after dam- age – to a greater or lesser extent depending on prevailing conditions – so as to permit the recovery of functional capabilities. Comparing CNS orga- nization to that of a computer rather than a telephone network, they see the possibility of messages flowing through the system by alternate routes in the event that some of the main transmission lines and message centers are damaged (1, 40). Thus, even the damaged nervous system has the potential of returning to a state of quasi-normal function in their view of a "plastic" (i.e., flexible, adaptable, modifiable) human brain. In fact, con- temporary anatomical and physiological studies have yielded information concerning the brain's capacity for functional repair that correlates well with the view of the computer scientists (20, 25, 34, 48). There have been documented observations of regrowth of neuronal processes after CNS tissue destruction, suggesting that reorganization occurs after damage to the brain even in the absence of any deliberate therapeutic attempts (79).

CNS plasticity is the potential for recovery of function after damage to the brain, based largely on redundancy or multiple representation of any given function. This is characteristic of the CNS both on the microlevel (i.e., large numbers of neurons are active simultaneously in carrying out each function) and on the macrolevel (i.e., there are multiple pathways and centers concerned with each function). The author's *multiple loop concept,* according to which all levels of the CNS are involved in mediating each and every function, rather than there being a separate "center" for each activity, deals with the latter aspect of the brain's organization (41). Imagine an individual carrying out a highly preferred (and therefore overlearned) activity. The brain initiates and mediates his movements through discharge of impulses by a particular interconnected set or circuit of neurons in a particular sequence of temporal pattern. The more skilled the individual grows, the more specialized and the more widespread become the neural networks that mediate this activity. Should the main "computation area" carrying out this program be damaged as the result of a stroke or mechanical brain injury, execution of this program may be switched to other neurons within the same region that escape injury, to those in neighboring regions, or even remote areas (such as the opposite hemisphere). As long as the process representing the concept of the activity (perhaps in terms of how it feels when that activity is correctly performed) and the intent to carry it out are preserved, the actual execution can be shifted to new "pathways"; given the opportunity for guided practice (therapeutic exercise), the patient thus has the potential to relearn any lost function. Since the actual execution of any voluntary act could be assigned to a number of different output mechanisms, there is no single "center" at which local damage could permanently halt all voluntary motor activity. This could only happen in the case of widespread diffuse damage, destroying all spinal and cranial motoneurons, which is extremely unlikely (or would not be survived).

It seems obvious, then, that therapy which aims at creating the kinds of conditions which prevailed during the original "programming" of an individual's motor circuitry—that is, provides repetitive practice of even the simplest motions, such as was necessary to initially establish the basic repertoire of human motion (not to mention specialized skills such as penmanship, graphic arts, muscial ability, etc.)—should maximize the probability of functional repair. It is also obvious that the patient's chances for rehabilitation depend not only on the anatomical and physiological substrates that tend to support recovery, but also depend on his therapist's enthusiastic application of treatment techniques that will optimally mobilize these mechanisms. The therapist's guidance of central repair processes is just as essential as the mechanical guidance to peripheral repair offered by millipore filter nerve-fiber bridging (88).

Practice

ANALYSIS OF THE MAJOR APPROACHES TO THERAPEUTIC EXERCISE

Space does not permit an analysis of all existing therapeutic exercise methods, nor even a detailed consideration of those most commonly used. Rather, those features most characteristic of each major method have been abstracted to permit comparison of the methods according to the various forms of facilitatory and inhibitory stimuli they utilize. The methods are discussed in alphabetical order, to avoid any implicit "ranking" according to the sequence in which they are introduced. All of the methods have certain elements in common, which is simply a reflection of the limits set by the realities of neuroanatomy and neurophysiology, on what will and what will not work. There are obvious differences in emphasis, however, and the author feels that it is possible to make objective value judgments about the methods based on the extent to which they: 1) incorporate particularly strong proprioceptive facilitatory stimuli, 2) involve calling upon the patient for voluntary effort, 3) promote the patient's involvement in sensory monitoring of his movements, and 4) generally adhere to the principles of motor learning as established by contemporary behavioral psychology.

Following the methodological discussions, a synthetic therapeutic approach is presented that incorporates features of all the major methods, as well as procedures that are new, experimental, and are dependent upon the use of electronic equipment. The latter are not in common usage at this time, but are at the forefront of rehabilitation research. Thus, the state of the art of therapeutic exercise today is portrayed in terms of showing the full range of options available to the "compleat ecclectic therapist."

BOBATH METHOD

The outstanding characteristic of the "neurodevelopment approach" (6–12), used primarily with juvenile cerebral palsy patients but also applicable in certain respects to dealing with adult stroke, is the use of involuntary responses to movement of the head and body (e.g., postural reflexes and equilibrium reactions) for purposes of modifying muscle tone or eliciting desired movements. The utilization of associated reactions is avoided, however, out of concern that the patient may learn to utilize these on his own to initiate "trick movements" of the affected limbs; such movements would hamper progress beyond the stage in which reflexes and reactions dominate toward performance of normal, discrete voluntary movements.

Supplemental proprioceptive stimuli (muscle stretch and "tapping") are used to facilitate and direct the patient's emerging responses to the head, neck, and body movement stimuli which elicit equilibrium reactions. The Bobath approach also includes procedures intended to suppress or inhibit neural activity producing spasticity in circumstances where the normal child would be relaxed, so that movement potential is freed from the restrictions caused by tight antagonists. Inhibiting or "breaking up" spasticity is accomplished by placing the patient in positions that lead to relaxation, involving both slow, prolonged stretch of tight muscles and establishment of particular patterns of vestibular stimulation (e.g., the pattern of vestibular stimulation in the supine position tends to inhibit extensor hypertonicity). Passive head-turning is also used in attempts to change the distribution of muscle tone throughout the upper extremities, or to elicit upper extremity movements, through the asymmetric tonic neck reflexes (ATNR). Trunk rotation and related lower extremity movements are encouraged by carrying head rotation past the point where the child responds with movements of the upper extremities and shoulders, so that he follows through with trunk rotation and appropriate leg movements to complete rolling over from supine into prone or vice versa.

One of the shortcomings of this approach is the exclusion of any attempts to enlist the patient's conscious effort toward making discrete voluntary movements. Since the Bobaths attribute the symptoms of cerebral palsy to dominance of the motor repertoire by primitive reflexes and pathological postural reactions mediated at spinal and brain stem levels (7, 10–12), therapists adhering to this approach have been instructed to avoid involvement of cortical mechanisms that are brought into operation in other methods through call for voluntary action or direction of the patient's attention toward stimuli with motivational properties (e.g., encouraging the child to reach for an interesting object).

It should be noted that while the Bobaths hypothesize that the cerebral palsied patient's movement repertoire is dominated by pathological reflex patterns and trick movements (e.g., production of elbow extension via the ATNR through deliberate head-turning), their rehabilitation procedures merely involve practice of additional reflex responses and equilibrium reactions, with no provision for helping the patient ultimately incorporate the normalized movement patterns he may learn through reflex training into his voluntary movement repertoire.

Thus, while the "neurodevelopmental approach" has obvious value by virtue of involvement of the patient in activities that increase the number and complexity of the movement patterns he can produce and/or experience (which in itself tends to counteract spasticity by preventing affected muscles from remaining in a shortened state for prolonged periods of time), the strict neurodevelopmental therapy adherent loses out on other valuable possibilities by virtue of failing to provide opportunities for learning skills necessary for discrete, functional movements—which could be accomplished through involvement of the patient in motivated volitional activities. This deficiency is an unfortunate consequence of the conception of the symptoms of cerebral palsy as being solely determined by altered reflex mechanisms. Interpretation of problems in cerebral palsy with abnormal muscle tone, postural stability, and control of phasic movements in terms of altered cortical sensorimotor mechanisms now seems a plausible alternative; it is more in accord with findings from postmortem neuropathological study of CNS specimens obtained from patients who had cerebral palsy. These show diffuse anoxic destruction of neurons throughout the somatic sensory and motor areas of the cerebral cortex and comparable damage in subcortical "relay nuclei" for the sensory pathways (19, 89).

BRUNNSTROM

There is no question concerning the efficacy of "central facilitation," which is probably mediated via intra- and interhemispheric connections at the cortical level, although the exact pattern of associated reactions may vary as a function of the patient's individually learned motor repertoire, particularly if the patient has had any specialized form of athletic training (e.g., he may simultaneously perform the same or the opposite movement of the upper extremities depending on whether he has been a boxing or rowing enthusiast) (37, 75, 91). While emphasizing the use of homolateral and bilateral associated reactions to recruit contraction of weak muscles through irradiation or overflow of activity from residually functional musculature during maximally resisted voluntary movement, the Brunnstrom approach to hemiplegia (15) is outstanding in terms of its broad incorporation of discrete proprioceptive and cutaneous stimuli as adjuncts for facilitation of individual muscles. Brunnstrom recognizes the importance of "shaping" or progressively refining the patient's recovering motor skills, advocating the initial use of synergies and reflex patterns to begin the recovery process and then continuing to modify these patterns into more complex functional movements.

Thus, after initiating mass reactions through call for maximal voluntary effort from the intact side against resistance, she utilizes tapping over the muscle belly and localized skin stimulation in order to facilitate the contraction of individual muscles that are not responding strongly enough. She also emphasizes calling the patient's attention to the sensations accompanying correctly executed movements, and recognizes the importance of cutaneous as well as muscle sensation for muscle control, thus incorporating an important aspect of sensory feedback therapy into her approach. However, her utilization of skin stimulation is different in detail from that by Rood. Drawing upon Hagbarth's studies of the γ efferent system (26, 38), she attempts to obtain facilitation of extensors (and reciprocal inhibition of flexors) by stimulating the skin overlying the extensors and overlying the joints.

In addition to the bilateral associated reactions of the upper extremities (which usually yield the same movement on both sides of the body) and of the lower extremities (which usually yield the opposite movements), Brunnstrom also uses tonic neck and tonic lumbar reactions in facilitating postural stability and mobility of the head and trunk. She also pays detailed attention to the hands, using traction, grasp, avoidance and Souque's extension phenomena to re-educate control of the fingers for manipulatory activities.

Thus Brunnstrom uses a combination of central facilitation, peripheral proprioceptive and peripheral cutaneous stimulation, to take the patient from an initial stage of mass synergistic reactions (which she interprets as dominated by spinal reflex mechanisms, but which most likely involve intra- and interhemispheric cortical interconnections) toward an intermediate stage of voluntary motion dominated by synergies; finally, she breaks away from the synergies to approach a final stage of refined, functional voluntary control of limbs, hands and fingers. Hers is the most ecclectic of the approaches considered, the combination of procedures she utilizes only stopping short of incorporating electronic equipment (i.e., electrical nerve and muscle stimulation, EMG biofeedback, or sensory feedback via artificial sense organs) as adjuncts to therapy.

KNOTT AND VOSS (PROPRIOCEPTIVE NEUROMUSCULAR FACILITATION)

Among the approaches we are considering, the PNF technique of Knott and Voss (50), as its name implies, makes the most explicit and precise use of true proprioceptive stimulation. The therapist utilizing this method attempts to facilitate the contraction of muscle groups in synergistic patterns. The patient executes diagonal-spiral movements, which begin with placing the muscles to be facilitated under maximal stretch and end with the muscles at the maximally shortened end of their range. The therapist applies graded resistance during the course of these movements so as to maintain facilitatory stretch afferent input and to recruit activity in the weak muscles through overflow from strong muscles during maximal effort. Thus we have the classical therapeutic exercise ingredients of sustained effort in performance of specially selected, repetitive motions, with facilitation initially applied through muscle stretch and sustained through resistance to contraction.

The PNF therapist is quite actively involved with the patient at all times, due to the complexity of the procedures — verbally cueing the initiation and controling the timing of movements, mechanically guiding the movements through the correct diagonal-spiral "track," and applying graded resistance matched to the patient's increases in strength.

The diagonal-spiral movements employed are patterns that have been adapted from functional activities including rolling over, rising from the floor to sitting, standing, walking, and daily self-care. Expositors of this method refer to "Beevor's axiom" to support the use of mass movement patterns rather than the facilitation of single muscles; however, as discussed previously, this no longer provides a sound rationale for the use of less-involved parts to promote activity of those weakened by CNS injury. We can account better for irradiation under conditions of maximal exertion against resistance according to the contemporary model of programmed cortical circuits which was mentioned in conjunction with the Brunnstrom method. Knott and Voss also advocate working for proper muscle balance and reciprocal relaxation through alternating contractions of agonist and antagonist.

Thus the PNF therapist places a "demand" on the patient, through calling for voluntary effort, guides this movement through a specific pattern toward a specific goal, and resists the movement while it is under way. The movement is facilitated at its onset through muscle stretch, which occurs as the limb is positioned at the extreme of the range of motion just before voluntary movement is called for. In addition, the therapist positions the patient to regulate the demands being made in terms of changing the direction of the gravitational force which the patient must overcome, and encourages visual tracking of the movements executed. The relative position of body parts are changed as treatment progresses, beginning by placing the joints in the strongest part of the range (i.e., with muscles under maximal stretch) and then progressing to the weakest part.

Discrete phasic motions (isotonic contractions), "holds" (isometric contractions while the patient holds a position against the therapist's attempt to displace the limb), and postural and righting reflexes are all utilized in the repertoire of repetitive exercise activities. While enough repetition of each activity is provided for the patient to re-learn the movements and develop endurance during their performance, there is sufficient variety of activity to sustain the patient's interest and prevent or reverse fatigue.

The procedures that the PNF therapist must carry out are among the most complex and most demanding of any method. They demand considerable ongoing involvement in physically handling the patient and additional responsibility for timing the movements, providing feedback and guiding the movements — all the while calling for an expenditure of energy in applying resistance in order to promote irradiation from activity of the strong muscles to recruit weaker ones. Careful selection of optimal patterns for each chain of muscles is needed so that each muscle goes through the maximal change in length during the fullest possible range of motion. And, attention must be paid to the balance of tension between agonists and antagonists so that the motion will not be limited by failure of reciprocal relaxation of the antagonists. The PNF therapist must be involved mentally with correctly timing all action commands, applying appropriate manual contacts, and verbally reinforcing the patient's efforts — all of this in addition to considerable physical exertion in applying graded resistance. (Learning to carry out all of these activities simultaneously is like learning to talk while playing the piano.)

A unique aspect of this method is that a number of procedures are employed strictly for promoting postural stabilization. Successive induction is among these; a series of rhythmic slow reversals of contractions between agonists and antagonists is used to build up a sustained co-contraction for joint stabilization. Joint compression (achieved through pressure loading of joints or weight-bearing to approximate the joint surfaces) is used to facilitate this state.

In addition to muscle stretch and joint compression, the PNF therapist also uses other forms of peripheral stimulation as adjuncts to the method. Deep cold (in the form of immersion or application of cold compresses) is used to produce a state of numbness in order to relax muscle spasm and eliminate pain. Selective superficial cold application is also used for facilitation of muscle contraction in a fashion similar to Rood's method.

ROOD

The distinguishing feature of Rood's approach (77, 78) is the application of cutaneous stimuli to discrete areas of the skin in order to modify the tone and promote the contraction of underlying muscles. The most effective modes of stimulus application are "brushing," utilizing a hand-held battery-powered cocktail stirrer with a rotary brush attached to the shaft, and "icing," through stroking with a popsicle-like icecube on the end of a stick. These rather odd details of stimulus application give the approach a "mysterious" aspect that some observers find questionable, but, as was pointed out earlier, there is a sound neurophysiological basis for this approach—namely, production of γ efferent activation through cutaneous stimulation—which behaves exactly in the human patient as one would predict from experimental studies with animals.

Mechanical and thermal stimulation of skin overlying a particular muscle leads to activation of the γ efferents innervating stretch receptors in that muscle. This in turn results in tuning up the stretch receptors in the muscle, by virtue of which its tone (i.e., baseline tension in the absence of deliberate movement) as well as its contractile response to stretch is enhanced. The essence of Rood's procedure, then, is the use of cutaneous stimuli to increase stretch receptor sensitivity, followed by proprioceptive stimulation—quick muscle stretch—which maximally facilitates the patient's voluntary contraction of the specific target muscles in which the stretch receptors have been "sensitized" through γ efferent activation.

The author's experience with this procedure indicates that it is reliably effective, although Rood errs in specifying that the therapist allow 30 minutes—a rather long time—to elapse between the cutaneous stimulation and the subsequent quick stretch facilitation attempt. Here is a situation where the therapist should experiment with the conditioning-testing interaction model in mind, in order to determine the optimal interval for each patient. There is no question that in some patients increased tone and brisker responses to stretch are noticeable immediately after cessation of the cutaneous stimulation. Were the therapist to wait even 5 minutes to apply stretch and call for voluntary action, the cutaneous facilitatory effect would largely have been lost.

Just as spinal reflex mechanisms do, the γ efferent system displays reciprocal innervation. Thus, it is possible to inhibit the activity of a given muscle (e.g., obtain relaxation from spasticity) by application of mechanical and thermal stimuli to the area of skin overlying that muscle's antagonist(s). Therefore, the full effect of brushing and icing is to increase tone of the underlying muscle and to decrease the tone of its antagonist; the therapist may make use of either or both of these effects as the patient's condition requires.

Rood's major contribution is in having extended therapeutic procedures beyond the traditional PNF complement, adding to the therapist's options the application of cutaneous stimuli that produce specific, localized changes in excitability of α motoneurons, muscle tone, and strength of volitional effort. Here again, methods using proprioceptive and tactile stimulation procedures should complement rather than compete with each other. The effect of muscle stretch can be maximized by "tuning up" the stretch receptors in the target muscles through brushing and icing. Cuta-

TABLE 4.1. *Procedures Utilized in Therapeutic Exercise*

Procedure	Effect Desired	Purpose	Patient Status
Electrical stimulation of nerve or muscle; electromyograph (EMG) recording and feedback to patient.	Facilitatory	Maintain tissue elasticity, prevent muscle atrophy, and demonstrate to the patient that potential for recovery is present in terms of artificially induced overt muscle contraction and electrically recorded manifestations or residual motor unit activity	Flaccidity or near zero muscle response
Recruitment of contraction, of weak muscles into synergistic action patterns (associated reactions and reflex responses) through overflow or irradiation	Facilitatory	To bring weak muscles into play under conditions of maximal voluntary effort with the residually functioning musculature, against resistance; for breaking up spasticity	Extreme weakness of important prime movers (elbow extensors, knee flexors)
Superficial skin massage, deep muscle vibration; passive manipulation through the range of motion; guiding very weak or erratic voluntary movements through the correct "track," providing enhanced sensory feedback, verbal feedback and cueing the patient's attention to sensations in the process	Facilitatory	To focus attention on the affected body parts while they are static, and help the patient attend to kinesthetic input while the body parts are in motion	Apraxic (i.e., capable of movement but inattentive to the affected extremities); or easily fatigued because of extreme weakness
Placement in "reflex inhibiting" positions (which involves utilizing vestibular stimulation to produce widespread modification of muscle tone) and/or slow, prolonged stretch of tight muscles	Inhibitory	To free patient from the restrictions that spasticity places on range of movement, and for altering tone to allow more normal resting postures	Prime movers moderately strong, but resting position and phasic movement limited by spasticity
Prolonged application of cold compresses; immersion of limbs in ice bath	Inhibitory	For localized, discrete reduction of spasticity limiting range of motion and hampering functional use of the extremity	Capable of movement and moderately strong in its execution, but range is limited and coordination poor
Movement of head and body so as to elicit tonic labyrinthine and neck reflexes, and equilibrium reactions of limbs and trunk	Mixed	For modifying the resting distribution of muscle tone; to give patient a wider range of postural and movement experiences	Muscles strong in isolated contraction, but muscle imbalance or lack of reciprocal relaxation influences posture and limits certain movements
Quick stretch (or, slow stretch of antagonists followed by quick stretch of agonist); repetitive tapping or vibration applied to the muscle belly	Facilitatory	Applied locally before and during the call for voluntary movement	Prime movers still relatively weak but delivering increasingly more contractile tension under volitional effort

Cutaneous stimulation (brushing and icing)	Facilitatory	For discrete facilitation of contraction of individual muscles, used as a refinement to maximize the effectiveness of proprioceptive stimulation	Same as above
Application of any of the facilitation procedures listed above to the antagonists of tight muscles	Inhibitory	To relax tight muscles through reciprocal innervation. This applies both to cutaneous and proprioceptive stimulation, since gamma efferent activation and spinal reflexes directly involving alpha motoneurons follow the same reciprocal innervation principle	Muscle tone requires local adjustment to normalize muscle balance and thus permit patient to assume more normal postures and perform smoother phasic movements
Kinesthetic sensory enhancement or substitution (i.e., the use of artificial electronic sense organs to provide position feedback and reinforce the patient for improved postural stability and control of phasic movements based on this information)	Mixed	For refining motor skills	Muscle tone is within normal range when patient is relaxed but fluctuates erratically when voluntary movements of any degree of complexity are attempted, as in athetoid cerebral palsy
Successive induction; rhythmic stabilization; joint compression	Facilitatory	To promote co-contraction of agonist and antagonist, for proximal postural stability	Generalized hypotonicity, ataxia and athetosis

neous stimuli can be applied for facilitation before the patient initiates a therapeutic exercise movement pattern, or during the movement, in order to alter the balance of muscle activity by further facilitating agonists or inhibiting antagonists.

While skepticism regarding this method still persists among physiatrists, based on what seems to them a questionable relationship between skin stimulation and muscle activity and/or the peculiarities of cutaneous stimulation utilizing "cocktail stirrers and popsicle sticks," it should be realized that neurologists customarily employ the very same mechanism in determining whether muscle tone can be increased during reflex testing by one of the many "Jendrassik maneuvers." In this instance, the patient is asked to interlock both hands and pull with one set of fingers against the other while the neurologist studies the knee jerk. This maneuver usually increases quadriceps tone and contractile strength, and it is no more mysterious than the effect obtainable with brushing and icing that a brisker knee jerk is elicited during the time that the patient is concentrating on efforts with his upper extremities (31, 32, 52, 68).

Finally, in a clinical research project where the procedure was almost identical to that involved in Rood's technique, Clarke (17) showed that the quadriceps stretch reflex was significantly increased in strength following application of a single, light scratch along the skin overlying this muscle. The results of this and similar experiments (30, 69) leave absolutely no doubt about the efficacy of cutaneous stimulation in modulating the tone of the underlying musculature. Thus, reluctance to utilize Rood's approach or insistence that the facilitatory effects thereby obtainable are too mysterious to be relied upon is quite unreasonable in view of the direct parallel between the effect as discovered in animal experimentation and these correlates demonstrated in human clinical experimentation. In fact, we have here an inspiring example of a therapist setting out to study a newly discovered neural mechanism which theoretically should lead to facilitation, and showing that it did in fact have that effect. Not only did she show that the theory actually worked in practice, she also formulated a set of procedures for capitalizing upon the beneficial effects available through utilization of this phenomenon in therapeutic exercise.

SYNTHESIS OF APPROACHES TO THERAPEUTIC EXERCISE

Having considered each of the major methods, it is possible for us to contemplate the full range of procedures which the contemporary rehabilitation team has available for application in therapeutic exercise activities (see Table 4.1). We must be willing to draw upon the contributions made by all of the major expositors of specific techniques and also to keep pace with newly emerging developments in the use of technological aids as adjuncts to traditional methods. (Specialized equipment would be required for some of these procedures—electrical nerve or muscle stimulators (74), EMG recording and display devices, and artificial electronic sense organs for feedback therapy — and such instruments may not be available to the therapist in private practice or in clinical settings outside of major hospitals and research laboratories. Still, these procedures are included among the list of activities since therapists have, in fact, been trained to carry them out.)

Therapists who have the inclination and capability to incorporate this entire "armament" of procedures in an ecclectic fashion, rather than being exclusive devotees of any one method, will be best equipped to deal effectively with the infinite variety of neurological symptoms encountered in rehabilitation practice (22, 23, 62). While the procedural details may require some alteration depending on whether the therapist works with adult or pediatric populations, the same principles clearly are applicable to both groups. If rehabilitation is viewed as an extension of adult learning, then motor learning in the child and neuromuscular re-education in the adult simply may be considered as different aspects of the overall development process. Regardless of the age range in the patient load, then, these procedures should all be of interest to every therapist and physician.

The list of procedures is arranged in a sequence corresponding to a scale of decreasing severity of symptoms, ranging from flaccid paralysis with spasticity of antagonists at the top (worst) end of the scale to very mild weakness and slightly impaired coordination at the bottom (best) end, in order to indicate in an approximate fashion the patient's status for which each activity would be appropriate. The specific purposes for which each activity would be used are also indicated.

Conclusion

Therapeutic exercise techniques demonstrably rest upon a sound theoretical foundation. Yet, in the author's experience many physiatrists and other physicians — who should view the services of the therapist utilizing these techniques as the major "prescription" they can dispense for treatment of neuromuscular disorders — appear to have little faith in this form of therapy. Contributing factors are the disputes between therapists who have become fanatical adherents of a single method or devotees of a particular expositor. The total refusal to relate practice and theory on the part of some therapists who prefer an empirical approach, undoubtedly has also contributed to this attitude among physicians. Perhaps the demonstration that a scientific basis for therapeutic exercise has been provided through classical and contemporary research in the neurosciences will influence physicians toward acceptance of these methods, as well as inspire therapists toward more explicit utilization of neurophysiological and behavioral principles in their application of therapeutic exercise.

REFERENCES

1. ARBIB, M. A. Distributed information processor — a computer and brain model. *Proc. Ann. Conf. Eng. Med. Biol., 8:* 31, 1966.

2. Asanuma, H., Stoney, S. D., Jr., and Abzug, C. Relationship between afferent input and motor outflow in cat motorsensory cortex. *J. Neurophysiol., 31:* 670, 1968.

3. Ashworth, B., Grimby, L., and Kugelberg, E. Comparison of voluntary and reflex activation of motor units. *J. Neurol. Psychiatry (Lond.), 30:* 91, 1967.

4. Basmajian, J. Control and training of individual motor units. *Science, 143:* 440, 1963.

5. Bates, J. A. V. The individuality of the motor cortex. *Brain, 83:* 654, 1960.

6. Bobath, B. Control of postures and movements in the treatment of cerebral palsy. *Physiotherapy, 39:* 99, 1953.

7. Bobath, B. A study of abnormal postural reflex activity in patients with lesions of the central nervous system. Parts 1-4. *Physiotherapy, 40:* 259, 295, 326, and 368, 1954.

8. Bobath, K., and Bobath, B. Treatment of cerebral palsy by inhibition of abnormal reflex action. *Br. Orthop. J. 11:* 1, 1954.

9. Bobath, B. The treatment of motor disorders of pyramidal and extrapyramidal origin by reflex inhibition and by facilitation of movements. *Physiotherapy 41:* 146, 1955.

10. Bobath, K., and Bobath, B. The facilitation of normal postural reactions and movements in the treatment of cerebral palsy. *Physiotherapy, 50:* 246, 1964.

11. Bobath, K. Tonic Reflexes. In *The Motor Deficit in Patients with Cerebral Palsy*, pp. 27-35. Clinics in Developmental Medicine #23. William Heineman Medical Books, Surrey, England, 1966.

12. Bobath, B. Motor development, its effect on general development, and application to the treatment of cerebral palsy. *Physiotherapy, 57:* 526, 1971.

13. Bossum, J. Time of recovery of voluntary movement following dorsal rhizotomy. *Brain Res., 45:* 247, 1972.

14. Bronk, D. W. Fatigue of the sense organs in muscle. *J. Physiol. (Lond.) 67:* 270, 1929.

15. Brunnstrom, S. *Movement Therapy in Hemiplegia*. Harper & Row, New York, 1970.

16. Chang, H.-T., Ruch, T. C., and Ward, A. A. Topographical representation of muscles in motor cortex of monkeys. *J. Neurophysiol., 10:* 39, 1947.

17. Clarke, A. M. The effect of stimulation of certain skin areas on the extensor motoneurone in the phasic reaction of a stretch reflex in normal human subjects. *Electroencephalogr. Clin. Neurophysiol., 21:* 185, 1966.

18. Clough, J. F. M., Kernell, D., and Phillips, C. G. Distribution of monosynaptic excitation from pyramidal tract and from primary spindle afferents to motoneurones of baboon's hand and forearm. *J. Physiol. (Lond.) 198:* 145, 1968.

19. Courville, C. B. Contributions to the study of cerebral anoxia. III. Neonatal asphyxia and its relation to certain degenerative diseases of the brain in infancy and childhood. *Bull. Los Angeles Neurol. Soc., 15:* 99, 1950.

20. Cowen, D., and Wolf, A. Healing in cerebral cortex of infant rat after closed-head focal injury. *J. Neuropathol. Exp. Neurol; 29:* 21, 1970.

21. Cratty, B. J. *Movement Behavior and Motor Learning*. Lea & Febiger, Philadelphia, 1973.

22. DeJong, R. N. *The Neurologic Examination*, Ed. 2. Hoeber-Harper, New York, 1958.

23. Denny-Brown, D. Disintegration of motor function resulting from cerebral lesions. *J. Assoc. Nerv. Ment. Dis., 112:* 1, 1950.

24. Denny-Brown, D. The extrapyramidal system and postural mechanisms. *Clin. Pharmacol. Ther., 5:* 812, 1964.

25. Eccles, J. C. The Effects of Use and Disuse on Synaptic Function. In *Brain Mechanisms and Learning*, pp. 335-352, edited by J. F. Delafresnaye. Charles C Thomas, Springfield, Ill., 1961.

26. Eldred, E., and Hagbarth, K. E. Facilitation and inhibition of gamma efferents by stimulation of certain skin areas. *J. Neurophysiol., 17:* 59, 1954.

27. Evarts, E. V. Representation of Movements and Muscles by Pyramidal Tract Neurons of the Precentral Motor Cortex. In *Neurophysiological Basis of Normal and Abnormal Motor Activities*, pp. 215-250, edited by M. D. Yahr and D. P. Purpura. Raven Press, New York, 1967.

28. EVARTS, E. V. Relation of pyramidal tract activity to force exerted during voluntary movement. *J. Neurophysiol., 31:* 14, 1968.

29. FETZ, E. E. Pyramidal tract effects on interneurons in cat lumbar dorsal horn. *J. Neurophysiol., 31:* 69, 1968.

30. GASSEL, M. M. The role of skin areas adjacent to extensor muscles in motor neurone excitability. *J. Neurol. Neurosurg. Psychiatry, 33:* 121, 1970.

31. GASSEL, M. M., AND DIAMANTOPOULUS, E. The Jendrassik maneuver. The pattern of reinforcement of monosynaptic reflexes in normal subjects and patients with spasticity or rigidity. *Neurology (Minneap.), 14:* 555, 1964.

32. GASSEL, M. M., AND DIAMANTOPOULUS, E. The Jendrassik maneuver II; an analysis of the mechanism. *Neurology (Minneap.), 14:* 640, 1964.

33. GILMAN, S., AND DENNY-BROWN, D. Disorders of movement and behavior following dorsal column lesions. *Brain, 89:* 397, 1966.

34. GLEES, P., AND COLE, J. Recovery of skilled motor functions after small repeated lesions of motor cortex in macaque. *J. Neurophysiol., 13:* 137, 1950.

35. GOODWIN, G. M., MCCLOSKEY, D. I., AND MATTHEWS, P. B. C. The contribution of muscle afferents to kinaesthesia shown by vibratory induced illusions of movement and by the effects of paralyzing joint afferents. *Brain, 95:* 705, 1972.

36. GUYTON, A. C. Organization of the Nervous System. In *Textbook of Medical Physiology,* Ed. 4, Ch 46, pp. 540–545. W. B. Saunders Co., Philadelphia, 1971.

37. HAERER, A. F., AND CURRIER, R. D. Mirror movements. *Neurology (Minneap.), 16:* 759, 1966.

38. HAGBARTH, K. E. Excitatory and inhibitory skin areas for flexor and extensor motoneurones. *Acta Physiol. Scand. 26(Suppl. 94):* 1, 1952.

39. HARRIS, F. A. Control of gamma efferents through the reticular activating system. *Am. J. Occup. Ther., 23:* 397, 1969.

40. HARRIS, F. A. The brain is a distributed information processor. *Am. J. Occup. Ther., 24:* 264, 1970.

41. HARRIS, F. A. Multiple loop input control of efferent activity. A physiological basis for facilitation techniques. *Phys. Ther., 51:* 391, 1971.

42. HARRIS, F. A. Inapproprioception: a possible sensory basis for athetoid movements. *Phys. Ther., 51:* 761, 1971.

43. HARRIS, F. A., SPELMAN, F. A., AND HYMER, J. W. Electronic sensory aids as treatment for cerebral palsied children. Inapproprioception, part II. *Phys. Ther., 54:* 354, 1974.

44. HAYMAKER, W., AND WOODHALL, B. *Peripheral Nerve Injuries,* Ed. 2. W. B. Saunders Co., Philadelphia, 1959.

45. HEBB, D. O. *The Organization of Behavior.* John Wiley & Sons, New York, 1949.

46. HUNT, C. C. The reflex activity of mammalian small nerve fibres. *J. Physiol. (Lond.), 115:* 456, 1951.

47. HUNT, C. C., AND PAINTAL, A. S. Spinal reflex regulation of fusimotor neurones. *J. Physiol. (Lond.), 143:* 195, 1958.

48. JANE, J. A., EVANS, J. P., AND FISHER, L. E. An investigation concerning the restitution of motor function following injury to the spinal cord. *J. Neurosurg., 21:* 167, 1964.

49. JANSSEN, K. S., AND MATTHEWS, P. B. C. The central control of the dynamic response of muscle spindle receptors. *J. Physiol. (Lond.), 161:* 357, 1962.

50. KNOTT, M., AND VOSS, D. E. *Proprioceptive Neuromuscular Facilitation,* Ed. 2. Harper & Row, New York, 1968.

51. KORNORSKI, K. Disintegration of skilled movements after lesions in premotor area 6. *Int. J. Neurosci., 1:* 39, 1970.

52. KROLL, W. Patellar reflex time and reflex latency under Jendrassik and crossed extensor facilitation. *Am. J. Phys. Med., 47:* 292, 1968.

53. KUKULKA, C. G., AND BASMAJIAN, J. V. Assessment of an audio-visual feedback device used in motor training. *Am. J. Phys. Med., 54:* 194, 1975.

54. LAITINEN, L. V. Neurosurgery in cerebral palsy. *J. Neurol. Neurosurg. Psychiatry, 33:*

513, 1970.

55. LANGWORTHY, O. R. *The Sensory Control of Posture and Movement.* Williams & Wilkins Co., Baltimore, 1970.

56. LASSEK, A. M. Effect of combined afferent lesions on motor function. *Neurology (Minneap.), 5:* 269, 1955.

57. LASSEK, A. M. Inactivation of voluntary motor function following rhizotomy. *J. Neuropathol. Exp. Neurol., 3:* 83, 1953.

58. LI, C.-L., AND TEW, J. M. Reciprocal activation and inhibition of cortical neurones and voluntary movements in man. Cortical cell activity and muscle movements. *Nature, 203:* 264, 1964.

59. LLOYD, D. Facilitation and inhibition of spinal motoneurons. *J. Neurophysiol., 9:* 421, 1946.

60. LLOYD, D. Reflex action in relation to pattern and peripheral source of afferent stimulation. *J. Neurophysiol., 6:* 111, 1943.

61. MEGIRIAN, D. Bilateral facilitatory and inhibitory skin areas of spinal motoneurons of cats. *J. Neurophysiol., 25:* 127, 1962.

62. MERRITT, H. H. *Textbook of Neurology.* Lea & Febiger, Philadelphia, 1957.

63. MIGLIETTA, O. Action of cold on spasticity. *Am. J. Phys. Med., 52:* 198, 1973.

64. MORRELL, R. M. Intracellular recording from spinal motoneurons following stimulation of the medullary pyramids. *Nature, 180:* 709, 1957.

65. MORTIMER, E. M., AND AKERT, K. Cortical control and representation of fusimotor neurones. *Am. J. Phys. Med. 40:* 228, 1961.

66. MOTT, F. W., AND SHERRINGTON, C. S. Experiments upon the influence of sensory nerves upon movement and nutrition of the limb. *Proc. R. Soc. Lond., 57:* 481, 1895.

67. NATHAN, P. W., AND SEARS, T. A. Effects of posterior root section on the activity of some muscles in man. *J. Neurol. Neurosurg. Psychiatry, 23:* 10, 1960.

68. OTT, K. H., AND GASSEL, M. M. Methods of tendon jerk reinforcement. *J. Neurol. Neurosurg. Psychiatry, 32:* 541, 1969.

69. OTT, K. H., AND GASSEL, M. M. Local sign and late effects on motoneurone excitability of cutaneous stimulation in man. *Brain, 93:* 95, 1970.

70. PAILLARD, J. The Patterning of Skilled Movements. In *Handbook of Physiology, Section I: Neurophysiology,* pp. 1679–1708, edited by J. Field. American Physiological Society, Washington, D.C., 1960.

71. PATTON, H. D. Spinal Reflexes and Synaptic Transmission. In *Physiology and Biophysics,* Ed. 19, pp. 153–180, edited by T. C. Ruch and H. D. Patton. W. B. Saunders Co., Philadelphia, 1965.

72. PETAJAN, J. H., AND PHILIP, B. A. Frequency control of motor unit action potentials. *Electroencephalogr. Clin. Neurophysiol., 27:* 66, 1969.

73. POWERS, W. T. *The Control of Perception.* Aldine, Chicago, 1973.

74. REBERSAK, S., AND VODOVNIK, L. Proportionately controlled functional electrical stimulation of the hand. *Arch. Phys. Med. Rehabil., 54:* 378, 1973.

75. REGLIA, F., FILIPPA, G., AND WIESENDANGER, M. Hereditary mirror movements. *Arch. Neurol., 16:* 620, 1967.

76. REINBERG, R. M., AND STUART, D. G. Servo-regulated electromagnetic system for muscle stretch and vibration. *Am. J. Phys. Med., 53:* 1, 1974.

77. ROOD, M. Neurophysiological reactions as a basis for physical therapy. *Phys. Ther. Rev., 34:* 444, 1954.

78. ROOD, M. S. Neurophysiological mechanisms utilized in the treatment of neuromuscular dysfunction. *Am. J. Occup. Ther., 10:* 220, 1956.

79. ROSE, J. E., MALIS, L. I., AND BAKER, C. P. Neural Growth in the Cerebral Cortex after Lesions Produced by Monoenergetic Deuterons. In *Sensory Communication,* pp. 279–302, edited by W. A. Rosenblith. MIT Press and John Wiley & Sons, New York, 1961.

80. ROSÉN, I., AND ASANUMA, H. Peripheral afferent inputs to the forelimb area of the cat and monkey motor cortex: input-output relations. *Exp. Brain Res., 14:* 257, 1972.

81. SALMOIRAGHI, G. C., AND VON BAUMGARTEN, R. Intracellular potentials from respiratory neurones in brain-stem of cat and mechanism of rhythmic respiration. *J. Neurophysiol., 24:* 203, 1961.
82. SCHWARTZ, A. S. Recovery from motor deficit under different motivational conditions. *Physiol. Behav., 4:* 57, 1969.
83. SHAMBES, G. M. Influence of the fusimotor system on stance and volitional movement in normal man. *Am. J. Phys. Med., 48:* 225, 1969.
84. SHERRINGTON, C. S. Flexion reflex of the limb, crossed extension reflex, and reflex stepping and standing. *J. Physiol. (Lond.), 40:* 28, 1910.
85. SHERRINGTON, C. S. *The Integrative Action of the Nervous System.* Yale University Press, New Haven, 1906 (reprinted in 1947).
86. SMITH, J. L., ROBERTS, E. M., AND ATKINS, E. Fusimotor neuron block and voluntary arm movement in man. *Am. J. Phys. Med., 51:* 225, 1972.
87. SPRAGUE, J. M., AND CHAMBERS, W. W. Control of posture by reticular formation and cerebellum in intact, anesthetized and unanesthetized and in the decerebrated cat. *Am. J. Physiol., 176:* 52, 1954.
88. THULIN, C. A., AND CARLSSON, C.-A. Regeneration of transected ventral roots submitted to monomolecular filter tubulation (millipore) — an experimental study in cats. *J. Neurol. Sci., 8:* 485, 1969.
89. TOWBIN, A. *The Pathology of Cerebral Palsy.* Charles C Thomas, Springfield, Ill., 1960.
90. TWITCHILL, T. E. Sensory factors in purposive movement. *J. Neurophysiol., 17:* 239, 1954.
91. WEISS, P. Self-differentiation of the basic patterns of coordination. *Comp. Psychol. Monogr., 17:* 1, 1941.
92. WIESENDANGER, M. Rigidity produced by deafferentation. *Acta Physiol. Scand., 62:* 160, 1964.
93. WIESENDANGER, M. Input from muscle and cutaneous nerves of the hand and forearm to neurones of the precentral gyrus of baboons and monkeys. *J. Physiol. (Lond.), 228:* 203, 1973.
94. WINSLOW, R., AND SPEAR, I. J. Section of posterior spinal nerve roots for relief of gastric crises and athetoid and choreiform movements. *J. A. M. A., 58:* 238, 1912.

5

Vicarious Motions (Trick Movements)

C. B. WYNN PARRY

When muscles are weak or paralyzed the movements they normally carry out may still be possible by the action of other muscles, which may be normal synergists of the affected muscles or may have an action quite different from them. The term "trick action" or "trick movement" is used to describe such a vicarious motion.

Trick movements can be divided broadly into two types—those which deceive the examiner into thinking that a muscle or muscle group is working when it is in fact paralyzed and those which successfully replace function lost by obvious paralysis.

An example of the first category is the ability of the long extensors to simulate abduction of the fingers in a complete ulnar nerve palsy. An example of the second category is the excellent abduction and elevation of the shoulder still possible despite total paralysis of the deltoid.

Physiologically, however, there is no logical distinction between types of trick action; in all, the body is attempting by using all means available to maintain as near normal function as possible.

Although a few workers, notably Sunderland (3) and Wood-Jones (5), have studied and described many trick actions, the subject is not well understood or widely known.

In this chapter an attempt will be made to describe and classify all the trick actions known to the writer. It must be realized, however, that the list will not be complete as much remains to be done in this field.

Classification

The different types of trick actions of muscles can be classified (an example is given in each case) as follows:

(a) **Direct Substitution of Favorably Placed Muscles.**
Example: The long heads of biceps and triceps, the clavicular

fibers of pectoralis major and the external rotators of the humerus can abduct the arm despite total deltoid paralysis.

(b) Accessory Insertion.

Example: A patient with a complete radial nerve palsy can still extend the terminal joint of the thumb (normally performed by extensor pollicis longus) because the abductor pollicis brevis and flexor pollicis brevis are inserted into the extensor expansion of the thumb.

(c) Tendon Action. Strong contraction of the antagonists of a paralyzed muscle can cause the appearance of contraction of the paralyzed muscle when there is inequality of length of the two muscles.

Example: When the finger flexors are paralyzed, wrist extension causes finger flexion as the flexors are shorter than the extensors. This is also known as a tenodesis effect. It is utilized to restore functional finger flexion in permanent flexor paralysis—e.g., in high median and ulnar nerve lesions, by advancing the origin of the flexors so that the degree of finger flexion is increased.

(d) Rebound Phenomenon. When the antagonist to a paralyzed prime mover contracts strongly and suddenly relaxes, it may look as if there is a contraction in the prime mover. In paralysis of the extensor hallucis as in lateral popliteal (common peroneal) nerve palsy, it may look and feel as if the muscle is contracting when the flexor hallucis strongly contracts and then relaxes. In testing in such a situation one asks the patient to make the opposite movement first—i.e. to flex the toe then relax completely and then attempt extension. When the prime mover is paralyzed, the opposite movement to that desired can be felt immediately.

(e) Anomalous Innervation. Abnormalities in nerve supply occur more commonly than is generally supposed. Seddon (2) indicated that one-fifth of all peripheral nerve injuries studied had some anomaly of nerve supply.

Example: A patient may have complete severance of the median nerve at the wrist and yet be able to oppose the thumb because the opponens and flexor pollicis brevis may be entirely supplied by the ulnar nerve.

(f) Gravity. Wood-Jones (5) stated that a muscle acting as a prime mover will not do its work if gravity will do it instead. Consequently the effects of gravity must be looked for when studying muscle action in patients with muscle weakness or paralysis.

Example: A patient with gross weakness of triceps may not be able to extend the elbow until the shoulder has been depressed sufficiently far for gravity to allow the elbow to straighten.

Trick Movements in Specific Lesions

PERIPHERAL NERVE INJURIES IN THE HAND

Radial Nerve Palsy

The interphalangeal joint of the thumb can be extended, despite the paralysis of the extensor pollicis longus, by the action of the short abductor, which has an insertion into the extensor expansion. Occasionally the short flexor also gains insertion into the expansion. The trick can be seen by applying slight resistance to the dorsal surface of the flexed terminal phalanx of the thumb. In the absence of action of the extensor pollicis longus the thumb is abducted away from the plane of the palm and rotated due to action of abductor and flexor pollicis brevis.

It is thus important to test for extensor pollicis action with the thumb lying against the index finger and not in palmar abduction. The slightest resistance to the interphalangeal joint will immediately demonstrate abduction.

The interphalangeal joints of the finger can still be extended normally, as this action is carried out by the interossei. The extensor digitorum acts only on the metacarpophalangeal joints except if these are firmly stabilized in extension, when its action is transmitted to the interphalangeal joints. If the extensor digitorum is paralyzed, attempting extension at the metacarpophalangeal joints results in flexion at these joints, due to the interosseus action extending the fingers and pulling down the extensor hood.

Thus extensor digitorum action should always be looked for with the fingers extended at the interphalangeal joints as there is at least 20° hyperextension at these joints. The wrist can seem to be extended despite paralysis of the wrist extensors when the wrist flexors contract by rebound when the wrist flexors relax after a sudden maximum contraction. This can be quite an impressive action and can be achieved against gravity.

The trick is detected by testing for wrist extensor action with the wrist almost fully extended passively. If the extensors are paralyzed the wrist and fingers can be seen to *flex* immediately.

Ulnar Nerve Palsy

Abduction of the fingers can be performed to a slight extent by the action of extensor digitorum.

Extensor indicis is a remarkably good abductor of the index and the extensor digiti minimi of the fifth finger. Although the movements of abduction are obviously accompanied by action of the extensors, it can be a most confusing trick action. To find out if the abduction is a trick or not, the patient should be asked to raise each finger in turn off the desk and then to move it from side to side. In a normal person the extensor stabilizes the metacarpophalangeal joint and the finger in the air while the interosseus abducts. In a patient with interosseus paralysis, once the finger has been raised off the desk it cannot be moved laterally, since the extensor is fully occupied in stabilizing the metacarpophalangeal joint. A very distinctive trick movement is then visible in which the whole palm and wrist move from side to side in an attempt to produce the movement.

Tests such as asking the patient to scratch the table with the palm flat or grip a piece of paper between the fingers, although helpful, are not, in our experience, as foolproof as that described above.

Adduction of the thumb is normally carried out by the adductor pollicis but in ulnar palsy can still be effected by a combination of flexor and extensor pollicis longus action. With the palm face up on the desk the thumb is brought down to the index finger in adduction mainly by gravity, assisted by the extensor pollicis longus. If resistance is offered to the movement, the interphalangeal joint of the thumb flexes at once, showing the trick action of the flexor pollicis longus.

This action becomes obvious without resistance when the patient is asked to adduct the thumb against gravity. In this case the arm is held in pronation with the radial border of the forearm facing the floor and the patient attempts to bring the thumb towards the index finger.

As a result of paralysis of the third and fourth lumbricals, the metacarpophalangeal joints of the ring and little fingers cannot be flexed except by action of the flexors sublimis and profundus, which cross these joints and therefore have some flexor action. Consequently the metacarpophalangeal joints cannot be flexed when the interphalangeal joints are extended, and attempts to hold the fingers straight with the metacarpophalangeal joints at right angles fail. When the patient is asked to bend the metacarpophalangeal joints with the interphalangeal joints extended, the interphalangeal joints immediately flex; this is a sure sign of lumbrical paralysis. It is now generally believed that the lumbrical's main function is to act as a brake to hyperextension.

Median Nerve Palsy

The main disability in a median nerve lesion at the wrist level is lack of opposition. This complex movement consists of four separate components — abduction in the palmar plane (perpendicular to the palm) by the abductor pollicis brevis (median supply), flexion across the palm by flexor pollicis brevis (median ulnar supply), rotation by opponens (median supply) and stabilization by adductor pollicis (ulnar supply).

There are numerous anastomoses between median and ulnar nerves in the thenar muscles. Only the abductor pollicis brevis is exclusively supplied by the median nerve. The importance of the short abductor has been shown in several patients studied in whom only this muscle was paralyzed. Despite an intact opponens, opposition may be impossible. When the patient attempts opposition, the long abductor pulls the thumb away from the index finger, but in a radial plane; as the thumb is carried across the palm, it collapses into the palm through lack of the short abductor. The thumb is carried across the palm by the long flexor, and the interphalangeal joint can be seen to bend as soon as the thumb starts to cross the index finger. Rotation is impossible.

Meanwhile the fifth finger is flexed at the metacarpophalangeal joint and extended at the interphalangeal joints to approach the thumb, and the flexor and opponens digit minimi elevate the fifth metacarpal in cupping the fifth finger. Should there be a combined median and ulnar palsy, the ability to elevate the fifth metacarpal is lost and the little finger is flexed at both metacarpophalangeal and interphalangeal joints due to lumbrical paralysis. In isolated opponens palsy the short abductor and adductor acting together can give a very confusing imitation of opposition.

Application to Re-education

In peripheral nerve injuries, and particularly those involving the hand, splints must be worn to prevent deformity. It is even more important that such splints also encourage function.

Movements, not muscles, are represented in the brain, and, during the long period while awaiting regeneration of the nerve, movement patterns must be preserved, not only to facilitate re-education in due course, but to effect daily functional tasks. As has been indicated, many so-called trick movements are available despite nerve palsies, and these trick movements can be used for function provided that correct splinting is applied.

The deformity to prevent in an ulnar palsy is hyperextension of metacarpophalangeal joints and flexion of interphalangeal joints – the claw hand. A lively splint should be given to the patient, not only to prevent this deformity, but to encourage flexion of metacarpophalangeal joints by the long flexors in order that the grip may be strong. The splint illustrated in Figure 5.1 (*bottom*) fulfills these requirements.

In ulnar nerve palsy the metacarpophalangeal joints of the ring and little fingers are hyperextended and the proximal interphalangeal joints flexed – the so-called claw hand. This prevents the long flexors from flexing these joints efficiently and so stability must be provided at the metacarpophalangeal joints.

The splint has a bar across the metacarpals and across the palm, and two cuffs round the proximal phalanges of the little and ring fingers joined by a hinge at the metacarpophalangeal joint. This not only prevents hyperextension at the metacarpophalangeal joints but allows full flexion and extension at these joints (Fig. 5.2). The palmar piece is small enough not to interfere with function.

A lively splint for thenar paralysis should bring the thumb away from the index finger in palmar abduction to imitate the action of abductor pollicis brevis (Fig. 5.3). This allows the long flexor to produce an imitation of opposition, pulling on the rubber of the splint. It is sometimes

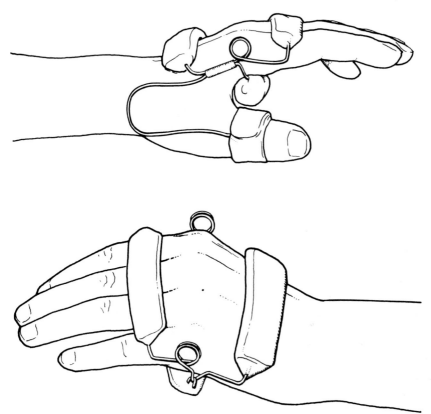

Fig. 5.1. Lively splint for ulnar palsy.

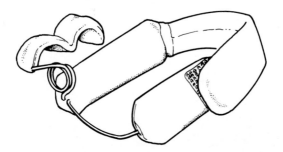

Fig. 5.2. Lively splint for medial-ulnar palsy.

not feasible to supply a splint that has a cuff round the wrist if there is
tender scarring or a neuroma on the median nerve. In this situation the
splint used for a combined median and ulnar nerve lesion is used.

Combined Median and Ulnar Nerve Lesion

Here function is prohibited both by the hyperextension at the metacarpophalangeal joints and the inability of the thumb to be brought away from the palm for opposition. When the lesion is at the wrist the long flexor can oppose if the thumb is held in palmar abduction. This is achieved by a cuff around the proximal phalanx of the thumb attached to a spring at the wrist. This is an integral part of a knuckle-duster with bars across the proximal phalanges and the metacarpals joined at the metacarpophalangeal joints by a hinge of piano wire at the metacarpophalangeal joint of the little finger (Fig. 5.1, *top*). Thus the stabilization effected at the metacarpophalangeal joints allows flexion at the metacarpophalangeal joints and the cuff and spring round the thumb concentrates the flexor pollicis longus as a rotator. The splint is light, easily cleaned, small enough to allow functional use and cheap to construct. Many of our patients have been able to service engines and work at electronics wearing such splints.

In radial palsies the wrist is held in flexion — the so-called dropped wrist. Grip is weak in this position and it is therefore necessary to support the wrist in dorsiflexion but wrist movements must be allowed.

The splint consists of a wire framework with a palmar pad fitting in the hollow of the palm well proximal to the metacarpophalangeal joints, the angle of which is arranged to provide dorsiflexion of 20–30°. Two supports fit firmly round the forearm, the distal support being closed round the distal forearm by velcro (Fig. 5.4). A piano wire hinge at the wrist allows active wrist movements. Full details for making these three splints can be found in Wynn Parry (6).

In a combined median and ulnar nerve lesion at elbow level the patient may have such good tendon action of finger and wrist flexors by wrist extensors that he can catch a bouncing ball. Often the abductor pollicis longus can provide a remarkable range of wrist flexion (in radial deviation).

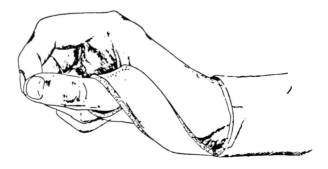

Fig. 5.3. Lively splint for thenar palsy.

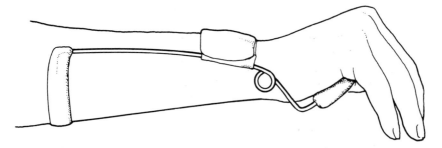

Fig. 5.4. Lively splint for radial palsy.

FOREARM ROTATOR PARALYSIS

There are certain clearly defined trick actions that can substitute for paralysis of pronators or supinators or stiffness of the radioulnar joints.

With the arm by the side and the elbow in extension, the forearm can be rotated in two ways—either by movement at the radioulnar joints or by internal and external rotation of the humerus. The latter is so deceptive that the forearm rotators or the mobility of the superior radioulnar joint must always be tested with the elbow at 90° and firmly held into the side. These remarks apply equally to the training of weak forearm rotators. In exercise therapy for these muscles or the superior radioulnar joint the patient must be prevented from abducting the shoulder to give spurious rotation.

PARALYSIS OF ELBOW FLEXION

In a complete musculocutaneous palsy the brachioradialis can effectively flex the elbow and in some patients weights of 3 kg (about 7 lb) or more can be lifted. In the absence of brachioradialis and conventional elbow flexors, elbow flexion can sometimes be achieved by adduction of the arm, pronation of the forearm, and combined contraction of the wrist and finger flexors and extensors. This is seen in upper trunk lesions of the brachial plexus.

The action of the wrist and finger flexors and extensors acting from their insertion to their origin is the basis of the Steindler procedure in permanent paralysis of elbow flexion. In this operation the origins of both the common extensors and flexors are advanced up the humerus, and powerful elbow flexion can be achieved. If the extensors are weak or paralyzed—as for example when the C.7 root as well as C.5 and C.6 are affected, this is not feasible and here the Clark-Brooks transfer is used in which the pectoralis major is inserted into the biceps. Functional elbow flexion may be hindered by the adductor action of the pectoralis and an external rotation osteotomy of the humerus is then needed.

PARALYSIS OF ELBOW EXTENSORS

Paralysis or weakness of triceps is not a grave disability except in heavy laborers or those who are dependent on crutches for ambulation. Weakness is common in this muscle, not only from poliomyelitis and other lower motor neuron disorders, but also following elbow fractures.

Gravity will allow elbow extension in normal function. Testing for triceps power, however, is often incorrectly performed, and thus misleading results are obtained. When testing, and indeed exercising, the triceps, the patient shoud be asked to flex his shoulder to 90 degrees and flex the elbow to its maximum.

When he attempts to extend the elbow, the shoulder will immediately be depressed to allow gravity to extend it. This becomes obvious if some resistance is offered. The elbow alignment must be carefully watched and, although the shoulder moves considerably, the angle between forearm bones and humerus does not alter.

However, patients have been seen in whom full elbow extension is possible with the shoulder abducted to 90 degrees and the elbow fully flexed. Here gravity cannot assist, and the active muscles are in fact brachioradialis and the wrist and finger extensors acting from their insertion.

Little resistance can be overcome in this movement, but it is certainly of functional significance. In one patient the movement became strong enough to dispense with a lively splint with spring extension aid.

SHOULDER PARALYSIS

Deltoid paralysis is common after axillary (circumflex) nerve lesions following fractures of the surgical neck of the humerus, and dislocation of the shoulder, and after C.5 brachial plexus lesions and poliomyelitis.

DELTOID PARALYSIS ALONE

There is a widespread belief that paralysis of the deltoid means loss of abduction of the arm. In 145 patients seen with paralysis of the deltoid alone, or a combination of teres minor and deltoid paralysis in an axillary nerve lesion, every patient has regained full function, including full abduction and elevation against strong resistance without any recovery being seen in deltoid. In every case the finding of clinical paralysis was confirmed by electromyography. The key muscles that must be present before this compensatory movement can be obtained are the external rotators of the humerus. In the absence of the deltoid, abduction is initiated by the supraspinatus, if present, and carried to about 70° by the long heads of the biceps and triceps. At the beginning of abduction, the humerus is externally rotated by the infraspinatus. At about 70° the clavicular fibers of the pectoralis major act as powerful abductors because the axis of the shoulder joint has not rotated externally. Thereafter, the serratus anterior elevates the arm through forward and upward pull on the scapula.

It is widely held that the supraspinatus must be working to allow this trick action. However, Watson (4) has observed complete rupture of the supraspinatus at operation in a patient who had full elevation of the arm. It is the infraspinatus that is vital.

It is our practice to teach patients this compensatory movement from the earliest stages after paralysis. First, it is essential to restore passive movements to the shoulder joint if these are absent. The re-education is carried out with the patient lying on his back and the arm supported in a sling with overhead suspension. Before any attempt is made to initiate abduction, the patient externally rotates the humerus. He is then asked to try to abduct the arm, and in so doing he will inevitably hitch up the shoulder by trapezius action. The therapist directs the patient's attention to this bad habit and encourages him to obtain the movement entirely at the shoulder. A certain degree of swing is allowed at this stage to give the patient the idea of movement.

In a small number of patients difficulty may be found in learning this trick. In these cases it is helpful to give specific resistance exercises to the long heads of biceps and triceps, and to break down the movements into isolated ones in each muscle involved. This is particularly helpful when there is associated weakness of the other muscles as in plexus lesions.

As the patient improves, the treatment couch is gradually inclined at an increasing angle so that gravity resists the movements more and more. A light weight (about $1/2$ kg or 1 lb) helps the patient to initiate and hold the movement. Patients usually learn full elevation in four weeks although one patient mastered the art in one half-hour session.

DELTOID PARALYSIS WITH OTHER MUSCLES INVOLVED

Often the deltoid is only one of a group of muscles involved. The typical upper trunk brachial plexus lesion results in paralysis of both spinati and deltoid. In this case patients do not develop trick abduction. Many learn the "arm fling." In this maneuver the arm is first adducted across the middle of the trunk. It is then suddenly sharply swung back with a quarter twist of the trunk. This carries the arm in pendulum fashion above the head. This fling is also associated in some cases with a marked arching of the back. It cannot be maintained for more than a few seconds, but patients with this disability find it very useful in reaching objects above their heads. It is certainly well worth while developing in all such patients.

If the biceps is intact, it is worth considering transplanting the teres major and latissimus dorsi to the back of the humerus, thus making them external instead of internal rotators. If these muscles are strong and the patient is cooperative, he can then be taught to abduct the arm by using the pectoralis and biceps and the new external rotators as abductors. This trick within a trick, as it were, has proved very successful in the right type of patient.

It is not essential that the biceps be intact for abduction to occur if some external rotator power is available. Patients have been seen in whom deltoid and biceps have been paralyzed but external rotators and pectoralis major were present. Extremely powerful abduction and elevation has been possible in these circumstances. It will be seen, therefore, that amazing shoulder function is possible despite considerable paralysis. It is thus vital that the patient be given every chance to learn substitution or "trick" muscle action under careful supervision. Arthrodesis of the shoulder should never be necessary unless a very large number of shoulder muscles is irrevocably paralyzed and even then at least 2 years must be allowed after plexus lesions for surprising recovery can occur even so late.

Patients with paralysis of the external rotators of the humerus attempt external rotation by extension of the wrist, fingers, and thumb. True external rotation should always be tested by asking the patient to keep the flexed elbow against the side, bringing the forearm out and away from the trunk. If extension of the wrist is the first activity seen, severe weakness or paralysis of the infraspinatus is certainly present.

TRICK MOVEMENTS OF THE LOWER LIMB

These are far less common. In a few cases trick action can substitute for efficient weight-bearing function, as is required in the leg. There are, however, certain trick actions that require discussion.

Hip

Trick actions of hip abduction and flexion may be seen in pareplegics who walk with their latisimmus dorsi and abdominal muscles. The latissimus dorsi acts by virtue of its pelvic origin and contracts from insertion to origin. The lateral abdominals, acting from the ribs, hitch the pelvis up, thus allowing the leg to clear the ground. The one muscle that must be present for walking to be possible is quadratus lumborum.

Hip extension is normally accomplished by the gluteus maximus; but, in its absence, the hamstrings (because they take origin from the ischial tuberosity) can extend the hip, acting from their insertion on the tibia to their origin. Isolated paralysis of the gluteus maximus without hamstring involvement is rarely seen, thus, the trick action is not observed often. In the absence of hip flexors the hip may be flexed in walking by the external rotators and the adductor magnus.

Knee

When the quadriceps is paralyzed, as is frequently the case in poliomyelitis and in femoral nerve paralysis, rebound action of the hamstrings results in a snap-forward extension of the knee. This is accompanied by exaggerated hip flexion and sudden relaxation of hip flexors to let the leg drop on the ground. Strong gluteal contraction stabilizes the pelvis as the weight is taken on the affected leg. This "trick" action allows the patient to walk but not normally to run.

Provided the glutei are fairly strong, paralysis of quadriceps on one side and even considerable bilateral weakness do not necessitate wearing a caliper. One patient has been studied carefully in whom both the quadriceps and all gluteal muscles of one leg were totally paralyzed. This patient could walk without calipers or canes for some miles—undoubtedly a highly unusual case but it illustrates the amazing function of which the human body can be capable.

Slow-motion cinema photography shows that the erector spinae, abdominal muscles and quadratus lumborum, by finely controlled reciprocal action, effected the pelvic tilt in the absence of the glutei—the patient going into momentary exaggerated lordosis as the weight was taken on the affected leg. The quadriceps paralysis was compensated by the usual rebound hamstring phenomenon.

Foot

In paralysis of the toe flexors, tendon action and rebound phenomenon by extensor contraction can give an impression of the flexor contraction. To be certain that it is not a trick the ankle and toe should be plantar flexed almost fully and the patient asked to bend the toes down. If the toe flexors are paralyzed, the toes will instantly extend slightly. Similarly in lateral popliteal palsies the action of the toe flexors and ankle flexors may suggest activity in the extensor muscles. Again when the ankle and toes are put into nearly full extension and the patient asked to extend the toes and ankle, they will flex immediately, indicating a trick action.

In paralysis of the peronei, strong inversion of the foot by tibialis posterior and sudden relaxation may give a spurious idea of peroneal contraction. To be sure that the action is a trick, the ankle is everted and, when the patient attempts to evert, the ankle immediately inverts.

In the early stages of reinnervation of a lateral popliteal palsy, the patient may not be able to evoke a flicker in the tibialis anterior when attempting to invert and dorsiflex the ankle but can do so when he contracts his quadriceps strongly. This is the principle of proprioceptive facilitation.

One patient has been reported in whom the peronei had been totally removed at operation for traumatic necrosis (1). Full eversion was, however, still possible by contraction of the gastrocnemius and the lateral toe extensors.

It has been found a most helpful rule that the earliest evidence of recovery in a lower motor neuron lesion is the cessation of the trick movement. For example, the earliest sign of recovery in the interossei is not the patient's ability to move the finger from side to side. When the patient raises the finger off a desk and attempts sideward movement, instead of the trick motion of the palm and hand on the finger, no movement at all occurs. This lack of trick movement indicates activity in the prime movers though in the early stages of recovery it may be so slight that no true movement may be seen. It is therefore important to know what trick movements to expect in lesions of the lower motor neuron, and, if they are not present when expected, early recovery may be assumed.

In summary, a knowledge of trick movements is of great value in the correct diagnosis of the extent of lower motor neuron lesions, in assessing recovery and in re-educating useful function in both temporary and permanent paralysis. Finally, in patients who are hysterical or malingering and affecting muscle paralysis, the absence of trick movements expected in the particular nerve lesion will be of diagnostic value.

REFERENCES

1. DARCUS, H. D. Personal communication.
2. SEDDON, H. J. In *Peripheral Nerve Injuries,* p. 5. M.R.C. Report (H.M.S.O.), London, 1954.
3. SUNDERLAND, S. *Aust. N. Z. J. Surg., 13:* 160, 1944.
4. WATSON, M. To be published.
5. WOOD-JONES, F. *Principles of Anatomy as Seen in the Hand.* Baltimore, 1942.
6. WYNN PARRY, C. B. *Rehabilitation of the Hand.* London, 1973.

6

Clinical Assessment of Joint Motion

_____ MARGARET L. MOORE

A knowledge of the range of motion of joints is important not only for physicians and therapists but for the anatomist, the physical eductor, and the engineering design analyst. The placement of foot pedals in automobiles, the design of seats for industrial workers and turret gunners as well as the design for maximum visibility in aircraft and automobiles is based on an analysis of the range of motion of the joints of the human body which participate in the operation of these devices.

An understanding of the normal and pathological motions in joints is the key to a comprehension of functional anatomy; it is the foundation for prescribing intelligently meaningful therapeutic exercises and knowing when to modify and terminate the treatment program.

Instruments of measurement of joint range of motion may vary from the complicated apparatus used by the research anatomist studying fundamental kinesiological problems to the simpler practical devices used in the clinic. For the busy clinic, measurements should be accurate and repeatable by the same observer and by different observers with similar training. The clinical instrument should be simple, durable, portable, and applicable to all joints, or to as many joints as feasible in persons with a variety of body builds and for different ages.

Much work on the fundamentals of joint range of motion assessment has been done since early in this century by persons of varied professional and academic backgrounds. Each world war has been accompanied by a burst of activity in the areas of physical disability measurement. Since the fairly comprehensive review of the literature by Moore (87) in 1949, there have been many publications which demonstrate increasing sophistication of design, in research methodology, and in instrumentation. In 1955, Salter (114) offered a good survey of the literature but did not include references from the United States in the fields of physical therapy and occupational therapy, each of which have contributed significant studies on joint mobility. Many physicians who deal with problems involving joint range delegate to the physical therapist the measurement and recording of range of motion.

Joint range of motion measurements often have a genuinely motivating effect on the patient, who learns by figures which are personal, vivid, and meaningful—especially when they progress in a desirable direction.

A determination of joint range of motion is a part of the education process for medical students as well as for students of physical therapy and occupational therapy. When properly integrated in the teaching program, students become aware of the changes in mobility related to age and occupation in addition to the effects of disease and injury. The fundamentals of gait, of activities of daily living (such as stair climbing and body transfer), and of self-help activities (such as feeding and dressing) are better understood if, along with an appreciation of the necessary strength, coordination and endurance, students become familiar with the joint mobility also required.

A well trained operator can obtain reliable measurements if he exercises enough care in the use of a carefully designed and constructed instrument.

Instrumentation

The most widely used and recommended instrument is the universal goniometer, sometimes called an arthrometer. Basically, it is a protractor, to the center of which two long slender arms or levers are attached. Usually, only one of the arms is movable, but many variations in design are possible as is evident from more than 30 publications cited at the end of this chapter (5, 6, 10, 13, 16–19, 26, 32, 33, 36, 53, 63, 66, 74, 83, 85–88, 94, 99, 100, 105, 110, 111, 115, 118, 126, 127, 129, 130, 132, 135).

COMMERCIALLY PRODUCED INSTRUMENTS

A universal goniometer should have the following characteristics: (a) A full-circle or half-circle protractor, depending upon the materials used in construction and on the personal choice of the operator. (b) A good draftsman's protractor marked *in graduations of one degree,* for accuracy. The graduations should be large enough to be read easily by the naked eye, or if necessary through an attached magnifying lens. If the instrument is made of metal it should have a keyhole indicator to reveal the area of motion measured (Fig. 6.1).(c) The protractor should be numbered in each direction—from zero to 180° and from 180° to zero. Two scales are needed on a metal instrument; one scale is adequate on a clear plastic full-circle instrument if well designed (Fig. 6.1). (d) The arms should be at least 12–16 inches long; for the measurement of finger joints, the arms have to be proportionately shorter. (e) The pivot rivet or fulcrum should permit free, smooth motion but should also be secure against slipping. (f) A prominent line should extend from the pivot to the distal tip of the moving arm. There should be a clearly marked extension of the baseline

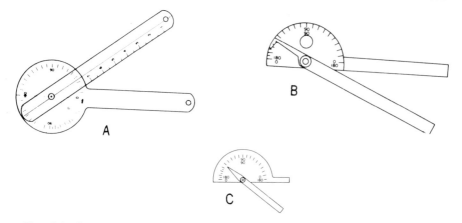

Fig. 6.1. Some commercially available goniometers. (A) Full circle, plastic; (B) half-circle, metal; (C) metal finger instrument.

of the protractor throughout the length of the stationary arm. (g) Each arm should be movable so that either may be the stationary or movable arm.

Protractors made of clear plastic are desirable but the coloring matter used to fill the marking grooves tends to "wash" out with time. Other universal devices have been designed with hinged arms, telescopic arms, adjustable stands, recording paper discs, water levels, and straps to secure them to the patients. While variations in instruments are great, *in each clinic, where more than one person uses goniometers, there should be a standardized device to reduce instrument and operator error.* Additional instruments may be needed to measure the spine and hand but all members of the staff should use the same instrument.

SPECIAL DEVICES

In 1914 Gifford (47) published what appears to be the first paper in the United States on instruments designed for specific joints. A few years later Fox (42) and Nutter (96) described several instruments for special joint studies which appear to have been based on apparatus designed in France by Amar and Camus. Albee and Gilliand (1) enlarged on these designs which were perfected by the U. S. Army during World War II (85, 87).

Upper Extremity. A weighted pendulum was designed by the U. S. Army for measuring the *shoulder joint* (85, 87). Albee and Gillian (1) and Rosen (111) described other instruments for this joint. One of the few *elbow* arthrometers was produced during World War II (85, 87). Special devices for the study of wrist motion have been designed for use in the laboratory and clinic (1, 24, 29, 57, 85, 87). Instruments to measure *pronation* and *supination* utilize handles to turn, platforms on which to rest the forearm, or drums with weighted pendulums to turn (6, 19, 29, 32, 42, 85, 87, 100). The *fingers* and *thumb* pose special problems for which a variety of solutions have been offered. Fox (42) described a fleximeter; Newman (93), a clear plastic full-circle. In addition, there have been tracings, radiographs, rulers, special finger goniometers, and clay or plaster impressions (2, 3, 5, 14, 42, 54, 81, 83, 93, 94, 96, 111, 123, 132).

Lower Extremity. Many instruments have been suggested for clinical measurement of the *hip joint* (1, 15, 52, 85, 87, 91, 111, 121); Ghormley (49) designed a research instrument which measured in three planes of motion simultaneously. Apparatus for studies on the *knee* closely resemble the universal goniometer with the addition of a pad that fits over the contour of the joint and adjacent parts (42, 85, 87). Some *ankle* devices fit under the foot, and some around the joint (7, 42, 62, 64, 85, 87). Barnett and Napier (7) used cineradiography while Karpovich (62, 64) designed an electric goniometer.

Head and Neck. Many techniques have been tried to measure the motion in the cervical region (9, 13, 37–39, 67–69, 77, 123). A group at the University of Minnesota used the bubble goniometer for mobility, and cinefluorography for more precise measurements. Defibaugh (31) claimed high reliability with a plastic pendulum of his design. Storms (123) described a way to measure the mobility of the temporomandibular joint. Pendleton studied the jaw with a ruler and calipers (102).

SPECIAL METHODS

Tracings. Manual tracings of large and small joints have been used by Gottlieb (51), Nutter (96), Rosen (111) and Pollock and Brooks (105).

Pendulum. A pendulum device said to be applicable to all joints was first described by Fox and van Breemen (43) and subsequently by others (50, 53, 74, 76, 85, 87, 129). The principle was reintroduced by Leighton (74, 76) in studies on healthy adults in a physical education assessment program. The device may rest on or be strapped to the part to be measured while a weighted pointer moves freely over a calibrated dial. Defibaugh (31) placed a similar device in the mouth of subjects to study mobility of the cervical region.

For all measurements utilizing the pendulum, the subject should be erect and the upright position must be maintained during measurements since the fixed reference point becomes the perpendicular initially indicated by the pendulum dial. As motion occurs, the dial rotates behind the pendulum, which comes to rest opposite the number indicating the excursion. At first it was used primarily on the hip, shoulder, and forearm but later it was recommended for all joints. Accuracy is dependent upon careful attention to a true perpendicular starting position of the pendulum. Additional error may be introduced because the contour of the part on which the instrument must be placed may vary.

Bubble Goniometer. Schenker (117) feels that the protractor (single plane) class of goniometer is totally unreliable because, in his opinion, there is no anatomic center of rotation in a joint. He applied the general principle of the bubble spirit level to goniometry. The bubble goniometer is small and light. It resembles a wrist watch with fluid between the face and the glass. A bubble in the fluid seeks the superior vault of the enclosed space (what would be 12 o'clock in a watch). The goniometer is strapped to the part to be measured. As the part moves, the bubble remains "horizontal" and the figures on the dial (in degrees rather than minutes) are rotated. When the part stops moving, the bubble comes to rest over the number of degrees of the excursion. Great caution must be exercised by the operator in the placement of the patient and in the maintenance of posture positions while the motions are executed. The same element of error would appear associated with this instrument as is found with pendulum devices. Many patients are unable to assume the standard body postures required for this and similar devices to obtain first, the zero reference position. Although the basic concept is good, until the idea can be incorporated into a device which is less expensive to manufacture and which lessens the errors inherent in routine clinical joint assessment, it will remain of limited usefulness. When enough care was exercised it was shown to be a reliable research tool, especially in the measurement of the cervical spine (9, 13, 31).

Most published articles on techniques of goniometry refer only fleetingly to measurements of the spine, either the dorsal lumbar area or the cervical region. This attests to the difficulty of a reliable measurement for this region of the body. A variety of techniques for measurements have been described from radiographs and a series of varied techniques (2, 5, 8, 21, 61, 69, 76, 77, 123, 128), to a very simple measurement of the inches from the floor reached by a patient performing forward flexion and lateral flexion (2, 3, 95). Motion pictures, x-rays, goniometers, bubble goniometers, and pendulum devices are among those described. A more precise analysis using a flexion curve rule was described by Israel in 1959 (61), but never became popular due in part to difficulties in placement. Orthopedists either estimate range of motion or use tape measures (3).

Electric Goniometers. These have been described by Karpovich (63), Moore (90) and Thomas and Long (125). Moore's instrument employs registration on the telemetry principle and tracings with it appear to be fairly similar to those obtained by Karpovich using an electronic device. The device of Thomas uses the principle of transduction.

Mathematical Determination. Williams (133, 134) offered an ingenious mathematical approach to the determination of joint range. Using the crease of the elbow as the pivotal reference, he marked the skin at equidistant points from it on the arm and forearm. The linear distance between the two points is measured in full flexion and extension.

Of the many other ingenious methods which have been recommended, we mention the photogoniometer of Zankel (139), the double exposure photographs of Wilson and Stasch (136), the optical goniometer of Wilmer and Elkins (135), and the use of xerography by Regenos (108). Flexibility tests used in France were reported by Myers (92).

Other Considerations. There have been many studies on the roles of the muscle strength, the speed of movement, the position of the parts, the dominant hand, and age. Most of the work has been concerned with the position of the joint and its effect on the muscle power (28, 113).

Handedness in conjunction with elbow position has been investigated by Provins (107) and Salter (114). The dominant hand was stronger when tested separately, but when both hands work together each is stronger than when either is working alone. Leighton (75) showed the range of motion decreases with increasing age especially in a group of young people between 10 and 18 years of age. Wright (138) presented a thoughtful analysis of different kinds of stiffness associated with a variety of joint lesions. Spilman and Pinkston (121) studied the position of the upper extremity and its effect on motion.

From all of these studies, it is evident *that techniques of clinical goniometry must be standardized by identifying the starting and posture positions with exactness* for correct use of instrumentation.

Numerical Expression

In 1948, Moore (85, 87) attacked the confusing state of numerical expressions which had been compounded over the years by proponents of different systems. Many attempts have been made since that time to arrive at a unified plan; in a 1956 report (86) it was evident that most physical therapists in the United States were taught the method based on the 0–180° scale later adopted by most medical groups (Figs. 6.2 and 6.3). First described by Silver (118) in 1923 but often attributed to Cave and Roberts (17) it was restated in a manual on joint measurement published by the American Orthopaedic Association (2, 3). The same numerical system was endorsed by a number of orthopedic associations throughout the world, the American Medical Association (5), and the Veterans Administration (104). It is so universally accepted that it should be utilized by all. According to this plan, in the upright, erect anatomical position, the joints are at 0° in motion; the foot is at a right angle to the leg and the palms are turned forward. The American Academy of Orthopaedic Surgeons calls this anatomical position a neutral position. The arc of motion begins logically, at 0° and progresses toward 180°. As motion progresses, the numerical expression is recorded in positive numbers; as a joint with restricted extension improves, the numerical expression of motion decreases.

There are authors (20, 33, 35, 71, 131) who prefer the system which is based on the geometric consideration that 180° is the true expression of the half circle or the sum of two right angles. In this system, flexion approaches 0° and extension is limited to 180°. As motion occurs, the numerical value decreases and progressive mobilization of a restricted joint yields diminishing values.

A third system using a full circle of 360° of motion, first described by

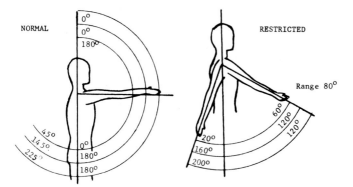

SYSTEM	NORMAL			RESTRICTED		
	Flex.	A.P.*	Ext.	Flex.	Ext.	Range
1. 0° - 180° (Moore, Cave, V.A., Amer. Acad. Ortho. Surg., Silver)	180	0	45	60	20	80
2. 180° - 0° (Krause, Dorinson and Wagner, Krusen, Clark)	0	180	145	120	160	80
3. 360° (Mundale et al, West, Ashhurst)	0	180	225	120	200	80

*Anatomical Position

Fig. 6.2. Three systems of numerical expression of range of motion for the shoulder joint.

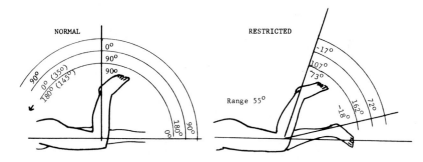

SYSTEM	NORMAL			RESTRICTED		
	Flex.	A.P.*	Ext.	Flex.	Ext.	Range
1. 0° - 180° (Moore, Cave, V.A., Amer. Acad. Ortho. Surg., Silver)	145	0	0	73	-18	55
2. 180° - 0° (Krause, Dorinson and Wagner, Krusen, Clark)	35	180	180	107	162	55
3. Right Angle (Conwell)	90	90	90	-17	72	55

*Anatomical Position

Fig. 6.3. Three systems of numerical expression of range of motion for the knee joint.

Ashhurst (6) and later advocated, at least for a time by others (35, 66, 83, 91, 130, 135), never achieved great popularity.

As opinion approaches unanimity, *it would be very wise and mutually helpful for all health profession to adhere to one goniometric plan and system of numerical expression — the one proposed by the American Academy of Orthopaedic Surgeons based on 0–180° (2, 3).*

NORMAL VALUES

There is much to be said for the advantages of tables of normal values for range of motion. They offer a basis for comparison of values not only to those who manage the patient but for medicolegal purposes. However, the manner of defining norms varies so much with variations in instruments and examiners that there are few common denominators with which to achieve a logical and universally acceptable set of appraisals.

TABLE 6.1. *Range of Joint Motion*

Joint	Action	Degrees of Motion
Shoulder	Flexion	180
	Extension	45
	Adduction	40
	Abduction	180
	Medial rotation	90
	Lateral rotation	90
Elbow	Flexion	145
Forearm	Pronation	80* to be changed from 90°
	Supination	85* currently listed
Wrist	Flexion	80
	Extension	70
	Abduction	20
	Adduction	45
Hip	Flexion	125
	Extension	10
	Abduction	45
	Adduction	(Air Force and Army list 40°)
	Medial rotation	45
	Lateral rotation	45
Knee	Flexion	140
Ankle	Flexion	45
	Extension	20
Foot	Inversion	40
	Eversion	20

Adapted from V.A. Standard Form 527 A — U. S. Government Printing Office.

TABLE 6.2. *The Spine and Its Motion*

	Cervical	Lumbar
Forward flexion	65°	95°
Extension backward	50°	35°
Lateral flexion	40°	40°
Rotation	55°	35°

Adapted from The Veterans Administration physician's guide: Disability, Evaluation, Examination, June 1963.

This does not mean that the study of normal range of motion is not informative and helpful. The continuous use of radiology, electromyography, and electronics draws us closer to "ideal" values.

Guide lines for normal range of motion have been suggested by many (5, 8, 16, 27, 32, 48, 88, 104, 114, 120). Since it is helpful for the clinician to measure the uninvolved joint as a basis of comparison, we produce here charts (Tables 6.1 and 6.2) based on recommendations of the U.S. Veterans Administration whose guidebook for physicians (104) does not state how the figures were obtained. They are presented for guidance only and should not be considered infallible. The American Academy of Orthopaedic Surgeons compares four sets of values for normal range of motion (2, 3) but they differ very little from those included in the Veteran's Administration chart. The actual manner in which the measurements were determined is not explained by the Academy in its publication.

The work of Inman and his associates (60) led to a more thoughtful and accurate analysis of upper extremity joint motions and made obsolete many estimates of shoulder range which had appeared previously.

Cobe (24) and Hewitt (57) measured the wrist joints in women with a device which precludes its use in studying other joints. They saw great fluctuations in "normal" range. Moore (55, 85) found measurement of the wrist less reliable than that of any of the upper extremity joints when measured by an experienced operator using two different types of goniometers.

Darcus and Salter (29) analyzed pronation and supination as related to the position of the elbow, to age and to different instruments. They found that range of motion decreases with age, and that apparatus utilizing grip devices were less dependable than those without a gripping handle. A similar analysis was made by Moore who studied the forearm with a universal goniometer and the U. S. Army instrument designed specifically for this motion (55, 85).

The University of Minnesota group (91) compared x-ray measurements and goniometric values of hip joint motion and found a discrepancy of only plus or minus 5°. Kottke and his associates (68, 69) studied motion in the cervical spine with cinefluorography and noted differences of as much as 50% between the norms accepted by the American Medical Association (5) and their own findings.

Recording Methods

For clinical use, any system for recording measurements should be rapid, accurate, and easily interpreted. Until there is unanimity in method and terminology, visual charts of joint range will remain desirable and important. Some clinics use a visual chart and others use charts which include joint diagrams as well as a tabular recording arrangement, as can be seen in Figure 6.4. Gerhardt and others (46) believe that with increased universality in numerical expression recordings can be more safely standardized and entered in charts in simple numerical experessions (Fig. 6.5). Recordings in three basic planes and combined creates a SFTR method of recording for sagittal, frontal, transverse, and rotation. Measurements can be simply entered as flexion and rotation. (Measurements can be entered as $0°-30°-120° = 90°$ range of motion or from $-30°$ to $120° = 90°$ range of motion. Shoulder motion may be recorded as $120°-0°-30° = 150°$ range of motion. The latter would indicate that motion is in both directions from the anatomical or neutral zero position.)

Freehand drawings and tracings have been used to record results, especially for the joints of the hand (51, 80, 97, 111).

Cumulative measurements have been plotted in graph form to show progression during the weeks in which the patient has been treated. Frequently these are associated with special studies, such as, for example, the charts of the Hand Rehabilitation Center of the University of North Carolina (Fig. 6.5). Additional tables and charts may also be used as well as photographs, which are clear but expensive and time consuming, and not easily applicable to daily departmental routine (136).

Nomenclature

We stongly recommend the standard nomenclature of the *Nomina Anatomica*. Terms of flexion, extension, medial and lateral rotation, abduction, and adduction are more appropriate than such terms as dorsi and plantar flexion, internal and external rotation, and radial and ulnar deviation. The term hyperextension is not standard and is reserved for the unnatural and unusual motion beyond the full range of ordinary extension. Cave and Roberts (17) proposed a satisfactory terminology in 1936 which was reviewed by Batch (8) in 1955 and again by Cave (16) in 1958.

The American Academy of Orthopaedic Surgeons did, however, redefine the motions of the shoulder, hand, and foot. The terminology for the foot was not changed very much but an attempt was made to identify the joints in which motion can be measured. The *tibiotalar* joint is responsible for flexion and extension; the *hind foot* can be measured passively for inversion and eversion at the *subtalar* joint; the *forefoot* at the *midtarsal*

NEW YORK UNIVERSITY MEDICAL CENTER
INSTITUTE OF PHYSICAL MEDICINE AND REHABILITATION
DEPARTMENT OF PHYSICAL THERAPY

NAME _____ AGE _____

DISABILITY _____ DIAGNOSIS _____ IN ___ OUT ___

RANGE OF MOTION TEST FOR LOWER EXTREMITY

1. Anatomical position is starting position. Range is measured with cauda as 0°, cranium as 180°. Rotating motions are from the midsagittal plane as 0° to lateral plane as 180°.

2. All ranges are expressed as passive range of motion. Check muscle chart attached for limitations caused by tightness, weakness, spasm, or contracture.

3. The scale is divided into units of 10°. Range of motion is recorded by filling in area of range

directly on attached sketch with date and examiner's initial.

4. Use of same sheet for subsequent tests is recorded in same color and dated accordingly.

5. Retrogression is marked by diagonal lines over area of previous test and dated.

6. If position is other than in sketch, indicate S for supine, P for prone.

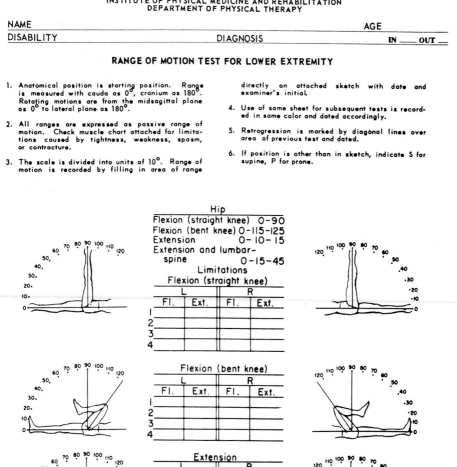

Hip

Flexion (straight knee)	0-90
Flexion (bent knee)	0-115-125
Extension	0-10-15
Extension and lumbar-spine	0-15-45

Limitations
Flexion (straight knee)

	L		R	
	Fl.	Ext.	Fl.	Ext.
1				
2				
3				
4				

Flexion (bent knee)

	L		R	
	Fl.	Ext.	Fl.	Ext.
1				
2				
3				
4				

Extension

	L		R	
	Ext.	E&L	Ext.	E&L
1				
2				
3				
4				

Hip

| Abduction | 0-45 |
| Adduction | 45-0 |

Limitations

	L		R	
	Abd.	Add.	Abd.	Add.
1				
2				
3				
4				

Fig. 6.4. Chart for recording joint range of motion measurements. (Reproduced with permission of the Department of Physical Therapy, Institute of Physical Medicine and Rehabilitation, New York University Medical Center.)

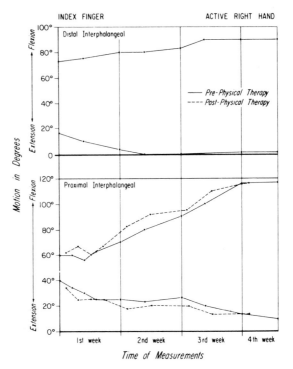

Fig. 6.5. Graphic record of change in range of motion in joints of the index finger during a four-week period. From, Hand Rehabilitation Center, School of Medicine, University of North Carolina at Chapel Hill.

joints of the *talonavicular* and the *calcaneocuboid* can be measured passively for medial and lateral rotation, and the abduction and adduction. The combined motions of active inversion and eversion occurring in the forefoot and the hindfoot can then be measured, frequently with a goniometer.

Starting Positions

The initial step in precise goniometry is to ask the patient to assume a specific body position, frequently called a *preferred starting position*. If carefully selected, these positions make it less difficult to isolate the desired arc of movement to be measured, and the instrument can be placed more accurately and its position maintained since the patient's position is less likely to deviate. The addition of motions in the same and adjacent joints other than the requested motion is more easily recognized and substitution avoided. The term "neutral position" is confusing and should not be used.

Preferred starting positions are identified for all test positions although they may vary depending on the physical ability of the patient. When standardized, it is more likely that measurements can be repeated by the same or different members of the staff. When deviations from the standardized positions are necessary because of the patient's physical disability, they should be recorded. The exact anatomical positions of all parts of the body which participate in the motion should be defined in the position to be utilized, such as identifying the direction of the hand in measuring motions of the shoulder.

Zero starting positions are essential to good goniometry (2, 5, 8, 16, 17, 32, 33, 88, 131).

Axis of Motion

Much has been written about the "axis of the joint" and "center of rotation." Some authors insist that the pivot of the measuring protractor can be centered on an anatomical landmark presumed to be an axis. Surely *no one specific landmark can accurately be called an axis of motion* for complex movements of the shoulder, ankle, wrist, knee, and hip, to cite perhaps the most obvious examples. The location of the axis or fulcrum is important but it has received far too much emphasis and incorrect description in the literature.

The ill defined axis of motion appears to shift as normal motion progresses. Consideration of the mechanics of movement indicate that the *intersection of the longitudinal projections of the two limbs or sides of the angle must coincide with the true axis of motion.* The acromial process, the lateral styloid, for example, are not in this intersection position throughout the full range of motion. To attempt to fix the protractor of the goniometer to any such specific anatomical landmark is open to real criticism and may indeed distort the motion actually present in the joint. If this specific part is identified first, it may then be impossible to adjust the arms of the instrument parallel to the limbs of the anatomical angle; *this should be the primary consideration in instrument placement.*

If the moving arm of the instrument is carefully placed as nearly as possible parallel to the long axis of the moving limb of the joint, and the stationary arm is placed parallel to the long axis of the apparently fixed side of the joint, then the axis of motion will fall where the two intersect and will automatically localize in the approximately correct position. Meticulous preliminary inspection of the relation of the fixed to the moving segment, prior to the placement of the goniometer was strongly recommended as a basic part of the technique as described by Moore (88). The U.S. Army and Air Force (32) and the American Academy of Orthopaedic Surgeons (2) avoid reference to a fixed axis of motion in goniometry utilizing a universal instrument. The fact that most other authors utilize a fixed axis of motion as a reference point for the placement does not make it correct. Schenker (116) sharply criticizes the use of the universal goniometer because of its frequent association with a fixed axis of motion. *Since no landmark is or can be a fixed axis, then a complete technique of goniometry should avoid reference to this in the application of the instrument to the joint.* Work done by others (40, 60, 138) lends credibility to the fact that no such landmark is or can be an axis of motion.

Karpovich (62) described a "center finder" to determine the location of the axis of rotation of the joint. If two arcs of a circle are given, the center of the circle will be found at the intersection of the perpendiculars erected at the midpoints of the two chords drawn through these arcs. Karpovich uses this geometric principle in determination of the axis of motion of joints in the body. He admits, however, that many of the joints of the body have migrating axes of motion and therefore the process he describes has to be repeated several times through consecutive parts of the range of motion of the joints in order to attempt to locate the axis. This is an interesting procedure and a fairly complex one; it should be studied further although at this time it would not be wise to include it as part of a standard technique of clinical joint motion measurement.

Techniques

Standardized and systematized techniques for clinical measurement must include specified and defined positions of posture of the body as well as of the individual joints under consideration. The instrument should be identified, and in an institution where more than one person is assigned to joint measurement, only one instrument should be utilized to reduce error. The same technique should be required of all staff members in order that the operator error be reduced. The part to be measured should be exposed and unrestricted, insofar as possible, by clothing or bandages. The range of passive motion is frequently of interest as it contrasts with the range of active motion; when recorded the difference between the two should be indicated in the record. The time that the measurements are taken should be identified as occurring before or after treatment.

The most complete description of the technique of goniometry was that by Moore in 1949 (88) although it did not include material on the spine, the cervical region, or the hands. Good general directions, in nomenclature, positioning and range appear in the 1963 and 1965 publications of the American Academy of Orthopaedic Surgeons (2, 3); but no technique for instrument placement is included in this material. In fact, a goniometer is not actually recommended by the orthopedist except by the most experienced surgeons. The omission of instructions in the application of the instrument seems to deny the reliability and validity studies which have been reported.

Less well defined directions given by Silver (118), West (130), Hellebrandt and Miles (56) and others (6, 20, 26, 83, 110, 111, 131) are considered inadequate for reliable clinical measurements.

Many of the special instruments previously described have specific placement requirements inherent in their basic construction. The following are the basic elements of the technique of goniometry for an instrument will a full-circle or half-circle protractor.

1. Begin by placing the patient in good body alignment — to simulate the anatomical position as closely as possible. Examine this position critically and prevent deviation from the initial alignment to the extent possible during the execution of the movement to be measured. Such deviation or substitution of motion may falsify results significantly.

2. Before starting to measure tell the patient simply and clearly what to do. If necessary, demonstrate the movement and urge the patient to execute as pure an anatomical motion as possible with no substitution or compensatory movements.

3. For ease in measuring and to isolate best the desired motion, the joints are measured from specific starting positions rather than in the true erect anatomical position. These will be referred to as "preferred positions."

4. All movements of extremities should be measured in degrees and from specified starting or 0° positions. Measurements in each arc of motion begin at 0° and progress toward 180°.

5. The zero starting position for any single movement of a joint is identical with the anatomical zero position except for the radioulnar joints, where the mid-position is selected as zero. Other positions are changed for convenience in measuring but the anatomical position of the part to be measured is not changed.

6. Having aligned the body, instruct the patient to swing the moving part rhythmically through the arc of motion to be measured and localize the approximate axis of rotation by inspection. If this cannot be done volitionally, move the part passively.

7. Always apply the goniometer to the lateral side of a joint except in measuring supination and a few other motions which will be explained below.

8. Instruments may vary considerably from one manufacturer to another. Frequently a commercial instrument cannot be placed so that zero on its scale is at the anatomical zero position of the joint; it often is 90° or 180°. The examiner must be aware of this and calculate the mathematical change himself so that he interprets his readings from a zero beginning.

9. In placing the stationary arm of the instrument parallel with the longitudinal axis of the fixed reference part, *attempt to sight over a considerable distance* and not just on a limited area.

10. To have both extremities execute the same movement simultaneously often aids balance, coordination and the maintenance of body position.

11. Since the true axis of motion is located at the intersection of the two limbs of the angle, this cannot be determined *until the end of the desired movement*. If the arms of the instrument *are fixed carefully at the end of the desired movement*, the nail head pivot of the instrument must fall in the region of the true axis of motion.

12. The instrument should be held loosely, away from or in light

contact with the patient's body. By trying to maintain the position of the goniometer against the moving part, the instrument position may be in error and the patient may be prohibited from executing his full range of motion.

13. Much depends on the steadiness of the operator in maintaining the position of the measuring instrument. If possible, the operator should steady his holding arm against his side or on a table top, depending on the position in which he has placed the patient.

14. Execute no force on the body in placing the instrument. To do so would destroy the accuracy of placement. Example: a slight pressure on the volar surface of the wrist might alter the result by 5–10° above true supination.

15. By finding the maximum degree of motion in both directions, the range of motion can be calculated. Example: flexion plus extension equals range of motion; pronation plus supination equals range of motion.

16. The elbow and knee are considered to be 0° extension joints since motion progresses normally in only one direction from the anatomical position. The range of motion is found by subtracting the lack of extension of the joint from the flexion degree obtained. Example: flexion 100°, extension −20°, equals range of motion 80°.

17. In all joints which move in two directions from zero position, the maximum motion in both directions is added to obtain the full range of motion. Example: shoulder, wrist, radio-ulnar; flexion and extension equals range of motion. In an abnormal joint in which a return to the zero anatomical position is not possible, the two figures are subtracted, as in the paragraph above.

18. The motions of the opposite extremity, if uninvolved, should be measured for comparison.

Standard procedure for the use of the universal goniometer is given for the shoulder, elbow, forearm, wrist, hip, knee and ankle. Placement of the instrument on selected motions is shown in Figures 6.6 to 6.11. Special instructions for measurements of the digits, the spine, and the cervical region will follow the section on standard procedure.

Standard Procedure

I. SHOULDER JOINT (Figs. 6.6 and 6.7)
    A. *Flexion:* 0° toward 180° anteriorly. The limb should travel forward with the palm of the hand facing the ceiling. Measure from the lateral aspect of the body.
        1. Preferred position: (a) The patient should be supine with good postural alignment. (b) The patient may be standing or sitting in a good posture if it is not desirable to have support from the firmness of the table top.
        2. Stationary arm — Place along the mid-axillary line of the trunk in line with the greater trochanter of the femur with no increase in lordosis permitted.
        3. Moving arm — Place along the lateral mid-line of the humerus in line with the lateral condyle of the humerus. (This will be out of line in full

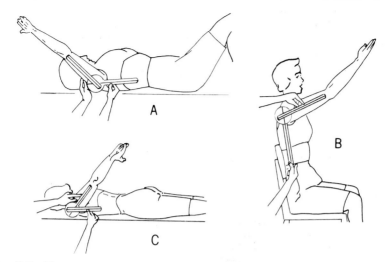

Fig. 6.6. Placement of goniometer for measuring shoulder joint motion (A) Flexion (supine), (B) flexion (sitting), (C) extension (prone).

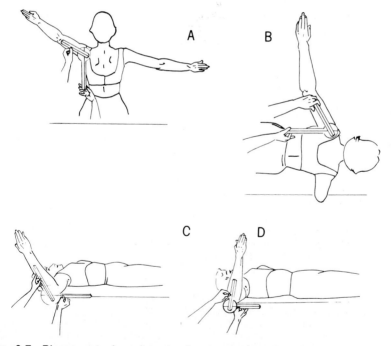

Fig. 6.7. Placement of goniometer for measuring shoulder joint motion. (A) Abduction (sitting), (B) abduction (prone), (C) lateral rotation, (D) medial rotation.

normal shoulder flexion since the humerus must rotate in order to assume this position beyond approximately 150–165°; use the olecranon process beyond this point.)

4. This axis will be somewhere in the vicinity of the acromion process but *do not sacrifice accurate placement of the arms of the goniometer* to secure the hinge of the instrument at this position.

5. Caution: Avoid extension of the trunk and abduction of the shoulder; keep the moving arm close to the body; avoid elevation of the shoulder.

B. *Extension:* 0° posteriorly toward 50°. Keep subject's hand facing forward.
   1. Preferred position: (a) The patient should be prone with good postural alignment. (b) As in I. A. 1 (b).
   2. Use the same reference points as in I. A.
   3. Caution: Avoid forward flexion of the trunk and abduction of the shoulder.
   4. Remarks: Extension can be measured with a straight elbow or with a flexed elbow to rule out action of the biceps, but always remeasure the same way.

C. *Abduction:* 0° toward 180° laterally. Measure from the posterior aspect of the body.
   1. Preferred position: (a) The patient should be standing or sitting with his back to the operator. The thumb should lead in the direction of the movement, with the palm of the hand facing forward. (b) The patient may be prone but in good alignment – or he may be measured in a supine position.
   2. Stationary arm – Place parallel to the spine but at the lateral aspect of the body; that is, in the posterior axillary line.
   3. Moving arm – Place on the posterior aspect of the arm parallel to the posterior mid-line of the humerus toward olecranon process.
   4. The axis will fall somewhere in the vicinity of the acromion process. Do not set goniometer by this.
   5. Caution: Avoid lateral flexion of the trunk, flexion or extension of the shoulder joint and elevation of the shoulder girdle.

D. *Adduction:* This is the return from abduction. Use the same technique as in I. C.

E. *Medial Rotation:* 0° toward 90°.
   1. Preferred position – The patient should be supine. Abduct the arm toward 90° with the elbow bent to 90° and the palm of the hand facing the body and the forearm perpendicular to the table top. The full length of the humerus should be resting on the table top; allow only the elbow over the edge of the table.
   2. Stationary arm – Place parallel to the floor with the nail head of the instrument at the olecranon process. Maintain this parallel zero position during movement of the part.
   3. Moving arm – At the completion of the executed motion set along the dorsal mid-line of the forearm between the styloid processes.

F. *Lateral Rotation:* 0° toward 90°.
   1. Preferred position – Use the same as in I. E.
   2. Placement – Use the same as in I. E.
   3. Caution: Watch for decrease or increase in abduction of the shoulder. The operator may steady the patient by placing a finger under the elbow (to keep a reference point of motion). This in no way hinders movement but it will rule out much substituted motion. Avoid flexion, extension, elevation or lifting the shoulder from the table.
   4. Remarks: (a) If this measurement is taken from a supine position, as is recommended, the humerus must be elevated with a pad to the plane of the acromion process. (b) If possible, note the degree of motion in both directions at the same time, as it is difficult to maintain the

position of the patient and the instrument. This can be done by setting the stationary arm parallel to the long line of the trunk.

II. ELBOW JOINT (Fig. 6.8)
   A. *Flexion:* 0° toward 145–160°. The palm of the hand is forward in the anatomical position.
      1. Preferred position – The patient should be supine or standing with the arm parallel to the lateral mid-line of the body and in the anatomical position.
      2. Stationary arm – Place along the lateral mid-line of the humerus toward the acromion process of the scapula.
      3. Moving arm – Place along the lateral mid-line of the radius toward the styloid process.
      4. The axis will fall somewhere in the vicinity of the lateral condyle of the humerus. Set the instrument arms first and do not sacrifice their positions to secure this one.
   B. *Extension:* This is the return from flexion and the same technique is used as in II. A.

III. RADIO-ULNAR JOINTS
   A. *Pronation:* 0° toward 90°.
      1. Preferred position – Measure in a sitting or a standing position. The elbow is flexed to 90° and the arm is held close to the side of the body. The thumb is directed superiorly. There should be no support under the forearm.

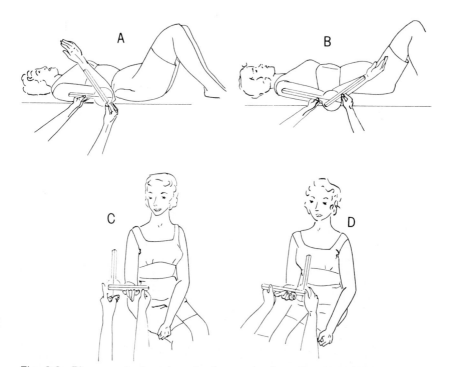

Fig. 6.8. Placement of goniometer for measuring elbow and forearm motion. (*A*) Elbow flexion (supine), (*B*) elbow extension (supine), (*C*) pronation (sitting), (*D*) supination (sitting).

2. Stationary arm—Place the instrument arm on the dorsal surface of the wrist parallel to the long axis of the humerus.

3. Moving arm—At the end of the executed motion place along the dorsum of the wrist on a level between the styloid processes of the radius and the ulna. Attempt to place the moving arm along the area of the styloid processes which is fairly flat and free from muscle or soft tissue.

4. Caution: Keep the elbow close to the side and do not allow abduction or any rotation of the shoulder. Keep the instrument proximal to the carpal region at the distal end of the radius-ulna. Avoid lateral flexion of the body toward the opposite side.

5. Remarks: (a) It is difficult to maintain the position of the stationary arm. There is no specific bony landmark on the wrist and the contour may change with edema or bandages. (b) Readings for a full-circle protractor instrument can be taken directly. To take a reading from a half-circle protractor the moving arm must be traced across the protractor with a card or a ruler edge and the degree for a corresponding angle taken. Some half-circle instruments have an extended pointer on the moving arm which accomplishes this purpose.

B. *Supination:* 0° toward 90°.

1. Preferred position—The same position is used as in III. A. 1.

2. The technique is essentially the same as in pronation but the instrument is placed on the volar surface of the wrist. Moving arm is adjusted to the widest, most flattened area just proximal to the wrist. Avoid lateral flexion of the body to the same side as the extremity being measured.

IV. WRIST JOINT (Fig. 6.9)

A. *Flexion:* 0° toward 90°.

1. Preferred position—The patient may be sitting or standing but should have no support under the length of the forearm with the elbow flexed. The forearm should be in pronation.

2. Stationary arm—Place along the lateral mid-line of the ulna toward the olecranon process.

3. Moving arm—This line parallels the mid-line of the fifth metacarpal.

4. The pivot of the instrument will fall in the carpal region of the wrist after the arms of the instrument have been adjusted.

5. Caution: Palpate the area of the hypothenar eminence in order to set the instrument arm along the line of the fifth metacarpal.

6. Remarks: Flexion can be measured on the radial side of the hand but the measurements of the two sides of the wrist will vary due to the anatomical structure of the wrist and the cupping of the hand on the little finger side. If measured on the radial side use the 2nd metacarpal for the distal landmark.

B. *Extension:* 0° toward 70°. The same placement is used as in IV. A., but the axis will shift. Place the arms of the goniometer correctly and the approximate position of the axis will be in a line perpendicular to the nail head pivot of the instrument.

C. *Abduction* or *Radial Flexion:* 0° toward 25°. The instrument is on the dorsum of the wrist.

1. Preferred position—Abduct the arm toward 90° with the elbow flexed and the forearm in mid-position of pronation and supination. The forearm may rest on a table top but there should be no support under the hand.

2. Stationary arm—Place along the mid-line of the dorsum of the forearm between the radius and the ulna toward the lateral condyle of the

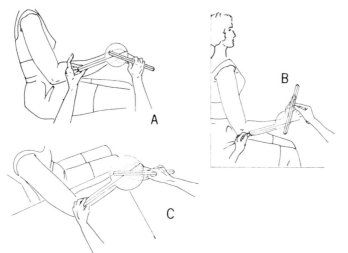

Fig. 6.9. Placement of goniometer for measuring wrist motion. (A) Flexion, (B) extension, (C) adduction.

humerus. Palpate to locate osseous reference points referred to. It is easier to place the instrument if the part is in 0° of pronation and supination with the arm abducted from the shoulder.

   3. Moving arm — Place along the third metacarpal toward the center of the metacarpophalangeal joint of the third digit.

   4. Caution: Avoid flexion or extension of the wrist or pronation and supination of the forearm. Do not use the phalanx for a point of reference due to movement of the metacarpophalangeal joint itself.

  D. *Adduction* or *Ulnar Flexion:* 0° toward 55° to 65°. The same placement is used as in IV. C.

V. HIP JOINT (Fig. 6.10)

  A. *Flexion:* 0° toward 115–125°. Measure from the lateral aspect of the hip.

   1. Preferred position: (a) The patient should be supine and in good alignment. (b) Measuring from a side lying position with the involved side uppermost is often a good check on observations made in the preferred position.

   2. Stationary arm — Place parallel to a line from the greater trochanter of the femur to the crest of the ilium. This would parallel the long axis of the trunk.

   3. Moving arm — Place along the lateral midline of the femur toward the lateral condyle.

   4. The axis will fall in the region of the greater trochanter.

   5. Caution: The musculature of the hip and thigh makes this measurement difficult. Palpate the part to be sure of placement.

   6. Remarks: The long axis of the trunk toward the mid-axillary region can be used as long as the back is not allowed to flatten. Allow the knee to bend if the question of tight hamstrings is not a problem. If measurements are taken with the knee bent, they should be repeated in the same position.

  B. *Extension:* 0° toward 10–15°. The patient should be in a prone position. The same landmarks and the same precautions should be used as in flexion, except that an arched back and an elevated hip will need to be controlled. It is often wise to measure from the side-lying position.

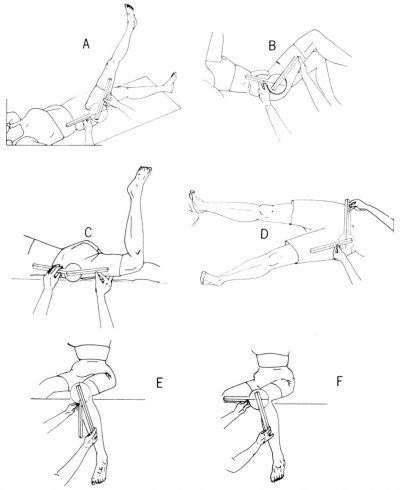

Fig. 6.10. Placement of goniometer for measuring motion of the hip joint. (A) Flexion (supine) with knee extended; (B) flexion, side-lying with knee flexed; (C) extension (prone); (D) abduction; (E) medial rotation with stationary arm vertical; (F) medial rotation with stationary arm horizontal.

    C. *Abduction:* 0° toward 45°. Measure from the anterior aspect of the pelvis.
       1. Preferred position—The patient should be supine and in good alignment.
       2. Stationary arm—Place on a line between the anterior superior iliac spines and maintain this line.
       3. Moving arm—The instrument is adjusted on the anterior surface of the thigh so that it parallels the dorsal mid-line of the femur toward the mid-line of the patella. The parallel position of the stationary arm should be maintained, however, it may need to be shifted on the line in order for the moving arm to be adjusted to the mid-line of the femur.
    D. *Adduction:* 0° toward 10–15°. The same landmarks and placements are used as in V. C. The uninvolved leg will have to be moved in abduction to allow for adduction of the involved leg.

1. Caution: The pelvis will drop but this need not interfere with the placement of the instrument or accurate measuremennt. The body may curl in the direction of motion and the hip may tend to rotate laterally for abduction and medially for adduction. Avoid this.

E. *Medial Rotation:* 0° toward 45°. Measure from the anterior position.

   1. Preferred position – (a) The patient should be sitting on a bed or table with the knee flexed to 90° over the edge of the support provided. Support the thigh over its full length. Sit erect and check the hip and leg line as follows: The anterior superior spine of the ilium, to the mid-line of the patella, the mid-line of the dorsum of the ankle, and the interspace between the second and third toes should be in the same sagittal plane. (b) Approximately the same position can be used with the patient supine and the knee flexed over the edge of the table.

   2. Stationary arm – From a starting position of 0° adjust the stationary arm parallel to the mid-line of the tibia with the nail head approximately in the mid-patella region. Maintain the instrument position approximately perpendicular to the floor, even though the leg will move from that position as in shoulder rotation.

   3. Moving arm – Place along the crest of the tibia to a point midway between the malleoli (anteriorly).

F. *Lateral Rotation:* 0° toward 45°.

   1. Preferred position – The same landmarks are used as in V. E.

   2. Caution: Avoid hip flexion, extension, abduction or adduction alone or in combinations of movement.

   3. Remarks: Both arcs can be measured with a single instrument placement if the stationary arm is parallel to the table top and the moving arm follows the crest of the tibia. However, most instruments cannot be read directly to secure the resultant value since the starting or anatomical position at 0° may be 90° on the protractor.

VI. KNEE JOINT (Fig. 6.11)

   Flexion: 0° for complete extension to 120–130° of flexion.

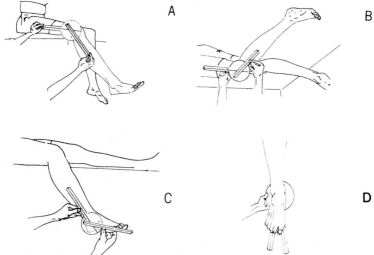

Fig. 6.11. Placement of goniometer for measuring motion of the knee and ankle. (*A*) Knee flexion and extension (sitting), (*B*) knee flexion and extension (prone), (*C*) ankle extension (sitting), (*D*) ankle eversion.

1. Preferred position—(a) The patient should be sitting on a treatment table with the thigh supported and the knee flexed over the edge of the support. (b) An alternate position is to place the patient prone with toes extending over the edge of the table when the knee is extended.
2. Stationary arm—Place parallel to the lateral mid-line of the femur on a line from the lateral condyle to the greater trochanter.
3. Moving arm—Place parallel to the lateral mid-line of the fibula toward the lateral malleolus.
4. The nail head or axis will fall in the region of the lateral condyle of the femur.
5. Caution: Do not attempt to keep the instrument pressed against parts of the lower extremity during motion since the contour changes too much to make this advisable. Palpate the thigh and leg before the procedure is begun in order to best avoid muscle bulk in the placement of the arms of the instrument.

B. *Extension:* This is the return from flexion and the same technique and placement are used as in VI. A.

VII. ANKLE JOINT

A. *Flexion and Extension:* Normal range—In the anatomical position, the position of the foot is like that in erect standing. At 0° the foot forms a right angle with the leg; extension to 45°, flexion to 20°. Use the lateral aspect of the joint.
1. Preferred position—Have the patient sit on the table with his knee flexed over the edge, or, have the patient lie down with his knee flexed.
2. Stationary arm—Place parallel to the lateral mid-line of the fibula on a line from the head of the fibula to the lateral malleolus.
3. Moving arm—Place parallel to the lateral mid-line of the fifth metatarsal. Palpate to be sure of the position.
4. The axis will shift considerably for the two positions of motion but shift the instrument superiorly or inferiorly until the two arms of the instrument parallel the reference landmarks given and do not attempt to set the nail head at any specific point
5. Caution: Avoid as much inversion and eversion as possible.
6. Remarks: (a) Measurements made on the medial aspect of the ankle will vary from those made on the lateral aspect of the ankle, mostly due to the longitudinal arch of the foot. Once a procedure is used, always repeat measurements with the same technique. (b) Ankle movements may be measured with the knee straight, but with the knee bent restrictions in motion due to a tight gastrocnemius are ruled out to a great extent. Again, always duplicate your first procedure.

B. *Inversion and Eversion* (of the Transverse Tarsal Joint): 0° toward 90° in both directions from the anatomical zero position (this is not the normal range of motion). Check the foot and leg line to be sure the patient is in a good starting position.
1. Preferred position—No specific position is recommended, except that the knee should be flexed to rule out hip rotation as this will introduce errors into the measurements.
2. Stationary arm—Place arm on the plantar aspect of the foot from the center of the heel to a line between the second and third toes with the nail head at the heel. The instrument should be maintained in this position after motion is begun.
3. Caution: Avoid rotation of the hip and flexion and extension of the ankle; do not attempt to hold the instrument tightly against the part.
4. Remarks: Only grossly quantitative measurements can be taken of

this motion due to the difficulty in ruling out partial flexion and extension.

Special Instructions

I. HAND MEASUREMENTS

A. *Fingers*

The metacarpophalangeal, proximal, and distal interphalangeal joints of all fingers may be measured in several ways. Three methods are most frequently used. One method requires the use of a universal goniometer (33, 93); the second one requires a special finger goniometer which rests over the joint (5, 59, 132); and the third utilizes a ruler (2, 14). Tracings and other devices may also be used, but are less frequently described in the recent literature. Passive motion measurements may be desired to contrast with active motion measurements.

1. *Universal Goniometer* (Fig. 6.12A).

A full circle plastic goniometer with a clear center is desirable. A half-circle device will need more adjustment to the new positions with the protractor directed toward the arc of motion to be measured. A metal instrument is more difficult to use for this lateral approach to joint measurement because of poor visibility and the smallness of the joint

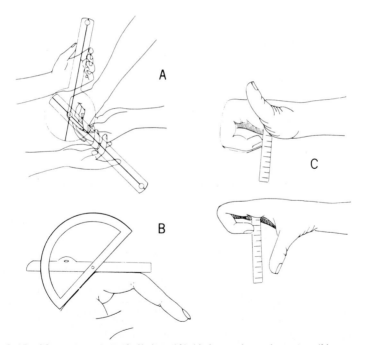

Fig. 6.12. Measurement of digits. (A) Universal goniometer (Newman [93]); (B) special finger instrument (reproduced with permission from H.S. Willard and C.S. Spackman, *Principles of Occupational Therapy*, Second Edition. J.B. Lippincott, Philadelphia, 1954); (C) with a ruler (reproduced with permission from American Academy of Orthopaedic Surgeons. *Measuring and Recording of Joint Motion*, 1963).

under study. Some plastic instruments have large dials and lack visibility which is necessary in this approach.

a. *Flexion:* 0° toward 90°.

    (1) Preferred position—(a) Hand should be relaxed with the wrist at 0° which is the anatomical position (AP). (b) If the effect of particular muscles or adjacent joints is of interest, the operator may wish to extend the wrist or flex it before measuring the fingers. The position used, if other than the anatomical position, should be noted on the record.

    (2) Stationary arm—Place or sight along the lateral mid-line of the proximal arm of the joint under study—either the metacarpal or phalanx.

    (3) Moving arm—Place or sight along the lateral mid-line of the distal arm of the joint under study—the phalanx.

    (4) The pivot will fall on the functional axis of motion after the arms of the instrument have been placed parallel to the arms of the two sides of the joint under study. Do not force the pivot to any special bony landmark.

    (5) The metacarpophalangeal joints of the third (long) and fourth (ring) fingers are most difficult to measure with the universal goniometer but with care in sighting, measurements can be obtained.

b. *Extension:* Return to the zero position. Lack of extension is recorded as minus degrees.

c. *Hyperextension:* Realign the instrument to measure motion in the hyperextension range beyond the mid-line. This realignment is not necessary with a full-circle clear plastic instrument.

d. *Abduction and Adduction:*

    (1) Preferred position—The hand is relaxed with the wrist in the anatomical position and with the palm down.

    (2) Stationary arm—Place on the dorsal surface along the mid-line of the metacarpal of the finger to be measured and extended along the mid-line of the first phalanx. (The AP for each finger can be determined in this manner.)

    (3) Moving arm—At the completion of the motion, place the moving arm on the dorsal surface along the mid-line of the first phalanx of the finger to be measured.

    (4) The pivot of the instrument will fall in the metacarpophalangeal joint *after* the arms of the instrument have been adjusted parallel to the longest line of the metacarpal and the phalanx.

    (5) Avoid flexion and extension of the fingers in any joint.

2. *Special Finger Instrument* (Figs. 6.1C and 6.12B).

a. *Flexion:* 0° toward 90°. Measure from the dorsal surface of each joint with the small goniometer designed for this purpose.

    (1) Preferred position. (a) Hand should be relaxed with the wrist at 0° or in the anatomical position (AP). (b) If the effect of particular muscles or adjacent joints is of interest, the operator may wish to extend the wrist or flex it before measuring the fingers. The position used, if other than the anatomical position, should be noted on the record.

    (2) Stationary arm—Place comfortably on the dorsal surface of the proximal arm of the joint at the mid-line of the metacarpal or phalanx.

(3) Moving arm — Place comfortably parallel to the dorsal surface of the distal arm of the joint under study and in the mid-line of the phalanx.

(4) Adjust the instrument until both arms are comfortably placed, and are as parallel to the mid-line of both bones making up the joint as possible. The axis will adjust itself to its appropriate position.

(5) Avoid pressure on the joint if only active motion is desired.

(6) The presence of edema, sutures, skin grafts, and bandages frequently restricts the placement of the instrument and makes it less satisfactory than the universal goniometer.

b. *Extension:* Return to the zero position from flexion. A lack of extension is recorded in a minus number of degrees.

c. *Hyperextension:* Cannot adequately be measured with the finger instrument as it requires placement on the very irregular surface of the palm of the hand.

3. *Measurements by a Ruler* (Fig. 6.12C).

a. *Flexion:* A composite view of the flexion action of the finger or fingers can be made with a ruler. The distance of the tip of the finger, at the edge of the nail bed, can be measured perpendicular to the 1) distal palmar crease, 2) mid-palmar crease, or 3) a point on the base of the palm. Action of the metacarpophalangeal joint is of course greatest with measurement to the base of the palm. Do not execute any pressure on the fingers or the palm of the hand unless the range of passive motion is desired. The contrast of active and passive motion is frequently informative.

b. *Extension:* Return to the AP of zero.

(1) Place a ruler or firm straight surface along the dorsal surface of the metacarpal of the finger under study. Extend it distally for several inches until it is beyond the length of the finger to be measured.

(2) Measure with a ruler the distance from the tip of the finger, at the edge of the nail bed, perpendicular to the surface of the extended straight surface or ruler.

(3) Be sure the ruler is held perpendicular to the extended surface.

c. *Opposition (abduction, rotation and flexion):*

(1) Measure the distance from the tip of the thumb, by the edge of the nail bed, to the base of the little finger.

(2) Measure the inability of the thumb to return to the AP by the same method.

(3) The contrast of active to passive motion is often informative.

B. *Thumb* (2, 3)

Similar measurements can be made of the thumb, for flexion and extension of the metacarpophalangeal joint and the interphalangeal joint, and extension and circumduction of the first metacarpal to the second metacarpal. Either the finger instrument or the univeral goniometer can be used. A ruler is best used for circumduction.

1. *Flexion and Extension:*

a. Metacarpophalangeal Joint — The metacarpal is the stationary arm and the first phalanx is the moving arm of the joint.

b. Interphalangeal — The first phalanx is the stationary arm and the second phalanx is the moving arm of the joint.

2. *Extension and Circumduction;* with the universal goniometer — the

second metacarpal is the stationary arm and the first metacarpal is the moving arm, but measurements on two planes of motion with a universal goniometer can be made.

a. Extension parallel to the plane of the palm.
b. Circumduction at right angle to the plane of the palm (a ruler may be used for this measurement).

Record all measurements in graphic and tabular form for permanent record.

II. SPINE (Dorsolumbar region)

X-ray and cinefluorography studies are recommended for more detailed studies of motion of the spine. It is doubtful that goniometric measurements are objective even though with good technique they may be repeatable and reliable.

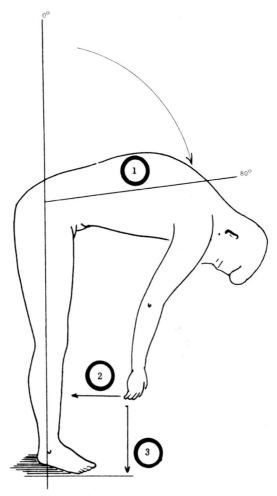

Fig. 6.13. Diagram illustrating flexibility of the spine. (Reproduced with permission from American Academy of Orthopaedic Surgeons. *Measuring and Recording Joint Motion*, 1963).

Several methods of measurements are proposed for routine measurements of the spine.

A. The distance of the finger tips to the leg or floor by a ruler (2, 95).
   1. *Flexion:* With the patient standing with feet together, or lying in a supine position in good posture, and with knees straight, measure the distance from the tip of the long finger to a spot in front of the great toe or to the knee or crest of the tibia (Fig. 6.13).
   2. *Lateral Flexion:* With the patient in a good standing position have him reach toward the floor on the lateral aspect. Measure the distance from the long finger tip to the floor at the level of the lateral malleolus.

B. Degree of motion of the trunk in relation to the pelvis with a universal goniometer (2, 5).
   1. *Flexion and Extension:*
      a. Preferred position—The patient should be standing in good alignment with his side to the operator.
      b. Stationary arm—Place parallel to the floor on a line with the crest of the ilium.
      c. Moving arm—Place at end of the motion and along the mid-axillary line toward the tip of the shoulder.
      d. Avoid rotation and the tendency to flex the knees.
   2. *Lateral Flexion:*
      a. Preferred position—Standing in good alignment with back to operator.
      b. Stationary arm—Place on a line between the superior iliac spines.
      c. Moving arm—Have patient bend to side. Place the instrument arm at the end of the motion along the mid-line of the back and spinous processes toward the spine of the seventh cervical vertebrae.
   3. *Rotation:* A reasonable estimate of the rotation of the shoulder to the pelvis is judged by the frontal view while the operator stabilizes the pelvis.

C. Bubble or pendular goniometers are recommended by Schenker (117) and Leighton (74), respectively. Refer to these references for specific instructions.

III. CERVICAL REGION
   A. With universal goniometer according to Lowman (77)
      1. *Flexion and Extension:*
         a. Preferred postion—The patient should be sitting or standing erectly with his side to the operator.
         b. Stationary arm—Place stationary arm on a line with the acromion process and on a line parallel to the floor.
         c. Moving arm—Place at the end of the motion on a line with the lobe of the ear.
      2. *Lateral Flexion:*
         a. Preferred position—The patient should be sitting or standing with his back to the operator.
         b. Place the stationary arm on a line with the spinous process of the seventh cervical vertebrae and on a line parallel to the floor.
         c. Moving arm—Place at the end of the motion on the mid-line of the cervical spine in line with the occipital protuberance.
      3. *Rotation:*
         a. Preferred position—Patient should be sitting or standing in good position facing operator.
         b. Stationary arm—Place stationary arm on a line with the jugular notch and on a line parallel to the floor.

      c. Moving arm—Place at the end of the motion in line with cleft of the chin.

      d. Avoid flexion and extension.

B. Head-Foot Goniometer, designed by Defibaugh (31) (NK Products, Santa Cruz, California).

  1. *Instrument*

      a. Place "O" point at either the left or right *edge* of the ball.

      b. When the motion is complete take your reading from the same edge of the ball (should enable you to obtain measures to 1 or 2° of accuracy with excellent reliability).

      c. Following use, the mouthpiece should be washed with soap and water and further cleaned with alcohol.

  2. *Investigated Method of Measuring Head Motion*

    a. *Flexion and Extension:*

Position:	Subject seated on straight chair with sacral and scapular areas against back.
Posture:	Elbows flexed, shoulders depressed and arms externally rotated and adducted in order to most effectively stabilize upper trunk.
Instrument:	Mouthpiece held firmly between teeth with goniometer in sagittal plane. Zero quadrant radius parallel to mouthpiece.
Action:	Subject actively flexes or extends his head as far as possible without moving his trunk.
Note:	Degrees of chair back slope must be added to flexion measurements and subtracted from extension measurements.

(Flexion and extension movements occurring primarily in the atlanto-occipital joint might be determined by seating the subject on a stool with his back against a wall. Under these conditions, when the subject flexes and extends with his head remaining in contact with the wall, most of the movement would probably be in atlanto-occipital joint.)

    b. *Lateral Flexion:*

Position:	Same as Flexion and Extension.
Posture:	Same as Flexion and Extension.
Instrument:	Mouthpiece held firmly between teeth with goniometer in frontal plane. Quadrant radius aligned with vertical center of face.
Action:	Subject actively bends head to the left or right as far possible.
Note:	Shoulders must remain stationary.

    c. *Rotation*

Position:	Subject supine.
Posture:	Same as above.
Instrument:	Mouthpiece held firmly between teeth with goniometer in transverse plane. Quadrant radius parallel to mouthpiece stem.
Action:	Subject rotates head to the right or left as far as possible.

Since these measurements are done actively, it is recommended that each measurement be repeated three times for accuracy.

C. Leighton Flexometer (74).

  1. *The Instrument*

    The instrument consists of a weighted 360° dial and a weighted pointer mounted in a case. The dial and pointer operate freely and independently; the movement of each is controlled by gravity. The instrument will record movement while in any position which is 20° or more off the horizontal. The zero mark on the dial and the tip of the pointer move freely to a position of rest and coincide when the instrument is placed in any position off the horizontal as indicated. Independent locking devices are provided for the pointer and the dial which stop all movement of either at any given position. In using the instrument, the flexometer is strapped to the segment being tested. The dial is locked at one extreme position (i.e., full flexion of the elbow); the movement is made and the pointer locked at the other extreme position (i.e., full extension of the elbow). Then the direct reading of the pointer on the dial is the arc through which the movement has taken place. The instrument has been titled the "Leighton Flexometer."

2. *Measurement Technique – Cervical Region*

    a. Flexion and Extension:

Starting Position:	Supine position on bench, head and neck projecting over end, shoulders touching edge, arms at sides. Instrument fastened to either side of head over ear.
Movement:	Count 1) head raised and moved to position as near chest as possible, dial locked 2) head lowered and moved to position as near end of bench as possible, pointer locked, 3) subject relaxes, reading taken.
Caution:	Shoulders may not be raised from bench during flexion nor back unduly arched during extension. Buttocks and shoulders must remain on bench during movement.

    b. Lateral Flexion:

Starting Position:	Sitting position in low-backed armchair, back straight, hands grasping chair arms, upper arms hooked over back of chair. Instrument fastened to back of head.
Movement:	Count 1) head moved in arc sideward left as far as possible, dial locked, 2) head moved in arc sideward right as far as possible, pointer locked, 3) subject relaxes, reading taken.
Caution:	Position in chair may not be changed during movement. Shoulders may not be raised or lowered.

    c. Rotation:

Starting Position:	Supine position on bench, head and neck projecting over, shoulders touching edge and arms at sides of bench. Instrument fastened to top of head.
Movement:	Count 1) head turned left as far as possible, dial locked 2) head turned right as far as possible, pointer locked, 3) subject relaxes, reading taken.
Caution:	Shoulders may not be raised from bench.

Reliability of Clinical Assessment of Motion

Until 1949 few articles appeared in the literature on critical assessment of the reliability of a goniometer as a clinical tool. The instrument had not been studied, the operators had not been studied, and only for special laboratory projects had the articulations of joints of the body been studied. It is gratifying to see that since 1949 (55, 85, 86) many more studies have been done in attempting to validate the reliability of both the tool and the operator. In the past, it has been said that the goniometric tool could not be considered reliable within ten degrees of error, but seldom if ever were statistics available to substantiate the statements.

INSTRUMENT

Several studies have indicated that *a well constructed goniometric instrument, either of universal or specialized design, is reliable whether the instrument is used by either one or several thoughtful and careful operators* (55, 85). Hellebrandt and associates (55) reported that the universal goniometer was as accurate in the hands of the careful observer as were the special devices designed for measurement of individual movements. The similarity in findings may be more apparent than real, and is in part dependent on the clinical significance of changes in mobility in various pathological conditions. The mean errors for movements in a single direction most difficult to duplicate were 4.3% and 3.9% respectively, for the two instruments. The lowest mean error for direction of movement more easily duplicated was 1.23% when made with the universal goniometer.

Total ranges of movement computed from the figures on the two arcs of movement fell in the majority of cases within three degrees on repeated trials. The computed range of shoulder flexion and extension, radio-ulnar pronation and supination, and wrist joint flexion and extension was within seven degrees when repeated. The coefficients of reliability were consistently higher and universally significant when the first and second trials of a two-trial procedure were compared, irrespective of the instrument used. The lowest coefficient of reliability was 0.85 and the majority were 0.99; 1,560 observations were made on thirteen motions in the upper extremity. To obtain the figures given, each motion was measured twice with each instrument. The coefficients of reliability for measurements in the wrist joint were moderate at 0.50 and 0.58 and indicate that while it is highly desirable for all measurements to be repeated with the same instrument, it is most necessary for this to be done at the wrist. The coefficients of reliability for measurements in other joints in the upper extremity were significantly high. No work was done on the lower extremity.

Hamilton and Lachenbruch (52) studied three instruments for measuring motion in the joints of the fingers. The three were the universal goniometer (Fig. 6.1*A*), an over the finger instrument (Fig. 6.1*C*) and an experimental instrument designed with a spirit level unit. Measurements were taken on joints of an unmoving hand which had been placed on a fixed plastic mold. Seven physical therapists with a random selection of the three instruments measured the same position 4 days in succession. Using an analysis of variance all three instruments were found to have the same degree of accuracy.

Karpovich (62) and Darcus and Salter (29) found that specially designed instruments, in one case for the knee and in another for the forearm, gave greater range of motion than the universal goniometer. These substantiate the findings in the 1949 report (55, 85), that in spite of high coefficients of correlation between trials for any two devices, the range of motion obtained from dissimilar instruments was quite different. Such data indicate that uncontrolled variables in instrument placement and patient positioning, when special instruments are used, are greater than with the universal goniometer.

Although few statistics are given, Schenker (116) states that his bubble goniometer is within 2° of accuracy on repeated trials. Glanville and Kreezer (50) claim that in three trials, a pendulum goniometer has a probable error of 0.5°, and Leighton (76) also claimed that a well constructed instrument when used repeatedly by a highly skillful person could give significant, reliable figures. In testing four groups of individuals the coefficient of reliability was 0.86 to 0.999 in his 1957 study, and between two tests with one operator and the same instrument carried out in 1956, the coefficient of reliability was 0.91 and 0.996. Karpovich's work (62) was interesting in that he found that the greatest error occurred in the maximum ranges of the range of motion such as in the 171–180° range rather than in the early stages of the movement. His figures also indicate that his electric goniometer had the highest degree of objectivity between operators but that all three instruments used by him—the universal goniometer, independently placed metal rods, and the electric goniometer—were statistically reliable. Kottke and Mundale (69) showed that x-rays gave 50% less motion than the norms recommended by the American Medical Association. Since methods of obtaining the above measurements were quite dissimilar, it is doubtful that it would be fair to compare the sets of measurements, for they may actually have been measuring different arcs of motion. Mundale et al. (91) compared the measurement taken by x-rays of the hip with external measurements of the hip and found plus or minus 5° of error with the external measurement being greater but with the lines of measurement being parallel.

OPERATOR

Several people have attempted to answer the question of whether or not the same operator, usually a physical therapist, should perform joint motion measurements for reliability, and whether or not the same physical therapist or operator should always measure the same patient. It would seem logical to assume that this should be the case, but few people have tested it statistically. In the claims of the Medical College of Virginia (55, 85), 220 measurements were made on 30 patients; each patient was measured twice by an experienced physical therapist, and twice by the average trained physical therapist. Only two trials per movement were permitted, and no external ink markings or indicators were permitted. These tests showed that the experienced physical therapist was accurate by plus or minus 3° on repeated trials, and that her measurements fell in this range 10.9 times more often than measurements by the average clinical physical therapist. The mean error for the experienced physical therapist was 3.76° and for the other physical therapist it was 4.75°. Again it was interesting that when the range of motion was computed from the two individual arcs of motion measurements the error increased to a plus or minus 7°. The mean error for the experienced operator was 5.3° and for the other clinical physical therapist it was 6.7°. Similar studies, by other individuals, have in some way substantiated these statements.

Bennett et al. (9) did four tests on patients and found plus or minus 5° of error between repeated tests as well as between two different operators in measuring the same motion of flexion and extension of the neck. In this instance the bubble goniometer was used for flexion and extension and the universal goniometer was used for rotation measurements. West (130) indicates that the operator should strive for the plus or minus 5° of error, but gives no figures on which this statement is based. These figures contradict the impressions of Wilmer and Elkins (135) who believe that measurements cannot be considered accurate within ten degrees of error.

Mundale (91) had two physical therapists in separate rooms repeat the same measurement on the same patients and found, in 108 pairs of observations, a 0.6° difference between the two operators. Of the measurements; 95% came within plus or minus 4° of error, and 99% came within plus or minus 6° of error. He then had 12 physical therapy students, with only a brief orientation of the procedure which was used, repeat the same motions. The measurements they obtained were favorable and parallel with those carried out by the experienced physical therapists.

The American Academy of Orthopaedic Surgeons states that an experienced surgeon may estimate the range of motion more accurately without a goniometer than with one but no data is available to support the claim (2).

Hamilton and Lachenbruch (52) in their work on the hand with 3 instruments and 7 operators determined that all were reliable with all 3 instruments. Variance for any one individual was not great but there was less reliability if several operators measured the same joint motion. The work of these two men supports the contention that one physical therapist well trained using a universal instrument should be reliable and that the same individual should continue to measure the same patient.

All of these studies indicate that the well informed physical therapist handling a reliable and well constructed tool can report highly reliable values. *No more than 3° of variance should be permitted on any two measurement trials.* To strive for at least this repeatability would increase reliability.

Several researchers have asked whether some joints are more accurately measured than others and found that this is the case. Moore (85, 86) and Hellebrandt et al. (55) indicated that when measuring the joints of the upper extremity, except for the wrist, all sources of error attributable to substitution, instrumental positioning and placement of the patient may be adequately controlled to a high degree by a careful observer. Movements of wrist motion are highly repeatable with either of two types of goniometers but are not comparable, as shown by a low coefficient of correlation, when the measurements of the two instruments are compared. This means that on certain joints (specifically, the wrist joint) one instrument is more reliable and valid than the other, but sufficient work has not been done to identify which instrument it is. The study did show that the measurements obtained by the experienced physical therapist did not have as great a range as those obtained by the less experienced physical therapist probably because the experienced physical therapist recognized substitution patterns earlier and stopped the motions sooner than did the less experienced individuals.

A similar discrepancy was found by Darcus and Salter (29) when measuring pronation and supination of the forearm. The simpler device without a handle control gave a much more reliable set of figures for the measurement of pronation and supination than did the special instrument designed similar to the Army World War II device. They did, however, find that there were extreme variations in measurements by the same individuals using the same instruments over a period of days, so that whether the variation was in the joints, in the operator's technique, or in the instruments, is still unclear. Hewitt (57) found that motions of the wrist varied as much as 100% in repeated trials over a period of days or weeks, but the instrument used in this study was a modified type somewhat similar to the World War II special device for the wrist motions. Defibaugh (31), using a modified pendulum device in measuring motion of the cervical region, found a coefficient of correlation between tests of suboccipital flexion and head rotation of 0.909 and 0.711, respectively, indicating a high to moderate reliability of the procedures he utilized. Equally high coefficients of correlation were obtained when the measurements by the author and alternate observers were compared. His study does indicate that reliability is high when repeat measurements are carried out on the *same* day rather than spaced several days apart.

Variations in age and the decrease in joint motion in increasing years have been substantiated in reports by Darcus and Salter (29) and by Leighton (75). The instruments used in these studies, however, were not identical, and studies should be done with conventional universal goniometers in order to compare results.

REFERENCES

1. ALBEE, F. H., AND GILLIAND, A. R. Methrotherapy, or the measurement of voluntary movement; its value in surgical reconstruction. *J.A.M.A., 75:* 983, 1920.
2. American Academy of Orthopaedic Surgeons. *Measuring and Recording of Joint Motion.* Detroit, 1963.
3. American Academy of Orthopaedic Surgeons. *Joint Motion. Method of Measuring and Recording.* Chicago, 1965.
4. American College of Surgeons, Committee on Trauma. *An Outline of the Treatment of Fractures.* Philadelphia, 1960.
5. American Medical Association. A guide to the evaluation of permanent impairment of the extremities and back. *J.A.M.A.* Special Number, February 15, 1958.
6. ASHHURST, A. P. C. The motion of the larger joints. *Int. Clin., 1:* 74, 1926.
7. BARNETT, C. H., AND NAPIER, J. P. The axis of rotation at the ankle joint in man. Its influence upon the form of the talus and the mobility of the fibula. *J. Anat., 86:* 1, 1952.
8. BATCH, J. W. Measurements and recordings of joint function. *U.S. Armed Forces Med. J., 6:* 359 (Feb.), 1955.
9. BENNETT, J. G., GERGMANIS, L. E., CARPENTER, J. K., AND SKOWLUND, H. V. Range of motion of the neck. *J. Am. Phys. Ther. Assoc., 43:* 45, 1963.
10. BERRESHEIM, F., McKOWN, E. R., AND SCHNAKE, E. Modified goniometer with practical improvements. *Phys. Ther. Rev., 29:* 513 (Nov.), 1949.
11. BOWMAN, E. Importance of measurement of movement in orthopedic cases. *Arch. Occup. Ther., 1:* 279, 1922.
12. BRADFORD, E. H. Case recording in spinal curves. *J. Orthop. Surg., 1:* 429, 1919.
13. BUCK, C. A., DAMERON, F. B., DOW, M. J., AND SKOWLUND, H. V. Study of normal range of motion in the neck utilizing a bubble goniometer. *Arch. Phys. Med., 40:* 390, 1959.
14. BUNNELL, S. *Surgery of the Hand.* Philadelphia, 1956.
15. CAMPBELL, S. K., AND KOHLI, M. A. Audio—tutorial independent study of goniometry. *Phys. Ther., 50:* 195, 1970.
16. CAVE, E. F., Editor: *Fractures and Other Injuries,* p. 10–11, 13–21. Chicago, 1958.
17. CAVE, E. F., AND ROBERTS, S. M. A method for measuring and recording joint function. *J. Bone Joint Surg., 18:* 455, 1936.
18. CHESHIRE, M. W. New apparatus: A device for measuring rotation of the neck. *Arch. Phys. Med., 38:* 592, 1957.
19. CLARK, W. A. A protractor for measuring rotation of joints. *J. Orthop. Surg., 3:* 154, 1921.
20. CLARK, W. A. A system of joint measurement. *J. Orthop. Surg., 2:* 687, 1920.
21. CLAYSON, S. J., NEWMAN, I. M., DEBEVEC, D. F., ANGER, R. W., SKOWLUND, H. V., AND KOTTE, F. J. Evaluation of mobility of hip and lumbar vertebrae of normal young women. *Arch. Phys. Med., 43:* 1, 1962.
22. CLAYSON, S. G., MUNDALE, M. D., AND KOTTKE, F. J. Goniometer adaptation for measuring hip extension. *Arch. Phys. Med., 47:* 255, 1966.
23. CLEVELAND, D. E. H. Diagrams for showing limitation of movements through joints, as used by the Board of Pensions Commissioners for Canada. *Can. Med. Assoc. J., 8:* 1070, 1918.
24. COBE, H. M. The range of active motion at the wrist of white adults. *J. Bone Joint Surg., 26:* 763, 1928.
25. CONGREVE, V. A simple finger goniometer. *Phys. Ther. Rev., 35:* 144, 1955.
26. CONWELL, H. E. Flexo-extensometer. *Surg. Gynecol. Obst., 40:* 710, 1925.
27. COULTER, J. S., AND MOLANDER, C. O. Therapeutic exercise (joints). *J.A.M.A., 104:* 118, 213, 1935.
28. DARCUS, H. D. The maximum torques developed in pronation and supination of the right hand. *J. Anat., 85:* 55, 1951.

29. Darcus, and Salter, N. The amplitude of pronation and supination with the elbow flexed to a right angle. *J. Anat., 87:* 169, 1953.
30. Davies, D. V. The anatomy and physiology of joints. *Physiotherapy, 49:* 3, 1963.
31. Defibaugh, J. J. Measurement of head motion. Part I. A review of methods of measuring joint motion. *J. Am. Phys. Ther. Assoc., 44:* 157, Part II: An experimental study of head motion in adult males. *J. Am. Phys. Ther. Assoc., 44:* 163, 1964.
32. Departments of the Army and the Air Force. Joint motion measurement. TM-8-640 AFP 160-14-1. Washington, 1956.
33. Dorinson, S. M., and Wagner, M. L. An exact technic for clinically measuring and recording joint motion. *Arch. Phys. Med., 29:* 468, 1948.
34. Duvall, E. N. Tests and measurements in physical medicine. *Arch. Phys. Med., 29:* 202, 1948.
35. Esch, D., and Lepley, M. *Evaluation of Joint Motion: Methods of Measurements and Recording.* University of Minnesota Press, Minneapolis, 1971.
36. Eve, F. C. Demonstration of clinical measuring instruments. *Proc. R. Soc. Med., 20:* 59, 1927.
37. Ferlic, D. The range of motion of the "normal" cervical spine. *Bull. Johns Hopkins Hosp., 110:* 59, 1962.
38. Fielding, J. W. Cineroentgenography of the normal cervical spine. *J. Bone Joint Surg., 39A:* 1280, 1957.
39. Fielding, J. W. Cineradiography of the normal cervical spine. *N. Y. J. Med., 56:* 2984, 1956.
40. Fish, G. H. Some observations of motion at the shoulder joint. *Can. Med. Assoc. J., 50:* 213, 1944.
41. Flatt, A. E., and Powers, W. R. Rheumatoid hand—physical therapy following insertion of the Flatt prosthesis. *Phys. Ther. Rev., 41:* 709, 1961.
42. Fox, R. F. Demonstration of the mensuration apparatus in use at the Red Cross Clinic for the physical treatment of officers. *Proc. R. Soc. Med., 10:* 63, 1917.
43. Fox, R. F., and Van Breemen, J. *Chronic Rheumatism, Causation and Treatment,* pp. 327–331. London, 1934.
44. Frescoln, L. D. Range of bodily movements. *Med. Times, 57:* 197, 1929.
45. Furey, J. G. Examination of the bones and joints of the extremities. *Med. Bull. U. S. Army, Europe, 11:* 208, 1954.
46. Gerhardt, J. J., and Russe, O. A. Instruction in application of the SFTR pocket goniometer in measuring joint motion with the neutral-zero method and SFTR recording. Orthopedic Equipment Company, Bourbon, Indiana, 1973.
47. Gifford, H. C. Instruments for measuring joint movements and deformities in fracture treatment. *Am. J. Surg., 28:* 237, 1914.
48. Gilliand, A. R. Norms for amplitude of voluntary movement. *J.A.M.A., 77:* 357, 1921.
49. Ghormley, J. W. Hip motions. *Am. J. Surg., 66:* 24, 1944.
50. Glanville, A. D., and Kreezer, G. The maximum amplitude and velocity of joint movements in normal male human adults. *Hum. Biol., 9:* 197, 1937.
51. Gottlieb, A. Graphic presentation of finger deformities. *Surg. Gynecol. Obstet., 29:* 420, 1919.
52. Hamilton, G. F., and Lackenbruch, P. A. Reliability of goniometers in assessing finger joint angle. *Phys. Ther., 49:* 465, 1969.
53. Hand, J. G. A compact pendulum arthrometer. *J. Bone Joint Surg., 20:* 494, 1938.
54. Harris, H., and Joseph, J. Variation in extension of the metacarpophangeal and inter phalangeal joints of the thumb. *J. Bone Joint Surg., 31B:* 547, 1949.
55. Hellebrandt, F. A., Duvall, E. N., and Moore, M. L. The measurement of joint motion. Part III—Reliability of goniometry. *Phys. Ther. Rev., 29:* 302, 1949.
56. Hellebrandt, F. A., and Miles, M. Vogel Report—inspection of training school by the Office of the Surgeon General, 1944, University of Wisconsin, Section of Physical Medicine. Principles of the technique of goniometry, p. 1–9 (mimeographed).

57. HEWITT, D. The range of active motion at the wrist of women. *J. Bone Joint Surg., 10:* 775, 1928.
58. HUPPRICH, F., AND SIGERSETH, P. O. The specificity of flexibility in girls. *Res. Q., 21:* 25, 1950.
59. HURT, S. P. Considerations in muscle function and their application to disability evaluation and treatment—joint measurement. *Am. J. Occup. Ther., 1:* 2, 4, 5, 1947; *2:* 1, 1948.
60. INMAN, V. T., SAUNDERS, J. B. D., AND ABBOTT, L. C. Observations of the function of the shoulder joint. *J Bone Joint Surg., 26:* 1, 1944.
61. ISRAEL, M. A quantitative method of estimating flexion and extension of the spine—a preliminary report. *Milit. Med., 124:* 181, 1959.
62. KARPOVICH, P. V., HERDEN, E. L., JR., AND ASA, M. M. Electrogoniometric study of joints. *U. S. Armed Forces Med. J., 11:* 424, 1960.
63. KARPOVICH, P. V., AND KARPOVICH, G. P. Electrogoniometer; new device for study of joints in action. *Fed. Proc., 18:* 79, 1959.
64. KARPOVICH, P. V., AND WIEKLOW, L. B. Goniometric study of the human foot in standing and walking. Ind. Med. Surg., 29: 338–347 (July), 1960.
65. KINZEL, F. J. et al. Measurement of the total motion between two body segments; I. Analytical development. *J. Biomech., 5:* 93, 1972.
66. KNAPP, M. E., AND WEST, C. C. Measurement of joint motion. *Bull. Univ. Minn. Hosp. Staff Meet., 15:* 405, 1944.
67. KOTTKE, F. J., AND BLANCHARD, R. S. A study of degenerative changes of the cervical spine in relation to age: a preliminary report. *Bull. Univ. Minn. Hosp., 24:* 470, 1953.
68. KOTTKE, F. J., AND LESTER, R. G. Use of cinefluorography for evaluation of normal and abnormal motion in the neck. *Arch. Phys. Med., 39:* 228, 1958.
69. KOTTKE, F. J., AND MUNDALE, M. O. Range of mobility of the cervical spine. *Arch. Phys. Med., 40:* 379, 1959.
70. KOVACS, R. *Electrotherapy and Light Therapy.* Philadelphia, 1949.
71. KRAUS, H. *Principles and Practices of Therapeutic Exercise.* Springfield, 1963.
72. KRUSEN, F. H. *Physical Medicine.* Philadelphia, 1941.
73. LEIGHTON, J. R. A simple objective and reliable measure of flexibility. *Res. Q., 13:* 205, 1942.
74. LEIGHTON, J. R. An instrument and technic for the measurement of range of joint motion. *Arch. Phys. Med., 36:* 571, 1955.
75. LEIGHTON, J. R. Flexibility characteristics of males ten to eighteen years of age. *Arch. Phys. Med., 37:* 494, 1956.
76. LEIGHTON, J. R. Flexibility characteristics of four specialized skill groups of college athletes. *Arch. Phys. Med., 38:* 24, 1957.
77. LOWMAN, E. W. *Arthritis.* Boston, 1959.
78. MCBRIDE, E. D. Disability evaluation. *Instruct. Lect. Amer. Acad. Orthop. Surg., 17:* 344, 1960.
79. MCBRIDE, E. D. Disability Evaluation; Principles of Treatment of Compensable Injuries. Philadelphia, 1953.
80. MARBLE, H. C. Application of curative therapy in the ward. *J. Orthop. Surg., 2:* 136, 1920.
81. MARBLE, H. C. *The Hand: A Manual and Atlas for the General Surgeons,* pp. 69–78. Philadelphia, 1960.
82. Medical College of Virginia, Clinics of Physical Medicine, Clinic charts for recording joint measurements. Richmond, 1946 (mimeographed).
83. MOCK, H. E., PEMBERTON, R., AND COULTER, J. S. *Principles and Practices of Physical Therapy,* Vol. III, Chapter 14, Molander, C. O. Therapeutic Exercise in Surgical Conditions, p. 1–69, Hagerstown, 1935.
84. MOLANDER, C. O., AND WEINMANN, B. Results of the "long arc" and the "short arc" treatment in the after care of poliomyelitis, *Arch. Phys. Ther., 24:* 74, 1943.

85. MOORE, M. L. Clinical measurement of joint motion. (Thesis) Medical College of Virginia. Richmond, 1948.

86. MOORE, M. L. Joint Measurement: Technic and Recording Methods. Proceedings of the Second Congress of the World Confederation for Physical Therapy. New York, 1956.

87. MOORE, M. L. The measurement of joint motion. Part I—Introductory review of literature. *Phys. Ther. Rev., 29:* 195, 1949.

88. MOORE, M. L. The measurement of joint motion. Part II—The technic of goniometry. *Phys. Ther. Rev., 29:* 256-264 (June), 1949.

89. MOORE, M. L. The technique of goniometry: Basic elements of technique and the goniometer. Section of Physical Therapy, School of Medicine, University of North Carolina, Chapel Hill, 1961 (mimeographed).

90. MOORE, M. L., FARRAND, S., AND THORNTON, W. The use of radio telemetry for electromyography. *J. Am. Phys. Ther. Assoc., 43:* 787, 1963.

91. MUNDALE, M. O., HISLOP, H. J., RABIDEAU, R. J., AND KOTTKE, F. J. Evaluation of extension of the hip. *Arch. Phys. Med., 37:* 75, 1956.

92. MYERS, H. Range of motion and flexibility. *Phys. Ther. Rev., 41:* 177, 1961.

93. NEWMAN, I. Physical therapy in the treatment of disabilities of the hand. Annual Conference, American Physical Therapy Association, 1963 (unpublished paper).

94. NOER, H. R., AND PRATT, D. R. A goniometer designed for the hand. *J. Bone Joint Surg., 40A:* 1154, 1958.

95. NORDSCHOW, M., AND BIERMAN, W. The influence of manual massage on muscle relaxation: effect on trunk flexion. *J. Am. Phys. Ther. Assoc., 42:* 653, 1962.

96. NUTTER, J. A. Reconstructive surgery; the problem of records. *J.A.M.A., 72:* 410, 1919.

97. NUTTER, J. A. The standardization of joint records. *J. Bone Joint Surg., 1:* 423, 1919.

98. O'NEILL, I. A simple light, inexpensive contact goniometer. *Phys. Ther. Rev., 33:* 639, 1973.

99. PARKER, J. S. Recording arthroflexometer. *J. Bone Joint Surg., 11:* 126, 1929.

100. PATRICK, J. Goniometer for measurement of supination and pronation. *Br. Med. J., 2:* 246, 1944.

101. PARTRIDGE, M., AND ABBOTT, W. Reproductibility of joint range of motion measurements using a universal goniometer. Contribution No. 12. Biomathematics Research Laboratory, Baylor University College of Medicine, 1963.

102. PENDLETON, T. B., COLEMAN, M. M., AND GROSSMAN, B. J. Jaw goniometer. *Phys. Ther., 54:* 23, 1974.

103. PERRY, J., AND BEVIN, A. G. Evaluation procedures for patients with hand injuries. *Phys. Ther., 54:* 593, 1974.

104. Physician's Guide: Disability, Evaluation, Examination. Department of Medicine and Surgery, Veterans Administration, Washington, 1963.

105. POLLOCK, G. A., AND BROOKS, G. An apparatus to measure muscle recovery and range of joint movement (fingers). *Br. Med. J., 2:* 220, 1942.

106. PROVINS, K. A., AND SALTER, N. Maximum torque exerted about the elbow joint. *J. Appl. Physiol., 7:* 393, 1955.

107. PROVINS, K. A. Maximum forces exerted about the elbow and shoulder joints on each side separately and simultaneously. *J. Appl. Physiol., 7:* 390, 1955.

108. REGENOS, E. M., AND CHYATTE, S. B. Joint range and deformity recorded by xerography. *Phys. Ther., 50:* 190, 1970.

109. ROBERTS, H. An inexpensive goniometer. *Phys. Ther., 53:* 766, 1973.

110. ROBINSON, W. H. Joint range. *J. Orthop. Surg., 3:* 41, 1921.

111. ROSEN, N. G. A simplified method of measuring amplitude of motion in joints. *J. Bone Joint Surg., 20:* 570, 1922.

112. RUSK, H. *Rehabilitation Medicine.* St. Louis, 1958.

113. SALTER, N., AND DARCUS, H. D. The effect of the degree of elbow flexion on the maximum torques developed in pronation and supination of the right hand. *J. Anat.,*

86: 197, 1952.

114. SALTER, N. Methods of measurement of muscle and joint function. *J. Bone Joint Surg., 37B:* 474, 1955.

115. SAYWELL, S. Joint measurement and muscle power. *Physiotherapy, 47:* 299, 1961.

116. SCHENKER, A. W. The accurate measurement of neuromuscular and musculoskeletal disabilities. *Milit. Med., 126:* 207, 1961.

117. SCHENKER, A. W. Goniometry—an improved method of joint motion measurement. *N. Y. J. Med., 56:* 539, 1956.

118. SILVER, D. Measurement of the range of motion in joints. *J. Bone Joint Surg., 21:* 569, 1923.

119. SMIDT, G. L., AND ASPREY, G. M. Relationship of the a-p spinal column deviation to the pelvi-femoral angle of extension. *J. Am. Phys. Ther. Assoc., 48:* 1345, 1968.

120. SNEDECOR, S. T. Muscle and joint examination charts. *Arch. Phys. Med., 27:* 33, 1946.

121. SPILMAN, H. W., AND PINKSTON, D. Relation of test positions to radial and ulnar deviation. *Phys. Ther., 49:* 837, 1969.

122. SPRAGUE, R. B., TIPTON, C. M., FLATT, S. E., AND ASPREY, J. M. Evaluation of a photographic method for measuring leg abduction and adduction. *J. Am. Phys. Ther. Assoc., 46:* 1068, 1966.

123. STORMS, H. A system of joint measurement. Phys. Ther. Rev., 35: 369, 1955.

124. TAYLOR, H. L., AND BROZEK, J. Evaluation of fitness. *Fed. Proc., 3:* 216, 1944.

125. THOMAS, D. H., AND LONG, C., II. An electrogoniometer for the finger. *Am. J. Med. Electronics, 3:* 96, 1964.

126. WAINERDI, H. R. An improved goniometer for arthrometry. *J.A.M.A., 149:* 661, 1952.

127. WAKELY, C. P. G. A new form of goniometer. *Lancet, 1:* 300, 1918.

128. WEDDELL, G., AND DARCUS, H. D. Some anatomical problems in Naval Warfare. *Br. J. Ind. Med., 4:* 77, 1947.

129. WEISS, M. A multiple purpose goniometer. *Arch. Phys. Med., 45:* 197, 1964.

130. WEST, C. C. Measurement of joint motion. *Arch. Phys. Med., 26:* 414, 1952.

131. WIECHEC, F. J., AND KRUSEN, F. H. A new method of joint measurement and a review of the literature. *Am. J. Surg., 43:* 659, 1939.

132. WILLARD, H. S., AND SPACKMAN, C. S. *Principles of Occupational Therapy.* Philadelphia, 1954.

133. WILLIAMS, P. O. The assessment of mobility in joints. *Lancet, 263:* 169, 1952.

134. WILLIAMS, P. O. Assessment of mobility in joints. *Rheumatism, 13:* 13, 1957.

135. WILMER, H. A., AND ELKINS, E. C. An optical goniometer for observing range of motion of joints; a preliminary report of a new instrument. *Arch. Phys. Med., 28:* 695, 1947.

136. WILSON, G. D., AND STASCH, W. H. Photographic record of joint motion. *Arch. Phys. Med., 26:* 361, 1945.

137. WRIGHT, R. D. A detailed study of movement of the wrist joint. *J. Anat., 70:* 137, 1935.

138. WRIGHT, V., AND JOHNS, R. J. Quantitative and qualitative analysis of joint stiffness in normal subjects and in patients with connective tissue diseases. *Ann. Rheumatol. Dis., 20:* 36, 1961.

139. ZANKEL, H. T. Photogoniometry, a new method of measurement of range of motion of joints. *Arch. Phys. Med., 32:* 227, 1951.

7

Resistance Exercise

DUANE A. SCHRAM

The relationship between work load and muscle strength has been known for a very long time. Until relatively recent times, most prescribed exercises have been of the resistance type since the part moved offers the resistance of its own weight when moved voluntarily and without planned assistance. Resistance and progressive resistance are not new concepts in exercise therapy, but it remained for DeLorme (2) to develop resistance exercises so thoroughly that wherever good medicine is practiced today resistance exercises are performed according to his system or a modification of it.

The first patients DeLorme treated with resistance exercises were soldiers suffering from muscle weakness following trauma. At the beginning, he applied the load directly to the part to be treated; for example, a boot to which weights could be added was strapped to the foot to exercise the quadriceps extensor of the knee (Fig. 7.1). The weight applied, the number of repetitions executed, and the tempo of the exercise remained constant during each week. The amount of weight used was the maximum which could be carried through the full range of motion for 10 excursions. This 10 repetition maximum (10 RM) was determined once each week; and a set of exercises of that value (10 RM) was repeated for from 7 to 10 times during each exercise session. Sessions were performed once on each of the first 5 days of the week; the patient rested on the last two. On the fifth, or last, exercise day of the week, the maximum weight for only one repetition (1 RM) was determined and recorded, and the 10 RM was established for the following week. DeLorme called this method "heavy resistance exercise" because the weights used were great when compared with those used in previous strengthening methods; an "all-out" effort was necessary to complete them. The muscles he treated were usually not diseased but had lost strength from disuse. Later, the same method of exercise was used for muscle weaknesss due to paralysis (as seen, for example, in poliomyelitis).

191

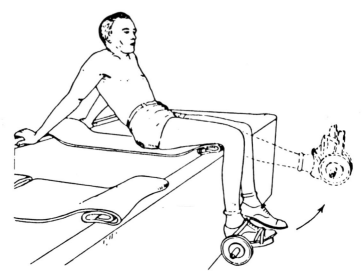

Fig. 7.1. Standard position for resistance exercise of the quadriceps femoris using a weighted boot. (From T. DeLorme, in *Physical Medicine in General Practice,* by W. Bierman and S. Licht, New York, 1952. Reproduced with the permission of the editors, and the publisher, Paul B. Hoeber, Inc.).

Progressive Resistance Exercise

In 1948 DeLorme (3) revised his original method and adopted the name progressive resistance exercise (PRE) because he believed the original name bore false implications since even muscles which could not contract against the force of gravity could be strengthened by this method. He exercised muscles of less than fair strength by counterbalancing the weight of the extremity with a cable and pulley arrangement and thus gave load-assisting exercise to muscle groups which could not perform antigravity motions (Fig. 7.2).

In the revised method, 20–30 repetitions were given in place of the 70–100 previously recommended. This permitted exercise with even heavier loads and thus enabled a more rapid gain in strength and in muscle volume. In the newer method, the initial one or two sets of repetitions were considered as a "warm-up" for the 10 RM exercises. Sample schedules for load-resisting and load-assisting exercises are:

Load-Resisting Exercise

First set of 10 repetitions—Use one-half of 10 RM
Second set of 10 repetitions—Use three-fourths of 10 RM
Third set of 10 repetitions—Use full 10 RM

Load-Assisting Exercise

First set of 10 repetitions— Use twice the 10 repetition minimum
Second set of 10 repetitions—Use one and one-half 10 repetition minimum
Third set of 10 repetitions—Use 10 repetition minimum

McGovern and Luscombe (7) advocated a reversal of the load-resisting schedule: they recommended using the full 10 RM in the first set and one-half RM in the third set. This variation stemmed from their experience with the "Oxford technique" introduced earlier by Zinovieff (12). In the Oxford technique the first set is 10 RM, and in each successive set the load is progressively lowered by about a pound while the 10 RM is increased each day by the same amount of weight.

Brief Maximal Exercise

Rose et al. (9), stimulated by the report of Hettinger and Müller (5) on the value of brief isometric contractions, tried still another variant of isotonic resistance exercise—brief maximal exercise (BME). They positioned subjects for weight loading of the quadriceps according to the manner popularized by DeLorme and determined the maximal lift which the quadriceps could support for 5 sec when the knee was fully extended from the position of 90° flexion. They learned that even healthy athletes found it difficult to lift successive 5-lb increments but that most subjects, including patients with weakened muscles, could raise successive increments of $1^{1}/_{4}$ lb. This they adopted as their unit of standard increment. Once a plateau of maximum strength was reached with progressive increments, strength could be maintained near peak for many months even when effort was expended with diminishing frequency. They felt that the measurement of the duration of strength maintenance without repeated exercise was probably beyond the limits of present experimental possibilities and were inclined to agree with Hellebrandt's theory that the persistence of strength might be related to the learned act.

Rose and his co-workers found that BME resulted in a cross-education strengthening of contralateral muscles in all normal subjects but not in a patient whose opposite unexercised extremity was immobilized in a cast.

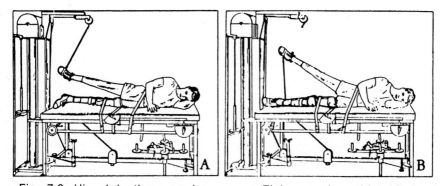

Fig. 7.2. Hip abduction exercises on an Elgin exercise table; (A) load-assisting (counterbalanced) exercise; (B) load-resisting exercise. (From T. DeLorme, in *Physical Medicine in General Practice*, by W. Bierman and S. Licht, New York, 1952. Reproduced with the permission of the editors and the publisher, Paul B. Hoeber, Inc.)

They also found that a muscle could gain in strength without increasing in bulk.

Weight Lifting

Resistance exercises using heavy weights are similar to those used in "body building." McQueen (8), in summarizing body-building techniques, makes a distinction between a regimen for producing muscle hypertrophy and one for producing muscle power.

The chief characteristic of the hypertrophy program is that all weight-lifting exercises are done in sets of lifts or repetitions; the weight is not released until the completion of a certain number of repetitions or sets. From answers to a questionnaire sent to 17 area finalists of the 1953 "Mr. Britain" (physique) contest, McQueen learned that nearly all contestants exercised on only 3 alternate days of the week and used, on an average, between 3 and 7 sets of 9–16 repetitions. It is important to note that the weight used was the maximum that could be lifted for the stated number of repetitions. In other words, every set of 10 repetitions was equivalent to 10 RM. Apparently, weight lifters and trainers had, in the past, started with a weight less than the 10 RM and then increased the load with each set of 10 repetitions until the actual 10 RM was reached. This method has become obsolete since it does not seem to produce as great an increase of muscle bulk as the system using the maximum weight which can be raised for every set of repetitions. Less weight is used only as a preparatory "warm-up." Experience has shown that if less than the 10 RM is habitually used for considerably more than 10 repetitions and for more than 4 or 5 sets on a muscle group, bulk may diminish. A high-repetition low-resistance exercise usually increases endurance or stamina but does not increase muscle bulk. The only muscle group which apparently does respond to a greater number of repetitions (between 20 and 30 but still a very small number of sets: between 0 and 4) is the gastrocnemius. Most of the finalists stated that they increased the amount of weight each week or fortnight and that after every 6–8 weeks they altered the lifting program by varying the type of motions and sets of repetitions to prevent boredom and "staleness" and to ensure continued progression.

McQueen lists refinements in the hypertrophy program such as "cramping," in which progressively more weight is added to the tired muscle, which continues to shorten so that finally a motion of only a few inches is executed in a muscle which is almost completely contracted. This procedure can be tolerated for only a few minutes; the muscle begins to ache intensely (ischemia), and the overlying skin often develops a mottled flushing with occasional small subcutaneous edematous blebs. Another refinement employs a mirror in which the parts are watched during contraction, thus enabling the weight lifter to concentrate intently on the performance of the exercised muscles. Some believe that this cortical awareness is very necessary for outstanding development and have learned to isolate muscle groups which they can contract at will.

Another refinement is based on the principle of peak contraction. By proper positioning, the greatest amount of weight can be saved for the final few inches of the range of motion. A good example is knee extension, in which the greatest force is at complete extension when the lever arm is longest and the weight is perpendicular to the pull of gravity. The refinement called "cheating" refers to the recruitment of neighboring muscle groups in completing a range of motion during an exercise. Knee extension also may serve as an example of this refinement. If a weight too heavy to complete knee extension is used, the athlete bends backward with his trunk and hip flexors, recruiting neighboring muscle groups to gain full extension.

The power program is a weight-lifting schedule practiced by weight lifters to prepare for competition. It consists of a decreasing number of repetitions performed with increasing resistance. Starting with 6–10 repetitions, the final lift is with 1 repetition maximum (1 RM). Weight lifters usually exercise more than body builders (5–7 days a week). The body builders believe that alternate days of rest are essential for muscle tissue anabolism. An example of a power program schedule is:

Weight in pounds	Set	Repetitions
90	2	4
100	2	3
110	2	2
120	2	1
130	1	1

Underwater Resistance

The principle of progressive resistance was applied to underwater exercises at the Georgia Warm Springs Foundation (10). An effective method was sought for developing strength in patients with moderate to severe poliomyelitic paralysis which would take advantage of density of water. Most muscles for which strengthening exercises were prescribed were graded between "poor plus" and "good minus." Some record of progression was necessary since previously only manual resistance had been applied.

Two devices were designed for underwater use: one for the lower and one for the upper extremity (Fig. 7.3). The advantages of this method included a desirable medium in which to work and a progression based on work per unit of time (power or horsepower). As seen Figure 7.4, the blade of the exercise boot is adjusted (for maximum resistance) to remain at a right angle to the arc of motion when advanced in one direction but to collapse on motion in the opposite direction (return motion). The patient is encouraged to repeat the movement cycles as rapidly as possible until signs of fatigue appear. The repetitions are executed at a regular tempo; the number of repetitions and the time consumed are recorded. Fatigue is evidenced by slowing of rate, diminution of range, gross incoordination or a complaint of muscle tiring. If there are no indications

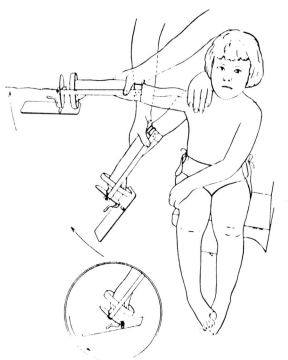

Fig. 7.3. Underwater resistance device. Illustration of abductor exercise of upper extremity. Blade approaches water surface but does not break through. Part is returned to starting position at even tempo. *Inset* shows collapse of blade on return motion. (Reproduced from *Archives of Physical Medicine, 32:* 221, 1951.)

of fatigue, a maximum duration is arbitrarily set at 3 min for one exercise series. For the record, the number of repetitions completed in 1 min is used as the time unit. Several muscle groups are usually exercised during a session. As the muscle group becomes fatigued, the therapist immediately readjusts the blade and repositions the patient, and exercise is begun on another group of muscles which requires strengthening. After all groups of muscles have been exercised to the point of fatigue, or for 3 min, the procedure is repeated beginning with the muscle group first exercised. The entire routine is repeated, and each time the patient is encouraged to push the blade through the water as rapidly as possible on each repetition and to check the number of repetitions against the moving second hand of a wall clock. As the muscle group becomes stronger, the patient will increase the number of repetitions per minute. Another advantage offered by this method is that a muscle group can pull the part through the full range of motion; this is true, for example, of the quadriceps, in which that part of the flexion range beyond 90° is lost when weights are lifted starting from a right-angle bend of the knee out of water. In underwater resistance exercise, the arc of motion begins with the quadriceps on a stretch (boot underneath the table) and ends after completing the full range of motion. As the part forces the apparatus through the arc of motion, there may be minor positive and negative accelerations, but the force required will be, if not constant, the maximum possible at any point in the arc. Both agonist and antagonist muscle groups may be exercised alternately and in the same cycle by locking the blade in the spread position.

Isometric Resistance Exercise

Weight lifters reject isometric or static exercises because they do not increase bulk, range of motion or endurance and because a plateau of strength improvement is reached fairly soon. Steinhaus (11) called attention to the work of Hettinger and Müller (5), from which it was concluded that isometric resistance exercise is the most rapid method of increasing muscle strength. These authors believe that, since the number of muscle fibers is fixed at birth, it cannot be increased by exercise. They believe further, that, regardless of how much it is used, a muscle will not grow

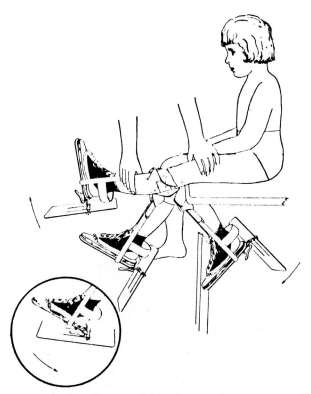

Fig. 7.4. Underwater resistance device. Illustration of a quadriceps exercise showing complete and free range of motion. On return motion (*inset*) the blade is partially collapsed with moderate pressure against spring. The force needed to push blade is near maximum at any point in the range of motion.

larger or stronger unless it is overloaded. This means that the intensity of work required must be increased above that to which it is currently accustomed: it must exert more power (foot pounds per minute) or work against greater resistance than previously. The stimulus for hypertrophy appears to be associated with a state of oxygen deficit within the muscle fiber. Contraction of a muscle to develop a tension of from somewhat less than one-third to two-thirds of its maximum strength for a period of only 6 sec a day diminishes the circulation enough to cause an oxygen deficit of all of its fibers and thereby speeds hypertrophy maximally. Rapid training induces only loosely "anchored" adjustment of the muscle to the increased demands made on it. If, however, this increased strength is maintained for a time, it becomes fastened or anchored in the muscle.

Clinical Application

The most important element in resistance exercise for strength gain is the persistent reinforcement of effort to limits beyond those easily met. Apparently neither a "warm-up" nor a "tapering off" period is necessary as long as the 10 RM are performed with the effort required by definition.[1] The evidence indicates that any form of resistance exercise properly pre-scribed, adequately supervised and performed with understanding and motivation will strengthen the exercised muscle.

The most skilled form of resistance exercise is that given manually by the therapist in the reeducation of neuromuscular segments weakened by lower motor neuron diseases such as poliomyelitis. This method is fre-quently prescribed early for those with "trace to poor" muscle strength and may be the treatment of choice during much of the convalescent period. Although it is doubtful whether normal muscle tissue can be injured by resistance exercises, some muscles will show loss of strength if over-worked. Knowlton and Bennett (6) have demonstrated the hazard of over-work in weak muscles. They believe that objective fatigue alone is not a reliable safeguard against overwork. The therapist must be alert to objec-tive and subjective signs of fatigue and must observe the day-to-day

---

[1] The 10 RM (repetition maximum) is the amount of weight a muscle can lift 10 times. It is determined by repeated trials, that is, the patient is asked to lift a weight of 10 lb 10 times. This determination is not easy for the newly referred patient, for, as DeLorme points out, he may not understand the meaning of maximum effort or he may be unwilling to exert himself because of pain or fear of injury. In fact, it may be unwise to demand maximum effort of a recently weakened muscle. For the muscle just recovering from trauma or disease, loads well below the 10 RM should be used and increased gradually for a week or more before the full 10 RM is reached. The frequency of exercise will depend upon the patient's response. DeLorme believes that one session of exercise on each of the 5 week days will usually be well tolerated, but he cautions that fewer periods are indicated by such reactions as fatigue or diminution of muscle power.

The 10 RM (repetition minimum) is the load that makes 10 lifts barely possible. The letters RM are used for both maximum and minimum since the former is used only in connection with load-resisting exercises and the latter with load-assisting exercises.

performance carefully to detect any decrement in muscle strength. The signs of fatigue as outlined above in the discussion of underwater resistance exercise may be used as a guide in avoiding fatigue in the poliomyelitic patient performing PRE.

The method of choice for strengthening normal muscle which has undergone disuse atrophy (without joint pathology) is heavy resistance with weights applied directly or indirectly (as shown in Fig. 7.5). Ideally, a progressive decrease of repetitions and an increase in load as practiced by competitive weight lifters are the most efficient approaches. Weight lifters have the time and assistants to carry out such a procedure, but such a method would be impractical for the average physical therapy clinic because of the time and cost factors. For practical purposes the 10 RM or some modification of it is adequate. In many clinics a schedule is used in which the weight is increased and the number of repetitions is decreased. For example, when a total of 15 repetitions has been reached in an exercise period, the weight is increased to the point where only 8–10 RM can be lifted. If after several daily sessions the patient is again able to perform 15 repetitions, the weight is again increased and the patient exercises with the new load until 15 repetitions are executed. Another modification in use is to complete the basic set of 10 RM in a shorter period of time. Greater

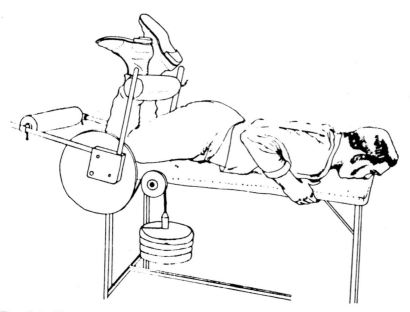

Fig. 7.5. Illustration of a body builder performing resistance exercise of hamstring muscles. Lower bar is used for quadriceps exercise in sitting position. Apparatus offers a constant resistance throughout available range. (From a photograph supplied by the Martin's Gymnasium Equipment Company of Oakland, California.)

power is needed to complete 10 RM in 6 sec than in 10. Thus, when the patient gains enough strength to do 10 RM in 6 sec, the load is increased to the point where 10 sec are required and the patient once more strives for the goal of completion of the set in 6 sec.

Several methods can and should be considered for patients with known pathology of the joint which will be moved during exercise. If the patient has a painful acute joint, isometric exercise will be indicated, at least initially, if the tension permits an "all-out" effort. Otherwise, a similar exercise of the unaffected side should be practiced until the acute condition subsides sufficiently to begin isotonic exercise. Hellebrandt (4) and Darcus (1) have shown that cross-education strengthens the contralateral part with this method.

REFERENCES

1. DARCUS, H. D., AND SALTER, N. The effect of repeated muscular exertion on muscle strength. *J. Physiol., 129:* 325, 1955.
2. DeLORME, T. L. Restoration of muscle power with heavy resistance exercise. *J. Bone Joint Surg., 27:* 645, 1945.
3. DeLORME, T. L., AND WATKINS, A. L. Technics of progressive resistance exercise. *Arch. Phys. Med., 29:* 263, 1948.
4. HELLEBRANDT, F. A., PARRISH, A. M., AND HOUTZ, S. J. Cross-education. *Arch. Phys. Med., 28:* 76, 1947.
5. HETTINGER, T., AND MÜLLER, E. A. Muskelleistung und Muskeltraining. *Arbeitsphysiologie, 15:* 111, 1955.
6. KNOWLTON, G. C., AND BENNETT, R. L. Overwork. *Arch. Phys. Med., 38:* 18, 1957.
7. McGOVERN, R. E., AND LUSCOMBE, H. B. Useful modification of programs. Resistance exercise technique. *Arch. Phys. Med., 34:* 475, 1953.
8. McQUEEN, I. J. Recent advances in the technique of progressive resistance exercise. *Br. Med. J., 2:* 328, 1954.
9. ROSE, D. L., RADZYMINSKI, S. F., AND BEATTY, R. R. Effect of brief maximal exercise on the strength of the quadriceps femoris. *Arch. Phys. Med., 38:* 157, 1957.
10. SCHRAM, D. A., AND BENNETT, R. L. Underwater resistance exercises. *Arch. Phys. Med., 32:* 222, 1951.
11. STEINHAUS, A. H. Some selected facts from physiology and the physiology of exercise applicable to physical rehabilitation. Read before the Study Group on Body Mechanics, Washington, D. C., Sept. 5, 1954, in (9).
12. ZINOVIEFF, A. N. Heavy-resistance exercises. *Br. J. Phys. Med., 14:* 129, 1951.

8

Brief
Isometric Exercises

_____ W. T.   LIBERSON

Following a study of the relationship between exercise and muscle training, Hettinger and Müller (9) found that in some of the subjects tested, final muscle strength and endurance were independent of the duration (2–45 sec) and frequency of repetition (1–7 times a day) of "static" exercises. They observed that the maximum strength increased in proportion to the cross section of the muscle. Although the number of subjects and controlled observations was very small, their results suggested the importance of a reevaluation of several problems of exercise regimen: Are isometric contractions more efficient than isotonic contractions? What is the optimal duration and frequency? What is the optimal stress in relation to the maximum strength of the muscle exercised?

The method of therapeutic exercise proposed by DeLorme and Watkins (5) appeared to be challenged by the observations of Hettinger and Müller. The progressive resistance exercises developed by DeLorme (4) are isotonic, are executed during relatively long sessions, and require different approaches for the development of maximum strength and endurance.

Rose and co-workers (27) attempted to apply the method of Hettinger and Müller clinically. They asked their subjects to lift with the quadriceps the greatest weight they could maintain for 5 sec (from 20 to 52.5 lb). Daily increments of $1^1/_4$ lb were added at consecutive sessions until a plateau was reached. Improvement in muscle strength ranging from 82 to 162% was observed over periods of from 39 to 90 days. When the method was applied to patients, the impression was gained that similar results could be obtained with either brief exercises or the DeLorme technique. The findings of Rose and his associates may be compared with those of Hettinger and Müller in relation to the following points:

1. No hypertrophy was found by Rose after brief exercises. Hettinger found a constant relationship between muscle strength and muscle cross section during the training period.

2. Rose obtained gains in symmetrical muscles of the unexercised extremities almost identical with those obtained in the exercised muscles (except when the unexercised extremity was in a cast). Hettinger used symmetrical muscles to check the results of different exercise schedules.

3. No attempt was made by Rose to evaluate the endurance factor in single brief muscle contractions.

We tried to analyze some of the factors involved in brief isometric exercises by studying the responses of the hypothenar muscle mass (especially the abductor digiti quinti) in 26 normal persons (14). Since these muscles are not used with great frequency in daily living their training is not contaminated by factors difficult to control in an experiment of long duration.

Normal Individuals

METHOD

Subjects. At first we divided our subjects into two groups of 13 each (ages varying from 20 to 45 years). Members of the first group (A) exercised the hypothenar muscles according to the method of DeLorme. The second group performed isometric exercises of the hypothenar muscles (as described below). After 9 weeks of training, the second group was divided into two subgroups, B and C. Group B (control) consisted of 7 subjects who continued with the same isometric exercises (once daily) as before until the end of the study (3 additional weeks). Group C consisted of 6 subjects who continued the same type of exercise as before, but instead of performing a single daily contraction for 6 sec, subjects repeated the exercise 20 times during each session. The subjects assigned to isometric exercises were divided into two groups in such a manner that at the end of the 9th week, the mean increase (percent) in muscle strength was the same for Groups B and C. Since the age range for Group A was different from that of the other groups, Group A was divided as follows: $A_1 - 6$ persons with the same age distribution as Groups B and C (20–30 years); and $A_2 - 7$ persons in the age range of 30–45 years.

DeLorme Exercises. Figure 8.1 illustrates the apparatus used for isotonic (DeLorme) exercises. The subject was asked to push a lever which raised a measured weight. The pushing movement was performed through the full range of motion (limited by a movable peg). Both the 1 RM and 10 RM were determined weekly. Each subject performed exercises on 4 days of the week: 10 with 50% of the 10 RM, 10 with 75% of the 10 RM and 10 with 100% of the 10 RM. The movements were executed at a rate of 10–15 per minute. The load was increased each week according to the recommendations of DeLorme.

Isometric Exercises. Figure 8.2 illustrates the apparatus used for isometric exercises. The subject was asked to exert a maintained maximal pull

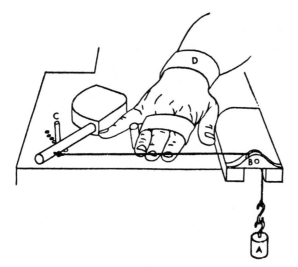

Fig. 8.1. Apparatus used to study isotonic (DeLorme) exercises; (A) weight, (B) pulley, (C) peg, (D) stabilizing strap.

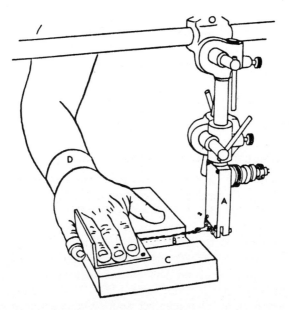

Fig. 8.2. Apparatus used to study isometric exercises; (A) transducer, (B) cable, (C) immobilizing device, (D) stabilizing strap.

for 6 sec on a cord attached to an isometric strain gauge myograph (Fig. 8.3). Figure 8.4 shows the calibration of the recordings. The subjects of Group B were asked to execute only one contraction a day; those in Group C repeated the contractions 20 times at 20-sec intervals.

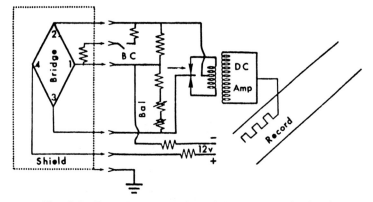

Fig. 8.3. Functional diagram of the myograph circuit.

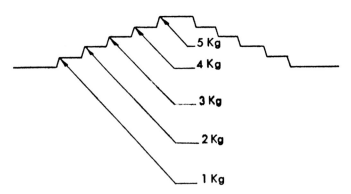

Fig. 8.4. Calibration of myograph; 5 mm equal 1 kg.

Muscle Strength and Endurance Testing

Each subject in every group was tested at the beginning of the experiment for: 1) maximal isometric contraction maintained for 6 sec (recorded on the myograph), 2) the 1 RM value, 3) the 10 RM value, 4) the circumference of the hand, and 5) the thickness of the hypothenar eminence (measured with calipers). At the end of the experiment, these five determinations were made again and, in addition, each subject was asked to maintain a pull on the isometric myograph cord with his hypothenar muscles until exhaustion. The time elapsed between the beginning of the pull and the moment that the myograph indicated 50% of the initial amplitude was taken as the index of endurance.

Contralateral Influence of Training

A determination of the 1 RM and 10 RM on the left (unexercised) hand was made on the 13 subjects who had exercised according to the method of DeLorme and on 5 subjects from Group B who had trained with brief isometric exercises. The remaining 2 could not be tested.

Results

INCREASE OF MAXIMAL MUSCLE STRENGTH

DeLorme Exercises. Table 8.1 shows that subjects in Group A increased their maximum muscle strength (1 RM) by 107% at the end of the experiment; they reached a plateau after 9 weeks. The increase of the 10 RM followed a parallel course with a final increase of 103%. Similar results were obtained in members of Groups A_1 and A_2 (respectively, 103 and 111% for the 1 RM; 101 and 104% for the 10 RM).

Isometric Exercises. The subjects in Group B (single exercises) increased their maximum strength to a higher degree (170%) and reached a plateau somewhat sooner—after 7 weeks (Table 8.2 and Fig. 8.5). Subjects in Group C (repeated isometric exercises) tripled their maximum strength (203% increase), as it continued to rise after a period of 9 weeks.

INTERGROUP COMPARISON

Time Factors. From Figure 8.5, which shows strength increase with time, it can be seen that members of Group B had a more favorable result than those of Group A. The results in Group C were even better, but Figure 8.5 does not express a real difference between Groups C and B. Indeed, the level for Group B is related to a single contraction, whereas the levels for Group C are related to the average amplitude for 20 consecutive contractions. It can be seen that at the beginning of the repeated exercises the mean amplitude for 20 contractions was below the level of the single contraction. However, with progression this average not only reached the level of the single contraction but exceeded it by about 10%.

Cross Testing. Table 8.3 shows that while Groups B and C show an increase of performance with isotonic exercises (for which they were not

TABLE 8.1

Groups	1 RM			10 PM		
	Pre-test gr.	Post-test gr.	Mean % increase	Pre-test gr.	Post-test gr.	Mean % increase
A_1	106	241	103	92	197	101
A_2	90	197	111	64	155	104

TABLE 8.2. *Isometric Exercise. Maximum Muscle Strength*

Groups	Pre-Test	After 9 Weeks		After 12 Weeks	
		gr.	Mean % increase	gr.	Mean % increase
B	1020	2700	165	2760	170
C	860	2360	174	2606	203

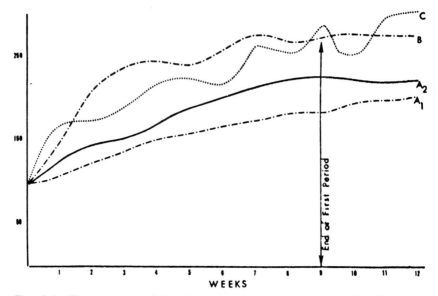

Fig. 8.5. Time course of the increase in muscle strength in all groups. Maximum muscle strength during consecutive weeks of training. After 9 weeks, the curve corresponding to Group C represents the average of 20 contractions. Letters A_1 through C are group designations.

TABLE 8.3. *Cross Testing. Mean Per Cent Increases*

1 RM (DeLorme) Test Groups	Strain Gauge Test	
	Mean % increase	
A_1	103	112
A_2	123	110
B	130	174
C	150	203

trained) comparable with or higher than Groups A_1 and A_2, the latter failed to reach the results achieved by either Group B or C under conditions of isometric exercise (112% instead of 174 and 203% respectively for Groups B and C).

Endurance. The most pronounced differences among the groups in relation to endurance are seen in Table 8.4. Those in Group C did best and those in Group A_2 performed most poorly. Figure 8.6 illustrates endurance curves for all four groups (at the end of the experiment).

Hypertrophy. Table 8.5 shows that only minimal changes of the muscle volume were found. In spite of the minimal change in volume, almost all persons reported a subjectively increased firmness of the exercised hypothenar eminence after the experiment ended.

Contralateral Findings. There were no significant training effects on the contralateral (unexercised) hand with either isotonic or isometric exercise. Thus the 1 RM in the right hand (exercised) was equal to twice the 1 RM found in the left hand at the end of training. Figure 8.7 illustrates similar findings for the brief contractions.

Extensive studies were made (14) on a few muscles of six patients — two with poliomyelitis, one with myotonia dystrophica, one with progressive spinal atrophy, one with rheumoatoid arthritis and one with toxic polyneuritis. Favorable results were obtained in all, although the improvement noted in the patient with progressive spinal atrophy was not functional (Fig. 8.8).

Gersten (6) employed isometric exercises in patients with weakened muscles and found comparable improvement to that produced by isotonic exercises. In a few instances where significant differences existed, the greater effect was seen in those who performed isometric exercises. Tepperberg (28) also found isometric exercises as effective in strengthening the quadriceps muscle as progressive resistance exercises. He feels they have the advantage of being less time consuming and less irritating

TABLE 8.4. *Endurance Index*

Group	Index of Endurance (in seconds)
A$_1$	69
A$_2$	57
B	101
C	170

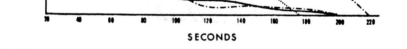

Fig. 8.6. Average endurance curves. Letters A$_1$ to C are group designations.

TABLE 8.5. *Hypertrophy*

Group	Tape Circumference (mm)				Caliper Measurement (mm)			Mean indiv. increase
	Total pre-test	Total post-test	Total gain	Mean indiv. increase	Pre-test	Final test	Total gain	
A$_1$	1310	1390	80	13	123	133	10	1.6
A$_2$	1610	1700	90	13	152	162	10	1.3
B	1485	1555	70	10	137	147	10	1.3
C	1187	1250	63	10.5	112	123	11	1.8

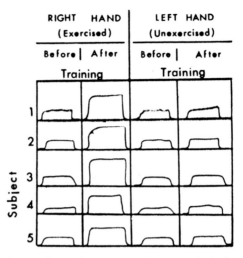

Fig. 8.7. Recordings of maximum muscle strength before and after single brief isometric exercise of both hands.

where there is joint damage. To improve muscle endurance, he uses repetitive isometric exercises.

Matthews and Kruse (21) found that isometric training was superior to the isotonic exercises. Magness, Lillegard, Sorensen, and Winkowski (20) did not find any significant difference between DeLorme and isometric exercises, although the latter were of shorter duration. The effectiveness of isometric exercises was also found by Moore (23).

Discussion

If the results described above express the fundamental pattern of muscle training, the following conclusions seem likely.

Daily single brief isometric exercises increase muscle strength more rapidly and at least as fully as classical isotonic exercises. Thus, the studies of both Hettinger and Müller and Rose and his co-workers seem to be confirmed by subsequent studies. In addition, our findings showed that such exercises increase the endurance to a higher level than the isotonic resistive exercises. Our data, however, show that some of the conclusions drawn from the work of Hettinger and Müller were premature. It is true that the increase of the maximal muscle strength is not much higher for those who perform the exercises 20 times a day instead of once daily. Yet Figure 8.6 shows that the stability of the performance continues to improve with the 20 times a day rate; Table 8.4 shows that endurance is much higher in Group C than in Group B. Group A (isotonic) shows a very low endurance in isometric exercises, while both Groups B and C have no difficulty in equaling or outperforming Group A in the exercises for which they did not have specific training.

Isometric brief single daily exercise may, however, lead to the same or a better level of performance and endurance than progressive isotonic exercises. We were not able to repeat the findings of Rose and his co-workers with respect to transfer in the unexercised hand.

The efficacy of brief repetitive isometric maximal exercises (BRIME) thus being established, the question arises: How to explain it? The original explanation of the efficiency of brief isometric exercises by Hettinger and Müller may be summarized as follows: Some unknown metabolic process initiates a chain reaction leading to an increase of muscle strength and hypertrophy. This chain reaction is set forth once a certain "threshold" is reached, for instance, when isometric contractions of a very brief duration and of relatively low intensity (of the order of 60–70% of the maximal effort) are performed. Our findings, showing that repetition of exercises is a contributory factor, suggest that this "threshold" is not attained by a single brief exercise. A search of more specific parameters explaining the efficacy of BRIME seems to be desirable.

Obviously, two aspects of the problem need to be considered while analyzing the efficacy of BRIME compared with the progressive resistive exercises (PRE): 1) their very short duration and 2) the presence of some specific "intrinsic" factor which makes them so efficacious.

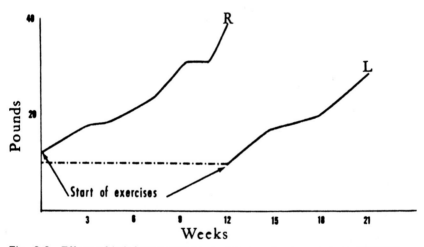

Fig. 8.8. Effect of brief repeated isometric maximal exercises (BRIME) on a patient with myotonia dystrophica, a 42-year-old man who complained of generalized weakness of 2 year's duration. At a 90° angle, the pull of the triceps surae was 5.039 g on the left and 5.972 g on the right. Three months after daily exercises on the right side (six repetitions of a 6-sec maximal isometric contraction) the triceps strength increased to 18.662 g; the opposite unexercised triceps remained at the initial test strength of 5.225 g. Treatments were then given to the left side and after eight weeks the muscle strength reached 13.883 g. After 6 months of exercise he was finally able to elevate his body on the balls of his feet. R, Right triceps strength; L, left triceps strength.

SIGNIFICANCE OF THE DURATION OF EXERCISES

Liberson et al. (15) analyzed in detail the factor of duration of exercises. Two points should be stressed. First, brief isometric exercise is preferable to a long isometric exercise because, in agreement with the classical observations, prolonged tonic contractions interfere with blood supply of the muscle. Second, the isotonic exercises, and for that matter the PRE, are not useful during the total duration of the muscle contraction insofar as their training effects are concerned. It has been known for almost a century that the muscle is more efficient when it is at its resting length than when shortened. On the other hand, the electromyographic (EMG) analysis of the isotonic contractions shows that the muscle potentials are not recorded with the same amplitude during the whole duration of the exercise. In certain phasic movements, a brief burst of electrical potentials may be responsible for a much more prolonged isotonic contraction. In other words, it is reasonable to assume that, during isotonic contractions, only certain limited periods of the exercise are contributory to the training effects, while the remaining part of the exercise is not. Conversely, one may assume that, during an isometric contraction, the entire duration of the exercise is contributory to the training effects, because this type of exercise may be conducted under the most favorable conditions as to the length of the muscle and its voluntary innervation. Viewed from this angle, it is possible that the differences between the effective durations of, respectively, BRIME and PRE are not as great as they appear to be on the surface.

We have studied the changes of the strength developed by four different muscles in several individuals as a function of the corresponding joint angle and confirm the loss of their tension when shortened. In our study the subjects were asked to develop maximal isometric contractions (Figs. 8.9 and 8.10). In view of this, it became desirable to determine the most favorable positions of the extremities in order to exercise isometrically each of their muscles.

INTRINSIC CHARACTERISTICS OF THE ISOMETRIC EXERCISES

Liberson et al. (15) compared the integrated electromyograms, recorded with skin electrodes, during PRE (10 repetitions) and BRIME in the same subjects. Integrated electromyograms (IEMG) summating the electrical potentials into smooth curves were found to be proportional to the muscle tension at a given length of the muscle. Figure 8.11 shows the amplitude of the IEMG in two subjects recorded from the biceps during a 10 RM exercise as compared with BRIME conducted at 130° of elbow flexion. It will be seen 1) that in general the electrogenesis is considerably lower during 10 RM exercises than during BRIME, and 2) that even at the *same length of the muscle* (130° of elbow flexion) the electrogenesis during 10 RM exercises was only 25% of that found during the BRIME. Therefore,

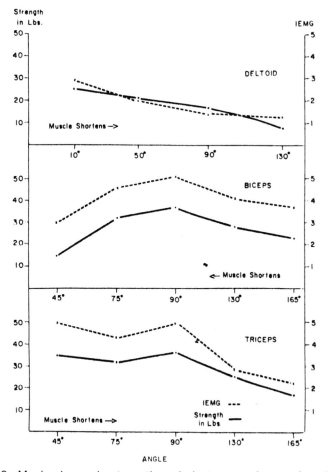

Fig. 8.9. Maximal muscle strength and electrogenesis as a function of the joint angle.

the degree of muscle innervation during BRIME is considerably higher than during PRE at the level of 10 repetitions. It seems reasonable to assume that this high degree of muscle activation constitutes a specific "intrinsic factor" of the efficacy of BRIME.

The relationship between an integrated EMG and muscle strength was considered by many authors, the EMG recording being used as an indicator of muscle strength (Basmajian and Latif (2); Nightingale (25); Inman et al. (12). Generally a linear relationship is found between them. However, Zuniga and Simons (31) found a slight deviation from a linear relationship.

Another factor in favor if isometric exercise is related to the speed of contraction: the higher the speed, the lower the maximal strength, according to Baer (1) and Buchtal (3).

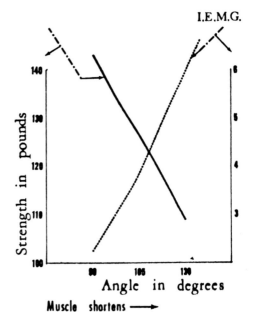

Fig. 8.10. Changes of muscle strength and the electrogenesis as a function of the ankle angle in the gastrocnemius.

OPTIMAL JOINT POSITIONS FOR BRIME

Classical tension-length diagrams show that when an isometrically contracting muscle is lengthened, the tension increases. However, this increase is for the most part due to the tension developed passively, and therefore the "contractile tension" is at a maximum for some intermediate value usually close to the "resting" length of the muscle. The highest dynamometric measurements do not necessarily indicate the optimal length of the muscle, although for some of the muscles this may be true. However, for some others, a high dynamometric value at a certain angle of the joint may indicate a mechanical advantage of the muscle pull rather than its intrinsic maximal efficiency. For instance, the contraction of the biceps characterized by a certain dynamometric reading with the elbow at 90° may be associated with a lower voluntary activation of the muscle than when the same dynamometric reading is obtained with the elbow at 180°. In the former case, the biceps pulls almost perpendicularly to the radius, while, in the latter, its pull is almost parallel to the long axis of this bone. Obviously, the dynamometric data may express both the influence of the muscle length and the mechanical advantage when the corresponding joint is at a certain angle. Besides, these two factors (muscle length and mechanical advantage) usually change in opposite directions.

As mentioned above, the level of the voluntary electrogenesis recorded in the muscle expresses the degree of muscle activation and therefore is a major factor affecting the efficacy of the muscle training. Integrated electromyography could provide, therefore, a method which would help us to determine the optimal positions for BRIME.

According to Inman et al. (12, 13), voluntary electrogenesis is considerably higher when the muscle is shortened than when it is lengthened, although the subject attempts in both cases to produce a maximal contraction. Some of these experiments were conducted on individuals subjected to cineplasty. However, Libet et al. (18) confirmed these findings on the gastrocnemius and tibialis anticus in normal individuals. It may be difficult to understand why the subject, attempting the same maximal voluntary effort, is unable to induce the same electrogenesis in his muscle, regardless of its length. In their study, Liberson et al. (15) confirm the observation of Inman et al. (12) as far as the gastrocnemius is concerned (Fig. 8.10). It was found that in this muscle and probably, although to a lesser degree, in the biceps, the differences in electrogenesis as a function of the muscle length are partially due to an artefact. Indeed, when the muscle was activated by a tetanizing current through the tibial nerve, the same differences in the amplitude of the induced electrical potentials, as in the case of the voluntary activation, could be observed for various degrees of ankle flexion. These differences could not, therefore, be ascribed to CNS mechanisms. The explanation seems to be the following one. When the gastrocnemius is relaxed, it takes a globular shape instead of a spindle-like one which it presents when it is stretched. More muscle tissue is then projected upon the recording electrodes and, therefore, the electrogenesis appears to be higher. In the biceps, the same occurs when the elbow is flexed at about 90°.

In flat muscles, such as deltoid and triceps, the observations of Inman et al. (12) could not be confirmed. In all the subjects without exception, the lowest electrogenesis was observed when their muscles were relaxed (Fig. 8.7); this was just the opposite of what was found for the gastrocnemius. However, Libet et al. (18) found that the decrease of electrogenesis

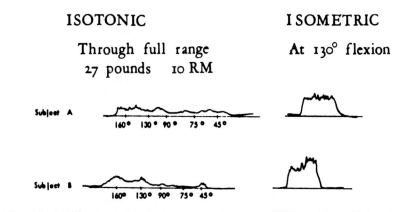

Fig. 8.11. Differences in electrogenesis between PRE and BRIME (see text).

on the stretched tibialis anticus can be avoided if the tendon is anesthetized. It therefore appears that complex mechanisms are involved in the relationship between the electrogenesis and the muscle length. A glance at Figure 8.9 will show that the curves of electrogenesis and those of dynamometrically measured tensions in the biceps, triceps and deltoid for different joint angles show essentially the same character. These data suggest that electrogenesis and the level of voluntary activation, which it expresses, are adapted, so to speak, to the mechanical potentiality of the muscle. When the latter is in an advantageous mechanical condition, for instance, when its length is close to its resting value or when it pulls at a right angle—in these favorable conditions—the innervation is at its maximum. Conversely, when it is in a poor mechanical condition, for instance, if shortened, the voluntary innervation correspondingly decreases.

The data in Figure 8.9 seem to be in apparent contradiction with the conclusions of Libet et al. (18). However, it is possible that the lengthened position of the muscle in our study was not associated with as pronounced a stretching of the muscle as in the case of Libet et al. (18). These authors also found that in the gastrocnemius there is an intermediary length of the muscle which seems to be most advantageous.

During the reported study, Liberson et al. (15) have found several examples of CNS regulation of the electrogenesis during the maximal effort of the subject: 1) when the individual is asked to make the maximum effort with his biceps during an isometric contraction and at the same time presses upon the table with his elbow, the electrogenesis is higher than if the effect of the biceps was not facilitated by an additional effort (Fig. 8.12); 2) when an experienced subject is told that the dynamometer shows a lower level of the maximal contraction than the one expected from him, his effort usually immediately increases by 10–20%; and 3) when a subject starts to tire and shows a decrease of the maximal voluntary contraction as a result of fatigue the electrogenesis increases (Figs. 8.13 and 8.14).

When a subject is asked to contract his biceps with a maximal effort against resistance, the triceps is almost "silent" electrically. However, if the subject is asked to maximally contract the biceps without any resistance, the triceps shows evidence of electrogenesis (Fig. 8.15). From the purely physiological point of view, new evidence concerning the functional feedback readjustment involving the spindle and Golgi apparatus in muscles and tendons suggests the explanation of why, despite a maximal effort by the subject, the maximum electrogenesis in the muscle may not be attained. According to Hufschmidt (11), a number of the motor neurons may remain in the "subliminal fringe" to the level of a fully activated pool of neurons.

According to Libet et al. (18), the above-mentioned results of a decreased electrogenesis in excessively stretched muscles may be explained by an

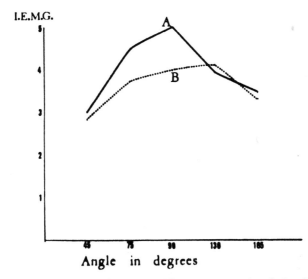

Fig. 8.12. Relationship between IEMG and strength of the biceps when subject is also pressing table with his elbow; (A) with stabilization, (B) without stabilization.

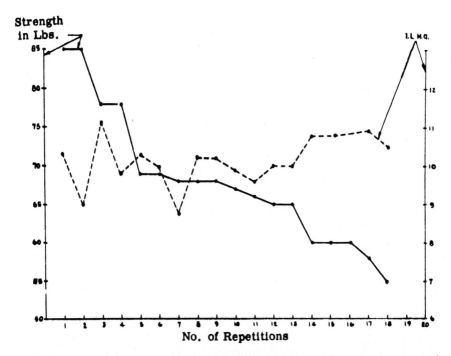

Fig. 8.13. Amplitude of IEMG increased slightly while muscle strength decreased as a result of repeated isometric exercises.

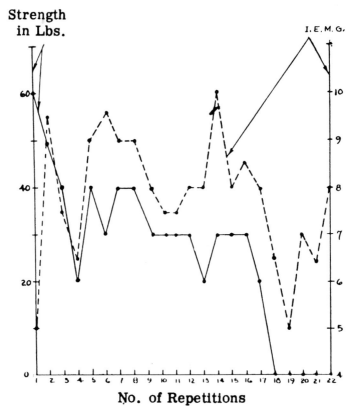

Fig. 8.14. Same type of experiment as illustrated in Figure 8.13. When muscle was virtually exhausted, amplitude of IEMG increased.

"autogenic inhibition" arising in the Golgi receptors of the tendons and decreasing the voluntary activation. The "autogenic inhibition" was considered by classical physiologists to explain the lengthening reaction. On the other hand, Hoffmann (10), Merton (22), Granit (7) and Hammond et al. (8) showed that, if during a voluntary contraction the nerve supplying the activated muscle is stimulated by a single electric shock, the contraction is suspended for 0.10 sec. Our studies not only confirmed these observations but also showed that a stimulus applied to a nerve supplying the muscle and the skin in the vicinity of the voluntarily contracted muscle is also able to inhibit, to a certain degree, the voluntary effort (Fig. 8.16). The original observations were amplified recently. (Liberson, 16, 17).

Thus, all these observations attest to the presence of a complex central mechanism of the control of the electrogenesis, which may permit us to understand the relationship between integrated EMG and the mechanical output of the muscle.

This discussion brings us, therefore, to the following conclusion. The efficacy of BRIME as to their training effects is probably due to a high level of muscle innervation associated with this type of exercise. In order to achieve this high degree of innervation, the exercise should be carried out at a joint angle which permits the highest mechanical output of the muscle and which is very easy to determine either by an adequate dynamometer or, in the absence of it, by a subjective evaluation by both the therapist and the patient.

Despite the merit of BRIME performed under the optimal conditions, it would be unreasonable to consider that its obvious advantages should prompt physiatrists to reject all but isometric exercises. Muscle training is an extremely complex and poorly understood process. In this process the increase of the muscle efficiency is due in part only to the changes in

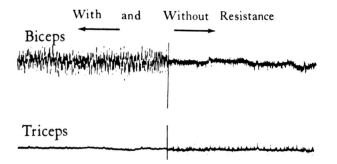

Fig. 8.15. When subject exhibits maximum biceps contraction the suppression of resistance against which he pulls elicits a diminution of electrogenesis in the biceps and its increase in the triceps.

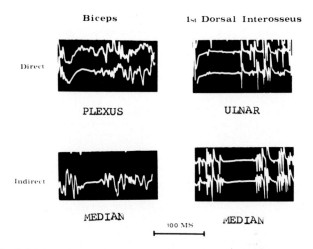

Fig. 8.16. Inhibition of the voluntary muscle contraction produced by brief stimulus applied to a nerve or plexus (at the beginning of each strip) either directly (to the nerve innervating this muscle) or indirectly (to a nerve which does not supply the muscle from which the recordings are made). (See Liberson (16, 17).)

muscle tissue itself. A readjustment of mental attitudes, a recoordination of the nervous centers, the adaptation of circulatory and metabolic processes—any of these extramuscular factors may play a dominant role. In our experiment these nonmuscular factors must have been of great importance, since the increase of performance was both considerable and rapid. On the other hand, therapeutic exercise in patients with different central and peripheral disorders raises a still more complex series of problems, which are discussed in other chapters. It would thus be unreasonable to consider that the reported facts concerning brief isometric exercises under optimal conditions should make them superior to isotonic exercises at all times; indeed, there are many instances in which movement through a complete range of motion is desirable. However, our results seem to justify a reconsideration of therapeutic exercises in the light of the present data and the introduction of brief isometric exercises with progresssively increasing repetition rate in patients for whom an increase of maximal muscle strength and endurance may constitute the link in the chain of therapeutic tools for muscle reeducation.

Recently several investigators raised questions as to the safety of isometric exercises because of the possible repercussions of these exercises upon cardiovascular function, particularly the diastolic pressure. Lind and McNichol (19) found dramatic cardiovascular changes following isometric exercises. Ramos et al. (26) state that static work consisting of squeezing a grip dynamometer at maximum effort produced a sharp rise in systolic and diastolic pressures during convalescence following myocardial infarction. These effects were less severe during dynamic exercises. Tuttle and Howath (29), Lind and McNichol (19) found analogous results. Whipp and Phillips (30) showed that it was the diastolic pressure which was particularly affected by these exercises. (See also Moore (24).)

It must be stressed that all these reported results concerned prolonged isometric exercises. The regimen which we suggested is related to *brief, repeated, isometric, maximal exercises* (BRIME), 5–6-sec duration with at least a 20-sec interval between them. We have checked several subjects before, during, and after such exercises, involving the small or large muscular groups, and have not found any significant changes in blood pressure.

REFERENCES

1. BAER, A. D., GERSTEN, J. W., ROBERTSON, B. M., AND DINKEN, H. Effect of various exercise programs on isometric tension, endurance and reaction time in the human. *Arch. Phys. Med. Rehabil., 36:* 495, 1955.
2. BASMAJIAN, J. V., AND LATIF, A. Integrated actions and functions of the chief flexors of the elbow; a detailed electromyographic analysis. *J. Bone Joint Surg., 39A:* 1106, 1957.
3. BUCHTAL, F., AND KAISER, B. Optimum mechanical conditions for the work of skeletal muscle. *Acta Psychiatr. Neurol. Scand. 24:* 333, 1949.
4. DELORME, T. L. Restoration of muscle power by heavy resistance exercises. *J. Bone Joint Surg., 27:* 645, 1945.

5. DeLorme, T. L., and Watkins, A. L. *Progressive Resistance Exercise.* New York, 1951.
6. Gersten, J. W. Personal communication.
7. Granit, R. *Receptors and Sensory Perception.* New Haven, 1955.
8. Hammond, P. H., Merton, P. A., and Sutton, G. G. Nervous gradation of muscular contraction. *Br. Med. Bull., 12:* 214, 1956.
9. Hettinger, T. and Müller, E. A. Muskelleistung und Muskeltraining. *Arbeitsphysiol., 15:* 111, 1953.
10. Hoffmann, P. *Untersuchungen uber die Eigenreflexe (Sehnreflexe) menschlicher Muskeln.* Berlin, 1922.
11. Hufschmidt, H. J. Zur funktionellen Organisation der Motorischem Einheiten eines Muskels. *Dtsch. Z. Nervenheilk., 178:* 583, 1959.
12. Inman, V. T., Ralston, H. J., Saunders, J. B., Feinstein, B., and Wright, E. W., Jr. Relation of human electromyogram to muscular tension. *Electroencephalogr. Clin. Neurophysiol., 4:* 187, 1952.
13. Inman, V. T., and Ralston, H. J. The Mechanics of Voluntary Muscle. In *Human Limbs and Their Substitutes.* New York, 1954.
14. Liberson, W. T., and Asa, M. M. Further studies of brief isometric exercises. *Arch. Phys. Med. Rehab., 40:* 330, 1959.
15. Liberson, W. T., Dondey, M., and Asa, M. M. Brief repeated isometric maximal exercises. An evaluation by integrative electromyography (unpublished).
16. Liberson, W. T. Monosynaptic reflexes and their clinical significance. *Clin Neurophysiol., Supp. 22,* 79, 1962.
17. Liberson, W. T. Widespread Inhibition and Silent Periods. Presented at the IVth International Congress of Electromyography, 1971.
18. Libet, B., Feinstein, B., and Wright, E. W., Jr. Tendon afferents in autogenetic inhibition in man. *Electroencephalogr. Clin. Neurophysiol., 11:* 129, 1959.
19. Lind, A. R., and McNichol, G. W. Cardiovascular responses to holding and carrying weights by hand and shoulder harness. *J. Appl. Physiol., 25:* 261, 1968.
20. Magness, J. L., Lillegard, C., Sorensen, S., and Winkowski, P. Isometric strengthening of hip muscles using a belt. *Arch. Phys. Med. Rehabil., 52:* 158, 1971.
21. Matthews, D. K., and Kruse, R. D. Effects of isometric and isotonic exercises in elbow flexor muscle group. *Res. Q. 28:* 26, 1957.
22. Merton, P. A. The silent period in a muscle of the human hand. *J. Physiol., 114:* 183, 1951.
23. Moore, J. C. Active resistive stretch and isometric exercise in strengthening wrist flexion in normal adults. *Arch. Phys. Med. Rehabil., 52:* 264, 1971.
24. Moore, J. C., Excitation overflow; an electromyographic investigation. *Arch. Phys. Med. Rehabil., 56:* 115, 1975.
25. Nightingale, A. Relationship between muscle force and EMG in standard position. *Am. J. Phys. Med., 5:* 187, 1960.
26. Ramos, M. V., Mundale, M. O., Awad, E. A., Witsoe, J. A., Cole, T. M., Olson, M., and Kottke, F. J. Cardiovascular effects of spread of excitation during prolonged isometric exercises. *Arch. Phys. Med. Rehabil., 54:* 496, 1973.
27. Rose, D. L., Radzyminski, S. F., and Beatty, R. R. Effect of brief maximal exercise on the strength of the quadriceps femoris. *Arch Phys. Med. Rehabil., 38:* 157, 1957.
28. Teppersberg, I. Personal communication.
29. Tuttle, W. W., and Howath, S. M., Comparison of effects of static and dynamic work on blood pressure and heart rate. *J. Appl. Physiol., 10:* 294, 1957.
30. Whipp, B. J., and Phillips, Jr., E. E. Cardiopulmonary and metabolic responses to sustained isonetric exercise. *Arch. Phys. Med. Rehabil., 51:* 398, 1970.
31. Zuniga, E. N., and Simons, D. G., Nonlinear relationship between averaged electromyogram potential and muscle tension in normal subjects. *Arch. Phys. Med. Rehabil., 50:* 613, 1969.

9

Biofeedback in Therapeutic Exercise

_____ J. V. BASMAJIAN

Teaching patients to control a wide range of physiologic processes can have amazing therapeutic results, but legitimate clinical use of biofeedback must be differentiated from its faddish popular image. In this era of exotic nonpharmaceutical treatments, physicians are rightly suspicious of novelties that they first read about in the public press. Biofeedback may appear at first to be just another such fad, and it is true that its popularity has been promoted by both self-serving and sincere adherents.

However, biofeedback's popular image masks its significance as a new tool in medicine, especially in rehabilitation of physically handicapped patients and in psychotherapy. Certain types of clinical biofeedback—almost wholly unrelated to the popular variety—have been proved at the scientific and practical level to be useful for alleviating serious neurologic symptoms, particularly in patients with upper motor neuron paresis and spasticity. The unfortunate and apparently unbreakable link of clinical biofeedback with the fad of the same name should not alienate physicians.

Biofeedback is the technique of using equipment (usually electronic) to reveal to human beings some of their internal physiologic events, normal and abnormal, in the form of visual and auditory signals and teaching subjects to manipulate these otherwise involuntary events by manipulating the displayed signals. The technique provides a feedback loop in which the person's volition is essential; unlike conditioned responses, the subject must want to produce the changes in the signals because they meet some goals.

The easiest form of do-it-yourself biofeedback—brainwave biofeedback—is the least understood scientifically. Alpha (α) waves are still a mystery for scientists to solve, not an acceptable treatment modality. More promising are electroencephalographic (EEG) feedback methods that emphasize willful manipulation of the theta (θ) wave content in the tracing as well as the sensorimotor rhythm. Several widely respected groups of investigator-clinicians have achieved modest but gratifying success in the control of epileptic seizures (1).

Biofeedback control of cardiac rates and blood pressure is under investigation, but less is known about the long-range efficiency and efficacy of biofeedback controls in actual hypertensive patients. Healthy people (and many hypertensives) can be trained to raise and lower their blood pressure voluntarily with appropriate apparatus that displays it visually and acoustically, calmly willing mean pressure changes in either direction of 10 mm Hg in a few minutes in a fairly reliable manner (2). Early reports are appearing of patients who maintained continued lower pressure over months. Blood pressure also can be willed upward. Paraplegic patients with postural hypotension can learn through biofeedback training to increase their pressure by as much as 30 mm Hg just before being raised to a vertical posture, thus avoiding a fainting spell.

With appropriate displays of cardiac tachometry, the ability of healthy subjects to raise and lower their cardiac rate at will has been applied in the clinic. Patients with premature beats can be trained to suppress their abnormal contractions (3).

If the subject is given direct readouts of the skin temperature, peripheral blood flow control mediated through the sympathetic nervous system can be altered dramatically. Changes of 5–10°C up or down can be achieved in the experimental laboratory with tiny thermistors on the fingers or toes. The problem for the physician is how to apply this to the treatment of peripheral vascular diseases. Temperature control of the extremities is more widely used in the treatment of migraine (4) where the results seem to go beyond the placebo effect, although that must also play a role.

Other kinds of pain also are being treated by psychotherapists with one form or another of biofeedback and these have been proved useful in the rehabilitation setting. Again, the placebo caution must be sounded, yet one cannot dismiss the success some clinics have achieved with biofeedback deep relaxation of muscles that are in spasm or hyperactive in the treatment of severe chronic tension headache (5). The results seem to go far beyond placebo effects, and they persist. Of course, deep relaxation strikes directly at the cause—muscle tension. Good psychotherapists quickly wean their patients from the biofeedback gadgets and teach them "self-control" for long-term treatment.

In the rehabilitation clinic, total body relaxation has been used along with exercise to reduce muscle spasms and associated pain, e.g., in patients with cerebral palsy and stroke in biofeedback relaxation enhances our subsequent training of motor performance.

In rehabilitation and therapeutic exercise, the most useful biofeedback approach is electromyographic (EMG). A premise of the technique has always been that patients can respond to a physician's request to alter the coarse level of activity of individual muscles that they could see as spikes on the cathode-ray oscilloscope and hear as popping noises on a loud-speaker (6). My demonstrations in the 1950s and 1960s of the possible application of EMG to myoelectric prostheses led to more intense studies with regard to how this control is exerted and how fine it can be.

The most dramatic application of EMG biofeedback in this decade has been in stroke patients (7). In about two-thirds of persistent cases, footdrop (which greatly hampers the swing phase of gait) can be alleviated by the addition of biofeedback to gait training. Alas, our techniques are still too primitive to salvage the remaining majority of patients. Neuro-muscular retraining methods for severe disabilities of muscle control and postsurgical disassociation, such as tendon transplants, also are being developed. EMG biofeedback is now a legitimate supporting rehabilitation tool for physicians and therapists, not a separate branch of medicine or science but a tool to be applied judiciously by professionals who treat and understand the medical problems of the whole patient.

Our group has published results obtained in controlled trials that substantiate the results in many patients treated without controls. Ther-apeutic exercise combined with biofeedback training produces greater increases in strength and active range of motion than therapeutic exercise alone. While much larger groups of patients need to be studied, the results achieved so far favor the rehabilitative use of biofeedback training when facilitation or inhibition of muscle activity is desired. Many hemi-paretic patients have a greater potential for rehabilitation than previously thought.

Foot Drop

The effectiveness of exercise therapy plus biofeedback training was compared with that of conventional therapeutic exercise in 20 hemiparetic patients with chronic foot drop (7). The 20 volunteers—10 men and 10 women aged 30–63 years—were randomly assigned to one of two equal groups. The tibialis anterior muscle was selected for study because of its primary function as the chief ankle dorsiflexor.

The increase in both strength of dorsiflexion and range of motion was about twice as great in the patients receiving biofeedback training as in the other group. Four patients in the biofeedback group achieved and retained conscious control of dorsiflexion. Three of these patients could walk without the use of their short leg brace at follow-up. While the overall response of the group receiving both forms of treatment was best, some good increases in strength and range of motion also were made by patients receiving physical therapy only. Our treatment schedule had been so abbreviated that we turned then to more thorough programs with even more gratifying results.

In our routine clinic, 39 patients have been treated with varying success for foot drop. About two-thirds had short leg braces (8). Our results follow.

Patients Previously Treated with Short Leg Brace. Twenty-five patients had been treated up to the time of biofeedback with a short leg brace which appeared to be reasonably efficient. All but one of these patients (who was age 70) fell into the age range of 31-64 with a good spread among the various ages. The shortest duration since the stroke was 3 months, but almost all of the patients had suffered their stroke many months or several years prior to biofeedback treatment, so the condition of their foot drop had stabilized. Of these 25 patients, 16 were able to discard their short leg brace entirely following 3-25 sessions (approximately $\frac{1}{2}$ hour) of biofeedback rehabilitation training. The remaining 9 patients showed little or no improvement, sometimes due to obvious reasons such as poor motivation, severe spasticity, early discontinuance of treatment, and intercurrent illnesses. Some of the patients were even able to discard their canes for the activities of daily living; several use their short leg brace intermittently when they are working for long periods of time on their feet.

Patients Previously Untreated with Short Leg Brace. Fourteen patients with footdrop had reasonably good function at the ankle and so they had not been treated with braces. Following from 3 to 17 sessions of biofeedback training, only 2 had no improvement of ankle function, while 6 had moderate to excellent improvement of strength and range of motion— greatly improving their gait.

Effects of Age, Sex, and Duration of Footdrop. No apparent direct relationship could be demonstrated for the effectiveness of biofeedback when it was compared (both successes and failures) with the age of the patient and the duration of the footdrop condition. Both patients who were in their 30s and in their 60s were among those who discarded short leg braces. The successful cases included male and female patients, in the same proportion as the general population of our cases. The duration of footdrop seems to have no relationship with successes among patients many years (e.g., $6\frac{1}{2}$ years) or 3 months after stroke; among the failures there were patients both early and late.

Subluxation of Shoulder

Our experience with shoulder subluxation has been uniformly good. Basing our approach on the hypothesis that subluxation is due to an unlocking mechanism (6) we have concentrated on improving the mobility of the scapula with the emphasis on restoring the proper glenoid cavity orientation. When the glenoid cavity is facing upward as well as forwards and laterally as in normal shoulders, the subluxation is eliminated. This is due to a tightening coracohumeral ligament and adjacent superior capsule of the glenohumeral joint.

Thirteen patients with subluxation in our early series (8) received muscle reeducation with biofeedback of the shoulder region. Clinical results have ranged from moderate to excellent reduction of the subluxation (including radiographic evidence) and an accompanying improvement of scapular and glenohumeral mobility.

Impaired Hand Function

Both relaxation techniques for spastic muscles and muscle reeducation of paretic muscles are employed for both the forearm musculature and for the intrinsic hand muscles. Severe spasticity can be moderately modified by targeted relaxation techniques where electrodes placed over the spastic group of muscles provide the patient through the biofeedback apparatus with instant feedback of his hyperactivity. A growing number of patients can be trained to relax spastic muscles by direct conscious effort. This in turn permits the voluntary use of the hand and the strengthening of grip and pinch without exuberant flexor synergies being evoked. Approximately a dozen sessions of personally tailored biofeedback rehabilitation therapy are needed. Perhaps a great part of the effectiveness of this therapy arises from the improved body image and motivation that the patient gains from the therapists. However, we have gained the impression that another part of the improvement is due to a restoration of motor controls through new or indolent cognitive and motor pathways.

Post-surgical patients have had their exercise regimen greatly shortened by intensive biofeedback (EMG and electrogoniometry) in our hand clinic (9, 10). Biofeedback permits a closer cooperation between the patient and the therapist also with post-traumatic hand-retraining programs.

Other Devices

In common with other rehabilitation centers we also use various forms of force and motion analysis that measure and display changes in the body—pressure transducers, joint angle devices, electrogoniometers, accelerometers, electronic "spirit levels," and others (10). The readout of these devices is fed back to the patient and therapist visually and acoustically. This permits them to work together to manipulate the readout by an effort of the patient's will to restore body balance or to achieve a desired pressure, angle, or motion. My occupational therapy colleagues have devised a host of gadgets that patients respond to with enthusiasm.

To motivate younger patients, some of the feedback is provided in the form of a desirable response, e.g., turning on and maintaining a television or radio program only by giving the desired performance. In a sense this is an addition of Skinnerian operant conditioning to the biofeedback technique. It certainly works in the Hand Clinic of Grady Memorial Hospital, where youngsters must move or squeeze their hands to play their transistor radios.

Of course, there are many conditions, such as complete spinal transection, in which biofeedback can act only on the obviously normal residuum of the patient's body. It would be folly to attempt to retrain muscles that are completely cut off along the control pathway from the brain. Yet even here there is a ray of hope: the patient with a spinal cord injury may not have a complete lesion; also, training to raise blood pressure voluntarily may prevent postural hypotension.

General Relaxation Therapy

We feel there is a major application of *generalized relaxation therapy* to the stroke patient and the cerebral palsy patient who obviously are under great emotional stress. A patient who is apprehensive and tense cannot cooperate to the fullest in therapeutic exercises. Thus, the therapist should not concentrate only on local relaxation (11).

Strategies

In the selection of strategies for applying biofeedback in the therapeutic exercise setting, the judgment of the supervising therapist and the realities of the situation result in great variation. Our actual management of patients has been described elsewhere (12). Outpatients are generally seen as often as possible, not less than twice a week being highly recommended. Sessions are of necessity rather short, 30–60 min.

In EMG biofeedback, electrodes are invariably "skin" or surface electrodes. For monitoring very weak muscles or for control of spasticity, large electrodes are used. Smaller Beckman silver-silver chloride electrodes are used for the control of finer movements or the training of larger muscles. For general relaxation therapy, standard forehead leads, widely used and described, are effective.

INITIATING CONTRACTIONS

Often a muscle will appear inactive and the patient will seem to have no means of knowing what he has to think or do to make the muscle contract. We have been using a very simple technique to help the patient initiate a contraction. The therapist supports the joint involved. As the patient thinks hard about the desired motion, the movement is passively performed. As the limb is returned to the initial position, the patient concentrates on relaxing and for maximal concentration, does so with eyes closed. After 5–10 passive motions, the motion is attempted unassisted. In the majority of cases this procedure has been successful in eliciting a voluntary contraction in the appropriate muscle, often with some visible joint motion. If, after several attempts, a voluntary response cannot be elicited, a repetition of the procedure may be of some benefit (12).

GAINING CONTROL OVER SPECIFIC MUSCLES

After applying the electrodes, the patient is asked to contract the muscles and try to perform the desired joint motion. Once the contraction is initiated, he is urged to work harder for a higher meter reading and to attempt a maximal effort for approximately 5 sec. Rest periods of 15–30 sec between contractions are important, because once the patient learns to reuse his paralyzed muscle, complete relaxation often is impossible. Therefore, maximal electrical activity during a contraction and minimal activity during the rest periods is stressed. The therapist should play a very active role during the session by 1) adding constant verbal feedback and encouragement, 2) setting slightly higher meter readings as the goal of the subsequent contraction, 3) making sure the motion produced is the appropriate one, 4) discouraging excessive muscle activity in the rest of the limb, 5) changing the position of the limb for better results, and 6) checking the electrodes to ascertain that they have not been displaced or pulled loose.

In the early training sessions, the stroke patient will very likely elicit the entire flexion synergy in both the upper and lower extremities as he attempts to dorsiflex the ankle. The therapist must decide whether to allow this pattern to continue. In the earliest sessions they may well be the only way the patient can contract the desired muscle. As strength increases, the associated muscle involvement must be discouraged by having the patient dorsiflex only to the point where the heel begins to move. The therapist must explain the importance of being able to dorsiflex without involving the other muscles (12).

CONTROL OF SPASTICITY DURING MOVEMENTS

Instead of working for a high EMG meter reading and a loud acoustic feedback signal, the patient is instructed to work on attaining silence and a null meter reading. The joint is positioned so that the muscle is electrically silent. The limb is then carried passively through a range which stretches the spastic muscle. The patient is instructed to relax completely. The verbal reinforcement is carefully administered throughout the session.

Once the control of spasticity through passive stretch has been learned, the patient is asked to contract the antagonist muscle(s), while keeping the spastic muscle relaxed and quiet. A slow contraction of the antagonist(s) lends itself to easier control of the spastic muscle. The main objective of the session is to help the patient become aware of the feeling of a tight, contracted muscle compared to a relaxed muscle. Awareness of this difference may take several sessions, but once the patient has mastered this concept he is often able to relax the spastic muscle upon command without the biofeedback reinforcement (12).

Sometimes the patient must learn to relax a spastic muscle before successful attempts can be made at strengthening the antagonist muscle, as in the case of a spastic gastrocnemius overpowering any attempts at dorsiflexion. Here again, emphasis is placed on the patient's recognition and control of the spasticity in the gastrocnemius. Once the relaxation of spasticity through passive stretch is learned, the electrodes are placed over the tibialis anterior to elicit dorsiflexion, as the therapist encourages dorsiflexion and reminds the patient to keep the gastrocnemius relaxed (12).

Conclusion

Biofeedback, especially EMG biofeedback, is a tool that may be used by physicians and therapists to improve many forms of therapeutic exercise.

Both to reeducate weak muscles and to relax hyperactive muscles (either local or general), the technique is the natural accompaniment of many procedures in the clinic aimed at improving cognitive and sensorimotor performance.

REFERENCES

1. STERMAN, M. B., MacDONALD, L. R., AND STONE, R. K. Biofeedback training of the sensorimotor electroencephalogram rhythm in man: effects on epilepsy. *Epilepsia, 15:* 395–416, 1974.
2. SCHWARTZ, G., AND SHAPIRO, D. Biofeedback and essential hypertension: current findings and theoretical concerns. *Semin. Psychiatry, 5:* 493–503, 1973.
3. WEISS, T., AND ENGEL, B. T. Operant conditioning of heart rate in patients with premature ventricular contractions. *Psychosom. Med., 33:* 301–321, 1971.
4. SARGENT, J. D., GREEN, E. E., AND WALTERS, E. D. Preliminary report on the use of autogenic feedback training in the treatment of migraine and tension headaches. *Psychosom. Med., 35:* 129–135, 1973.
5. BUDZINSKI, T. H., STOYVA, J. M., ADLER, C. S., AND MULLANEY, D. J. EMG biofeedback and tension headache: a controlled outcome study. *Psychosom. Med., 35:* 484–496, 1973.
6. BASMAJIAN, J. V. *Muscles Alive: their Functions Revealed by Electromyography,* Ed. 3. Williams & Wilkins Co., Baltimore, 1974.
7. BASMAJIAN, J. V., KUKULKA, C. G., NARAYAN, M. G., AND TAKEBE, K. Biofeedback treatment of foot drop after stroke compared with standard rehabilitation technique: effects on voluntary control and strength. *Arch. Phys. Med. Rehabil., 56:* 231–236, 1975.
8. BASMAJIAN, J. V., REGENOS, E. M., AND BAKER, M. P. Rehabilitation biofeedback for stroke patients. 2nd Joint Conference on Stroke. American Heart Association, Miami, 1977.
9. KUKULKA, C. G., BROWN, D. M., AND BASMAJIAN, J. V. Biofeedback training for early finger joint mobilization. *Am. J. Occup. Ther., 29:* 469–470, 1975.
10. BROWN, D. M. Biofeedback in occupational therapy: new horizons in upper extremity rehabilitation (Cassette tape, Cat. No. T-81). In *New Methods in Physical Rehabilitation* Series, edited by J. V. Basmajian. Biomonitoring Applications, Inc., New York, 1976.
11. FAIR, P. L., AND BASMAJIAN, J. V. Relaxation therapy in physical rehabilitation (Cassette tape, Cat. No. T-82). In *New Methods in Physical Rehabilitation* Series, edited by J. V. Basmajian. Biomonitoring Applications, Inc., New York, 1976.
12. BAKER, M. P., REGENOS, E. M., WOLF, S. L., AND BASMAJIAN, J. V. Developing strategies for biofeedback; applications in neurologically handicapped patients. *Phys. Ther., 57:* 402–408, 1977.

10

Crutch and Cane Exercises and Use[1]

_____ MORTON HOBERMAN

The origin of crutches[2] and canes as aids to the disabled and infirm is unknown. In all probability it dates back to the era when man became a biped and began to use his fore-extremities for specialized purposes (11, 17, 18, 25).

Construction

Until the seventeenth or eighteenth century, the crutch was a single stick with a crosspiece at or close to the top. About that time drawings and paintings began to depict crutches with a hand piece between split uprights, held together on top by a crosspiece. In essence, this is the wooden crutch still in greatest use (Fig. 10.1A). A number of variations of this crutch have appeared in the last 50 or 60 years. In some the materials used were different; in others variations of the crutch top or tip were made. In most instances the variations were usually recommended and made with some specific disability or infirmity in mind (crab or plate tip for athetoids, "Canadian crutch" top for patients with triceps weakness, "Kenny crutch" or "English cane" for poliomyelitis patients).

The standard underarm or axillary crutch is made in two styles. One is adjustable in total length as well as in the height of the hand piece (Fig. 10.1A). The other style, known as the permanent or plain split crutch (Fig. 10.1B), is not adjustable as to total length or position of the hand

[1] We wish to express our thanks to The Williams & Wilkins Company and to the editors of the _American Journal of Physical Medicine_ for permission to rephrase material on parallel bar activities and to the editors of the _Physical Therapy Review_ for permission to rephrase material on mat activities.

[2] "Crutch (Old English—_cryce;_ Old Teutonic—_krukja_ or _krukjon_—to bend. A staff for a lame or infirmed person to lean upon in walking, now one with a cross piece at the top to fit under the armpit." _Oxford Universal Dictionary._

piece. A variation of this style is known as the spring-top underarm or axillary crutch. In this model (Fig. 10.1C) the wooden axillary crosspiece is replaced by a rubber or hair filling covered by leather and nailed or riveted to the two uprights. It is usually recommended for those individuals who use crutches to a considerable extent for ambulation and must carry some of the body weight on the shoulders as well as on the hands.

Wooden crutches are usually made of selected hardwoods such as birch, ash, hickory or maple. Custom-made crutches are usually made of Brazilian rosewood, hard-rock maple, or lemon wood. The latter woods are usually more resilient, less likely to splinter or crack, and take a better finish. In every wooden crutch the grain of the wood should run lengthwise to minimized possible breakage (10).

The adjustable crutch is heavier than the permanent crutch of the same size because of the additional piece of wood (the extension) and because the shafts are usually thicker to compensate for the lesser resiliency. The hand piece and extension piece are fixed to the uprights by means of bolts and winged nuts. The extension piece and shafts have numerous holes at regular intervals so that the total length of the crutch can be varied and so that the hand piece can also be raised and lowered (the many holes also decrease the strength of the crutch).[3]

In the variations of these crutches, where the wooden shoulder piece is removed and the uprights are cut down to midarm or forearm length, the uprights are usually joined together by a circular leather cuff two to three inches wide, which is nailed to the wood (Fig. 10.1D), or by a piece of metal (Fig. 10.1E). These have the disadvantage of usually not fitting the arm when a jacket and an outercoat are worn. At the New York State Rehabilitation Hospital the cuff is split, and then the ends are secured with a buckle and strap (Fig. 10.1F) so that it can close over a coat sleeve.

With the advent of aluminum alloys which have good tensile strength as well as lightness, metal crutches came into vogue. Both bar metal and tubular metal (stronger ounce for ounce than bar metal) are in use. The bar aluminum is most frequently used to reproduce the wooden crutches previously described. The one distinct advantage the aluminum crutch has is its lightness. The tubular aluminum is used almost exclusively for single upright crutches. Those with protruding handgrip and crosspiece for the axilla (Fig. 10.2A) resemble the ancient crutch. They are usually adjustable in total length as well as in handgrip length. In this model, the lower piece can be telescoped into the upper piece, reducing the overall length to cane size and offering the advantage of easier storage (in cars, theaters, planes). A very popular single upright crutch is an adjustable forearm style, made of tubular aluminum with the upright bent out 30° above the handgrip. Two models are available, one with the

---

[3] The shoulder piece in both types of crutches is usually joined to the uprights by a mortise and tenon joint, frequently without glue, and held in place by a small wire brad on each side. Since the brads tend to loosen with extensive use, they should be replaced by small woodscrews (6).

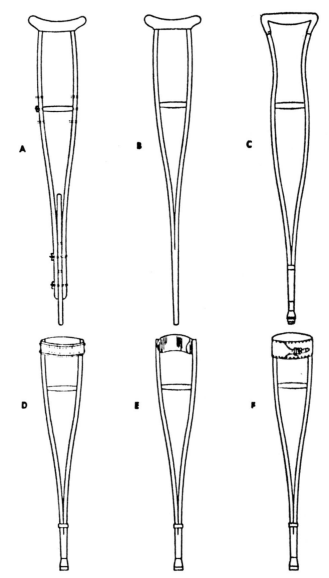

Fig. 10.1. (A) Adjustable underarm or axillary crutch; (B) permanent underarm or axillary crutch; (C) spring-top axillary crutch with Whittemore tip; (D) forearm crutch with closed circle cuff (leather); (E) forearm crutch with U-shaped cuff (metal, may be covered with leather); (F) forearm crutch with open circle cuff, closed by strap and buckle (leather). The crutches shown are wooden, but similar models are made of aluminum.

forearm piece stationary (Fig. 10.1D), the other adjustable (Fig. 10.1E). The crutch is held to the forearm by a cuff of spring steel (usually attached to the upright by a swivel joint) similar in shape and purpose to

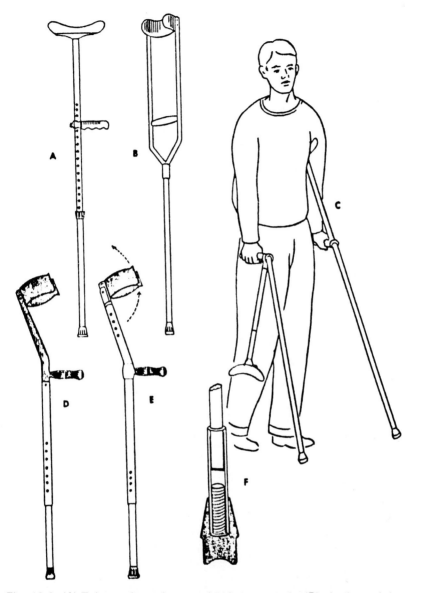

Fig. 10.2. (A) Telescopic underarm aluminum crutch; (B) single upright arm aluminum crutch with U-shaped cuff; (C) wing aluminum underarm crutch (and cane); (D) forearm aluminum crutch with stationary forearm piece; (E) forearm aluminum crutch with adjustable forearm piece; (F) detail of recoil spring in base of crutch. (Not shown is the Everett crutch which is similar to the crutch pictured in B above and has a triceps cuff 4 cm (1½″) below the elbow.)

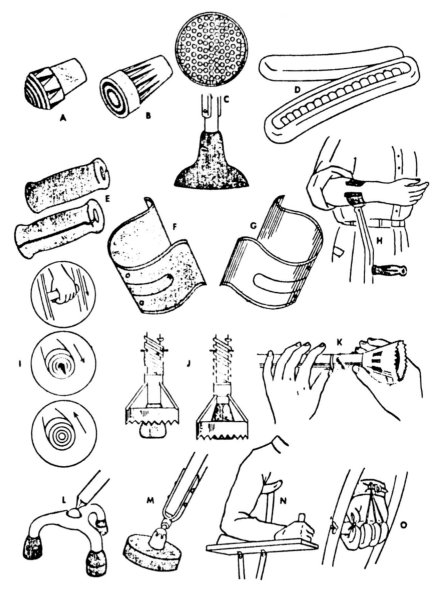

Fig. 10.3. (A) Crutch tip, small — unsafe; (B) crutch tip, suction type; (C) crutshoe tip, large size, suction bottom (D) shoulder pad of latex or sponge rubber; (E) handgrips, rubber; (F) forearm cuff, rubber-covered; (G) forearm cuff, plain steel; (H) forearm cuff, side opening (I) all-weather crutch tip, retractable metal tip; (J) nonslip crutch (or cane) tip; (K) non-slip crutch (or cane) tip; (L) crab foot tip; (M) disc tip (universal joint); (N) platform crutch; (O) glove to hold paralytic hand on hand piece.

a greatly enlarged bicycle clip. The cuff can be rubbed-covered (Fig. 10.3F) or plain steel (Fig. 10.3G). This crutch allows for greater freedom of use of the hands since the handgrips can be released without losing the crutch. The opening of the forearm cuff can be placed on the side (Fig. 10.3H). In this position there is even less likelihood of loss of the crutch when the user has to flex the elbows forcibly, or falls accidentally. Another model of this crutch incorporates a shock-absorbing recoil spring at the end of the lower tube to decrease impact (Fig. 10.2F). This has not become very popular, possibly because of the recoil impact on the elbow and shoulder joints. Another type of single upright aluminum crutch has as its outstanding feature the ability to fold down the part of the upright above the hand piece (12) (Fig. 10.2C) and presumably to allow its use as a cane as well as a crutch. However, since this is accomplished by turning the hand piece, it can be accidently dropped and is therefore not safe.

The cane now used for medical reasons is most frequently made of a hardwood such as maple or ash, or of bamboo, and usually has a curved or crook top (Fig. 10.4A), less frequently a T-shaped (Fig. 10.4B) or a ball top (Fig. 10.4C). More recently, aluminum canes have also been used. These are usually adjustable (Fig. 10.4D, F) in length. (This is an advantage in institutions where such a cane can be used to determine the proper size for a particular patient.) Another aluminum cane has four contact points and is known as the four-legged cane (Fig. 10.4E) or as the cane-glider when small wheels replace the two inside tips. In some institutions these are used in the transitional stage when progressing from ambulation with crutches to ambulation with canes. The four points of contact give greater stability and sense of security. The wheel type is used when difficulty is experienced in advancing the cane with each step (the cane can be pushed forward rather than picked up and placed forward).

A number of accessories for crutches and canes have been devised. While known as accessories they are, for the most part, essential for the person using the crutch or crane. In this category may be mentioned rubber crutch tips, rubber axillary pads and handgrips, triceps bands, wrist straps, "weather tips" and "crab foot tips."

The rubber crutch tip is probably the most important accessory and should be carefully selected. Since its purpose is to provide good contact with the ground to prevent slipping no matter at what angle the crutch is placed, it should be made of good rubber, of the suction design (Fig. 10.3B, C) and 1½ to 2 inches in diameter. Smaller tips (Fig. 10.3A) and those made of hard rubber do not provide an adequate surface contact and wear excessively. The Whittemore tip (Fig. 10.1C) is still used on some wooden crutches (especially the axillary spring-top type). This is a metal base to which is screwed a small rubber tip. The presumable advantage of this tip is that it will not come off even with vigorous use of the crutch. However, the Whittemore tip is usually too small and too hard to provide adequate contact and stability for the average crutch user.

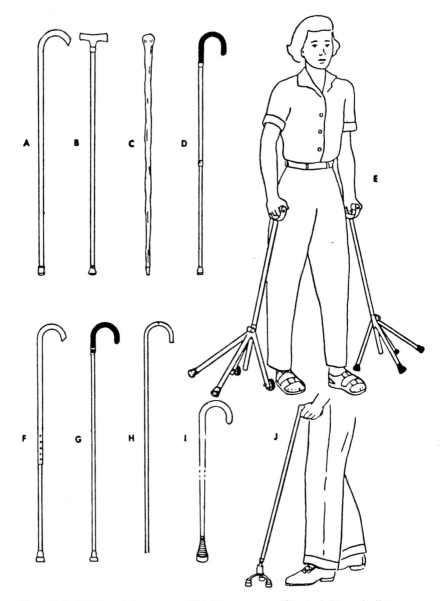

Fig. 10.4. (A) Crook-top cane; (B) T-top cane; (C) straight or ball-top cane; (D) adjustable aluminum cane, rubberized handle (E) cane glider, two types— with and without wheels; (F) adjusted aluminum cane; (G) aluminum cane with rubberized handle, nonadjustable; (H) nonadjustable aluminum cane, type used by the blind; (I) crook-top cane with ice gripper (J) crook-top cane with crab foot attachment.

The rubber axillary pad (Fig. 10.3D) is usually made of latex or sponge rubber shaped to fit the axillary crosspiece. Its original purpose was to relieve underarm pressure and thus prevent undue compression on nerves and blood vessels in the axilla (21, 26, 27, 29). In some institutions its use is forbidden because it is said to encourage weight bearing on the shoulders instead of the hands, or because it causes the upper part of the crutch to stick in the axilla, which results in greater difficulty during some activities (preparatory to sitting down, falling, elevation). While for most crutch users this is true, there are some patients who do not have adequate strength to hold crutches against the chest wall, and for these persons rubber crutch tops are quite necessary for adequate performance of activities.

Rubber handgrips are also made of sponge rubber and will fit the hand pieces of all standard crutches. They are usually recommended for persons who develop pain or numbness of the hand as a result of great pressure on the hand piece. Unfortunately, the rubber grips tend to rotate on the hand piece. Furthermore, the addition of a rubber grip frequently makes the hand piece too large for comfortable handling. To overcome these difficulties, where it is necessary for the patient to have the cushioned effect, the wooden hand piece can be replaced by a narrow metal tube covered with sponge rubber and leather of identical size as the original hand piece. Occasionally, the length of the hand piece must be increased to accommodate a very broad hand. We have not found specially shaped or positioned hand pieces to be of any marked value (24). Some provide for a "better grip," others for a "better anatomical angle of the wrist." However, they then present problems during elevation activities and whenever the crutch is turned out of the axilla to be used as a means of pushing up from the seated position. Such hand pieces also tend to make crutches definitely "right handed" or "left handed."

The triceps band is extremely valuable for the crutch user who is unable to maintain the elbow in extension under weight bearing. It usually consists of a metal band or cuff shaped to fit the arm approximately 3–4 inches above the elbow, covered with leather and fixed to the posterior upright of the crutch (Fig. 10.5A). Occasionally a forearm band is needed to stabilize a weak extremity (Fig. 10.5B). The triceps band needs a pectoral stop on the superior aspect of the anterior upright to prevent the crutch from slipping posteriorly as the weak triceps gives way and exerts pressure against the cuff.

The wrist strap is used for those patients who have weakness of the wrist extensors and are unable to prevent the wrist from going into flexion on weight bearing. The strap may be of leather or cloth webbing. It is usually buckled around both uprights, and the hand is inserted between the strap and the hand piece so that the strap produces pressure on the dorsum of the wrist (Fig. 10.6C).

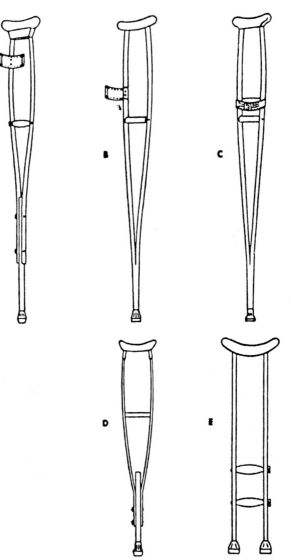

Fig. 10.5. (A) Adjustable underarm crutch with triceps band; (B) permanent underarm crutch with forearm band; (C) permanent underarm crutch with strap to hold wrist in extension; (D) adjustable underarm crutch for small child, made of bar aluminum uprights and tubular aluminum extension piece (New York State Rehabilitation Hospital); (E) mat crutch with additional hand piece for elevation activities.

One of the most frequent complaints of the crutch user is the difficulty encountered during snowy and icy weather (or on wet tile, wet leaves, highly polished floors, slippery mud, etc.). In an effort to aid the crutch or cane user, several devices have been developed and are available (4). For

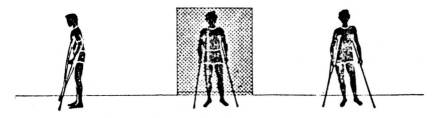

Fig. 10.6. Silhouettes of crutch balancing positions. Standing erect, leaning backward against a wire screen, shifting weight to one crutch. (This figure and the two which follow are reproduced from and with the permission of the journal *Modern Medicine.*)

the most part they are best suited for snowy or icy surfaces. In one crutch a pointed retractable metal tip has been built into the wood tip. The metal tip juts through the rubber tip when the handgrip is turned (Fig. 10.3*I*). (It is also made in an aluminum crutch.) Because it is activated by rotating the handgrip, the possibility exists that the metal tip can be accidentally protruded while the user is walking on a nonslippery wooden or concrete surface and cause him to lose his balance (besides scratching the surface) (6).

Two other types of nonslip tips (Fig. 10.3, *J* and *K*), which can be mounted on any crutch or cane, are also available. In these the gripping surface is a circle of serrated steel teeth, which is held above the rubber tip when not in use (usually by springs). When needed, the gripper surface is manually lowered to a point just below the rubber tip. Unfortunately, the suction rubber tip is too large and cannot be used with most ice and snow grippers.

The crab foot tip was designed to aid those patients who were unable to adequately control the angle at which the crutch struck the ground (athetoids and ataxics for the most part) (1, 30). The use of a universal joint with the crab foot (Fig. 10.3*L*) ensures the user that at least one tip, and in most instances two tips, will strike the ground at a proper angle to prevent the crutch from slipping. In a few instances where the crab foot has not been satisfactory, a rubber-covered round metal disc (10 cm or 4 inches in diameter) has been substituted for the crab foot with good results (Fig. 10.3*M*) (6). Such tips (crab foot or round disc with universal joint) can also be put on canes when indicated. A suction rubber tip incorporating a swivel joint between the tip and the crutch attachment has become available. We have found that the tip has a tendency to detach at the swivel joint whenever heavy angular pressure is brought to bear on the cane or crutch.

Two other crutch types are sometimes listed under accessories. One is the mat crutch; the other is the platform crutch. The mat crutch (Fig. 10.5*E*) is an ordinary crutch which has been cut off below the hand piece (distance depends on the sitting and kneeling height of the individual using the crutch) (15). It is usually used for patients who have paralysis of both lower extremities and who will eventually have to use bilateral long leg braces as well as crutches for ambulation. The patient can begin to learn the fundamentals of crutch management and use in the long sitting position on a mat (or floor) before he is permitted to stand. Patients who have poor trunk-hip balance should always be started on mat crutches in the sitting position and progressed to longer mat crutches in the kneeling position before attempting standing balance with regulation crutches.

The platform crutch was developed to aid the person with flexion contractures at the elbow or severe wrist fractures or deformities who needed crutches to ambulate (Fig. 10.3N). Instead of body weight being borne on the hands, it is carried on the forearm, for the most part. The handgrip frequently is made to fit the contractures and deformities of the hand.

Fitting of Crutches and Canes

Many methods have been described to properly fit a patient with crutches (8, 19, 20, 23, 31). One thing is certain: only rarely will the "dry measurements," taken by any method, result in crutches which fit exactly. Fortunately, adjustable or expansion crutches are available in most rehabilitation centers and hospitals. The "dry measurements" serve as a starting point at which the adjustable crutches are set so that the patient may begin his standing balance activities. In most instances crutch length and hand piece position will be altered depending on the upright posture, type and degree of disability, body type and size, upper extremity strength, balance and coordination.

The initial measurements can be taken with the patient supine (preferably on a hard surface such as a floor or a table top), or on a tilt table or standing upright. In any position it is important that the shoulders and shoulder girdle be relaxed. Measurement is made from the anterior axillary fold to the bottom of the shoe heel (if the patient is measured in bed, without shoes, add 2–3 cm (1 inch) for men and 4 cm (1½ inches) for women). This is the length of the crutch from the middle of the axillary crosspiece to the bottom of the rubber tip of the crutch (if a rubber shoulder piece is to be used, this must be part of the measurement). Since crutches should be held against the chest wall at least 3 cm (or 1 inch) below the axillary folds, the crutch should touch a point approximately 5–8 cm (2–3 inches) to the side and also in front of the mid-lateral aspect of the foot. At first, crutches are used with a broad base for balance. This base is narrowed with confidence born of experience.

The correct position for the hand piece is best determined when the crutch has been adjusted to the proper total length. The crutch is then placed in proper position (see last sentence, previous paragraph). Again with the shoulder and shoulder girdle relaxed, the elbow is flexed 30°, the wrist is dorsiflexed to its maximum position, and the fingers are formed into a fist. The hand piece should be placed in line with the fist. It is again emphasized that for the vast majority of patients further adjustment as to total length and hand piece position will eventually have to be made. This is especially true for the so-called permanent crutch user (for example, paraplegic and poliomyelitis patients), as distinguished from the temporary crutch user (post-fracture patients, lower extremity amputees prior to prosthetic fitting). It is of course also true for the child who uses crutches for any length of time.

Many elderly patients who use crutches temporarily because of hip and knee disability find it more convenient to have the elbows extended rather than flexed at a 30° angle. Since they are rarely called upon to perform elevation activities during the period of their disability, it is advisable to permit the more convenient hand position. Some brace and crutch walkers also prefer the extended position of the elbows for ambulation. They can add a second hand piece to the crutch (higher to produce elbow flexion) to be used for elevation activities (see mat crutch with two hand pieces, Fig. 10.5E).

Most adjustable crutches are now made in three sizes: child, youth, and adult. However, since not all crutch manufacturers agree as to crutch sizes for these three groups, it is best to order the crutch by actual length required rather than as child, youth, adult, or small, medium, large.

If the patient has attained adult growth and has become proficient in the use of his crutches, consideration should then be given to obtaining for him a pair of permanent nonadjustable crutches. These are not as heavy, nor as bulky, as the adjustable type and are frequently more acceptable in appearance.

CANES

Measuring a patient for a cane is comparatively simple. In most instances the patient is able to stand. Measurement is made from the top of the greater trochanter of the femur to the floor (patient wearing shoes). It will be noted that in the normally proportioned individual, when the clenched fist with extended wrist is placed at the top of the greater trochanter, the elbow will be flexed to approximately 30–40°. The measurement made above is for the length of the cane from the highest point of the handle to the bottom of the rubber tip. Canes also are made in three sizes, and each size usually has a specific diameter. The shortest cane is usually 2 cm (⁵/₈ inches) in diameter; the medium cane, 2.2 cm (⁷/₈ inches) in diameter; and the longest, 2.5 cm (1 inch) in diameter. These canes can, of course, be cut down to required size. It should be remembered that the diameter of the cane is also the diameter of the cane handle. Canes of longer length or greater diameter can usually be obtained on special order. In passing it should be noted that canes for the blind (Fig. 10.4H) are frequently longer (by up to 30 cm) than those used for orthopedically or neurologically handicapped persons.

Kinesiology of Crutch and Cane Walking

In essence, a crutch or a cane is an extension of the upper extremity, used to provide support, balance, and weight bearing normally provided by an intact functioning lower extremity. Theoretically, the loss of use (due to pain, instability, or paralysis) of one lower extremity should be compensated for by one crutch (moderate or total loss) or one cane (little loss). In practice, one crutch is seldom advised unless the patient has considerable weakness in one upper extremity or has excellent balance and coordination. It may also be useful in unilateral disabilities (hip arthritis, hemiplegia).

It is a rather simple task to enumerate the muscle groups which should be present and active for good crutch walking (8, 19). Normal musculature of the upper extremities and shoulder girdles is the ideal situation. Normal upper extremity muscles are essential for good ambulation if the patient has complete paralysis below the tenth thoracic segment. An accurate manual muscle test is therefore an important prerequisite to crutch instruction and training. Weaknesses or muscular imbalance thus found in the upper extremities should be corrected, if possible, by proper exercise prior to intensive crutch practice. The more strength, coordination and endurance the patient can attain in the muscles of the upper extremities and shoulder girdles, the less difficulty will he have in ambulating with crutches.

The more important crutch-walking muscle groups of the shoulder girdle and upper extremity, listed from proximal to distal, are: 1) scapular depressors (latissimus dorsi, lower trapezius, pectoralis minor), to stabilize the upper extremity and prevent hiking of the shoulder on weight bearing; 2) shoulder adductors (pectoralis major and latissimus dorsi), to hold the crutch top to the chest wall with the arm; 3) flexors, extensors and abductors of the arm at the shoulder (deltoid), to enable placement of the crutch forward, backward and sideward respectively; 4) extensors of the forearm at the elbow (triceps and anconeus), to stabilize this joint in weight bearing by preventing flexion or buckling (these, plus the shoulder depressors, are most important in raising the body from the floor to allow the lower extremity to swing); 5) wrist extensors (extensor carpi radialis and ulnaris), to hold the wrist in proper position to bear weight on the hand piece (although the position of extension is more important than the muscle action); 6) finger and thumb flexors (flexor digitorum sublimis and profundus, flexor hallucis longus and brevis), to adequately grasp the hand piece so that the crutch can be moved to the desired position. Weakness or paralysis of any of these muscle groups will compromise the eventual gait pattern. A few weaknesses can be aided by accessories (triceps cuff, wrist extensor strap, forearm platform and finger flexor glove) (Figs. 10.7 and 10.8).

It is difficult to say which muscle groups are most important for crutch ambulation since much depends on the pattern of paresis or paralysis in

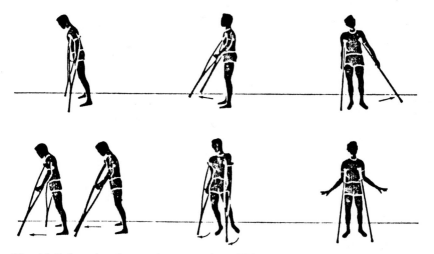

Fig. 10.7. Leaning forward on crutches, lifting crutches off floor, lifting one crutch off floor, leaning forward, turning, "no hands."

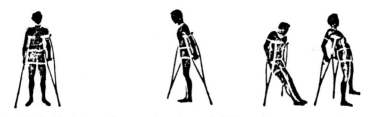

Fig. 10.8. Variations in crutch grip and shifing the center of gravity.

all the extremities and trunk. The presence of even "poor" hip extensors and flexors can greatly enhance the ambulatory potentials of one crutch walker over another who has no voluntary control of hip musculature. Poor quadriceps, in contrast to "zero" or "trace" quadriceps, may mean that the patient can use short-leg braces rather than locked long-leg braces, and so develop a smoother, less awkward gait. It should be noted that the biceps is not listed as an essential muscle group for crutch walking. This is mentioned because so many bed patients are urged to "exercise" on an overhead or trapeze bar where the biceps receives the major strengthening effect.

There are several other factors which are equally or more important than muscle strength and upon which the success of crutch walking frequently depends. First and foremost is the will, desire or motivation of the patient to be able to walk with crutches (and braces when indicated). Unfortunately there are many persons who experience a profound emotional upset with the onset of physical disability. To them crutches (and braces) are constant reminders that they are cripples (a term used frequently by such patients to indicate the degradation of the physical status in which they find themselves). They usually need psychological as well as physical aid and assistance.

Depending on the degree of depression and feeling of degradation, support can be supplied by the physician and therapist in the milder forms, but patients with more severe forms of such feelings may require psychological and psychiatric counseling and guidance. It is therefore essential that the physician explain to the patient (and frequently his family) the reasons for the use of crutches (and braces). It is our firm belief that no physician should ever tell a patient he will never be able to do without crutches in the future. Only time and experience can do this for the patient.

The other factors, referred to above are frequently grouped together as "techniques" or "performance methods." They include balance, coordination and timing. It is well known in sports, crafts, and muscial activities that some people seem to be endowed with a better sense of balance, coordination, and timing than others. However, most of the less fortunate can improve their balance, coordination, and timing with conscientious, diligent, regular practice. Crutch walking is no less a learned skill which needs constant repetition and attention to detail if it is to be perfected. Of the three factors, balance is the most important to attain to the maximal level before routine ambulation with crutches is permitted.

Patients who are permitted to ambulate at will before maximal balance is achieved rarely walk well or securely. The patient must make the same determined effort to learn balance, coordination, and timing in crutch walking that he would to learn a new tennis stroke or a new technical piece for the piano. It cannot be repeated too often that only daily practice with attention to detail will provide the necessary work to make the crutch walker skillful (2, 7, 8, 13, 20, 22, 23, 28, 31).

Exercise to increase strength, balance, coordination, and timing can and should (if possible) be started while the patient is still confined to bed. Most normal persons rarely develop their voluntary musculature to its maximal level of strength. It is of distinct advantage to the potential or actual crutch walker that his upper extremity (and scapular) muscles are developed to maximal strength since he will be using them for weight bearing. In the patient who has had no involvement of the upper extremities, weight-resistive exercises are taught in bed (the weight or resistance can be of any material, or springs of graduated resistance or even body parts which are lifted or elevated).

The important features are that all exercises be taught properly and that the patient be advised how many times to perform each exercise during each period and how many exercise periods are to be completed each day. The physician should prescribe the exercises to be performed and give the therapist an estimation of the patient's present exercise capacity and potential. The therapist is requested to report to the physician untoward reactions to exercise (pain, extreme shortness of breath, fainting, extreme fatigue, etc.) as well as the patient's progress.

The physician and the therapist should repeatedly emphasize to the patient the importance and necessity of each exercise in the eventual role of crutch walking and other daily activities. The latter, daily activities, are actually more important to most severely disabled individuals. However, the greatest concern of most disabled persons is "Will I be able to walk again?" In order to increase strength and endurance, exercises must be of a progressive nature both as to amount of resistance overcome and number of repetitive movements performed. Each of these elements, resistance and repetition, has a beneficial effect on the other. The best results are obtained when both are increased gradually.

Specific details of exercises to be performed in bed, on mats, in wheelchairs, standing in parallel bars and standing with crutches have been reported by Deaver and Brown (8), Sanders (28), and Hoberman, Cicenia, Dervitz, and Sampson (15). In most instances these include exercises without apparatus as well as with apparatus. What is important is the realization that the exercises should be started as soon as possible, that they be performed daily, and that they be prescribed to meet the needs of the particular individual as well as of the disability. All exercises are learned with greater ease if they are first described (verbal and written cue), demonstrated by the physician or therapist (visual cue), then attempted by the patient, with the assistance of the physician or therapist (tactile and kinesthetic cues), and finally performed by the patient alone (proprioceptive cues) under supervision.

Another educational method that can be used to improve exercise performance is to have the patient teach or supervise other less advanced patients. This will occasionally make the indifferent patient take stock of how and for what purpose he is performing a certain exercise or group of exercises. It will frequently make him turn to the therapist to ask, "Why is this done this way and not another way?" or "That patient performs the exercise easier or better than I do; why? What am I doing incorrectly?"

Whenever possible, each patient should be given personal instruction at the beginning of an exercise program. As he improves in understanding and performance, he should join other patients performing the same or similar exercises (group exercises and activities). Here the patient can be instructed how to assess successes and failures in others and so be guided in his activities. Here he will also have the opportunity to socialize with others similarly afflicted and actively working toward their recovery of function. Here he is able to compete with fellow trainees rather than with the "all too perfect teacher."

Virtually all exercises without apparatus listed for bed or mat can be performed in either location. The mat is much to be preferred to the bed for active exercise since it is lower (less fear of falling), usually larger (more room, especially for rolling and turning exercises), and firmer (better exercise performance).

Balance exercises can also be started in bed with the patient sitting at the edge, at first with support, and then without support. If the latter is possible, the patient is suddenly but gently thrown off balance by the therapist. In this way the patient has an opportunity to regain his righting and positioning sense. Progression in this activity is thence to the mat for balance activities with and without support in the long sitting position, and then in the kneeling position. The final progression for the potential crutch walker is in the upright position with support (crutches and wall) and without support (just crutches).

In many institutions an intermediate step between mat balance and crutch balance is given: parallel bar standing and balance activities. These are usually desirable since it is best to introduce only one new factor to be achieved at each progression. In going from the mat to the upright position with crutches, the patient has two factors to overcome: standing and manipulation of full-length crutches. Patients who are slow in learning or severely disabled so that balance at best is precarious should be advanced from parallel bar activity to a combination of one bar and one crutch.

The rate of progression from bed to upright position is determined by the extent of disability, the patient's ability to learn and retain what he learns, and the amount of physical strength and endurance he has attained. Whenever possible, individuals should be grouped with others of comparable degrees of involvement, learning capacity, and stamina. In this manner, frustration is reduced to a minimum.

The patient should practice balancing with crutches while leaning against a wall or wire netting. He should also practice placing crutches in different positions and shift his body weight while standing with them (Figs. 10.6–10.8) before crutch gait is taught.

The type of crutch gait to be taught to the disabled person will of course depend on several factors: type, extent and degree of disability, and the residual patterns of weakness. These will vary from patient to patient, and each one should be evaluated individually. However, there is a progression in gaits from the simplest to the most difficult and from the slowest to the most rapid. It is our opinion that anyone who is going to use crutches for any length of time should be progressed through as many gait patterns as is possible. Of course the patient with the least amount of disability will find even the so-called "difficult gaits" easy to perform, while the severely disabled will find the simplest gait difficult. The simplest gaits are the "tripod drag-to," the "rocking chair gait," and the "tripod alternate step" (8, 9). These are "simple" only in that they are not as complex in the motion pattern necessary to produce movement or forward advancement. For the most part they are direct continuations of the standing crutch balancing exercises, without support. The crutches are advanced a few inches in front of the patient, who then leans forward and either drags both feet to the crutches, or rocks forward and back until his feet advance to the crutches, or brings first one foot to the crutches and then the other. In the first two, the feet rarely leave the floor, so that a "tripod" is constantly maintained which gives considerable balance and stability. In the third gait, the tripod is momentarily disturbed as each foot is advanced. Slightly better balance is needed for this gait to accommodate the minor shifting of weight from one side to the other and back.

There are two other types of gait for forward progression: the point gait (four-point and two-point) and the swing gait (swing-to and swing-through). The point gaits are somewhat more stable since at no time are both feet or both crutches off the ground at the same time. By the same token, point gaits produce a slower rate of progression than the swing gaits. Both types require good balance and timing.

Point gaits are most easily performed by persons having hip hikers (elevators) and lateral abdominals. The presence of hip muscles (flexors, extensors, abductors), while necessary for the two-point gait, is not essential for the so-called four-point gait in which progression is accomplished by successive forward advancement of each point (that is, right crutch, left foot, left crutch, right foot, repeat). The two-point gait can be accomplished in two ways: either the crutch and foot on the same side advance together, or the crutch on one side advances with the foot on the other side. The latter is theoretically more stable since weight is still borne on both sides. However, this gait is apparently more awkward for most patients to perform.

The swing gaits are actually progressions of the "tripod" gait: tripod — swing to — swing through. In the swing-to gait, both crutches are brought forward together. The trunk and lower extremities lean forward as one, weight is transferred to the uppers, and both lowers are lifted and swing up to the crutches. At the end of the "step," the patient should be in normal crutch stance, ready to take the next "step" or stop.

The swing-through gait is probably the most difficult of all gaits because it requires the best balance and timing. It is also the fastest means of ambulation with crutches. With each "step" the individual actually unbalances himself and then recovers. It begins exactly like the swing-to gait, but, instead of lifting both lower extremities and bringing them to the crutches, they are brought through the crutches, landing in advance of the crutches. As a result, the crutches are behind the individual when his feet touch the ground. He must, therefore, be able to bring the crutches forward again rapidly before hip and trunk balance is upset, resulting in jackknifing and a fall. Jackknifing can be prevented by complete hip extension.

Walking with crutches backward, or to the side, or turning is also accomplished by the point or swing type of gait. These are practiced as part of crutch management so that they are perfected prior to actual ambulation.

Mention must be made of a gait used by some temporary crutch users who are not permitted to bear weight on one lower extremity (post-trauma, post-surgery, acute inflammatory reactions, Perthe's disease, amputations). Their stance is truly tripod. They usually use a swing-to or swing-through gait, moving the affected extremity with the other and landing on the nonaffected foot. Some of the patients are permitted "partial" weight bearing on the affected extremity. Here a modified point-swing gait is used since the affected extremity moves forward with both crutches and then the unaffected extremity is brought to or through the crutches.

Cane walking, for some reason, has been comparatively neglected by most medical practitioners. The probable reasons are public opinion associating the use of a cane with "foppishness and dandyism," plus the inadequate realization of the amount of relief which cane use can afford an affected lower extremity. Blount (3), in a Presidential Address to the American Academy of Orthopedic Surgeons, urged his colleagues to reconsider the use of the cane to aid their patients. There is no doubt that even partial weight bearing on one or two canes will greatly relieve pain and irritation of an affected hip, knee, ankle or foot. In addition, the use of a cane will prevent undue pressure and use of the unaffected extremity.

The question is frequently asked, "In which hand should a cane be carried: on the same side as the affected lower extremity or on the opposite side?" Theoretically, since it is an extension of the upper extremity for weight bearing, the cane should be carried in the opposite hand. In this position it will automatically be brought forward with the affected lower extremity (normal pattern of alternate hand-foot movement in walking). The patient must be taught to bear down on the cane when the unaffected lower extremity begins the swing phase. When successfully performed, this will prevent lurching or tilting of the trunk over the affected extremity and will result in a more normal gait pattern. Successful cane users will frequently report greater endurance as well as less pain and fatigue. In part this is due to restoration of a more normal gait pattern and consequently more efficient muscle use.

Practically speaking, many patients cannot use the cane in the opposite hand. This is especially so in patients who have considerable instability in the hip and knee due to weakness and pain. These people receive more assistance when the cane is carried on the same side and advanced simultaneously with the affected lower extremity, acting almost like a splint as well as a weight-bearing surface. We have also noted that persons who are decidedly one-handed have greater difficulty manipulating a cane in the nondominant hand than even a crutch. When a cane is indicated for these people it is best to teach them the proper use of the cane in the dominant hand regardless of the side of disability. Occasionally a patient will have weakness or pain in opposing upper and lower extremities (poliomyelitis, traumatic injuries, arthritis). Here, too, it will then be necessary for the patient to use the cane in the hand on the same side as the affected lower extremity.

Two canes are frequently used by patients with bilateral amputations, arthritis, poliomyelitis residuals, multiple injuries to the lower extremities, multiple sclerosis and other similar disabilities. The gait used with two canes will depend on the type of disability, degree of involvement of each lower extremity, and age. With canes, however, only the "point" gaits are feasible. The four-point and two-point gaits with canes are exactly like those with crutches (see above). Where two canes are used because of severe involvement of one lower extremity, the gait used will be like that of the "temporary" crutch user. That is, both canes and the affected extremity are advanced together, and weight bearing is taken principally on the canes while the unaffected extremity is carried forward.

A number of the accessories used on crutches can also be used on canes. Every cane used for medical purposes should have a good rubber tip (Fig. 10.3, B) The ice and snow tips can be added if necessary (Fig. 10.3, J and K). The crab foot tip and disc tips (Fig. 10.3, L and M) can also be used for patients who have difficulty with placement (athetosis, ataxia, multiple sclerosis). In some institutions the glider canes are used for patients who are being progressed in ambulation from walkers. Most patients are able to grasp the ordinary crook-top cane without difficulty. Some patients with hand weakness can grasp a T-top cane better and obtain more weight bearing on the straight surface. We have yet to see a patient who can handle a straight- or ball-top cane better than the crook- or T-top cane.

Exercises Preparatory to Crutch Walking

The exercises which follow are presented as examples which can be performed in various situations, prior to actual ambulation with crutches, to improve balance, strength, endurance, and coordination. They are not the only exercises which may be necessary. Some may not be applicable to some patients, and some may even be contraindicated in others. The physician must decide what exercises he wishes his patient to perform and also indicate how much exercise the patient should perform. Many of these exercises can and should be performed daily by the crutch walker even after he learns to ambulate. Walking, per se, does not exercise sufficiently the many muscle groups needed in daily activities which the crutch user usually has to perform in addition to ambulation.

We shall not discuss here progressive resistive exercises for the muscles of the upper extremities, but rather the more complex movements.

Crutch activities have been resolved into their component motions. It is our opinion that it is best to begin with the more simple movements, learn them well, and increase endurance before going on to the next more complex movement.

These exercises, dealing essentially with those movements pertaining to eventual crutch use, have been taken from a larger group of exercises designed to give the disabled individual practice in motions for all the activities of daily living (5, 6, 8, 15). They do not represent the sum total of exercises to be performed by any one patient.

Mat and Bed Exercises

These are grouped together because they can all be performed on a mat, and many can at least be started in bed.

1. *Pelvic Tilter:* Patient supine, legs extended, arms at side. Patient attempts to flatten the lumbar spine, pressing it into the bed or mat. This motion is used many times a day by the crutch walker to prevent "jacking" (acute flexion of the trunk at the hips) during daily activities. It teaches the patient how to roll his pelvis forward when doing swing gaits, going up and down elevations and getting up from the seated position.

2. *Hip Hiker:* Patient supine or prone, legs extended, arms at sides. Patient attempts to lift the iliac crest to the lower ribs on the same side. Repeat on opposite side. Alternate sides rhythmically. This exercise develops coordination and skill for point gaits and elevations.

3. *Sitter-upper:* Patient supine, legs extended, arms at sides. By pressing down on the mat or bed with the upper extremities, the patient raises the head and trunk to a semireclined position (the elbows are now flexed). By extending the forearms at the elbow, the patient comes to the long-sitting position. This is a functional exercise to strengthen the shoulders and elbow extensors, which are so important in crutch walking.

4. *Sitting Push-up:* Patient in long-sitting position, palms flat on mat or bed, close to hips. Patient extends the forearms at the elbows, attempting to lift the buttocks clear of the mat or bed. Blocks or sandbags may be used under the hands to produce a greater lift. This is a preliminary exercise for all activities where body weight must be lifted by the upper extremities.

5. *Trunk Twister and Hip Raiser:* Patient in long-sitting position, hands on knees. Patient twists trunk to one side and places both hands on the mat or bed next to the hip faced. By extending forearms on elbows the patient attempts to raise the buttocks from the mat or bed. This is another exercise to lift the body weight with the upper extremities in a varied position found in many daily activities.

6. *Sitting Hip Hiker:* Patient in long-sitting position, hands on knees or hips. Patient attempts to approximate the iliac crest to the lower ribs on the same side. In so doing he moves the buttocks backward. He repeats the same movement on the other side. He then attempts to move forward by the same movement (not as easy as backward because the lower extremities must be pushed forward).

7. *Sitting Swing-Through:* Patient in long-sitting position, palms on mat or bed. Patient places the hands posterior to the hips and extends the forearms at the elbow. As the buttocks are raised, the patient swings them backward through the hands as much as possible. To move forward, patient places hands anterior to the hips, extends the forearms at the

elbows and slides the lower extremities forward when the buttocks clear the mat or bed. These are preliminary motions for the swing gaits and elevations.

8. *Prone Push-up:* Patient prone, arms abducted, elbows flexed, hands flat on mat or bed. Patient attempts to lift the head and upper trunk by extending the forearms at the elbows, while stabilizing shoulders and scapulae. A good exercise to further strengthen almost all upper extremity muscles used in crutch walking.

The following exercises should not be attempted on a bed.

9. *Hip Swayer:* Patient balanced on hands and knees. Stabilizing the trunk with the upper extremities, patient sways his hips first to one side and then to the other. A good exercise to develop balance and coordination of the trunk and hips.

10. *Camel and Cat:* Patient balanced on hands and knees, head extended, lower back in lordosis (camel position). By flexing the head and contracting the abdominal muscles (resulting in forward pelvic tilt), patient attempts to round the back (cat position). Another good balance and coordination exercise for the trunk and hips.

11. *Forward Reacher:* Patient balanced on hands and knees. Patient attempts to raise one arm until it is horizontal to the mat, while retaining his balance on the knees and other arm. Repeat with other arm. A preliminary balance and coordination exercise for many activities in which balance is maintained on both feet and one crutch while the other is raised for forward placement.

12. *Backward Reacher:* Same as above except that the arm reaches backward toward the buttock. Preliminary for activites where one crutch will be placed behind the patient.

Mat Exercises with Crutches and Benches

Some of the following exercises are direct carry-overs from exercises described above. In those given below the patient begins his training in crutch management in the long-sitting position. The patient learns how to handle crutches without combating total body balance at the same time. The patient then progresses to kneeling upright balance utilizing small benches. Here again, balance is learned first (trunk on the hips), and then crutch management is taught at this level. The value of the exercise is usually the same as that given above.

1. *Shifter:* Patient in the long-sitting position, mat crutches in the axillae, elbows flexed, wrists extended, hands grasping the hand pieces (this will be called "crutch position" in the following exercises). Patient shifts trunk first to one side and then to the other. This is preliminary balance exercise and in addition provides the first indication of what weight bearing on the upper extremities feels like.

2. *Crutch Raiser:* Crutch position. Patient shifts his trunk weight to one side. The crutch on the opposite side is lifted laterally without

displacement of the axillary position. Repeat on other side. A progression in balance, coordination, and crutch management.

3. *Sitting-Crutch Push-up:* Crutch position. Patient pushes down on his hands (in so doing, he extends the forearms at the elbows and depresses the shoulder girdles), raising the buttocks from the mat.

4. *Sitting Four-Pointer:* Crutch position. Patient shifts weight to crutch on one side (right), hip hikes on the opposite side (left), moving that hip backward. Then the patient moves the crutch on that side (left) in line with that hip, shifting body weight to that side (left), and hip hikes the other hip (right) backward and brings that crutch in line with the hip. The same motions are then performed in a forward direction. In this direction it is advisable to place the crutches slightly in front of the hips. This is the preliminary four-point gait with crutches.

5. *Sitting-Crutch Swing-Through:* Crutch position. Patient places the crutches just posterior to the hips, and pushes down on his hands (see 3, above). As buttocks clear the mat, the patient swings backward as far as possible. Crutches are again placed behind the hips and movement repeated. This motion can also be performed in a forward direction by placing the crutches anterior to the hips and swinging the trunk forward.

Kneeling Bench Exercises

Many patients experience difficulty balancing the trunk on the hips while kneeling. These patients should progress to kneeling bench exercises before kneeling crutch exercises. The bench (stool, box, chair, or bar) should reach to the greater trochanter when the patient is held upright in the kneeling position.

1. *Getter-Upper:* Patient balanced on hands and knees, bench between or just in front of hands. Patient shifts weight to one hand and places the other on the bench. The weight is then shifted to this hand, and the other hand is placed on the bench. With both hands on the bench he extends the forearms at the elbows, rolls the pelvis forward and comes to the erect (trunk) kneeling position. While primarily a balance exercise, this motion is used many times in daily activities.

2. *Bench-Shifter:* Erect kneeling position, slight flexion at elbows. By alternatively extending the forearms at the elbow, patient shifts weight from side to side.

3. *Dipper:* Erect kneeling position. Patient lowers chest to the bench and then returns to erect position.

4. *Four Pointer:* Erect kneeling position. Patient balances weight on both knees and one hand (right). With the other hand (left) he slides the bench forward several inches. He then rests his weight on both hands and slides the opposite knee (right) forward. Repeat, alternating hands and knees. This exercise may also be performed in a backward motion.

Exercises with Kneeling Mat Crutches

1. _Scooper:_ Patient balanced on hands and knees. Crutches placed on top of each other alongside of patient, axillary end level with knees. Patient shifts body weight to the hand on the side opposite the crutches. He "scoops" up the crutches with the other hand (grasping the hand pieces from backward forward). The crutches are placed vertically in front of the shoulder. Repeat with crutches on the other side. This is a basic exercise in learning how to handle both crutches with one hand as well as how to manage pick up and placement.

2. _Climber:_ Patient in position at end of "Scooper." He shifts weight to the hand on the crutches and then places the other hand on the lower part of the crutch shaft. By extending the forearms at the elbows, patient "climbs" up the shaft until both hands are on the hand pieces and the trunk has assumed the erect kneeling position.

3. _Kneeling-Crutch Stance:_ Patient in position at end of "Climber." Patient takes the uppermost crutch with the "Climber" hand and places it under the axilla on that side. After shifting body weight to that side, the other crutch is positioned in the axilla.

4. _Kneeling-Crutch Shifter:_ Kneeling-crutch stance position. Crutches slightly in front of knees, axillary portion held close to chest wall, weight carried on hands. Patient shifts weight from side to side.

5. _Kneeling-Crutch Lifter:_ Position as above (exercise 4). Patient shifts weight to one side, then lifts opposite crutch clear of mat. Repeat on opposite side.

6. _Kneeling-Crutch Forward Placer:_ Position as above (exercise 4). Patient shifts weight to one side, raises other crutch and places it forward several inches. Repeat, advancing other crutch. Return to starting position by reversing movement.

7. _Simultaneous Forward Crutch Placer:_ Position as above (exercise 4). Patient balances on knees, lifts both crutches at one time and places them several inches forward. Patient leans forward, pushes off and then places crutches in original position. Exercises 6 and 7 can also be performed in a backward direction. However, in both exercises the patient must roll his pelvis forward to prevent sudden trick-hip flexion.

Wheel Chair (and Armchair) Exercises

Occasionally some patients are unable to get on a mat or are excluded from mat exercises for various reasons. If the patient is permitted to sit up in a wheel chair or an armchair, several useful exercises can still be performed.

1. _Sitting Push-ups:_ Similar to mat push-ups except that knees are flexed.

2. _Sitting Balance:_ Patient leans forward in chair and balances trunk without holding chair arms.

3. _Sitting Balance Twister:_ Patient, in addition to leaning forward, twists first to one side and then to the other. As balance is learned with ease the exercise is progressed by placing the hands first on the chest and then on the head as twisting of the trunk is performed.

Parallel Bar Exercises

In parallel bars the patient is standing on his feet. Total body balance must be mastered before the patient can advance to crutch activities outside the parallel bars. Here the patient has the opportunity of locating his point of balance (center of gravity). The center of gravity of the body changes when there is considerable paralysis or weakness of the lower extremities and trunk. Here too, ambulatory motions without crutches can be initiated.

1. _Stancer:_ Parallel bars are raised to a height which permits the elbows to flex slightly when the hands grasp the bars. If indicated, the lower extremities are braced or placed in splints (14). Feet are placed 4–6 inches apart. Heat is held erect (chin in); trunk is balanced on the hips (as in kneeling erect). The hands are on the bars, several inches in front of the hips. Weight bearing is distributed on hands and feet.

2. _Parallel Bar Shifter:_ Stance position. Patient leans forward, placing body weight on hands, and returns to the starting position by pushing down on the bars. Patient may also shift weight to one hand and then to the other and can also shift body weight from side to side.

3. _Parallel Bar Arm Raiser:_ Stance position. Patient leans forward and places weight on both hands. After pushing off to return to starting position, one hand is raised from the bar. Patient leans forward, again replacing the hand, and repeats, lifting the other hand. Later, both hands are lifted simultaneously.

4. _Parallel Bar Push-up:_ Stance position. Patient pushes down on bars simultaneously, lifting feet clear of floor. He then lowers feet to floor and reestablishes point of balance.

5. _Parallel Bar Hip Hiker and Leg Swinger:_ Stance position. Patient shifts weight to one hand and foot (right), extends the opposite forearm (left), clears the floor with the left foot. Return to balance position. Repeat on opposite side. Later, the extremity which is hiked is swung back and forth (either with intrinsic hip musculature or by displacement of body weight) before being replaced on the floor.

6. _Four-Point Gait Drill:_ Stance position. Patient moves the right hand forward on the bar, places weight on right hand and foot, hikes the left hip and places the left leg forward. The left hand is now placed forward and body weight is shifted to the left extremities, while the right hip is hiked and the extremity advanced. Patient must push off (not pull) with the hand on the same side as the leg being advanced. Sliding handgrips can be used on the parallel bars to discourage the patient from "pulling" rather than "pushing off."

7. _Drag-to Gait Drill:_ Stance position. Patient places both hands forward several inches on the bars, leans the trunk forward so that the elbows flex slightly. Bearing down on both hands, the elbows straighten and the body is lifted sufficiently to permit dragging the feet to hand position.

8. _Swing-to Gait Drill:_ Stance position. Patient goes through the same motion as in above. However, this time the body is lifted clear of the floor and feet are swung to the hand-position.

9. _Swing-Through Gait Drill:_ Stance position. Patient performs same motion as above, however, this time as legs are swung forward they go beyond the hand position. As the feet touch the floor the pelvis must be rolled forward and the hands brought up to or in front of the feet.

10. _Sideward Gait Drill:_ Stance position, facing one bar, with both hands on the same bar. Patient places right hand several inches to the right, bears weight on both hands and left leg, hikes right hip and moves right leg to the right. Body weight is now placed on both hands and right leg, left hip is hiked and left leg moves to the right. Left hand is moved to the right to assume stance position. This should also be practiced moving to the left.

11. _Backward Four-Point Gait Drill:_ Stance position. Patient shifts body weight to the right side, hip hikes on the left and moves the left leg backward. Weight is shifted to the left side. The right hand is moved backward, followed by hiking the right hip and moving that leg backward. Displace body weight to the right and move left hand backward to assume stance position.

12. _Backward Swing Gait Drill:_ Stance position. Patient places both hands slightly behind hips, carrying body weight on the hands as the trunk "jacks" slightly. By pushing down forcibly on the bars, the body is lifted from the floor and swung backward. Depending on strength of the uppers and coordination, the patient may swing the feet to or through the hands.

13. _Ascending Forward Drill (Leg-Swing):_ Stance position facing a small stool or platform (5 cm or 2 inches at first). Patient shifts body weight to the right, hikes the left hip and swings the left leg until it clears the platform edge. Weight is then shifted forward on both hands. By pushing down on the bars some of the body weight is transmitted to the left leg. As a result, the right leg is free of the body weight. The right hip is hiked, and the leg is swung forward onto the platform. In actual practice, the hip with the strongest hiker and flexors is the one first elevated to the platform.

14. _Ascending Forward Drill (Swing-up):_ Stance position facing platform. Distance of patient from platform depends on height to be ascended and strength of hip flexors. Patient shifts body weight to both hands; elbows flex slightly. By bearing down forcibly on hands, body is raised from the floor and the legs are swung onto the platform. As the body

continues forward (momentum of swing) both hands are brought forward on the bars.

15. *Ascending Backward Drill (Leg Swing):* Stance position, facing away from platform. Patient shifts weight to the right side, hikes the left hip and swings the left leg backward until it clears the platform edge. Hands are worked backward alternately until body weight is on the left leg and the right leg hangs free. The right hip is hiked and swung backward onto the platform. In practice the side with the stronger hip hiker and extensors is the one first placed on the platform.

16. *Ascending Backward Drill (Back-Jack):* Stance position, facing away from platform, though heels may touch platform. Patient places hands slightly in front of hips, trunk leans forward and elbows flex. Keeping head down, patient bears down forcibly on the bars so that hips are raised upward and backward, clearing the platform edge with the feet. As soon as feet land on the platform patient releases hands, brings them back and rolls pelvis forward.

17. *Descending Forward Drill (Hip Hiking):* Stance position on platform at edge. Patient places hand ahead of hips, flexing trunk. Shifting weight to right side, patient hikes the left side until the heel rests on the platform edge. He then shifts weight to left side and hikes the right hip, bringing the right foot forward until it clears the platform edge. Shifting weight to both hands, he hikes the left hip till the left foot also clears the platform edge and lowers the body slowly until both feet touch the floor. Patient then rolls pelvis forward and assumes stance position.

18. *Descending Forward Drill (Stepping-off):* Stance position on platform at edge. Patient places hands ahead of hips, flexing trunk. He then shifts weight to right side, hikes left hip, swings the left foot forward until it clears the platform edge and places it on the floor. The patient bears down forcibly on both hands and hikes the right hip, the right foot is swung until it clears the platform edge and is placed on the floor. Pelvis is rolled forward and patient assumes stance position.

19. *Descending Forward Drill (Swing-off):* Stance position at platform edge. Patient places hands ahead of hips, flexing trunk. Body weight is shifted forward on both hands. By pushing down forcibly on the hands the body is lifted clear of the platform edge and is swung forward to or through the hands.

The foregoing drills for gaits and elevation activities are basic and fundamental. The usual progression from the parallel bars is to one crutch and one bar, and then to two crutches in wide parallel bars. The final progression is to two crutches, at first with the support of a wall, a cyclone fence or a bar, and later without any support. In each of these areas of training, the drill progression repeats itself from balance to strength and endurance through coordination and the performance of a skilled activity.

REFERENCES

1. BACHYNSKI, B. A mechanical aid to walking. *J. Bone Joint Surg., 35A:* 1013, 1953.
2. BLODGETT, M. L. The art of crutch walking. *Occup. Ther. Rehabil., 25:* 27, 1946.
3. BLOUNT, W. P. Don't throw away the cane. *J. Bone Joint Surg., 38A:* 695, 1956.
4. BUHLER, J. Safety device to prevent sliding of crutches. *Wein. Klin. Wochenschr. 63:* 801, 1951.
5. CICENIA, E. F., AND HOBERMAN, M. Parallel bar activities in physical therapy and rehabilitation. *Am. J. Phys. Med., 34:* 591, 1955.
6. CICENIA, E. F. Crutches and crutch management. *Am. J. Phys. Med., 36:* 359, 1957; Crutch management drills. *Modern Med., 26:* 86, 1958.
7. CULLINAN, J. F. A new formula for teaching crutch ambulation to paraplegics. *Occu. Ther. Rehabil., 26:* 85, 1947.
8. DEAVER, G. G., AND BROWN, M. E. The challenge of crutches. I., II., III., IV., V., VI., *Arch. Phys. Med., 26:* 397, 515, 573, 747, 1945; and *27:* 141, 683, 1946.
9. DEAVER, G. G. What every physician should know about teaching crutch walking. *J.A.M.A., 142:* 470, 1950.
10. Editorial. Crutch mastery. *Am. J. Surg., 73:* 404, 1947.
11. EPSTEIN, S. Crutches of yesterday. *Hebr. J. Med., 1:* 201, 1938.
12. GINGRAS, G., AND WHALLEY, G. A new metal folding adjustable crutch. *Treat. Serv. Bull., 3:* 40, 1948.
13. HARRIS, D. M. Crutch balancing. *Phys. Ther. Rev., 30:* 424, 1950.
14. HOBERMAN, M., AND CICENIA, E. F. A simple splint with knee cap as an aid in precrutch training. *Phys. Ther. Rev., 30:* 378, 1950.
15. HOBERMAN, M., ET AL. The use of lead-up functional exercises to supplement mat work. *Phys. Ther. Rev., 31:* 1, 1951.
16. HOBERMAN, M. Rehabilitation techniques with braces and crutches. I., II., III. *Occup. Ther. Rehabil., 30:* 203, 282, 377, 1951; and IV., V., VI., *Am. J. Phys. Med., 31:* 21, 82, 373, 1952.
17. HOLLIDAY, R. C. *Walking Stick Papers.* New York, 1918.
18. LESTER, K. M., AND OERKE, B. V. *Accessories of Dress.* Peoria, 1940.
19. LOVETT, R. W. The tripod method of walking with crutches. *J.A.M.A., 74:* 1306, 1920.
20. MAHONEY, H. T. The after-care of poliomyelitis. III. Teaching coordination and balance. *Am. J. Nurs., 32:* 14, 1932.
21. MILANES, M., McCOOK, J., AND HERNANDEZ, A. L. Thromboarteritis due to crutches. *Angiologia, 4:* 37, 1952.
22. NELSON, D. Crutch walking, or how to teach a patient to use crutches. *Am. J. Nurs., 39:* 1088, 1939.
23. OLMSTED, L. Crutch walking. *Am. J. Nurs., 45:* 28, 1945.
24. PARK, H. W., MALONE, E. W., AND STREGLICH, R. Tilted crutch handpiece. *Arch. Phys. Med., 33:* 731, 1952.
25. REAL, A. *The Story of the Stick in All Ages and Lands.* New York, 1875.
26. ROLLING, A., AND BINDA, B. A case of thromboarteritis due to crutches. *Angiologia. 2:* 145, 1950.
27. RUDIN, L. N., AND LEVINE, L. Bilateral compression of radial nerve (crutch paralysis). *Phys. Ther. Rev., 31:* 229, 1951.
28. SANDERS, E. M. Mobilization of paraplegics. III. Crutch walking. *Occup. Ther. Rehabil., 30:* 61, 1951.
29. VALLS-SERRA, J. Arteritis due to crutches. *Angiologia, 3:* 59, 1951.
30. VINEBERG, A. M., AND BOWEN, H. B. A self-stabilizing triple grip base crutch. *Can. Med. Assoc. J., 52:* 613, 1945.
31. WRIGHT, W. Crutch-walking as an art. *Am. J. Surg., 1:* 372, 1926.

11

Gait and
Gait Retraining

PAUL J. CORCORAN AND
M. PESZCZYNSKI

The purpose of this chapter (now extensively revised by P.J.C.) is to present the scope of normal and abnormal gait, and the problems connected with both, and to discuss the limitations of the exact knowledge in this area. We shall also concentrate on *gait pathology*—how to examine for it, how to evaluate the results of the examination and to prognosticate—and on the principles of *gait retraining*. The emphasis will be on gait problems of the adult and the aged rather than on the normal and abnormal locomotor development of children.

For didactic reasons, pathological gaits resulting from weaknesses of single muscles in the lower extremities will be presented as well as abnormal gait patterns which are not covered in other chapters in this book but which are problems frequently encountered in physical medicine departments.

We should like to begin by reviewing briefly and mentioning some of the milestones in the historical development of research on the subject of gait. Some excellent observational studies in the analysis of gait were done by the Weber brothers as early as 1836 (59). Marey's (30) photographic method of analyzing movements of the extremities laid a basis for Braune and Fischer's (22) 1895 mathematical calculations of velocities and accelerations, and the computation of forces involved in lower extremity movement. During the span of time between World Wars I and II Scherb (51) contributed a great deal of basic information in the myokinetics of gait. He evaluated the role of individual muscles and the sequence of muscle activities during ambulation. Schwartz (52), among others, added methods of evaluating the reaction from the floor and measuring ground pressure. More recently Inman and the University of California group (56) refined electromyographic (EMG) data on the functioning of particular muscle groups during the normal ambulation process, and shed some light on the function of the hip and the forces rotating the long axis of the lower extremities.

Steindler (55) made an extensive review of existing knowledge in the area of pathological gait, especially orthopedic types of disorders. He also included many of his own findings in this review, particularly in the area of indications for and prognosis of surgical interventions to gain ambulation or to improve gait function. Drillis (17) reported an extensive biomechanical analysis of a number of pathological gaits. Morton (15) studied the distribution of forces between segments of the foot and the floor, particularly their influence on disorders of the foot. He also discussed some of the concepts of the role of developmental factors in the functioning of the lower extremities. Taylor and his group (57) investigated the influences of rest and movement, including gait, on different factors, with special attention to the cardiovascular system. Shortly after World War II, Leithauser (27) made his well-known contribution of the value of early ambulation following major surgical interventions. Basmajian (3) has reviewed the EMG data on normal locomotion. In the past decade, a number of gait laboratories (10, 25, 54) have increased the sophistication of gait analysis and added to the basic understanding of how people walk.

Around the time of World War I groundwork was laid by Benedict and Murschhauser (4) in energy expenditure during different variations of normal gait. Later Gordon and Vanderwalde (23) as well as Bard and Ralston (2) presented data on the energy expended by patients with certain disabilities during ambulation. Passmore and Durnin (39) reviewed the energy cost of a variety of human activities and McDonald (32) reviewed and collated the world literature on the energy expenditure of normal human locomotion as it related to a variety of physical parameters. Corcoran (11) reviewed methods of measuring energy expenditure and results of studies of handicapped ambulation. Murray (36) and Shoup (53) reported on the effects of crutches and canes on the biomechanics of locomotion.

It has long been known that mood and personality influence gait; it is becoming more and more evident that, in addition to the still fairly unknown factors enabling neurological control of muscle activities during ambulation, the different levels of sensory functioning, especially those of the person's image of his own body, his concept of his body in space, and the degree to which he is actually able to perceive space correctly, are all of paramount importance in understanding normal and abnormal gait.

Biomechanics of Gait

Biomechanics was the first aspect of ambulation to be analyzed thoroughly, and hence most of the exact knowledge about gait pertains to this area (18).

Each leg alternately goes through a stance phase and a swing phase during the ambulation process. The stance phase (also called the support phase) begins at the moment the heel touches the ground when the leg is advanced and ends the moment the toes leave the ground after the push-off and when the leg is still behind the body. The span of time that both legs are simultaneously in the supporting phase is called the period of double support. The center of gravity of the trunk rises and falls an average of 5 cm (2 inches) with each step. Normal adult males average 110 steps/minute (17, 20) at an average speed of 3 miles/hour (11, 17, 20, 45). Thus, a 70-kg (155-lb) man walking at 3 miles/hour does 310 inch-pounds of work with each step, or 2,842 ft-lb/minute. Since 3,086 ft-lb/minute are equal to 1.0 kcal/minute, and assuming 23% efficiency (112), 4 kcal/minute are required to raise and lower the center of gravity of the trunk during normal ambulation. This alone accounts for about 90% of the 4.3 kcal/minute energy cost (11, 45) of walking at 3 miles/hour. The remaining 10% may be attributed to the work of accelerating and decelerating the limb segments and trunk, and overcoming the internal viscosity of the tissues.

If the lower extremities and their connection to the trunk via the pelvis are represented by rigid poles with only one axis through the hips (50), forward movement of the center of gravity of the body would proceed along a path characterized by a series of arcs with high amplitudes and a marked sinusoidal lateral displacement. The continuous marked changes of elevation, lateral direction, and velocity would require a great deal of energy to produce a movement. Instead of this extravagant inefficiency there are different determinants which allow the center of gravity of the human body to move with an almost even velocity along a complex but mild spiral curve and produce movement with the least expenditure of energy. These determinants are (50):

1. The movement of the swinging hip, which is faster than that of the stance hip, that is, pelvic rotation in a horizontal plane.
2. The lowering of the pelvis on the side of the swinging leg (pelvic tilt in the frontal plane).
3. Slight flexion (15°) of the knee of the supporting leg shortly after the heel-strike (between the so-called double lock of the knee).
4. A shifting of the axis of the radius of the supporting leg from the heel to the forefoot.
5. The knee flexion associated with the heel-rise at the end of the stance phase.
6. The lateral displacement of the pelvis toward the weight-bearing side.

Interference with these determinants may result in either physiologically borderline gaits or definitely pathological gaits.

The young adult is very efficient during his normal walking pace. The comfortable walking speed of 3 miles/hour corresponds to the speed at which the energy cost *per unit of distance* (i.e., the work of walking) is minimal (13, 45). It also falls in the range of speed where EMG activity in the lower extremities is minimal (34), and where the natural pendulum periodicity of the lower limb is approximately the same as the optimal cadence. In different moments of the stance and swing phases of the lower extremities much of the actual work of moving the body forward is performed by gravity and inertia instead of propulsion produced by muscle contractions. Superimposition of EMG and electrogoniometric data (23, 49) demonstrates that most of the muscular activity is occurring while the muscle is lengthening, or eccentric, contractions, which provide greater force and efficiency than shortening, or concentric, contractions (26).

In summary, then, the forward movement of the main mass, i.e., the trunk, is produced by inertia resulting from previously imposed velocities (preceding steps, among other factors), by the work of gravity permitted to occur during the controlled loss of balance and to a lesser degree by propulsion produced by the contracting muscles of the extremities.

Normal and Abnormal Myokinetics

This description of the action of specific muscle groups of the lower extremity during the ambulation of an average, normal, young adult has been extracted mainly from the findings of the University of California group (56), while the simplified description of pathological gaits due to weaknesses of single muscle groups essentially follows analysis of Long's (28) presentation of the subject (Fig. 11.1).

The most pronounced activity of the pre-tibial group (lengthening contraction) is noted immediately after the heel-strike. This group controls

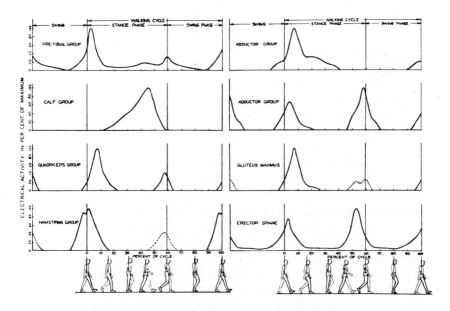

Fig. 11.1. Idealized summary curves representing phasic action of major muscle groups during level walking. Derived from EMG studies of 10 adult males walking at the rate of 95 steps per minute. (———) Consistent activity; (-----) less consistent activity. Reprinted with permission from the University of California publication *Prosthetic Devices Research*.

the plantar flexion of the foot at that time and prevents slapping of the forefoot on the ground. The second most prominent activity occurs about the time of take-off in dorsiflexing the foot (shortening contraction) so that the toes clear the ground during the swing phase.

Paralysis or marked weakness of the pre-tibial group produces such symptoms as a slapping of the forefoot immediately after the heel-strike and a foot drop during the swing phase. Excessive knee and hip flexion (steppage gait) is usually used to compensate for the foot drop. Occasionally if the hip flexors are too weak to produce the high steppage gait, the foot may instead be dragged, with the entire lower extremity externally rotated. This type of gait is also seen in patients with plantar flexion spasticity for whom a steppage gait is not feasible because of extensor spasticity of the whole lower extremity. Moderate weakness of the dorsiflexors of the foot may not produce a foot drop at all during the swing phase, but a foot-slap will definitely be evident. Mild weakness of the dorsiflexors may be noticed, as foot slapping, only when the subject is tired or is walking rapidly.

The muscular activity of the calf group builds up from mid-stance and controls (lengthening contraction) the forward fall of the body. It gradually stabilizes (isometric contraction) the angle between the shank and the foot after the axis of rotation has shifted from the heel to the center of the metatarsal heads and permits the heel to be lifted off the ground. Finally, at the last moment of the propulsion phase, the calf muscles contract (shortening contraction), thereby maintaining the height of the pelvis at the end of the stance. At the same time they assist the shift from the gravitational energy of the forward falling (dropping of the center of gravity) as the phase of double support is reached, into the kinetic energy of the forward translation or propulsion.

Paralysis or weakness of the calf muscles may be characterized by both dropping of the pelvis on the affected side and slowing of its forward movement at the last moment of the stance phase. At moderate speeds, a patient may compensate both features by contracting the abductors and rotators of the opposite hip at the phase of double support. In contradistinction to the medius limp, where the drop and lag of the hip occur on the side opposite to the muscle weakness, these occur on the same side in the calf muscle limp and are of a more momentary character. The medius limp diminishes with quicker gaits, while the calf muscle limp is accentuated with rapid walking.

The major activity of the quadriceps is noted shortly after heel-strike and is associated with the cushioning effect of the mild knee-bend which occurs between the double locking of the knee. The second most prominent activity of this muscle may be noticed at the transition from the stance to the swing phase, and it probably acts as a hip flexor to initiate the swing.

When the quadriceps in paralyzed, extension of the knee on weight bearing is produced by contraction of the hip extensors, which drive the distal femur, and thus the knee; backward. A secondary role in the extension of the knee on weight bearing can be ascribed to the plantar flexion activity of the calf muscle group, which similarly may drive the proximal tibia, and thus the knee, backward. Some patients enhance their backward knee movement by pressing against the anterior thigh with the hand; often this is done quite unobtrusively with the hand in the pants pocket. Thus the quadriceps limp is characterized by forcible extension of the knee at heel-strike concomitant with the forward drive of the involved hip. Constant hyperextension of the knee as a stabilizing and compensating mechanism in the early stance phase eventually results in a genu recurvatum.

During a normal walking pace the activity of the hamstrings occurs at about the time of heel-strike. Just prior to heel-strike at the end of the swing phase the hamstrings, acting as knee flexors decelerate (lengthening contraction) the forward swing of the leg. At the time of heel-strike and immediately afterward, acting as hip extensors they decelerate and eventually prevent the pelvis and trunk from flexing forward on the femur (inertia). At the beginning of the stance phase the functions of the hamstrings are reinforced and taken over by the activity of the gluteus maximus.

Isolated weakness of the maximus is rare. When we talk about the "maximus gait" we actually mean weakness or paralysis of the hip extensors as a group. The hip extensor gait ("maximus gait") is characterized by an apparent anterior protrusion of the affected hip immediately after the heel of the involved extremity strikes the floor. It is produced by a forcible backward thrust of the trunk to counteract the inertia-produced forward movement of the trunk and to keep the center of gravity behind the hip joint. A tightly extended knee in mid-stance is also typical of the "maximus gait."

The major activity of the hip flexors occurs at the beginning of the swing phase, and was discussed in connection with the function of the quadriceps (rectus femoris). It is typically most pronounced in the isolated iliopsoas weakness resulting from poliomyelitis but is not too rarely seen in some severely handicapped hemiplegic patients who are unable to initiate the swing phase of the involved leg by flexing their affected hip. If the patient is not able to shorten the involved lower extremity during the swing phase, a backward thrust of the trunk is associated with circumduction, a lateral movement of the trunk toward the unaffected side which elevates the hip to enable the affected leg to clear the ground during the swing phase.

The main activity of the hip abductor group occurs as the body weight is assumed by the stance leg, and it gradually diminishes (lengthening contraction) while controlling the downward list (gravity) of the opposite side of the pelvis.

Weakness of the hip abductors produces the so-called gluteus medius gait. When uncompensated, this gait is characterized by a greater than normal dropping of the pelvis on the unaffected (opposite) side during its swing phase, an apparent lateral protrusion of the affected hip on weight bearing, and most distinctly by a lateral sliding of the upper two-thirds of the trunk and the head toward the affected side, caused by movement of the lumbar spine. This movement brings the center of gravity of the main mass of the body closer to the axis of the supporting affected hip without excessive dipping of the affected shoulder. A forward swinging of the shoulder on the unaffected side may accompany the stance phase of the affected limb, reinforcing the weak rotatory functions of the medius by carrying the unaffected hip forward at the termination of the arc of stance of the affected limb. If the gluteus medius weakness results from a lesion of the motor roots of L.4 and L.5, the pretibial group will also be weak and a steppage gait may also be present.

The so-called compensated gluteus medius gait is seen in patients with a severely weakened gluteus medius. It may occur when the patient who usually walks with an uncompensated gait experiences discomfort or pain, or wishes to avoid the cosmetic or social stigma associated with excessive pelvic movement. The "compensated gluteus medius gait" is characterized by an apparent medial deviation of the hip on the affected side during weight bearing to bring the axis of rotation of the supporting hip beneath the main mass of the body. This apparent medial deviation occurs simultaneously with a marked bending of the entire trunk sideward over the affected hip on weight bearing, and a resultant dipping of the shoulder on the affected side. The thrust of the trunk toward the affected side lifts the opposite hip, and thereby makes clearance of the ground possible during the swing of the unaffected lower extremity.

The function of the hip adductor mass during ambulation is complex, and the details are less well known. The major activity of the group occurs during the early swing phase and is considered to be related to the abrupt external rotation of the femur at the end of the stance phase as an expression of some of the main forces of propulsion of the body. When this external rotation cannot be absorbed by the foot (lifting of the longitudinal arch) at this phase, the patient may show a marked movement of the heel inwardly along a circle, the center of which is the ball of the forefoot. A minor activity of the hip adductors occurs at the beginning of the stance phase and is thought to assist the hip abductors in stabilizing the hip.

The increased energy required in the presence of joint immobilization was studied by Ralston (46). Hip immobilization at 150° caused less of an energy increase than either 180° or 120°. Knee immobilization caused significant increases at fast walking speeds or when the angle of flexion was 135° or greater. Ankle immobilization caused negligible increases.

Pain on weight-bearing causes a characteristic "antalgic" gait which appears similar whether the pain arises from the hip, knee, ankle, or foot. The patient minimizes the duration of the stance phase, and abruptly jerks the head, arms, and upper trunk downward at the onset of stance. The decreased pain resulting from a decrease in the downward force of gravity on the painful lower extremity can be appreciated by anyone who has had to walk with a stone in the shoe.

General Considerations

Biomechanical data on the gait changes occurring with age or pathology of the locomotor or neurological systems are beginning to accumulate in gait laboratories. The little information which does exist about the maturing of the neuromuscular and locomotor systems during the first years of human life is derived primarily from clinical observations. The high degree of efficiency which the young adult demonstrates in his normal gait is developed during the second decade of life. Robinson (48) found that prior to age 17 the rate of energy expenditure is higher (i.e., less efficient) for a given walking speed; thereafter it is relatively stable well into old age. Burnett and Johnson (9) reported on a detailed study of the development of gait in childhood, and found adult gait patterns appearing as early as 2 years.

In a study of gait patterns Murray (37) found that men over age 60 tended to show slower free walking speed, shorter stride, wider base, slower cadence, lower swing-to-stance time ratio, and greater floor-to-foot clearance. In another study of normal women (38), she found (in agreement with Finley and co-workers) (20, 21) that women walk slower than men, due almost entirely to shorter stride lengths related to shorter stature and limb length. Women walking in high heels (33, 38) show still slower velocity and shorter stride length, and a 10–15% increase in energy expenditure (31).

Curiously, mean pedestrian speed and pedestrian density are inversely related (6); i.e., people walk faster in crowded places. Individuals in a crowd tend to walk at fairly uniform speeds, creating difficulties for the disabled pedestrian who must walk slower due to the higher energy cost of handicapped ambulation. Even in crowds, women normally walk somewhat slower than men (5).

Any study of the effects of ageing is complicated by the difficulty of differentiating between physiological and pathological ageing. In his search for psychological tests which can be used to differentiate between physiological aging and the effects of brain damage, Hallenbeck (24) found that accuracy and speed of motor performance are both impaired with the former while poor behavior in novel situations is a result of the latter.

Describing the neurological changes of age, Critchley (15) stressed the fact that the aged person's gait has features of an involutional process which primarily affect the extrapyramidal system. The aged have an attitude of general flexion. They hold their heads and necks in a forward flexed position and show a gentle dorsal kyphosis. In addition, their hips and knees are slightly flexed. The mild rigidity of the muscles is more noticeable in the proximal segments of the extremities than in the distal segments, in the legs more than in the arms. There is general poverty of automatic movements, and associated movements are reduced in amplitude and speed. Strangely enough, the old motor system seems to be more affected than are the pyramidal and cerebellar systems.

When we try to translate some of Critchley's clinical observations of the gait of the aged into what we know about biomechanics, it can be said that their gait is characterized by the least expenditure of energy possible within the remaining abilities of the locomotor apparatus. The old person is less able to use gravity and inertia in ambulation and therefore must resort to actual muscle work. There is diminished ability to use adequately the determinants of gait which allow saving of energy. People of advanced age have an increased likelihood of tripping over small objects, and they have great difficulty in regaining their balance once they have started to fall. The aged person takes short steps because he does not have enough accuracy and speed, especially in control of the hip musculature, to be able intermittently to lose and recover the same amount of balance the young adult can lose and recover during the swing phase of ambulation. Shorter steps are also an adaptation to the decreased rotation of the pelvis. Probably the degree to which the aged bend their knees while walking is almost the same as the optimal degree of flexion in which knees should be fused and still permit the most efficient gait for a patient.

Danowski and Wratney (16) have published a list of averages of muscle strengths according to age and sex. They discussed the probable influence endocrinological factors have on strength changes occurring in different muscle groups throughout the lifespan, but they did not include a discussion of how these age- and sex-produced changes in muscle strength are related to the characteristics of the gait in each of the groups under consideration.

Controlled data pertaining to the influence of metabolic changes such as fatigue, moods, and intake of drugs (alcohol) on gait are very limited, as are those describing the effects of sleepiness, body build, posture and awareness of posture, education, and professional and vocational habits. Steindler (55) listed and briefly described some of the physiologically borderline types of gait. His review of pathological gaits deals predominantly with such factors as the influence of one shortened leg, joint fusions or limitations of joint motion, pain within the locomotor system and adjustments of the organism to such individual and complex muscle weaknesses as those most commonly produced by poliomyelitis.

Even the most superficial discussion of pathological gait and gait retraining would be inadequate if the different levels of sensory functioning, the influence of the organization of neuromuscular functioning, energy expenditures and the ability of the cardiovascular system to adjust itself to energy requirements of different types of locomotion were not touched upon.

We are very gradually learning more about the distortions of our perception of the space around us as well as our concept of the position of our bodies in this space. Bruell (7) found a high statistical correlation between the degree of a hemiplegic patient's inability visually to judge deviation from upright in a dark room and this same patient's inability to learn to walk independently and safely. A particular example of a patient's disorganized concept of his position in space is his feeling that he is upright when he is really leaning backward (43). This happens in younger patients after they have been bedfast for a prolonged period and in old people after even short bed confinements.

Bruell (7) found that with physiological aging the ability visually to judge deviations from upright is diminished markedly. Other postural information, including proprioception, is similarly impaired in the aged. There are good reasons to believe that the aged are even more handicapped when they have to judge the upright while walking than when standing still.

Some elderly people with brain injury can attain limited independence in walking only when they stop after every other step to regain their balance (intermittent double step gait) (42).

Very little has been learned about the higher functions involved in ambulation. Most of the available neurological information about motor ability pertains to posture or to righting reflexes, but data about the neurophysiology of ambulation itself are very scarce. For example, in patients with far-advanced Parkinson's disease, the problem is more in the area of the "volition" to initiate walking for a given distance. Very often just approaching this patient and ordering, "Stand up and walk," are enough to elicit a satisfactory motor response. It is well known that under conditions of extreme stress, such as the threat of fire in the home, parkinsonians are able to get up and run.

Some degrees of apraxia of the lower extremities are not too different from the above-described patterns. On the other hand, there are apraxias in which the ability to perform a meaningful complex movement is lost. For instance, some hemiplegic patients have lost or have an impaired foot placing reaction and its application in the transition from the swing phase to the stance phase of the hemiplegic leg. Another form of apraxia of ambulation is characterized by the fact that the patient can walk automatically only when he is not concentrating on the movement of his legs.

Although very little is known about the sudden collapses of either the legs or the whole body which are rather commonly seen in the advanced age groups, the blame is tentatively placed on abnormal functioning of the higher levels of the gamma motor system. A large percentage of the cases in which dizziness interferes with older people's ability to walk is also blamed on disorders of the nervous system (43).

Gordon and Vanderwalde (23) and Clinkingbeard and Gersten (10) studied the energy cost of paraplegic ambulation. They drew attention to the value of objective information about energy expenditure when patients with different degrees of impaired neuromuscular functioning ambulate with and without assistive devices. It would appear from their preliminary data that there is a close relationship between the amount of energy expended while walking and the amount of nonfunctioning of the neuromuscular apparatus. They point out that the ceiling for sustained paraplegic ambulation (or, for that matter, for normal ambulation) (11) is an energy expenditure 5–6 times higher than the basic metabolic rate of the individual. The energy cost for paraplegic ambulation is 2–4 times that for able-bodied persons walking at the same speed. It increases rapidly with small increments in speed, limiting paraplegic crutch-walking to 1.0–1.5 miles/hour. Wheelchair ambulation, by contrast, requires no more energy than normal walking at the same speed (25). Gordon and Vander-walde (23) suggest that in addition to the degree of disability, energy expenditure is modified by age, weight, degree of spasticity and the patient's inherent agility and coordination as shown in his economy of motion and in his stride pattern. Clinkingbeard and Gersten (10) found that 4–6 weeks of paraplegic gait training were required to reduce energy costs to their lowest level and that they rise significantly again after a few months of nonwalking.

Energy expenditure depends on:

Erdman et al. (19) and Traugh et al. (58) found that elderly above-knee amputees expend 60–70% more energy than able-bodied walkers, whether using a prosthesis or walking on crutches without a prosthesis. Other studies have shown lower energy costs for younger above-knee amputees. Locking or unlocking the knee produced only small changes, and amputees had lower energy costs with the knee lock set in their preferred mode, whether locked or free. A hydraulic knee joint produced a 10% savings of energy at fast walking speeds (2.7 miles/hour), but not at the 1–2 miles/hour speeds which are ordinary for above-knee amputees (44).

Below-knee prosthetic ambulation requires negligible (10%) increases in energy cost with adequate stump length and greater increases (40%) with short stumps. Even bilateral below-knee amputees, however, require less energy to walk (40–45% above normal) than unilateral above-knee amputees (12). This underscores the importance of salvaging the knee joint, if possible, during amputation surgery. Bilateral above-knee amputees require energy expenditures of more than twice those of able-bodied ambulators, and are limited to speeds of less than 1 mile/hour. Their speeds and energy costs are comparable to those of paraplegics. Patients with hemiplegia expend 65% more energy than normal subjects, but this can be reduced to 52% by use of an ankle-foot orthosis to control the equinovarus deformity (14). Their speeds and energy costs are comparable to those of unilateral above-knee amputees. Thus the energy cost and speed implications are about the same for prosthetic lower limbs as for paralyzed, braced lower limbs.

It should be remembered that persons walking with gait disorders are not ordinarily expending energy at a greater rate than the 4–5 kcal/minute of normal subjects; instead, they are purchasing less speed for the same expenditure of energy. However, with very severe locomotor disabilities (e.g., paraplegia or bilateral above-knee amputation) the energy costs do become higher than this, even at their extremely slow walking speeds.

The ability of the cardiovascular system to adjust itself to the requirements of being upright changes markedly after a prolonged period in bed. Taylor et al. (57) found that young adults needed 7 weeks of recovery to regain the degree of cardiovascular response to posture they had prior to 3 weeks of recumbency. There are good reasons to believe that in the aged the recovery of the cardiovascular system is more delayed after even shorter periods of being bedfast.

Examination of Gait

As in all other aspects of a clinical examination the physician who describes a patient's gait must have an adequate knowledge of this field. He must know the principles of the mechanics of normal gait, be able to analyze physiological borderline variations of gaits, be familiar with the classical pathological gaits caused by single muscle paralyses or limitations of range of motion, and have a good mental picture of the locomotion disorders found in different neuromuscular impairments, including those which are a reaction to pain. Sometimes awareness of the existence of a variety of causes for an excessive or asymmetrical movement of body parts is essential.

When examining a patient having an abnormal gait pattern, certain principles must be adhered to. After having taken the patient's medical history, the examiner should have the patient demonstrate his gait several times so that he can try to pinpoint the primary abnormal characteristic. It is essential that the patient be asked to change the pace of his ambulation several times, since some disorders may be noticed only during quick walking and others are pronounced only during very slow ambulation. Similarly, standing up, sitting down, walking uphill and downhill or climbing stairs may bring out the abnormalities of his gait. While the patient is walking, each joint should be watched separately and a mental comparison made with normal function. Special attention should also be directed to the swing of the upper extremities. The first impression will not be complete unless the patient is asked to stop suddenly, to make turns, to pass objects and other persons and to go through a doorway.

The possibility of an accumulation of imbalance during consecutive steps must be considered, and the examiner should determine whether a patient who needs mild assistance while walking will be able to walk without the assistance if asked to stop after every other step (42). Hopping on one leg is one of the more sensitive tests for evaluating the patient's ability to recover his balance. The complete examination should include asking the patient to walk with his eyes closed. This will not only enable differentiation between different ataxias but will also give some picture of the patient's orientation in space. A simple screening test that can be used for a more detailed examination of the strength of the muscles is to ask the patient to walk on his tiptoes or on his heels. Quadriceps and gluteus maximus strength may be assessed by asking the patient to arise from a chair using only one lower extremity. Stair ascent and descent also indicate the strength of these muscles as well as general stamina and balance. The patient should also be asked to walk barefoot, or the soles and heels of his shoes may be checked for areas of marked wear.

It is best to analyze the patient both while he is walking as relaxed and automatically as possible and while he is asked to concentrate on giving his best walking performance. Patients having some disorders may, when asked to concentrate, be able to stop shuffling, to shorten the swinging leg properly or to dorsiflex the foot in which a tendon transplant has recently been performed.

In disorders of the central nervous system it is essential to determine whether any differences exist between performance of particular motor functions while the patient is lying down and when walking, to indicate the degree to which postural reflexes and patterns assist or hamper the patient's ability to walk. While lying down a hemiplegic patient may show no voluntarily active flexion of the hip, but while he is walking he may be able to initiate the swing of the lower extremity with his hip flexors. Another patient may be able to dorsiflex his involved foot while in bed or sitting, but will drag this foot in a plantar flexed position during the swing phase of ambulation (40). A patient with some knee flexion spasticity when in a supine position may demonstrate a strong, well-supporting extensor thrust when standing or walking. Impaired proprioception reaction may be the reason a patient who has fairly adequate voluntary movements of the involved foot when sitting is not able to strike the floor automatically at the end of the swing phase of the involved lower extremity.

A patient who uses assistive devices such as canes or crutches should be asked to walk with and, within reason, without these devices. For example, the patient with a right gluteus medius weakness may walk almost normally if he uses a cane in his left hand, but without the cane he may revert to the classical gluteus medius gait. Occasionally a patient must be ambulated between parallel bars to ascertain the degree of his unawareness that he is not maintaining an upright position while walking (7).

Bizarre gait patterns which fit no known syndrome should make the examiner suspect a hysterical gait, which should be differentiated by individual muscle examination and observation of the patient when he is not aware of being watched. Worden and Johnson (60) have described five characteristic signs of hysterical paralysis: 1), cogwheel response, a jerky relaxation of the muscle being tested; 2), inconsistencies, when apparently flaccid muscles contract during functional activities; 3), bizarre gaits which lack a pattern consistent with known pathology; 4), slow-motion effect, in which movements are done in a slow and more laborious fashion; and 5), overflow of activity into unrelated areas such as the trunk or upper extremities.

Once the patient's main problems have been identified or several probable diagnoses are suspected, he is subjected to a more thorough examination, such as measuring the length of the extremities, checking for limitations of range of motion, evaluating the strength of certain muscles, evaluating and localizing etiology of pain or discomfort, and performing a thorough neurological examination. After the physician has accumulated all the pertinent information during the physical examination, he will often repeat his examination of the patient's gait.

Principles of Gait Training

Most of the principles of gait training are so simple that they are considered obvious, and so, unfortunately, their application is not always adequately controlled. Some of the basic functions of rehabilitation are to give the patient encouragement, an opportunity to prevent the development of locomotor disuse and the possibility of learning or relearning to walk.

Often gradual development of the patient's abilities may be necessary for him to produce his best possible performance in ambulation. A patient may need to be placed on a graduated sitting tolerance program; tilt table routine; graduated standing up exercises, sometimes weight bearing on one leg only; balancing exercises; muscle strengthening exercises for the upper extremities for good control of crutches; progressive resistance exercises for specific weak but key muscles, such as the quadriceps; active or passive stretching of tightnesses or contractures; and reinforcement of proprioception by visual training.

In many instances the prescription for gait training will include measures to protect the patient. The types of temporary or permanent protection will differ and may include the stabilizing support of parallel bars; orthoses to protect bones, joints or muscles; a walker, crutches or canes; or assistance and supervision by the therapist.

In many instances gait training does not improve the patient's locomotor performance, because he has not had an adequate amount of assisted or supervised ambulation. This is particularly true for the aged patient (41, 42). It is wise to place some patients who have not improved or who have stopped improving in their gait training on a 2–3-week trial period of walking for 2 or 3 min of every 15–30-min period throughout their half or full day treatment session. Satisfactory cardiovascular and neuromuscular adjustment to ambulation needs may not otherwise occur for some patients.

Evaluation and Prognosis

While examining a patient for gait problems and when summarizing our findings, we should continuously ask ourselves what recovery can be expected with guidance or whether enough recovery will occur without our intervention; how long will the expected recovery take or how long will therapy be needed; and finally, the most essential question, how can the patient reach the goal we have set for him.

Comprehensive care (43) is one of the basic factors in treating chronic disease or disability. It is hardly necessary to elaborate here on the fact that the patient's ability to improve his locomotor functioning depends heavily upon his general well-being and the degree to which some of his concomitant diseases are treated successfully.

Although the philosophy of rehabilitation imposes a fair degree of optimism on the part of the patient, the physician and the therapist, we must be realistic. Often pronunciation of unrealistic goals is, in the long run, damaging to the patient.Heroic efforts to restore walking ability in high paraplegics, bilateral above-knee amputees, and similarly severely disabled persons may sometimes be inappropriate. The patient's expressed wish to walk again usually reflects a broader desire to get about, to do things and have a meaningful, rewarding life. A wheelchair, a car with hand controls, and a vocational rehabilitation or independent living plan, may address real needs more effectively. The lower energy cost, greater speed and safety, and ability to carry objects when using a wheelchair should be weighed against the benefits of walking for each individual. The responsibility of the health professional is to educate the patient to the available options and their relative merits; the well-informed patient will ordinarily make the best decision for himself.

The paraplegic who masters crutch-walking early in his rehabilitation program, only to discard his braces and use a wheelchair, should not be considered a therapeutic failure. The period of gait-training may have had important benefits: the psychological sense of having "made a come-back"; the upper-extremity strengthening; and the more positive accept-ance of the wheelchair as the optimal mode of ambulation. Terms such as "wheelchair-bound" or "confined to a wheelchair" should not be used by rehabilitation personnel. The wheelchair should be looked upon, not as a confining device, but as a liberating device which may open up new horizons for the severely gait-impaired person. This becomes more true as architectural barrier removal-programs make homes, public buildings, and transportation more accessible. The physician should also not be reluctant to prescribe an electric wheelchair in the presence of severe upper-extremity deficits or when special occupational or avocational interests require long or hilly travel.

The evaluation is greatly influenced by our knowledge of the natural history of the disabling disease. The patient will be handled differently depending upon whether he is in a period of recovery, has reached a permanent level of disability or has a progressing disorder. The time lapse between the catastrophic episode and the commencement of treat-ment plays an important part in the prognosis. The patient's age has a definite bearing on our treatment aims as well as the time within which we expect them to be accomplished. Gait training of a disabled child may take years. On the other hand, the average period of gait training for an old person who has suffered a stroke (40) or sustained a fractured hip (41) is 2–4 months. (To extend gait training beyond a period of 6 months is rarely justified in this age group.) In patients who reached their optimum gait years earlier, ageing or overwork may lead to losses in muscle strength and endurance, and a new period of gait training may be called for, while the patient learns a safer gait with more bracing or ambulation aid (1).

In establishing ambulation goals we must consider the safety of the patient after the goal has been reached, although on the average we have to expect the risk of the reambulated patient's suffering the traumatic consequences of a fall to be greater than for the average able-bodied person. It is not unusual to discharge a patient from actual gait training and "throw him into deep water," because such a trial short cut is often the only way to assess the patient's abilities to attain independence in ambulation.

Often it is very difficult to decide whether our gait training goals should satisfy such conventions as a normal or nearly normal appearance or whether we should concentrate on ease and safety in ambulation. This issue can become confused if we do not adequately understand the complex problems of ease and safety associated with the different abnormal gait patterns.

It is not uncommon that on initial examination we are not able to assess fully the patient's problems and his capabilities. In such instances a trial period of therapy is justified so that the patient can be observed during treatment.

The physician who has a good knowledge of and experience in gait training will usually prescribe a graduated ambulation program, and the details of such a program should not be left to chance. In addition to assuring or improving the adjustment of the cardiovascular and neurological systems to the requirements of being upright and ambulating, special attention should be concentrated on a judicious program of prevention of contractures and strengthening exercises for some key muscle groups. It should be stressed here that permitting the patient to ambulate frequently enough may in many instances be an adequate method of preventing some contractures and may take the place of a formalized power building exercise program.

It is the responsibility of the physician who is prescribing and supervising the treatment program to decide on the basis of his knowledge and experience whether and when bracing is necessary for the lower extremities.

The physician in charge of the ambulation training of a disabled person should of course consider the practicality and the gamut of surgical procedures which may improve the patient's performance or make his locomotor abilities safer.

As in other areas of applied science, it is difficult to assess the degree to which the physician who is prescribing and supervising a patient's gait training program should rely on a detailed gait analysis and to what degree his general impression should dominate his decisions. Knowledge of details is essential, but awareness of the limitations of our knowledge of the different factors involved in ambulation (8) places a higher price on our personal experiences in this field of therapy.

REFERENCES

1. ANDERSON, A. D., ET AL. Loss of ambulatory ability in patients with old anterior poliomyelitis. *Lancet, 2:* 18, 1972.
2. BARD, G., AND RALSTON, H. J. Measurement of energy expenditure during ambulation with special reference to evaluation of assistive devices. *Arch. Phys. Med., 40:* 415, 1959.
3. BASMAJIAN, J. V. *Muscles Alive: Their Functions Revealed by Electromyography,* Ed. 3. Williams & Wilkins Co., Baltimore, 1974.
4. BENEDICT, F. G., AND MURSCHHAUSER, H. Energy Transformations During Horizontal Walking. Carnegie Inst. Publ. 231. Washington, 1915.
5. BOWERMAN, W. R. Ambulatory velocity in crowded and uncrowded conditions. *Percept. Mot. Skills, 36:* 107, 1973.
6. BRUCE, J. A. The Pedestrian. In *Traffic Engineering Handbook,* pp. 108–141, edited by J. Baerwald. Institute of Traffic Engineers, Washington, D.C., 1965.
7. BRUELL, J. H., AND PESZCZYNSKI, M. Perception of verticality in hemiplegic patients in relation to rehabilitation. *Clin. Orthop. 12:* 124, 1958.
8. BRUELL, J. H., AND SIMON, J. I. The development of objective predictors of recovery in hemiplegic patients. *Arch. Phys. Med., 41:* 564, 1960.
9. BURNETT, C. N., AND JOHNSON, E. W. Development of gait in children; I. Method; II. Results. *Dev. Med. Child. Neurol., 13:* 196, 1971.
10. CLINKINGBEARD, J. R., GERSTEN, J. W., AND HOEHN, D. Energy cost of ambulation in the traumatic paraplegic. *Am. J. Phys. Med., 43:* 157, 1964.
11. CORCORAN, P. J. Energy expenditure during ambulation. In *Physiological Basis of Rehabilitation Medicine,* Ed. 1, Ch. 10. W.B. Saunders Co., Philadelphia, 1971.
12. CORCORAN, P. J. Energy expenditure of bilateral lower extremity amputees. In preparation, 1977.
13. CORCORAN, P. J., AND BRENGELMANN, G. L. Oxygen uptake in normal and handicapped subjects, in relation to speed of walking beside velocity-controlled cart. *Arch. Phys. Med. Rehabil., 51:* 78, 1970.
14. CORCORAN, P. J., JEBSEN, R. H., ET AL. Effects of plastic and metal leg braces on speed and energy cost of hemiparetic ambulation. *Arch. Phys. Med. Rehabil., 51:* 69, 1970.
15. CRITCHLEY, M. Neurologic changes in the aged. *J. Chron. Dis., 3:* 459, 1956.
16. DANOWSKI, T. S., AND WRATNEY, M. J. Age and sex related muscle weakness. *Arch. Phys. Med., 40:* 516, 1959.
17. DRILLIS, R. J. Objective recording and biomechanics of pathological gait. *Ann. N.Y. Acad. Sci., 74:* 86, 1958.
18. EBERHART, H. D., INMAN, V. T., AND BRESLER, B. The Principal Elements in Human Locomotion. In *Human Limbs and their Substitutes,* Ch.15, edited by P. E. Klopsteg and P. D. Wilson. Hafner, New York, 1968.
19. ERDMAN, W. J. ET AL. Comparative work stress for above-knee amputees using artificial legs or crutches. *Am. J. Phys. Med. 39:* 225, 1960.

20. FINLEY, F. R., AND CODY, K. A. Locomotive characteristics of urban pedestrians. *Arch. Phys. Med. Rehabil., 51:* 423, 1970.

21. FINLEY, F. R. ET AL. Locomotion patterns in elderly women. *Arch. Phys. Med. Rehabil., 50:* 140, 1969.

22. FISCHER, O. Der Gang des Menschen. *Abh. Koenigl. Saechs. Gesellsch. Wissensch, Bd. 21-28,* 1898-1904.

23. GORDON, E., AND VANDERWALDE, H. Energy requirements in paraplegic ambulation. *Arch. Phys. Med., 37:* 276, 1956.

24. HALLENBECK, C. E. The Comparative Effects of Old Age and Brain Damage on Intellectual Functioning (thesis). Western Reserve University, Cleveland, 1959.

25. HILDEBRANDT, G., ET AL. Energy costs of propelling wheelchair at various speeds: cardiac response and effect on steering accuracy. *Arch. Phys. Med. Rehabil., 51:* 131, 1970.

26. KNUTTGEN, H. G. *Neuromuscular Mechanisms for Therapeutic and Conditioning Exercises,* pp. 97-102. University Park Press, Baltimore, 1976.

27. LEITHAUSER, D. J. *Early Ambulation and Related Procedures in Surgical Management.* Springfield, 1946.

28. LONG, C. Pathological Gait: A Discussion of Pathological Gait Due to Muscular Weakness (mimeographed).

29. MAGORA, A., ROZIN, R. ET AL. Investigation of gait; 1. A technique of combined recording. *Electromyography, 10:* 385, 1970.

30. MAREY, E. J. *La méthode graphique dans les sciences expérimentales.* Paris, 1885.

31. MATTHEWS, D. K., AND WOOTEN, E. P. Analysis of oxygen consumption of women while walking in different styles of shoes. *Arch. Phys. Med., 44:* 569, 1963.

32. McDONALD, I. Statistical studies of recorded energy expenditure of man; II. Expenditure on walking related to weight, sex, age, height, speed and gradient. *Nutr. Abstr. Rev., 31:* 739, 1961.

33. MERRIFIELD, H. H. Female gait patterns in shoes with different heel heights. *Ergonomics, 14:* 411, 1971.

34. MILNER, M., BASMAJIAN, J. V., AND QUANBURY, A. O. Multifactorial analysis of walking by electromyography and computer. *Am. J. Phys. Med., 50:* 235, 1971.

35. MORTON, D. J. *Human Locomotion and Body Form.* Baltimore, 1952.

36. MURRAY, M. P. A survey of the time, magnitude and orientation of forces applied to walking sticks by disabled men. *Am. J. Phys. Med., 48:* 1, 1969.

37. MURRAY, M. P., ET AL. Walking patterns in healthy old men. *J. Gerontol., 24:* 169, 1969.

38. MURRAY, M. P., ET AL. Walking patterns of normal women. *Arch. Phys. Med. Rehabil., 51:* 637, 1970.

39. PASSMORE, R., AND DURNIN, J. V. G. A. Human energy expenditure. *Physiol. Rev., 35:* 801, 1955.

40. PESZCZYNSKI, M. Ambulation of the severely handicapped hemiplegic adult. *Arch. Phys. Med., 36:* 634, 1955.

41. PESZCZYNSKI, M. Rehabilitation of the elderly patient with a pinned fracture of the hip. *J. Chron. Dis., 2:* 311, 1956.

42. PESZCZYNSKI, M. The intermittent double step gait. *Arch. Phys. Med., 39:* 494, 1958.

43. PESZCZYNSKI, M. Post-traumatic Rehabilitation. In *Trauma in the Aged,* edited by E. Bick. New York, 1960.

44. RADCLIFFE, C. W., AND RALSTON, H. J. Performance characteristics of fluid-controlled prosthetic knee mechanisms, Report No. 49, University of California Biomechanics Laboratory, San Francisco, 1963.

45. RALSTON, H. J. Energy-speed relation and optimal speed during level walking. *Int. Z. Angew, Physiol., 17:* 277, 1958.

46. RALSTON, H. J. Effects of immobilization of various body segments on the energy cost of human locomotion. Proceedings of the Second International Ergonomics Association

Congress, Dortmund, 1964, Suppl. to *Ergonomics*, pp. 53–60, 1965.

47. RALSTON, H. J., AND LUKIN, L. Energy levels of human body segments during level walking. *Ergonomics, 12:* 39, 1969.

48. ROBINSON, S. Experimental studies of physical fitness in relation to age. *Arbeitsphysiologie, 10:* 251, 1938.

49. ROZIN, R., ET AL. Investigation of gait; 2. Gait analysis in normal individuals. *Electromyography, 11:* 183, 1971.

50. SAUNDERS, J. B., INMAN, V. T., AND EBERHART, H. D. The major determinants in normal and pathological gait. *J. Bone Joint Surg., 35A:* 543, 1953.

51. SCHERB, R. Ueber myokinetische Probleme in der unteren Extremitaet. *Beilageheft Ztschr. Orthop. Chir., 67:* 101, 1938.

52. SCHWARTZ, R. P., ET AL. Kinetics of human gait. *J. Bone Joint Surg., 16:* 343, 1934.

53. SHOUP, T. E., ET AL. Biomechanics of crutch locomotion (91 refs.). *J. Biomech., 7:* 11, 1974.

54. SMIDT, G. L. Methods of studying gait. *Phys. Ther., 54:* 13, 1974.

55. STEINDLER, A. *Kinesiology of the Human Body.* Springfield, 1955.

56. Subcontractor's Report: Fundamental Studies of Human Locomotion. (University of California) Berkeley, 1947.

57. TAYLOR, H. L., ET AL. The circulatory changes in man induced by bed rest and alterations in activity. *Fed. Proc., 4:* 71, 1945.

58. TRAUGH, G. H., CORCORAN, P. J., AND REYES, R. L. Energy expenditure of ambulation in patients with above-knee amputations. *Arch. Phys. Med. Rehabil., 56:* 67, 1975.

59. WEBER, W., AND WEBER, E. *Mechanik der menschlichen Gehwerkzeuge.* Göttingen, 1836.

60. WORDEN, R. E., AND JOHNSON, E. W. Diagnosis of hysterical paralysis. *Arch. Phys. Med. Rehabil., 42:* 122, 1961.

12

Exercises in Water

___ J. B. STEWART AND J. V. BASMAJIAN

During the last century and the early years of this century, European spas pioneered in the treatment of locomotor and rheumatic disorders. As a result of experience gained in the treatment of poliomyelitis after the First World War and of orthopedic patients during the Second World War with underwater exercises, the method has become an accepted part of rehabilitation programs in many centers not associated with naturally occurring hot springs. The development in these centers has caused the emphasis to pass from hydrotherapy (chemical and thermotherapy) to therapeutic exercise.

Exercises in water give the patient an opportunity to perform movements in a medium which not only provides buoyancy to the body and its members but also allows movement with so much less effort that seriously weakened parts may be moved and exercised in a manner not possible without support. In addition, group activities, both exercises and games, in a deep pool have been found to be of great benefit to patient morale.

The average specific gravity of the body with air in the lungs is approximately 0.974 (1). Assuming that the specific gravity of the body is uniform throughout, the amount of floating body seen above the surface is the difference between unity and 0.974 or 0.026. The effect of buoyancy, therefore, on the almost wholly immersed body is sufficiently great to almost overcome the effects of gravity. The patient's weight on his joints is thus minimal when he stands in his maximum depth of water. This fact is of great value in the execution of walking exercises in water for patients whose weight-bearing joints would not be able to support them in air.

Minimum muscular effort is required of the patient when his limb is moved gently in the horizontal plane, since the forces of gravity and buoyancy balance each other. But it is also important to stabilize the body or some part of it. Stabilization may be achieved with the support of a surface such as a table or chair; with grips or a rail, if the patient has the strength to grasp them; with canvas straps, which must not be applied too tightly; or by the therapist's hands, e.g., by stabilizing the patient's pelvis when movements of the legs are desired, giving the patient a fixed point from which to work.

The effects of buoyancy may be used to assist or resist the movement of the limb. As progress in muscle power increases, the effect of buoyancy may be used to help the patient begin a limb movement which partially ends above water level. When the pelvis or shoulders are stabilized by the therapist or the support of an appropriate device, the patient is assisted by buoyancy to raise the arm or leg in its fully extended position. Similar movements of abduction and adduction of the limbs, with stabilization of the shoulders or pelvis, are also used to gain maximum assistance from buoyancy. As function improves, the limb is made to resist the effects of buoyancy in its initial movement. The same principles apply for trunk exercises, in which case the hip joints (with legs held extended) are used as the fulcrums; or the shoulders may be stabilized by using the arms as the rigid levers, with fulcrums at the shoulder joints.

A third use of underwater exercise resides in its temperature. The warmth of the water acts to relax the part and the body. Another value of hydrogymnastics is psychological: even the smallest amount of voluntary motion (not possible in air) helps the patient retain a "body image" of movement and gives hope of one day moving the part without the help of water.

Selection of Patients

The chief indication for underwater exercises is muscle weakness of such degree that motion in air is difficult, but in which there is reason to believe that there is the possibility of increasing strength through voluntary motion. This is seen most commonly in partial peripheral nerve lesions, especially in poliomyelitis and polyneuronitis. Lowman and Roen (2) also recommend them for strengthening muscles and stretching contractures of the amputated stump; following joint injuries; after abdominal fascial transplants; in paraplegia; and in certain cases of cerebral palsy. Still other conditions for which underwater mobilization is often recommended include extensive skin burns and rheumatoid arthritis in the convalescent stage.

The selection of patients suitable for hydrogymnastics is of the greatest importance. Those with very high or very low blood pressure should be excluded, as should patients with infective skin lesions or open wounds. Patients with an elevated temperature from any cause should not be treated in warm water until it has subsided to normal for at least 72 hours.

Seriously debilitated patients are not usually suited for this treatment, but where, for some reason, treatment is considered desirable it may be given for short periods (up to five minutes at first) on alternate days. In all cases, the reaction of the patient should be observed, not only when in the pool, but also on the day following. If there is undue lassitude or fatigue or a loss of appetite, the duration of treatment and the amount of work done during treatment should be reduced.

Treatment

The temperature of the water will depend upon the condition to be treated. Where relaxation is one of the principal objects of treatment, as in spastic paralysis, a high temperature of from 98° to 100°F is most suitable. When the primary objective is exercise, the patient will be able to work for longer periods without fatigue at water temperatures of from 92° to about 95°F, depending upon the amount of muscle activity.

In the early days of underwater treatment, the therapist usually entered the pool for closer supervision and for better audibility. Therapists who remained in the warm chlorinated water for long periods sometimes experienced considerable weight loss; others were inconvenienced by skin maceration or irritation. Lowman and Roen (2) advise the use of a waterproof coverall (fishing wader) for therapists who work with patients in the pool. When the pool edge is built up to the waist level of the therapist, guidance for most exercises may be given from outside the pool.

Treatments should not be given immediately after meals, nor is it wise to give them too long after meals. The patient should be asked to empty his bladder before immersion, since a warm bath often has a diuretic action.

When the patient arrives for underwater exercise, he should be given a cleansing shower, dried and given shorts or, in the case of female patients, a proper bathing suit. Ambulatory patients will walk down the steps of the pool, supporting themselves with the handrails. Other patients may be lowered into the pool with a manually or electrically operated hoist, the hooks of which have been attached to a canvas stretcher onto which the patient has been transferred.

The general principles of therapeutic exercise are applied to exercises under water in relation to those special considerations which apply to the principles of hydrodynamics.

Assistive motion is achieved by moving the part in the direction it seeks when placed in water; this will depend upon the specific gravity of the part and is determined by placing the part in the horizontal position. Buoyancy may be increased by supporting the part with floats made of cork or wood or with inflated sacs of rubber or plastic. Resistance can be increased by applying a weighted splint to the part or by having the patient move an object with a wide (resistant) surface. It may also be increased by decreasing the depth of water through which the part moves; for example, in walking retraining, the patient walks in shallower water as he improves.

For detailed descriptions of underwater exercises the reader is referred to the excellent manuals of Lowman and Roen (2) and Bolton and Goodwin (4).

Equipment

Where there will be mostly adults in need of group activity, a large pool, deep at one end, will probably prove to be the best choice. In an orthopedic hospital or a hospital with many physically disabled patients, a large but shallower pool is indicated; where the patient population is limited to children, the pool may be smaller and shallower still. For the smaller hospital, where the number of patients referred for underwater exercise is small, a Hubbard tank will prove sufficient.

Any container of water of sufficient size will permit underwater exercises. The "keyhole" shape of the Hubbard tank offers probably the most useful design for the greatest range of body motions in a limited space (Fig. 12.1). A platform of aluminum may be suspended from four standard hydraulic jacks fixed to the outside of the tank (Fig. 12.1). The platform may be raised as the muscle power of the patient improves, thereby reducing the assistance to movement given by the water buoyancy. An inclined plinth made of canvas, stretched on a tubular frame, may be used inside the tank in the same manner as the Lowman plinth mentioned above.

Several other pieces of apparatus are desirable; some of these will remain stationary, and others will be moved. In addition, many smaller auxiliary devices are useful. Parallel (walking) bars of adjustable height and width, about 25 cm below water level, are advantageous for ambulation exercises as well as for strengthening the muscles of the extremities

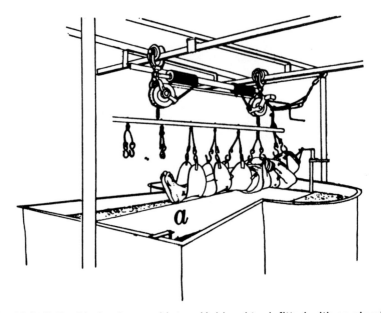

Fig. 12.1. Patient being lowered into a Hubbard tank fitted with an aluminum platform (a) which can be fixed in a raised or lowered position.

and trunk. Clip-on canvas slings, made to fit the bars, are used to support the shoulders, trunk or pelvis when free movement of the arms or legs is desired. A pair of detachable bars may be fitted to one end of the bars, projecting above water level, to carry a small canvas sling on which the patient may rest the head when lying prone above the bars.

The circumferential handrail at water level (Fig. 12.2*C*) helps support the patient in many exercises. When supine, the patient may grasp it in the manner of a horizontal bar and exercise elbow flexors. The toes may be hooked under it for stabilization or it may be grasped in the supine position for trunk flexion exercises.

A flat working surface, sloped into the water so that the lower part of the body may rest on it under water, offers many advantages. Best among these is the submerged (Lowman) plinth (3), on the surface of

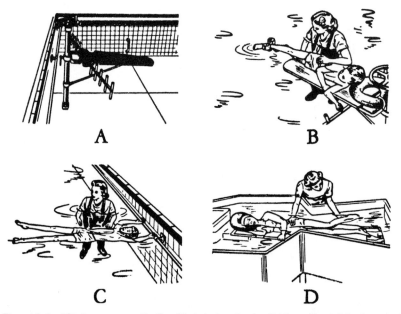

Fig. 12.2. (*A*) Lowman plinth. Stainless steel plinth adjustable for various depths of water and degrees of inclination. Crossbars with rubber-covered handgrips are adjustable in an arc toward or away from table and for inward and outward rotation of upper extremity. The narrow tapered end supports the sacrum centrally. (*B*). Flexion-extension exercise of hip. Patient alternately contracts flexors and extensors of under hip with knee extended as therapist stabilizes pelvis, resists flexion and assists extension. Note use of cork floats under right ankle. (*C*). Illustration of stabilization by handrails. (*D*). Illustration of a flexion-extension knee exercise with patient side-lying on a tank platform. Therapist stabilizes pelvis and hip, assists patient in extension and resists flexion. (From C. L. Lowman and S. G. Roen. *Therapeutic Use of Pools and Tanks.* Philadelphia, 1952. Reproduced with permission of Dr. Lowman and the W. B. Saunders Company, publisher.)

which the body may be wholly or partly supported by adjustment of its inclination (Fig. 12.2*A*). It is fitted with adjustable arms which allow handgrips in different positions of the forearms and adaptation to varying arm and shoulder lengths and deformities.

The submerged bench or seat (3) permits exercises in the sitting position; the steps at the shallow end of the pool may also serve the same purpose for foot and leg exercises.

Devices with strong buoyancy are very useful to give additional support to some part of the body. These devices depend upon the buoyancy of air, tree trunk or bark. In the first group are inflated rubber rings of different sizes which may support a foot, head, pelvis or trunk and the type of mat floats used at beach resorts. Wooden planks may be used to support parts of the upper extremities. Cork may be used in a variety of ways to support almost any part of the body (Fig. 12.2*B*). Thick discs of cork are drilled through their centers and joined to one another by lengths of heavy cord or rope. By uniting several such pairs of cork, large areas of the body may be supported on the ropes between the cork buoys.

Other wooden objects useful in pool exercises are paddles and wands. Resistance to arm motions can be increased when the blade of the paddle is turned to offer more surface as it advances through the water. Small wands are used by the patient with hands under water to increase resistance and to observe his progress in supination and pronation.

Lightweight plastic splints may prove useful in certain cases, for example, where hip movement is desired with the knee kept in full extension. Weighted boots may be made from waterproofed plywood, cut to the size of the patient's foot and fitted with lead heels and crossbars held firmly in place by a canvas strap applied as a figure of eight around the ankle and forefoot. The weighted boots lower the patient's center of gravity and give him a feeling of stability while walking in the deep pool, without sacrificing the buoyant effect of the water.

REFERENCES

1. DUPERTINS, C. W., PITTS, G. C., et al. Relation of specific gravity to body build in a group of healthy men. *J. Appl. Physiol., 3:* 678, 1951.
2. LOWMAN, C. L., AND ROEN, S. G. *Therapeutic Uses of Pools and Tanks.* Philadelphia, 1952.
3. LOWMAN, C. L., ROEN, S. G., et al. *Technique of Underwater Gymnastics.* Los Angeles, 1937.
4. BOLTON, E., AND GOODWIN, D. *An Introduction to Pool Exercises.* Edinburgh, 1956.

13

Therapeutic Exercises for Cerebral Palsy[1]

———————————— DANIEL HALPERN

Cerebral palsy is a term that refers to a group of conditions which have the common characteristics of (a) impairment of motor control, (b) resulting from disturbed function of the brain, (c) originating in the period of growth and development of the brain (up to 8 years of age), (d) and which are not progressive in character (1). The symptomatology may vary depending upon the central nervous system structures whose function is impaired, and their role in the acquisition, maintenance, and control of motor activity.

The etiological background for the impairment of function is important from the point of view of epidemiological, nosologic, or prophylactic considerations. An appropriate understanding of etiology may be essential to the general management and counseling of the patient and family. However, once the static nature of the lesion is established, the important problems from the therapeutic point of view are to define the motor repertory of the individual; to make an estimate of the ability to learn new motor activities where they are deficient, and to acquire control over undesirable, adventitious motor activity. Since the characteristic clinical problem in cerebral palsy is a deficiency of motor control, the purpose of therapeutic exercises is to assist the individual with cerebral palsy to acquire, or learn, new motor abilities, and to develop them to a functional level of performance.

[1] This study was supported in part by RT-2 Grant: 16-P-56810, of the Rehabilitation Services Administration of the Department of Health, Education, and Welfare. The author wishes to acknowledge with appreciation the invaluable comments and suggestions of Frederic J. Kottke, M.D.

It should be recognized that cerebral palsy is a complex condition that has effects not only on the physical growth and development but also on skills, personality, the cognitive ability, personal and social attitudes of the patient, the emotions, attitudes, and interactions of the family. Management of the individual with cerebral palsy must include professional attention to all these aspects of human function. This discussion will confine itself to the single subject of therapeutic exercises, since the question of total care of patients with cerebral palsy is outside its scope.

A noxious process which gives rise to brain damage or dysfunction in the specific area of motor activity is likely to disrupt function in other areas as well (2). Thus, while the specific function of motor control has been chosen to define cerebral palsy, many patients with this condition have disturbance of other functions such as impaired cognitive functions, speech, attentiveness, emotionality, or convulsive disorders. These factors, together with personality factors such as self-esteem, ability to persevere, rapport, and the ability of the family to support, reinforce, and carry over a therapeutic regime all need to be considered in the total therapeutic management program. Often they will constitute strong determinants of the basic content of the program since they will modify significantly the conditions under which learning can occur best, as well as the ultimate level of achievement.

Development and Motor Organization

Gesell and his colleagues have established firmly based principles of growth and development proceeding in a regular sequence of motor abilities (3). Paine et al. (4) have shown that in normal children, motor development is marked by a regular sequence in which reflexes appear, mature, and disappear when others mediated at a higher level become evident. In children with motor abnormalities the relationship between specific reflexes remained, but there was a great tendency for earlier reflexes to persist, and for higher level reflex activity to be delayed in appearance. McGraw (5), much earlier than this, showed also that a specific motor function first appeared as a reflex, then gradually weakened as maturation occurred. As volitional control asserted itself, the strength of the activity or its effectiveness increased again, as it was used in a functional context, and eventually exceeded the original reflex levels.

These studies highlight the fact that reflex activity represents a simplified component, or subroutine of motor activity that is elicited by exposure to a specific sensory stimulus. As the individual matures, repeated experiences provide opportunities for utilization of these activities in a functional role; and for their suppression in nonpurposeful situations. The subroutine is maintained as a component of functional activity, but its obligatory elicitation by a specific stimulus is inhibited. In essence, this may be seen as a process in classical conditioning, where a specific activity is elicited in response to a new stimulus through experience; and the inhibition of the response to specific stimulation represents habituation to a nonsignificant or nonrewarded stimulus.

Bruner (6) has shown that in order to carry out a skillful motor act all of the components necessary need to be available before they can be integrated into the total praxis. In the development of motor skill gradual improvement occurs by shaping of the components of the movement with continued trial and experience. The integration of these existing multiple components into a single organized movement may occur quite suddenly, in a stepwise fashion, rather than gradually. The basic unitary components originate from innately structured patterns that are used in the course of spontaneous or stimulated movements. These gradually evolve into exploratory activity when consequences result. As the repertory increases, combinations develop which acquire additional functional attributes contributing to the formation of skilled motor patterns.

It follows from this work that, where subroutines or components of skilled motion are not available because of the inherent defect in exploratory ability, specialized training procedures need to be carried out to establish smaller, unitary motions which are achievable, and build, by combination of these units, in an instructed learning situation the components which the patient has not been able to develop in the absence of the spontaneous exploration that occurs normally.

The motor components used by the developing individual include gross generalized motor patterns previously engaged randomly, spontaneously, or in the course of the constant exploration of the normal child. They would also include developmentally organized reflexes elicited by appropriate stimulation. Bruner's work also suggested that after these unitary activities are synthesized or integrated into a functional activity, a child engages in repetitive performances, as in play, in which the new complex pattern is mastered, and speed, strength, and accuracy are achieved as a gradual improvement in skill or dexterity.

The acquisition of useful motor function then, is a process by which individual motor components are made available through innate reflex, and voluntary exploratory activity. The initial repertory of a child is composed of a limited selection of gross or mass movements and reflexes which become modified with normal experience. New reflexes appear, to supervene over more primitive ones. Components of the early gross activity are individually explored and brought under voluntary utilization. Repetition increases the ability through the learning process of volitional initiation, maintenance, or termination. Synthesis of unitary components evolves into skilled motion through gradual shaping and refinement. It appears that the synthesis of components occurs as the result of a process of trial or exploration and is a stepwise event rather than a gradual improvement, suggesting a form of insight.

Symptomatology and the Therapeutic Problem

The motor disturbances seen in cerebral palsy are related to the systems of motor organization involved and have their effects on the process of motor development outlined above. The most frequently observed abnormality of motor control in cerebral palsy is that of spasticity. This is usually characterized as a form of muscular hypertonia in which there is excessive activity of the deep tendon reflexes associated with the velocity-responsive monosynaptic Ia reflexes (7) of the muscle spindle. In many individuals there is also associated a persistent dystonia, giving rise to contractures and deformity. This dystonia is not present in all individuals with spasticity and, where present, is not at all uniform in all individuals, or in all areas in the same individual. This dystonia is responsive to the length of the muscle and has been ascribed to excessive activity of the secondary muscle spindle afferents (8).

The excessive activity of the muscle spindle reflexes is the result of impaired inhibition by cerebral cortical control of muscle spindle reflexes. As a result of the impaired selectivity of motor components, these patients show stereotyped motor patterns in which activation of one muscle group is consistently associated with that of other groups in ways unrelated to function. As a result of impaired activation, there is a weakening in specific muscle groups, usually those antagonistic to the hypertonic muscles such as the wrist extensors and supinators, finger extensors and intrinsics, hip abductors, anterior tibialis and peroneal muscles. Finally, as Hughlings Jackson indicated, spastic individuals show a "poverty of movement" as a result of limited variety, adaptability, and modulation of motor activities.

The second commonest disturbance represents an impairment of inhibition manifested by more or less continuous, purposeless movements, worse on effort, manifested as choreiform or dystonic writhing movements. These are recognizable frequently as uninhibited spinal or supraspinal reflex patterns. Athetosis is thus characterized by poor selectivity of individual specific motor patterns. However, the stereotyping seen in spasticity though present is not as prominent. In patients with athetosis, there is more frequent evidence of individual fine motor activity in the intrinsic muscles of the fingers, supinator and extensor muscles of the upper extremity, and abductor and extensor muscles of the hips, and the anterior tibialis and peroneals in the legs. This fine motor activity is often present as adventitious excessive movement or tone, and is one of the components to be evaluated to determine to what degree training should emphasize utilization or inhibition.

Two important factors appear to be operative in patients with athetosis. There is a defect in inhibition of many of the spinal and supraspinal reflexes, as well as what appears to be nonspecific individual adventitious muscular activity. There also appears to be difficulty in maintenance of postural activity which is normally carried out on an automatic basis (9). There is often deficiency in the supporting function of the lower extremities for standing and balancing, or in the upper extremity at the shoulder, elbow, and wrist when necessary to hold the hand poised for useful function. The same problem is often observed in the trunk and head control where appropriate posture is insufficient to provide an adequate foundation for the functional activities of sitting, reading, or observing the surroundings.

In addition to inhibition of irrelevant motor activity, and activation of the essential muscle groups, normal motor activity requires spatial, temporal, and force-related modulation. Deficiency in this area is referred to as dysmetria when control of position or direction or distance is deficient. Impaired control of speed or timing in terms of having different muscle groups contracting in proper sequence is referred to as dyssynergia. These deficits are subsumed under the general term ataxia and are commonly ascribed to impairment of cerebellar function. It should be recognized, however, that these symptoms of impaired control can occur as a result of damage outside the cerebellum in the cerebro-cerebellar pathways, or in the pathways receiving cerebellar projections. In addition, many patients with athetoxis exhibit dysmetria and dyssynergia which on close observation appears to be based on proprioceptive inattentiveness. This is really a form of habituation, since proprioception is meaningless to an individual whose every moment is unpredictable because of adventitious movement. Under spontaneous, uncontrolled conditions, proprioceptive feedback becomes irrelevant information.

It has been traditional to recognize the roles of injury to cerebral cortex, basal ganglia, cerebellum, and the vestibular system (10, 11) in the symptomatologic configurations presented in cerebral palsy. Recent studies (12) are beginning to expose the roles played by the limbic system, hypothalamus and reticular system in learning, attentiveness, memory, and retrieval. In the extensive literature now accumulating in this area, there are strong indications that damage to these structures interferes with the ability to respond appropriately to relevant cues necessary to achieve well organized motor sequences, to inhibit or habituate previously acquired maladaptive motor or behavioral patterns, or to respond effectively to positive or negative rewards. It is necessary therefore to observe whether the patient attends appropriately to relevant stimuli, responds appropriately to reward stimuli, and can maintain attentiveness in the learning situation for a period of time necessary to achieve adequate learning. Where these are deficient, alteration in the training program, techniques, and goals will have to be made. At the same time, where these functions retain some degrees of effectiveness, they should be identified and their ability to enhance learning or new motor activity exploited.

Motor Evaluation

The training of motor activity in patients with cerebral palsy requires a description of the motor repertory of the patient in terms which lend themselves to an appropriate task analysis and setting of goals.

The motor repertory can be described in terms of:

1. Volitional Activity
2. Involuntary Activity
3. Control

Volitional activities are those which the patient is able to initiate, follow through, or maintain on specific command.

Voluntary motion can be described according to three parameters which may coexist at any moment in time. The parameters of voluntary motion are:

1. Specific vs. Stereotyped
2. Conscious vs. Automatic
3. Prime Mover vs. Postural

The *specific* aspects of motion refer to the capacity of the individual to execute a single, precise movement, at will, or any selected joint or muscle, unaccompanied by any other motor activity. This quality is contrasted to the stereotyped motion in which an individual joint motion, or muscle action is always associated with movement of another joint or muscle. A common example is elbow flexion associated with shoulder abduction in the hemiplegic patient. *Stereotyped* activities are usually not considered as learned activities but rather as whole or partial components of a reflex activity which the individual activates voluntarily. The essential element to be recognized is the degree of selectivity open to the patient.

The distinction between *conscious* and *automatic* activity represents the level of attention required in effecting the activity. Normally, attention is directed only to a small segment of motor activity. Most often, only certain aspects of a particular motion are observed, such as speed, target, force, or direction of a motion while many of the postural foundations, or supportive motions are carried out automatically without direct attention. Normally, automatic motor activity is accessible to the individual. There is awareness of the action, and, within limits, it may be sensed, altered, or interrupted at will most of the time unless the speed is too great. Automatic activity represents a high level of learning or training. Other terms describing automatic activity which connote better its real meaning are "pre-programming," or "feed-forward" mechanisms. These signify the idea that the movement pattern or sequence, sometimes referred to in neurophysiologic terms as the engram, is so well established that feedback mechanisms are no longer continuously operative. Their intervention has been reduced to a level of periodic sampling for overall guidance.

Because this type of activity is often carried out without the conscious awareness and attention of the individual to each detail, it has often mistakenly been considered as activity in which the cerebral cortex does not participate. There is no evidence that this is so, and considerable evidence that the cerebral cortex takes part in the learning, and, in the effective processing of automatic activity. Present neurophysiological concepts of motor organization conceive of the central nervous system operating as an integral unit in which the cerebral cortex, where it is intact, dominates subcortical activity; organizes and modulates it by inhibition or facilitation of various components as functionally determined (13). By selectively influencing the lower levels of the central nervous system, the cortex sets a bias so that selected stimuli may elicit responses at those levels without the need for the messages to be transmitted to the higher centers before any action occurs.

In the presence of cortical damage, the uninhibited, unmodulated activity of lower centers of the central nervous system is considered as reflex or stereotyped activity rather than automatic. It is possible to train activity which does not include residual intact cerebral cortex only with the greatest difficulty. Subcortical learning of motor activity has been demontrated to occur, but such learning occurs with great difficulty and is at best at a most primitive level (14).

Postural activity is motor activity which maintains a body part of limb in a specific spatial orientation. In normal functioning, postural activity provides support for specific goal-oriented or *prime mover action*.

Involuntary motor activity represents reflex activity as a stereotyped response to specific sensory-receptive stimulation, or adventitious, uninhibited activity in response to nonspecific stimulation. From the ontogenetic point of view, reflex activity represents the action of certain innate structural pathways at different levels of the neuraxis. For higher level reflexes, as in the static and kinetic labyrinthine reflexes, there appear to be elements of experience and learning necessary to prompt, effective functioning. Also, these reactions disappear, or develop inadequately with injury to higher centers. Other involuntary motor activity relates to nonspecific, generalized excitation or activation. This process represents a basic deficiency in inhibition and is commonly referred to as "overflow" activity. It is especially observed in normal individuals in poorly coordinated, insufficiently learned activities or unfamiliar or difficult situations. In particular, this kind of activity is observed in athetoid individuals although it is rather frequently seen in spastic persons as well.

The important observation required with regard to involuntary activity is the position along the spectrum ranging from *obligatory* to *facultative* which is represented by the ability of the individual. How much control of the reflex can be exhibited? If a reflex is obligatory, and there is no possibility for a patient to learn to inhibit or activate it purposefully for a functional goal, then a training program would not be warranted; and either medications, surgery, or other assistance must be offered to diminish the strength of the stimulus or the response (intramuscular neurolysis, tendon lengthening, etc.).

On the other hand, if some degree of control exists, then a training program may be attempted to increase the patient's ability to inhibit the reflex when desired, and to activate or modulate it as needed. Often both measures may be necessary. Medications such as diazepam, phenothiazines, dantrolene, or others may aid in diminishing specific or general motor responsiveness. A therapeutic environment at a low level of noise, both visual or auditory, may be helpful in aiding patients to maintain their responsiveness within useful limits of control. As control improves, the environmental milieu may be enlarged and allowed to be noisier to approach more normal situations. Reinforcement is given for successful achievement in the new circumstances.

Involuntary reflex activity is not necessarily abnormal. In fact, normal motor activity utilizes such reflex activity as a basic substrate for certain categorical, low skill activities. The abnormality is measured by the difficulty in inhibition of the reflex as required by function. Involuntary reflex activity has been described by Sherrington (15), and more recently by Fiorentino (16), and Kottke (8). The chronology of reflex activity and appearance in patients with cerebral palsy has been described by Paine et al. Reference to these works would be essential in the understanding of these activities.

Control is defined as the mechanism by which the distance, direction, and speed of motion are regulated to a degree appropriate to the functional requirements. The accuracy of control determines the effectiveness of any motion with regard to the following components: (a) *spatial*, e.g., direction and distance; (b) *temporal*, e.g., velocity; and (c) *synergic*, e.g., regulation of force. Failure of the mechanism of control of distance and direction is recognized as dysmetria, while failure in the control of speed or strength is referred to as dyssynergia. When the difficulty is in measuring accurately, with sufficiently rapid feedback to maintain a smooth motion or a steady posture, these terms are conjointly subsumed under the term ataxia.

Other defects are also referred to as dyssynergia. They are recognized as the inability to coordinate different muscles, or motor patterns to effect a functionally well-organized motion. These problems may vary in complexity. Simpler examples are the nonspecific impairment of inhibitory ability that occurs with "overflow" types of motor activity, or of the specific inhibitory activity where identifiable reflexes are activated abnormally, interfering with the ultimate functional motion. This is what is frequently seen in athetosis.

In another context, dyssynergia is represented by an inability to properly coordinate the force, timing, or sequence of a number of different components of motion into an effective pattern, merging into the entity of dyspraxia. The words dyssynergia and synergy are therefore applied in the literature to a number of different entities, and an effort must be made to define the meaning of the terms whenever it is used.

The qualities of dysmetria and dyssynergia attributable to cerebellar disorder respond to specific training activities only to a limited extent. However, in children, prolonged exposure to controlled successful experience appears to be associated in a significant number of individuals with a general improvement in functional ability, and sometimes, in the recently acquired ataxias, though not as often, even with improvement in the neurological signs, e.g., finger-to-nose test. The dyssynergia of the inhibitory or praxic deficit does respond to specific training, and an appropriately organized training program should be offered.

The fundamental descriptors of the motor repertory, namely the voluntary, involuntary, and control characteristics must be organized into a developmental as well as a functional framework in order to be able to evaluate their significance and to establish appropriate goals for training which can be quantitatively measured to record progress.

Motor functions are organized into basic activity classifications for convenient identification and analysis. Each function should be analyzed with respect to volitional, involuntary, and control characteristics. The speed, strength, shortness of latency, and duration represent measures of volitional ability. The degree of volitional coordination of multiple muscular or skeletal components of a motion in correct temporal and force relationships should be described as objectively as possible. Deficiency in this voluntary component represents dyspraxia, or apraxia. The appearance of adventitious movements, or hypertonia in the form of nonspecific or reflex activity representing involuntary activity may be measured or estimated in quantitative terms. Inaccurate movements with ataxic tremor may also be represented quantitatively, and means should be sought to establish as objective measures of these parameters of motion as possible.

Task Analysis for Motor Training

In order to consider systematically the complex organization of motor activity, each of the basic motor functions may be subdivided into component tasks. These can then be analyzed and defined in terms suitable for quantitative description and well-defined goal-setting. Specific therapeutic objectives can be established in this way.

A. *Posture*
   1. Head control – duration of erect posture, response to tilting
   2. Sitting balance – including equilibrium responses for head, trunk, upper extremities, lower extremities to tilting
   3. Quadripedal balance including equilibrium responses
   4. Standing balance including equilibrium responses
B. *Ambulation*
   1. Support reaction – hip extensor, knee extensor, triceps surae
   2. Reciprocation – associated adduction or abduction, rotational motions
   3. Dynamic equilibrium – body shift over line of support

 4. Segmental control — ankle, foot, knee, pelvis, spinal control, upper extremity coordination, head and neck control

 5. Gait sequence

C. *Upper Extremity*

 1. Reach — shoulder flexion, adduction, elbow extension, wrist extension

 2. Grasp — intrinsic-extrinsic coordination, thumb-finger coordination, palmar, opposed grasp, prehension, fine prehension

 3. Positioning — pronation, supination, wrist extension versus flexion, shoulder rotation, abduction

 4. Placement

 5. Release

 6. Withdrawal

 7. Manipulation — thumb-finger oppositional adjustment

  a. Individual finger mobility

  b. Pronator-supinator adaptive motion

  c. Shoulder rotation adjustment

D. *Oral Structures*

 1. Mastication

  a. Chewing — jaw opening and closing

  b. Lateral motions of the jaw

  c. Protrusion and retraction

 2. Lips and cheek

  a. Closure

  b. Opening

  c. Sensory awareness

 3. Tongue

  a. Protrusion and retraction

  b. Lateral deviation

  c. Supraversion, infraversion

  d. Bolus management

  e. Placement for phonetic production

 4. Pharyngeal musculature

  a. Velo-pharyngeal closure

  b. Swallowing mechanism

 5. Glottal function

  a. Laryngeal closure-opening

  b. Fine control

 6. Respiratory motor control

  a. Inspiratory volume

  b. Expiratory volume

  c. Force and duration

Motor function in each area should be assessed individually. These functions, as listed above can be identified and their level of accomplishment determined. Those carried out only with assistance or facilitation, but not spontaneously, should be choosen for training if adequate maturation of the supportive functions have been achieved.

Motor Training

The acquisition of new motor function in individuals, who do not develop it spontaneously, requires training of motor activity in a context of learning. New motor activity places the same demands on the motor organizational process as the acquisition of skill in any individual. Because they have not been attained spontaneously, unitary motor components have to be introduced by demonstration, facilitation, or passive motion with appropriate feedback to provide the correct sensory criteria for adequate guidance and control. Feedback for correctness of motion is a complex process that encompasses an evaluation of accuracy, appropriate control of hypertonia, as well as effective strength, and, above all, integration of individual components to become an organized functional unit. The correct processing of all these sensorimotor activities is called coordination. Tactile cues, pressure, gentle manual resistance with verbal and visual supplements can be used to elicit or demonstrate the appropriate body part and its position, motion, or tone. For special purposes, where sensory awareness is deficient, or where reception is embedded in a complex of competitive stimulation, assistive devices providing "biofeedback" may be used to provide figure-background contrast, or special interest by novelty.

To be accessible to the learning process, a unitary component of a functional movement, e.g., elbow extension as part of reaching, wrist extension as part of grasp, hip extension as part of ambulation, must be available to the individual in some form. The role of the "facilitation" techniques described by a number of authors (17–21) is to elicit a motor activity and render it available to the central nervous system so that it may participate in the learning process. Motor activity in this sense, includes inhibition as well as activation according to the patients' requirements for performance in each specific instance. A review of the techniques proposed by Brunnstrom, Bobath, Rood, and their followers, demonstrate a number of maneuvers designed to encourage inhibitory as well as facilitatory activity. All the so-called facilitation methods are based on the principle that some form of somesthetic stimulation will elicit a desired muscular response which then, by repetition, will become integrated into the motor repertoire of the individual.

When specific motor goals for any movement pattern are identified, it becomes necessary to train each of the three motor components: activation, inhibition, and accuracy. A motor activity to be trained is identified as absent, ineffective, or weak. It is selected because it is required for improved function, and because there is a clinical judgment that improved function may be possible. When a contraction is absent or very weak, it may be facilitated using the techniques of the authors referred to above. A few of the maneuvers have been most frequently useful in my experience, are simple to apply, and results are observable immediately. It is therefore worthwhile trying them before going into other complex procedures which may elicit adequate responses only after some delay.

Vigorous, but brief manual skin effleurage over the desired muscle group, either singly, or together with manual percussion of the muscle belly in a series of short taps with the tips of the fingers held in a flexed position will often elicit a muscle contraction spontaneously as a result of the myotatic and associated gamma (γ) reflexes. The command is given to move the joint during the effleurage or during the percussion, or immediately afterward. If reflex movements are observed, they are pointed out to the patient, and the instruction is given, "Now you do it while I help you."

A few passive movements of the limb are useful as a demonstration of the motion that is desired. This provides physiological afference which can be used as a model for voluntary activity the patient is to attempt. The passive movement can be followed by a command to attempt an active motion with manual assistance. Reinforcement should be given promptly when the desired muscle activity is felt along with the assistance. The assistance is diminished with repetitions as the responses of the patient allow. Often, in one session, not usually the first, it is possible to progress from passive movement to active-assisted, active, and active-resistive contractions. When possible, this progression is extremely motivating, and full utilization of this sequence should be made. Retention of new motor patterns is often difficult in patients with motor impairment of this type, and forgetting occurs from one day to the next; and therefore the procedure must be repeated regularly. Eventually a transition is made from facilitatory and training techniques to inclusion in useful functional activity and specific training exercises to be carried out at home.

Passive placement of the limb in a desired position with the instruction to "hold it there" is another useful maneuver to achieve both contractile and inhibitory activity. The task is made more or less difficult by placing the limb at angles stretching the spastic or dystonic muscle group to a greater or lesser degree. Assistance can be given to this activity, and reinforcement for any detectable correct muscle contraction. Of course, strong reinforcement is given to a successful hold. A facilitatory maneuver to assist this action is a series of four or five rapid stretches of the flaccid or weaker muscles, followed immediately by passive placement in the desired position with the command to "hold it there."

An electrical stimulator as described by the Ljubljana group (22) can also be used as a facilitation device and is often extremely effective. The only real objection to its use is the anxiety or mild discomfort which a child may not be willing to tolerate. However, with appropriate management most children can be induced to use it successfully. The stimulator is useful if it can deliver square wave pulses at a width of 0.1–0.7 msec, at a frequency of 25–70 Hz and a voltage ranging from zero to 100 volts. The output impedance of the stimulator used at the University of Minnesota is 1,000 ohms. The device is battery-operated and can be used at home when the patient or a number of his family has been instructed in its use. The technique for using the stimulator is to use the highest frequency, the shortest duration, and the lowest amplitude necessary to obtain effective contraction. The frequency and duration are allowed to remain constant once the most useful level is determined. The amplitude is turned down to zero or below the effective level and the patient is instructed to attempt the desired movement. As the patient tries to contract, the amplitude is raised gradually until an active contraction is seen. The procedure is repeated, with reinforcement for each contraction especially when it is noted that the amplitude does not have to be raised as high as originally. Often, in one session it is possible to obtain effective contractions without any stimulation at all after 10–15 electrically assisted ones. The number of repetitions should be governed by the degree of success the patient has. It is best to stop before the point is reached that attention flags, and the contractions become weaker.

Inhibition of muscle activity is trained by asking a patient to contract the muscle, providing resistance just sufficient for the patient to be aware of the contraction and by allowing some movement. The patient's attention is directed to the sensation of the movement or the sensation of the resistance both within the muscle and at the skin, and/or the visual consequences of any movement permitted. Mechanical or electrical devices, such as electromyographic displays may be used at this point to enhance the perception of the motor activity. The patient then is asked to stop the action, relax, or loosen up. The words used should be clear, short, familiar, and meaningful to the patient. By resisting the motion, or feeling the muscle or tendon, the therapist is aware of even momentary reductions in tone. These correct responses should be immediately identified and positively reinforced, with immediate feedback without reinforcement when the tone returns if not at the therapist's command. From time to time, the patient should be informed of the return of abnormal tone to provide feedback and improve awareness. Repeating this feedback too often, however, becomes frustrating, since it carries negative value signifying failure. By knowing how long the patient can maintain relaxation, the therapist can forestall this failure by instructing the patient to contract the muscle, or simply to let it do whatever it will do. The implication here is that a clear message is given indicating appropriate expectations, and the ability to maintain inhibition for even a moment or two can be regarded as a success since that is all that was demanded. An exercise would consist of alternate sequences of "contract" – "hold" – "relax" responses. Again, the words used here should be appropriate to the patient's language level. For some patients it may be necessary to say simply "move it" or "push my hand." The therapist should be aware also of extraneous muscular activity in other parts of the body and by direct instruction, reduce the intensity of effort. Also, by diminution of unnecessary stimulation, as in using a quiet room, one can allow the attention of the patient to be concentrated on the one activity being trained. It may be necessary to make a minimum of demands for activity on the patient. This can be done by providing support for any postural activity the patient requires, or by allowing him to lie on a mat in a side-lying or supine position so that he is totally supported and attention needs to be directed only to what is being asked for without any need for other postural or voluntary activity to intervene.

The implications of this concept with regard to learning motor activities have been discussed above; but there is one further aspect of learning functional motor activities that needs to be considered. As has been observed previously, an essential aspect of maturation is the association of reflex motor activity to a new and goal-oriented stimulus. Thus, if the patient had strong extensor thrust in a lower extremity in the sitting position, this could be inhibited by a Marie-Foix maneuver, i.e., stretching of the extensor muscles of the toes by passive flexion of the toes at the metatarsophalangeal joints. This is a somesthetic stimulus giving rise to flexor activity of that lower extremity. The association of the flexor activity then with attempted voluntary flexion on command would be a functional association. The result of such repeated practice where reflex facilitation reinforces volition, is to make the ongoing flexor activity available to the voluntary control.

When this control of the flexors has been developed, if the extensor thrust is initiated by a stimulus, the voluntary flexor activity will be associated with inhibition of extensor thrust, which can then be specifically trained voluntarily. While a particular motor activity can be elicited and developed through repetition alone in response to a specific somesthetic stimulus, the important element required for functional purposes is the ability to carry out the motor activity in response to a functional stimulus. It therefore follows that as soon as a motor activity becomes available on the basis of somesthetic stimulation, the appropriate functional stimulus and context should be introduced. This stimulus may be a command, the previous motion in a functional sequence, as in walking, dressing or feeding. Or, the stimulus may be a previously unused sensation which is made by the therapist to substitute for the usual one which is not available to the subject. An example would be the use of visual guidance for head control, or sitting balance, substituting for proprioceptive or vestibular sensation. Another example would be a verbal signal, even one spoken by the subject himself, or visual feedback to substitute for deficient reflex support reaction. Because of the difficulty which many individuals with brain damage have in unlearning old and learning new material, it is essential that a movement pattern not be learned as a reflex pattern in too rigorous a manner before making the transition to functional stimuli.

Since the achievement of new motor patterns is a function of learning ability, methods of training should utilize procedures which have been shown to be most effective for learning. Among the most powerful techniques for teaching is that referred to as instrumental learning or behavior modification (23). There is a large body of literature documenting the effectiveness of the principles of reinforcement of a desired activity as a means of obtaining its repetition in desired circumstances (24). Careful application of the principles of behavior modification to the motor problems of the patient with cerebral palsy will achieve a maximum level of new functioning.

An important factor in the application of learning theory to motor training in cerebral palsy is that precise definition of functional goals is an essential element in achieving successful learning. In much of the literature describing the use of instrumental learning or behavior modification principles, the goal for training is a gross behavior with the expressed or implied assumption that all of the motor components were within the usual repertory of the subject. In cerebral palsy this assumption is not true. Goals therefore have to be directed first at subsidiary components of functional movements which in themselves, may be achievable so that they can be utilized as building units to be synthesized into a useful functional motor act at a later time (25, 26).

Functional movements may be broken down into convenient motor components or into extremely small sections of discrete joint movements, or even single muscle contractions depending upon the level of achievement of the child. For example, head control can be trained by tilting the child to 10°, or 15° of tilt in any or all of the directions, and reinforcing him for making the appropriate adaptive correction by head movement. A child who has severe disability in head control can be trained by placing his head in the erect position, assisted by passive support, and reinforcing him for maintaining it for a few minutes to several hours. The support can be manual, a soft collar, a plastic orthosis, or even a Boldrey type head support, as is required. Progress can be recognized by the diminishing amount of support needed and the increasing time of erect posture. The training process needs to be coordinated with splinting, or bracing, to maintain the head in the correct position passively during most of the day to accustom the child to a new erect "normal" posture. Assistive training devices should be used to supplement therapeutic exercises. Since the manual support is interactive, it can be associated with demand for responses for erect head position which can be reinforced.

An example of training of motor components in the upper extremity would be to divide the reaching motion into shoulder flexion, or abduction, as required, where the shoulder abduction is reinforced for increased duration at different angles, since this is a postural activity. The shoulder flexion is reinforced for accuracy and control of direction because this is a specific voluntary action. Elbow extension and flexion are trained separately, concomitantly, but not simultaneously, in a limited range which gradually extends as skill is improved. Reinforcement can be given for the accuracy of elbow motion with inhibition of adventitious shoulder, wrist, or hand motion. When there is great difficulty, shaping is used to proceed from crude motion with much overflow to precise motion with minimal overflow. Where the shoulder support is severely impaired, only the requirement of controlled elbow motion is taught while the therapist provides the necessary support and restraint manually until the elbow motion is learned.

To provide support and adequate feedback, the patient's forearm should be held in one hand by the therapist, so that the hand is supported by the therapist's fingers and the palm is under the volar surface of forearm. The other hand may be free to guide other parts such as the middle or lower arm. In this way, changes of position of the wrist, elbow, or shoulder can be felt, and assisted, or resisted by the therapist. Changes of tone in the muscles of the shoulder, arm, or forearm can be detected by the therapist who informs the patient immediately, thus providing feedback. In this way, the therapist directs the attention of the patient, increasing awareness of both the sensory and the motor components of the muscular activity. Reinforcement, or reward is accomplished when correct responses occur through this feedback technqiue, and by the clear approval accompanying the correct motion.

When there is ability to maintain a position which has been initiated passively, volitional control should be introduced by requiring a voluntary termination of the holding position. Rather than allowing the activity to fade with fatigue, a timed duration of hold is selected that is uniformly successful and a response is required to alternating commands of "hold" and "let it go." Manual assistance is given by passive motion, if voluntary release is not forthcoming. Verbal, or other meaningful reinforcement is given for any relaxation felt by the therapist during the passive motion. Shaping for increased relaxation and promptness of response to command is carried out through this reinforcement so that inhibition, or voluntary relaxation occurs more and more promptly, and completely at the appropriate command. These components can then be integrated, or synthesized into the complex motion. Wrist dorsiflexion can similarly be trained by reinforcing for active dorsiflexion when function is already available, or by initially providing some rapid stretch to the wrist flexors, placing the wrist in a neutral or extended position, as feasible, and reinforcing for increasing long duration of maintenance of the position, to the command "hold it." Assistance may be given manually, or by electrical stimulation, and withdrawn as needed as long as the duration is recorded.

A program for training upper extremity control would include the following exercises as an example, where these components were found clinically to be deficient, insufficient, or lacking control of accuracy:

1. *Shoulder abductor maintenance at 90°, 45°, 135°*
    a. With elbow flexed
    b. With elbow extended
        Reinforce for increasing endurance up to 5 min and graph daily results. Establish limits for allowable adventitious rotation, and flexion-extension of shoulder and elbow. As improvement occurs, narrow the limits of overflow and start a new graph. Reinforce for accuracy. Record time scores daily, or weekly (Fig. 13.1).

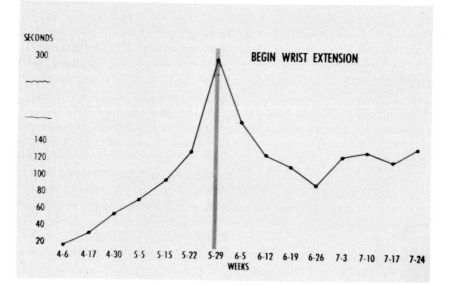

Fig. 13.1. Graph of shoulder abduction endurance. Note the improvement to a maximum is followed by a decline in ability that continues several weeks after new conditions of difficulty are introduced, until the process of synthesis is mastered.

2. Shoulder flexion and extension

Active flexion or extension is performed on command. Reinforce for accuracy according to therapist's observations, e.g., anything less than 10° of adventitious rotation, abduction or adduction, to improve smooth motion in the proper direction. If undesired abduction, adduction, or rotation accompanies the motion, clues should be given by tactile and verbal means, with reinforcement for gradually improving inhibition of these components. Other limits may be set depending on the ability of the patient. Record either the number of sequential successful extensor-flexor cycles achieved, or the percent of the set as a practical goal.

3. Elbow extension-flexion

Reinforce for accuracy throughout the full range. Provide shoulder support if needed for accurate motion. Remove shoulder support as skill improves. Record the number of successful trials, or the percentage of the target performance. The patient's reaction to the mode of recording is a factor in the selection. Do not push performance to a maximum each day, since this always terminates as a final failure, and patients become demotivated. End each therapy on a successful performance. Increase goals regularly as achievable, so patient is maximally successful.

4. Wrist extension goals

a. Reinforce active flexor inhibition
1. On command after passive placement
2. On command after active extension
b. Reinforce active extension
1. With facilitation

2. Without facilitation *when capable*. Record the number of repetitions successfully completed

Therapist's fingers in palm, feel for flexor activity, observe flexor tendons for evidence of tension. Reinforce for active maintenance of flexor relaxation, or extension of the wrist. Record the duration of extension and the angle. As the angle improves, start new graphs.

5. *Resynthesize*
   a. Shoulder-elbow simultaneous active flexion-extension. Support the wrist and fingers in relaxed neutral position. Therapist's fingers in patient's palm, volar forearm facing volar forearm. Instruct and reinforce for smooth, accurate motion of both joints. Give feedback as soon as there is detected any adventitious motor activity or tone other than the desired combination. Reinforce for correct motion immediately
   b. Elbow-wrist
   c. Shoulder-elbow-wrist

This may not have to go in the same combinations or order. Decisions are clinical depending upon the relative control and success of the individual motions. Where a component is still unsuccessful, the therapist should assist that component during the voluntary activity of the other components.

6. *Grasp and release*
   a. Finger flexion and release—count repetitions. The therapist feels the patient's fingers with his/her own fingers and reinforces immediately for the appropriate activity, or inhibition. Record the number of successful motions, or the duration of either a successful grasp, or an inhibition of reflex grasp.

7. *Thumb abduction, and adduction-opposition*
   a. Voluntary pinch and release with reinforcement for each activity. Shape by gradual approximation toward opposition if feasible.

These exercises can be done in a functional context, with play activities, or in occupational therapy, as well as in physical therapy. Electromechanical or the therapist's signals may be used, or modified toys provided to maintain interest and novelty.

The task of ambulation can be subdivided for training purposes into the components of:

1. Support Activity
2. Reciprocation
3. Dynamic Equilibrium
4. Segmental Coordination
5. Gait Sequence

In analyzing the motor repertoire for ambulation, each of these subsidiary functions should be looked at, and defined individually, baseline records made, and regular measurements taken of the response to training. Periodic evaluations will highlight the kind of progress being made which will justify either continuation of the program, its alteration, or discontinuance.

The *support activity* should be distinguished from the reflex support reaction, and while reflex activity can and should be used as a means of making available the motor activity for learning, the essential needs for training are to bring it under voluntary control both in the initiation, and in the inhibition phases. To the extent that the reflex activity is facultative, it can be useful. When it is obligatory, means will have to be found to diminish its strength so that effective inhibition can be achieved to accomplish ambulation. If this can not be done, then effective ambulation is not possible. Similarly, for totally inadequate support activity, especially in the presence of obligatory flexor dystonia, the prognosis for ambulation is poor, unless means can be established for diminishing the flexor dystonia.

The support activity should be initiated by improving extensor activity at the hips, knees, and trunk. In patients with flexor hypertonia, the first necessity would be the training of inhibition of flexor activity. The principles involved are the general principles of training inhibition anywhere, described above. A number of maneuvers proposed by Bobath, such as the gentle, rhythmic, rotatory rocking of the pelvis in the prone position over a padded log with hips abducted, have been observed to be associated with general relaxation. This provides a useful response for reinforcement, so that it can be assumed voluntarily. It provides a base, therefore, for proceeding to the necessary extensor activity under conditions of flexor relaxation. Other techniques including electromyographic biofeedback have been proposed by a number of authors. Use of biofeedback should be accompanied by some measurement of the response to determine its effectiveness. This sensory feedback should be incorporated into the voluntary control system by using established principles of learning.

When inhibition of hypertonic motor activity is introduced by such maneuvers, this is quite similar to the elicitation of any motor activity by reflex facilitation. The activity, inhibitory as well as facilitatory, becomes available to the central nervous system. Through identification of the response and its visual, tactile, and proprioceptive sensory correlates the attempt is made to convert the response to a specific volitional activity. Later, with emphasis on repetition, such activity can be developed in some individuals as an automatic behavior. Very frequently, in spastic patients, training methods may not be sufficient to effect inhibition of hypertonia unless surgical lengthening or intramuscular neurolysis are carried out.

Muscle relaxants, or tranquilizers may be helpful in this situation as an assistive device to learning. As voluntary control begins to develop, it may be possible to diminish the dosage of the medication.

To facilitate the support reaction, and at the same time provide assistance by increasing vestibular stimulation and plantar contactual stimulation the individual can be placed in an upright or tilted back position on a tilt table set at 65–85°. The supporting straps across the knees and pelvis can be loosened as the support reaction improves. Assisted standing next to a table with a buttocks strap and padded knee support is extremely useful since the degree of independent support can be monitored more easily and the strap support can be loosened with greater assurance that there is active participation by the patient. In both situations, the patient should be given activities which require movement, or shifting of balance as feasible. A game of catch or tetherball, or manipulative-craft activities in occupational therapy are good examples. When appropriate, balance shifts are made, or extensor activity is elicited, reinforcement is given and is scored for the success.

From the point of bilateral support progress can be made to initiate and develop unilateral support. At first the patient learns to lean forward or backward or tilt sideways while standing on a stable platform; and then later as ability develops he proceeds to tilting from one side to the other on a rocking platform maintaining the support alternately on the right and left legs. This may also be done as a crutch drill if appropriate, or in parallel bars with and without the assistance of the therapist. The essential element again is to provide immediate verbal, visual, and/or tactile feedback relative to the activity of the hip and knee extensors and the degree of extension of the knees and hips. Strong reinforcement usually through verbal approval needs to be given to the successful achievement of the upright posture and the support reaction. Rewards should be directed to success in controlling individual segments when this is meaningful, and progress to reinforcement for coordination of the whole body posture as it can be achieved. The erect spine is as important as maintained extension and support at the hips and knees. Establishment of control of an erect spine is most often necessary before extension and support of the hips and knees can be learned.

Further progression can be made to a more dynamic exercise of standing up from a seated position starting with assistance for hip or knee extension as needed, and ultimately diminishing that assistance and working for increased numbers of repetitions as an active effort; and then to increase duration of standing balance. The use of assistive play material, such as a "jolly-jumper" and other similar devices are·welcome additions, both in terms of the demand for activity which can be repeated for long periods of time, and the reinforcement they develop. Their use also can and should be coordinated with a recording of the length of time and the number of repetitions that they are successfully used. The patient should not be required to be operating them for periods longer than they can master successfully.

Reciprocation may be introduced passively, by manual manipulation with the patient in the supine position, similar to some of the exercises proposed originally by Phelps. However, reinforcement should be given for active participation in activity for even the briefest instance as soon as it is sensed by the therapist. The therapist should attempt to elicit the activity both verbally and by any facilitatory techniques that are clearly successful. Reinforcement should be given verbally, as promptly as possible for even the briefest active response. A tricycle or stationary bicycle is a useful device for obtaining reciprocal lower extremity motion in the seated position. It should be remembered, however, that the specific motions and rhythms of the hips and knees in cycling activity differ considerably from those in walking; and attention will be necessary to having the patient learn the new pattern when walking training becomes indicated, and unlearning the cycle patterns for this activity.

Many children with cerebral palsy have difficulty in making these discriminatory responses. It, therefore, is useful to proceed to some form of assisted ambulation with reciprocation in order to clarify the learning of the specific motor sequence appropriate to each activity. In other words, if the child learns reciprocation as a form of knee flexion associated with hip flexion alternating with knee extension associated with hip extension, it becomes difficult for a number of children to alter this pattern to that of ambulation where hip flexion is associated with knee flexion only in the initial phase of swing, whereas in the later phase of swing knee extension supervenes. The same thing is true with the hip extension where hip extension is associated with knee extension in the initial phase of stance and knee flexion becomes associated with hip extension in the later phase. This rigidity in learning is a problem in children with different varieties of motor control and intellectual deficiencies. Reciprocation can proceed to assisted ambulation where the balance and equilibrium requirements are provided by the therapist's assistance. As improvement occurs if upper extremities will need to be used, they can be introduced into the program through the use of a weighted cart with a low center of gravity, then parallel bars which introduce the concept of reciprocation of the upper extremities, and finally four-point crutch ambulation. In each case, records can be kept of the distance walked, the rate of walking, the regularity of rhythm. The motion elicited, and reinforcement should be given promptly and regularly for each of these characteristics when reciprocation is the main object to be trained.

Dynamic equilibrium consists of maintenance of the center of gravity of the body, as well as each of its segments between or over points of support during active movement. The forces involved include those of acceleration and deceleration, as well as gravity. They are opposed by muscles, frequently of abnormal strength or tone in patients with cerebral palsy. Analysis of the motor repertory of each patient will indicate the specific areas of concern for individual patients. Examples of common problems are the excessive forward or lateral placement of the foot in stepping during ambulation. This of course gives rise to inadequate support because the hip extensor mechanisms are inadequate to continue to accelerate the body forward while being required to support against gravity where the changed force vector relationships around the hip joint require muscle strength in the normal, or even athletic range depending upon the angle. A similar problem is observed for crutch placement. If normal strength existed, a long step would be feasible. Thus, patients should be instructed and reinforced for utilizing a step length or crutch placement distance appropriate to their abilities. Identification of the problem, followed by specific verbal, or nonverbal means to limit and direct a patient for accurate placement with reinforcement when the patient does it independently or spontaneously are important elements in training.

An example of lateral dynamic dysequilbrium is the frequent problem of inadequate hip abductor activity leading to scissoring. Often, even after spastic hip adductors have been lengthened surgically and good passive range of motion is demonstrable, patients continue to have scissor gait because of pelvic drop on the swing side. This problem is the result of weak hip abductors. They may not be able to improve in strength to be independently adequate. Instruction of the patient to carry out a voluntary, compensated Trendelenburg maneuver helps place the center of gravity of the upper portion of the body over, or lateral to the stance hip joint. Dynamic stability is acquired in this manner, and the swing limb is free to move forward.

In contrast to the child with a lower motor neuron lesion, many children with cerebral palsy have difficulty learning this maneuver, and much effort must be expended in training it. This weight shift coordinates naturally with crutch placement. A rhythmic verbal call can be used to instruct each patient. Often assistance is required initially in carrying out the maneuver. To give cues adequately, the therapist should sit on a rolling stool behind the patient. One hand is placed over the stance trochanter, the other just below the axilla over the lateral thorax, and as the patient makes the step forward, pressure is applied with each hand, and verbal directions to shift are given. By the amount of resistance experienced, the therapist can know when the patient is participating in the activity; and reinforcement can be given appropriately and promptly, and the assistance reduced accordingly.

Segmental coordination describes the temporal relationships of the motor patterns executed by each of the body segments. Kinesiologic analysis should be made of the dynamics of each of the body segments during ambulation. A decision must be made to set a goal for the optimum pattern for each segment, based on the realities of the patient's potential. Some regard for normal segmental relationships should be accorded, but in many cases these are not achievable, and other patterns will have to be accepted.

The sequence that is observed during stance phase of ambulation immediately after the foot is flat on the ground is that of hip extension, body progression, lateral body shift, back extension, return body shift, and toe support. The degree of hip abduction and rotation, knee extension, and ankle dorsiflexion that occurs during the progression from heel strike to toe-off are important elements in the effectiveness of the walking pattern. In particular, the behavior of the pelvis around the hip joint and the shift of body weight including back extension, as the center of gravity approaches the vertical alignment of hip, knee, and ankle joints; and then, as the hip and knee progress forward ahead of the ankle joint, each may require special adaptation, or training to achieve the most effective and esthetic ambulation. Similarly, during the swing phase, the sequence and amount of knee flexion, ankle dorsiflexion before, during, and after toe-off; the timing and degree of knee extension and hip rotation during swing, and prior to foot strike should be observed and recorded; and specific attention and training directed to these elements to the end that they are functioning at maximum strength and effectiveness, and in correct, useful temporal relationships to the rest of the gait pattern. Finally, the degree of ankle dorsiflexion during swing, and the character of foot placement, i.e., whether it is heel strike, flat foot placement, toe touch or toe strike should be included in the establishment of specific training goals.

An attempt should be made to train these segmental, phasic motor activities to be carried out at appropriate strength levels in the correct temporal patterns to produce ambulation of the greatest effectiveness, and hopefully efficiency. Unfortunately, these are not identical criteria, and a balance must often be established between them.

As in previous sections, those segmental components that are deficient in strength or effectiveness, may be improved by the use of facilitatory measures, and when effectively carried out can be introduced into the gait sequence. One example here, is the use of synkinetic motor activity of the hip flexors to facilitate ankle dorsiflexion. This is a well-known technique and can be used to introduce ankle dorsiflexion by starting in the sitting position, if dorsiflexion cannot be elicited in any of the other positions.

The patient is asked to flex the hip with knee flexed against manual resistance, the ankle dorsiflexes often spontaneously; but, sometimes a command or prior rapid stretch to the tibialis anterior is required. When the contraction occurs it is pointed out, with strong reinforcement, the skin over the tendon of the tibialis anterior is touched, and pointed out to distinguish it from the flexor hallucis longus which often contracts also.

The maneuver is repeated several times during each training session, and the patient is asked to try to dorsiflex the ankle without resistance against the hip flexors, and, if successful, with resistance against the tibialis anterior. Gradually increased knee extension is allowed, and decreased hip flexion, reinforcing for repetition, diminished latency, and strength of tibialis anterior contraction. Measurements of each can be made depending upon the particular parameter that is of greatest importance in the walking pattern for that patient. The technique can then be transferred to the walking situation, where the therapist, seated on a rolling stool, resists forward stepping (hip flexion) with straight knee of the swing leg; providing visual and tactile feedback, and reinforcing anterior tibialis contraction during the swing phase and heel strike.

When this is mastered, one may progress to reinforcement of eccentric contraction of the anterior tibialis to prevent foot slap. This, however, is much less usual within the capability of the average patient with cerebral palsy.

Similar synkinetic motor patterns can be used for hip abduction and rotation, although their use is not as frequently successful. A search must be made for facilitatory techniques which will elicit adequate response before determining that the activity is not feasible. Other facilitatory techniques may be used in a similar manner to elicit the desired motor activity and make it amenable to learning process.

The *gait sequence* is the resynthesized or integrated performance of the individual subsidiary components of the ambulation process. During the early learning periods, each of the components of support, reciprocation, dynamic equilibrium, and segmental coordination are individually trained. As the ability to carry them out is acquired, each of these components are introduced into the walking pattern in its appropriate phasic relationship to the gait pattern as a whole. It should be noted that there is no purpose in waiting until total mastery of each component is achieved before resynthesis into the whole pattern is carried out.

As was discussed previously, learning is extremely specific, and while isolation of a motor act is required for proper identification of the important relevant feedback criteria for effective performance, the most useful learning is in the situation in which the act is to be used. Isolated and synthesized training should proceed concomitantly as soon as the basic ability to effect the desired component with reliability and effectiveness has been demonstrated.

When effective execution of the target movements required for optimum ambulation in a specific patient has been achieved, the movements should be included in the ambulation training program in appropriate sequence. Manual, visual, and verbal cues should be established so that communication of commands and feedback can be accomplished with facility and in the proper phase. Often these can be organized into a rhythmic sequence of commands. For example, in an athetoid patient with problems in hip abduction, knee extension, and ankle dorsiflexion, the commands to be given might be the series such as: "crutch," "lean," "step" (forward), "heel" (dorsiflexion), "knee" (straighten), "crutch," "lean," etc. Additional cues can be given by pushing the trochanter and the opposite mid-axillary thoracic wall, to aid in shifting body weight; alternatively, touching over the quadriceps tendon or anterior thigh when the knee should be straightened; stroking over the shin or the anterior compartment during swing phase or before heel strike when dorsiflexion is desired. The correct foot with which to step can be indicated by a nudge with the therapist's foot, or hand as required.

Measurements may be carried out by recording the number of steps, or the distance walked that met criteria for component performance in the appropriate gait sequence. Care should be taken to place criteria for components performed in the gait sequence at a different level than when individually performed. Most frequently there is a decline in skill achieved when an activity is carried out as part of a larger group of activities. Further training in the synthesized mode is required to reestablish the highest ability of component performance in the new complex total activity.

After initial learning of any motor activity is accomplished, a therapeutic program needs to be organized to provide regular repetitive exercise of that action. Circumstances that call for repetition as specific voluntary activity as often as possible are required. However, the guarantee of useful level of skill is its incorporation into regular functional daily activity. It should be the aim for anyone involved in training motor activity in patients with cerebral palsy to develop as soon as possible, a series of functional activities, whether required daily care, or recreational in character, which will require the performance of newly learned activities over many repetitions for a long period of time. In this way, specific voluntary activities can be incorporated into the motor repertory on an automatic level, provided the central nervous system mechanisms for automaticity are available.

The requirements for optimum learning make it necessary for a therapist to give immediate sensory feedback to an instructed motion in order to direct attention of the patient to the motion or to the events surrounding it for informational purposes, as well as for reinforcement or reward. The stimulus in this cases becomes the somesthetic or visual sensation of the position or movement. Reinforcement techniques serve to direct attention, and therefore enhance awareness of the motion, its correctness or incorrectness, with gradual refinement of the skill being demanded subsequently, as more sensitive criteria for success are developed. Reinforcement, as reward, also serves to attach value or significance to a particular performance, assisting in definition of what should be recognized by the patient as success.

REFERENCES

1. MINEAR, J. A classification of cerebral palsy. *Pediatrics, 18:* 841, 1956.
2. TOWBIN, A. *The Pathology of Cerebral Palsy.* Charles C Thomas, Springfield, Ill., 1960.
3. KNOBLOCH, H., AND PASAMANICK, B. (Eds.) *Gesell and Amatruda's Developmental Diagnosis*, Ed 3. Harper & Row, Hagerstown, Md., 1974.
4. PAINE, R. S., BRAZELTON, T. B., DONOVAN, D. E., DORBAUGH, J. E., HUBBELL, J. P., AND SEARS, E. M. Evolution of postural reflexes in normal infants, and in the presence of chronic brain syndrome. *Neurology, 14:* 1037–1048, 1964.
5. McGRAW, M. B. *Neuromuscular Maturation of the Human Infant.* Hafner Publishing Co., New York, 1963.
6. BRUNER, J. The Growth and Structure of Skill. In *Mechanisms of Motor Skill Development*, edited by K. Connolly. Academic Press, New York, 1970.
7. MATTHEWS, R. B. C. Evidence that the secondary as well as the primary endings of the muscle spindle may be responsible for the tonic stretch reflex of the decerebrate cat. J. Physiol., *204:* 365–393, 1969.

8. Kottke, F. J. Reflex patterns initiated by secondary sensory fiber endings of the muscle spindles: a proposal. *Arch. Phys. Med. Rehabil., 56:* 1–7, 1975.
9. Jung, R., and Hassler, R. The Extrapyramidal System. In *Handbook of Physiology,* Section 1, Neurophysiology, edited by J. Field. Washington, American Physiological Society, Washington, D.C., 1960.
10. Christensen, E., and Melchior, J. *Cerebral Palsy, A Clinical and Neuropathological Study.* Spastics International Medical Publications, 25, London, 1967.
11. Lucey, J. F., Hibbard, E., Behrman, R. E., Esquivel de Gallardo, F.O., and Windle, W. F. Asphyxiated newborn monkeys. *Exp. Neurol., 9:* 43, 1964.
12. Isaacson, R. *The Limbic System.* Plenum Press, New York, 1974.
13. Towe, A. L. The Motor Cortex and the Pyramidal System. In *Efferent Organization and the Integration of Behavior,* pp. 67–97, edited by J. D. Maser. Academic Press, New York, 1973.
14. Buchwald, J. S., and Brown, K. A. Subcortical Mechanisms of Behavioral Plasticity. In *Efferent Organization and the Integration of Behavior,* pp. 99–136, edited by J. D. Maser. Academic Press, New York, 1973.
15. Sherrington, C. *The Integrative Action of the Nervous System.* Yale University Press, New Haven, 1947.
16. Fiorentino, M. *Reflex Testing Methods for Evaluating Central Nervous System Development.* Charles C Thomas, Springfield, Ill., 1963.
17. Bobath, B., and Bobath, K. *Motor Development in Different Types of Cerebral Palsy.* Heinemann Publishing Co., London, 1975.
18. Knott, M., and Voss, D. *Proprioceptive Neuromuscular Facilitation in Therapeutic Exercise.* Hoeber Inc., New York, 1963.
19. Brunnstrom, S. *Movement Therapy in Hemiplegia, a Neurophysiological Approach.* Harper & Row, New York, 1970.
20. Gillette, H. *Systems of Therapy in Cerebral Palsy.* Am. Lect. Series #762. Charles C Thimas, Springfield, Ill., 1969.
21. Pearson, and Williams, C. E. *Physical Therapy Services in the Developmental Disabilities.* Charles C Thomas, Springfield, Ill., 1972.
22. Gracanin, F., Krac, J., and Rebersek, S. Advanced version of the Ljubljana functional electronic peroneal brace with walking, rate-controlled tetanization. *In Advances in External Control of Human Extremities.* Belgrade, Yugoslav Committee for Electronics and Automation, 1970.
23. Skinner, B. F. *Science and Human Behavior.* Macmillan, New York, 1953.
24. Michael, J. L. Rehabilitation. In *Behavior Modification in Clinical Psychology,* edited by C. Neuringer and J. L. Michael. Appleton-Century-Crofts, New York, 1970.
25. Meyerson, L., and Kerr, N. Behavior Modification in Rehabilitation. In *Child Development: Readings in Experimental Analysis,* edited by S. Bijou and D. Baer. Appleton-Century-Crofts, New York, 1967.
26. Touchette, P. E. The effects of graduated stimulus change on the acqustion of a simple form discrimination in severely retarded boys. *J. Exp. Anal. Behav., 11:* 39–48, 1968.

14

Exercise in Paraplegia

_____ ARTHUR S. ABRAMSON

Rehabilitation, together with antibiotics and surgery, has given the paraplegic an opportunity for a longer and better life. Perhaps the most important therapeutic tool in rehabilitation is exercise; it has a role in preventing complications, maintaining health and improving function; it is maximally effective when done at the right time, in the proper form, and in sufficient quantity.

Three stages of function are recognized: bed to wheelchair to ambulation. The nature of and rationale for the kind of exercise designed to take the patient through these stages will be outlined. The model will be the patient who has lost sensation and motor power due to traumatic transverse myelopathy, permitting modification for incomplete cord transection or cauda equina lesion.

Similar principles are applicable to the tetraplegic, but in this case the extent of the neurologic lesion will limit the functional goal. They are also applicable to the paraparetic whose paralysis is slower in onset, as would occur in expansion of a spinal tumor. In this case the clinical picture may be somewhat different in that the state of spinal shock may not occur, the potential for recovery after surgery is often better, and the paralysis may not become as profound as in the case of trauma.

The First Stage

The initial response to acute injury to the contents of the spinal canal is complete flaccid paralysis below the level of the injury. This is called the state of diaschisis, more commonly but less accurately known as "spinal shock."

Where the lesion is below the level of the first lumbar vertebra, that is, in the region of the cauda equina, flaccidity and areflexia remain permanently unless recovery of voluntary function occurs. When the injury is to the spinal cord, that is, above the level of the conus of the cord, spasticity develops after the state of diaschisis passes off. The exception to this latter rule occurs in the rare case when the spinal cord below the level of the lesion undergoes degeneration because of ischemia resulting in permanent flaccidity. Diaschisis lasts for varied periods of time ranging from hours to weeks and occasionally months. If the state of flaccid paralysis passes off within a few hours, or, at the most, in a few days, the recovery of voluntary function is usually better than when the paralysis lasts for weeks or months.

During this period the patient may be in negative nitrogen balance and will develop muscle atrophy rapidly (1). Although the atrophy is particularly severe in the area of paralysis it also occurs to some extent in all muscle groups which remain normally innervated, since this is a time of bed rest and disuse for the entire organism (2).

Osteoporosis will develop below the level of the lesion because there is reduced stress on the skeleton (3). A major factor in this reduction is loss of muscle contraction. Weight bearing, once thought to be a major factor, apparently has only a minor effect on preventing metabolic losses from bone (4). Calcium loss from the bone is greater than its deposition, and this metabolized calcium is excreted largely through the urinary tract. High calcium content of the urine predisposes to the formation of calcium urinary stone, especially in the presence of alkaline infected urine. There is also a tendency to the rapid formation of soft tissue ossifications, especially around the hip joint (5). These may also begin to occur early and, together with the development of soft tissue contractures due to prolonged maintained inactive postures, may produce deformities with restriction of range of motion which is often permanent.

The negative nitrogen balance associated with atrophy of muscle and bone is usually aggravated by poor protein intake (6). There may be loss of appetite potentiated by a reactive depression. This leads to a state of malnutrition and, thus, reduced viability of tissues. Moderately prolonged pressure over bony prominences, which is likely to occur because of the patient's difficulty in turning himself and because of the loss of sensation, may lead to the formation of decubitus ulcers.

During diaschisis, the bladder is atonic or hypotonic and in the past was managed by continuous or tidal drainage through an inlying catheter. The prolonged presence of the catheter and the need to change it frequently predisposed to urinary infection and a high incidence of stone formation and vesicoureteral reflux. More recently, intermittent catheterization has become the treatment of choice and this has led to a reduction in the incidence of infection, stone, and reflux (7).

Malnutrition, muscle atrophy, osteoporosis, urinary infection, urinary stone, reflux, soft tissue ossification, contracture and decubitus ulcer are complications which occur during this early period and which may result in prolonged ill health and may act as barriers to rehabilitation. Most can be prevented or at least minimized (7); exercise is of the utmost importance in achieving this goal, directly or indirectly.

Muscles which are under voluntary control should be exercised to supply the stimulus for retaining dietary protein; this will help reduce the negative nitrogen balance, prevent or retard disuse atrophy in muscles which remain under voluntary control, and maintain a better overall state of nutrition and viability of tissues (8). Exercise can be given to the muscles of the upper extremities and shoulder girdle and to the spared abdominal and back muscles when the lesion is of the cauda equina. All available muscle groups should be shortened through their full range against resistance supplied by weights through pulleys while in bed (Fig. 14.1) or by the use of dumbbells. Such resistance should be applied at least once or preferably twice a day if this can be tolerated by the patient. The resistance should be increased from day to day but should not be so great as to present the patient from having a fairly prolonged exercise period. The limiting factor in this routine is the patient's subjective feeling of fatigue. However, exercises to the point of fatigue are not contraindicated unless there is a coincidental disorder such as severe heart disease. Experience has shown that the patient who is thoroughly tired as a result of planned activity usually sleeps and rests better and develops a better appetite. There have been studies tending to show that such prolonged regimens of resistive exercises are not necessary for developing muscle strength. It may be that only few movements against maximum resistance performed once or twice a day will strengthen muscle (9). However, the intent is not only to increase strength but also to improve nutrition and to train dexterity, endurance, and speed of substitutive movements, which will be of use in improving capacity to perform activities of daily living. Repetition is at least as important as resistance in accomplishing these objectives. In fact, the physiologic processes underlying strength, endurance, speed and coordination differ

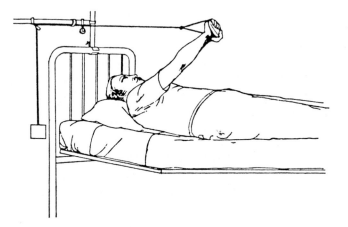

Fig. 14.1. Use of pulley in bed as conditioning exerciser.

from each other and each requires its own form of exercise for development. In addition, there are great psychological benefits to be derived from working hard toward a goal.

Conditioning exercises should be continued until the patient is completely active and ambulatory to his full capacity. Although the latter activity is then sufficient to maintain full metabolic and functional benefits, a continued daily conditioning program is insurance against unforeseen crises with sudden increased demands on energy reserves.

At the beginning, only passive exercises are possible in the lower extremities. All joints, including the hips, knees, and ankles, are carried through their full range but not beyond the point where resistance to movement is encountered. Such resistance may be due to the early formation of soft tissue ossifications. Forcible stretching may result in fractures and hemorrhages within these ossifications, producing still more heterotopic bone. However, there is some evidence that persistent passive motion may create pseudoarthroses in the ossification permitting the retention of range of motion (10). X-ray films of joints should be examined before a program of stretching is instituted.

Passive stretching of the lower back in flexion is indicated as long as spinal fracture is not present or there is no condition such as herniated nucleus pulposus where manipulation might result in aggravation of the neurologic condition. Stretching the patient's back while he is in bed or on a mat with legs fully extended also permits stretching of the hamstring muscles, counteracting their tendency to shorten as a result of spasticity or of prolonged sitting in a wheel chair.

When and if voluntary movement begins, active assistive exercise must be used through full range for those groups showing trace movement. Active movement with gravity eliminated and with the use of powder boards and skates should be used where there is poor contraction, active motion against gravity where there is fair contraction, and contraction through full range against resistance in higher grades of muscle strength (Fig. 14.2). There are many special exercise regimens which have been advocated for stimulating, capturing and improving returning voluntary function, especially in the spastic (11). Some of these are based on the notion that involuntary reflex patterns when repeated often enough aid

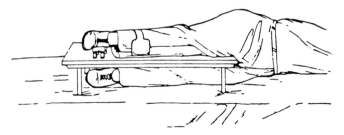

Fig. 14.2. Exercise with skate and powder board eliminates effect of gravity.

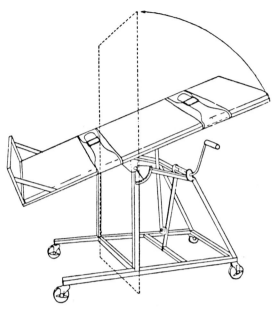

Fig. 14.3. Tilt table is used in conditioning by changing angle of table top.

in the return of voluntary functions. It seems illogical to assume that involuntary movements will have any effect in improving volition since each is subserved by different central nervous system mechanisms. In addition, it is difficult, if not impossible, to predict if and how much voluntary return will occur in any one patient. To attribute such return to any special form of exercise is unwarranted in our present state of knowledge. It is better to assume that return of voluntary function is spontaneous and that it can be improved and rendered more useful by training.

As early as is feasible and with the state of the skeleton (such as absence of fractures) permitting, the patient should be started on standing exercise. This consists of placing him in a supine position on a tilt table which is then tilted for 30 min at an angle of 45° or less, a position which the patient should be able to withstand without syncope (Fig. 14.3). This should be repeated twice a day, increasing the angle each time until he is able to stand in the upright position for at least ½ hour. The neurologic lesion disturbs central control of the sympathetic nervous system and causes temporary peripheral vascular paralysis and pooling of blood in the lower extremities on standing. This pooling effect is aggravated by the prolonged bed rest. Autoregulation of the vasoconstricter apparatus usually occurs, sooner or later, when the system is challenged by postural exercise. Besides conditioning the vascular system, standing also aids in urinary drainage.

The combination of passive, active, resistive and standing exercises, when given at the proper time in the proper combination and in the proper quantity, is instrumental in minimizing many of the complications mentioned earlier.

When in bed, the patient should have an overhead trapeze, permitting him to shift his weight from place to place easily and frequently. In addition to the added exercise this affords, it also prevents prolonged pressure on any one bony prominence. He should also be taught to turn in bed without the use of the overhead bar, as this is the beginning of training in activities of daily living and prepares him for the successful use of a bed.

The Second Stage

When the patient has become adapted to the standing position he is ready to use the wheelchair, to exercise on mats, and to stand between parallel bars. This may or may not take place before diaschisis disappears. Its passing, in the case of spinal cord injury, will herald the onset of spasticity, which with time may become increasingly severe, especially if excessive complications such as decubiti, urinary infection, and stone have facilitated the spinal cord because of feedback of noxious stimuli in the early phase during which the cord is reorganizing itself. In order for the patient to participate more easily it may be necessary to relieve him of some of his spasticity prior to the institution of the above-mentioned activities. The technique most commonly used is that of passive stretching through full range of motion (Fig. 14.4). Relief of spasticity results when excessive contractions are stimulated through the stretch reflex. The reflex must be continually stimulated by stretching the muscles slowly and repeating the maneuver over and over again until the extremity is made less spastic. The relative laxity of the extremity may last from 30 min to many hours and permits the patient to undertake activities which in themselves may delay return of the spasticity. Such stretching also has the advantage of preventing deforming contractures. While stretching must be done by the therapist at the beginning, the patient himself will

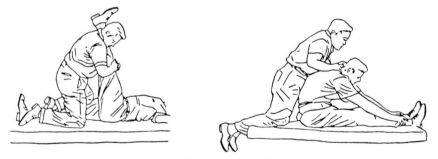

Fig. 14.4. Passive stretching for spasticity.

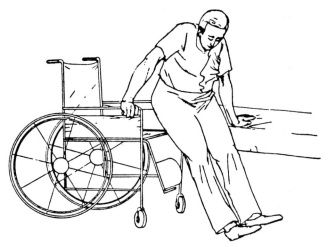

Fig. 14.5. Patient transferring to wheelchair.

gradually learn to do this in both the sitting and the standing positions. This is important, since stretching to reduce spasticity may have to be used by the spastic throughout life.

Preparation for transferring to a wheelchair must be preceded by training in moving from place to place in bed in a sitting position. This is done on outstretched arms with palms flat on the bed, elevating the trunk with the shoulder girdle muscles (depressing the shoulders). When he has become adept at this maneuver, the patient places his feet over the edge of the bed, and, with one hand on the bed and the other on the outer arm of the wheel chair, he raises his body and brings it from the edge of the bed onto the seat of the wheelchair (Fig. 14.5). He then places his feet on the footplates of the chair. The reverse of this technique is used for getting into bed, although some prefer to get into bed by using the overhead trapeze for lifting. There is nothing to choose between these techniques except that the individual may occasionally be in a position where he must use a bed without an overhead trapeze.

In the wheelchair the patient should do push-ups on the arm rests to strengthen the triceps and shoulder depressors and to habituate him to relieve the pressure on his buttocks often. Bedsores most commonly form over the sacrum and trochanters in the first or bed stage but may occur over the ischial tuberosities after prolonged sitting in the wheelchair has begun. Besides the use of a pressure dissipating cushion they can be prevented by standing at frequent intervals, by frequent changes of the sitting position, and by push-ups.

The next step is that of mat exercises. Exercise mats are customarily placed on the floor, and the patient is taught how to get from the wheelchair onto the floor (mat) and back again. Since it is likely that he will have to transfer himself more often from chair to chair rather than from chair to floor, it is preferable to place mats on a platform of the same height as the seat of the wheelchair (Fig. 14.6). The use of such platforms makes it easier for the patient to transfer and practice by himself and simpler for the therapist to work with the patient without back strain. Special exercise sessions should be devoted to learning the technique of getting down to and up from the floor. A series of two to four stools of graduated heights in front of the wheelchair seat are used for this purpose. The stools are removed alternately and then are eliminated as the patient improves his ability to lift himself (Fig. 14.7). On the mat the patient not only continues reconditioning exercises started in bed and those exercises permitting him to turn over but also learns to crawl and begins training for crutch walking.

Intact flexors of the hips are thought to be necessary for the act of crawling, but crawling is possible even with the paralysis of paraplegia. If, in the hand and knee position, the patient places his outstretched arms and hands forward and then advances his trunk forward as he flexes the elbow on one side, the extremity on the opposite side will slide forward (Fig. 14.8). By reversing this procedure the other leg will advance. Such training is necessary since crawling may be an important means of locomotion on emergent occasions when crutches and braces or wheelchair are not available.

Exercises in preparation for crutch walking are done with cut-down crutches. These are sufficiently long so that when sitting on the mat depression of the shoulders will permit the trunk to be raised between the crutches (Fig. 14.9). Preliminary crutch gaits are then practiced by advancing each crutch alternately and moving it backward or sideways. This not only strengthens the shoulder depressor muscles which are so important in ambulation but also trains other muscle groups used in crutch gaits. Practice in tilting one side of the pelvis and then the other is good preliminary exercise for a four-point gait. This is possible in a patient with a cauda equina lesion.

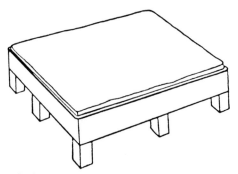

Fig. 14.6. A mat platform with mat. Two 5-foot-square platforms may be joined to receive a mat of 5 by 10 feet. Height of platform from floor is 18 inches.

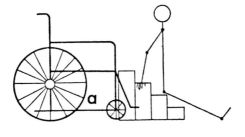

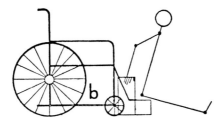

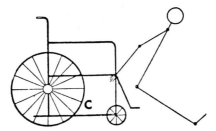

Fig. 14.7. Method of getting up to and down from wheelchair: (a) with four benches of graduated heights, (b) alternate benches, and (c) without benches.

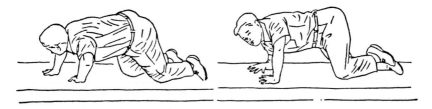

Fig. 14.8. Crawling.

An upright position between parallel bars is attained by splinting the knees. For this purpose padded boards or knee cages, stocked in a number of sizes, may be used. Because of drop foot, ambulation between parallel bars is not easy, but the patient can exercise his shoulder girdle muscles by doing push-ups. The most satisfactory push-up technique uses a double maneuver – straight up and then tilting forward. Progressively, the num-

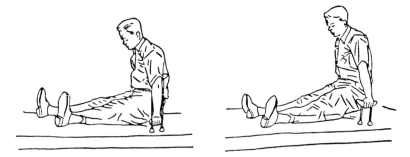

Fig. 14.9. Two types of cut-down crutches.

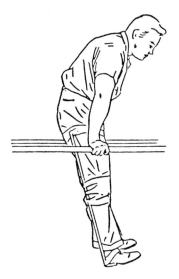

Fig. 14.10. Patient performing a push-up in parallel bars.

ber of push-ups should be increased day by day in order to increase endurance(Fig. 14.10). He can also stretch the hamstrings and calf muscles by bending to the floor while standing (Fig. 14.11). If the abdominal muscles are flaccid an abdominal binder may be used during the first attempts at standing to restore the diaphragm to the full expiratory position. Elastic bandages may be applied to the legs to prevent venous pooling.

If clinical progress has been satisfactory, the patient is now in good nutritional state and has developed powerful and well-coordinated muscles, especially in the arms and shoulder girdles. He has become proficient in transferring himself, in moving from the wheelchair to the floor and back, in crawling and in stretching himself. He has adapted his vascular system to the upright position. The favorable functional and metabolic effects of his activities have prevented or reduced the incidence of compli-

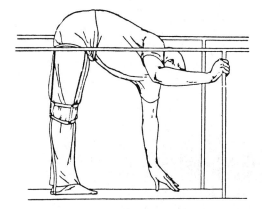

Fig. 14.11. Stretching between parallel bars.

cations. He has learned to move around in his wheelchair at a satisfactory speed for satisfactory distances. He is ready for crutch and brace ambulation.

The Third Stage

Rehabilitation programs up to the end of World War II established goals of total brace and crutch ambulation. The results of these programs were less successful than hoped for. This was at first attributed to lack of motivation, but certain physical factors were found to be important. The patient with a flaccid (low) lesion could be taught to ambulate with a greater degree of success than one with a higher transverse cord lesion who was spastic. The intensity of energy expenditure is dependent on residual functioning muscle mass; the more muscles that are paralyzed the less the ability to expend energy (12).

Walking is largely performed by the upper extremities and shoulder girdle, which are mechanically inefficient for this function. Even with long training, which in itself gradually reduces the energy costs of performance, energy expenditure eventually remains higher than for walking in the normal individual (12). Loss of sensation also forces many muscles under voluntary control to work harder in order to maintain balance. Obesity, weight of braces, and spasticity add to energy costs (12). The margin between ability to expend and expenditure in the paraplegic is so greatly reduced that even slow walking is comparable to running in the normal person. Obviously, paraplegics cannot do this all day long, and, even if they could, it would be at the expense of energies required for full vocational and other functions.

Ambulation has its advantages. It reduces spasticity in some and exercises all muscles under voluntary control; it prevents contractures. In the spastic, it may prevent osteoporosis and calcium loss, bone fragility, stone formation, and soft tissue ossifications reflexly by stimulating the contraction of paralyzed muscles. In permanent flaccid paralysis these may not be prevented by ambulation because muscle contraction cannot be reestablished (4) but metabolic losses from bone are self-limiting. These losses lasting a shorter time for low lesions than for those at a higher level (13). Ambulation also aids in urinary drainage by relieving sphincter spasticity as part of the overall relief of spasticity. Ambulation also enables the paraplegic to get to places which are inaccessible to a wheelchair (14). It is especially useful in perpetuating the overall reduction in spasticity which occur following neurectomy and tenotomy (15). Thus ambulation training in the paraplegic is useful if combined with wheelchair locomotion. With this in mind, it is clear that braces should be fitted to most paraplegics.

Long leg braces attached to pelvic band or body brace are most frequently prescribed (16). This type of brace is somewhat difficult to put on, is worn with some discomfort, and adds to the weight the individual has to carry. Its purpose is to prevent spontaneous flexion of the hips while standing, due to either instability or spasticity. They also prevent outward rotation of the lower extremities and lumbar lordosis, the latter occurring because the paraplegic, to be stable in the standing position, must lock his hips against the anterior pelvi-femoral ligaments. In addition, spasticity with flexion contracture of the ilio-psoas muscles may also render the fully upright position difficult to attain. One theory is to supply the full bracing as described and to reduce the amount of bracing as the patient develops the need for less. The other view is to supply only long leg braces in the belief that this is all that is necessary to substitute as much as is possible for loss of function (14). In spinal injuries as high as the upper thoracic region there still remain some very important and powerful muscles which are normally innervated and lie below the lesion level. They are the latissimus dorsi, the lower portion of the trapezius, the pectoralis and serratus anterior muscles. They receive their innervation from the brachial plexus, bypassing high thoracic lesions and even low cervical ones. These muscles, if made adequately strong by training, can control stability of the trunk and hips (14).

The latissimus dorsi under normal circumstances will adduct, extend, and internally rotate the humerus. When the insertion in the humerus is fixed, the mobilizing end of the muscle is transferred to its origin in the lower back and pelvis. If the feet are on the ground and the knees splinted, this action extends the hips. The patient can do this by clamping the axillary rests of the crutches between the humerus and the body, thus fixing the shoulders. Besides this forward pull, these muscles afford equal and opposite lateral pulls as long as the axillary rests of the crutches are held with equal pressure on both sides (Fig. 14.12). These maneuvers give active extension of the hips, locking of the hips in extension against the anterior pelvifemoral ligaments and lateral stability of the hips.

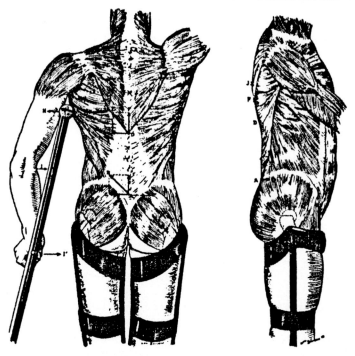

Fig. 14.12. Analysis of forces of muscle pulls created by contraction of the latissimus dorsi and lower trapezius muscles. At left, forces Ac and AC' are equal and opposite lateral thrusts at the pelvic level. When shoulders are equally fixed by static contraction these thrusts are equal and establish conditions for lateral stabilizing of the trunk. Force FD pulls upward at the D 12 level. In the lateral view at right, force AC thrusts the pelvis forward, which counteracts hip flexion due to instability or spasticity. The curved upper posterior thigh bands hug the gluteal curve which permits the buttocks to act as soft tissue hindrance to external rotation.

The lower portion of the trapezius will follow the same general rule; with fixation of the shoulders, the scapulae are fixed (14). The mobilizing end of this muscle is now transferred to its origin, exerting an upward pull from the region of the twelfth dorsal vertebra, which is the upper end of the lumbar curve, and thus straightening the lumbar lordosis (Fig. 14.12). In addition to the latissimus dorsi and trapezius muscles, other muscles of the shoulder girdle play their roles in stabilizing the trunk. The pectoralis and serratus anterior muscles tend to pull the upper part of the trunk backward as the latissimus tends to pull the lower part forward.

The integrated action of all muscles of the shoulder girdle is potentially capable of stabilizing the trunk of the paraplegic in the absence of pelvic band or back brace. Only training will permit these muscles to act effectively in this fashion. Such training is best obtained in the functional or standing position. The patient stands between parallel bars, holding them with his hands in front of him. He repeatedly pulls himself from the hip-flexed to the upright position by tightening the shoulder girdle muscles while maintaining the elbows at a fixed 30° angle with the position of the shoulders unchanged in space. This effort is gradually increased by progressively increasing the resistance to the movement. This can be done with a simple apparatus consisting of a padded belt around the pelvis attached to a cable carrying weights over a pulley at the end of the parallel bars (Fig. 14.13). The progress of training can be measured daily by observing the optimum weight the patient can carry 10 times from the flexed to the upright position (Fig. 14.14). Maximum strengthening of the movement can be accomplished within 2 or 3 weeks in a well-motivated person (17).

External rotation of the extremities can be minimized by using a curved upper posterior thigh band which permits the buttocks to act as soft tissue blocks to rotation. Using stirrups instead of calipers permits the foot to remain flat on the ground, helping to prevent rotation by friction. Such stirrups can be made to be as easily removable as calipers.

For maintenance of trunk stability during ambulation, the lessons learned between parallel bars must be carried over to crutches. The intermittent elevation of ambulation is done by the piston-like action of the trunk through the shoulder girdle, the elbows being kept at a fixed angle or extending only slightly. Throughout this procedure the muscles are never completely relaxed, and the long periods of exercises previously

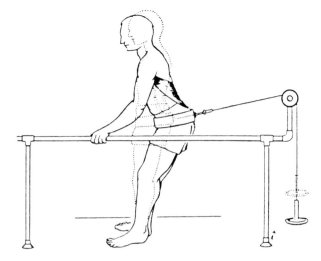

Fig. 14.13. This patient should be wearing long leg braces. Only the pelvis is thrust forward by tightening the shoulder girdle. The weight can be increased daily to provide progressive resistance exercise.

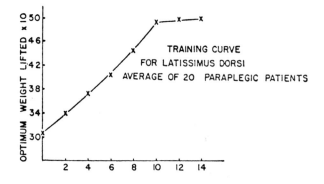

Fig. 14.14. Training curve for latissimus dorsi.

devoted to strengthening shoulder depressors and triceps will now show their value. It is probably true that pelvic bands and back braces slightly reduce the energy costs of ambulation by permitting more relaxation of the shoulder girdle muscles (12); they still do not reduce costs sufficiently to permit total crutch and brace ambulation. The slightly added costs seem to be of little consequence in the limited type of ambulation advocated. Ultimately, ambulation with crutches will be used only as a special exercise regimen by the greatly motivated and rarely as a method of total ambulation. The latter is more likely to occur in the very young teens where the energy costs seem to be less and the energy reserves seem to be greater.

CRUTCH GAITS

There are three fundamental types of gait available to the paraplegic. They are: 1) the alternate gaits, 2) the shuffle-to and swing-to gaits, and 3) the swing-through gait (16).

The first alternate gait is the four-point gait, in which one crutch is advanced, then the opposite foot, then the other crutch, and then the other foot (Fig. 14.15). This is very stable gait, always leaving three points on the floor at one time. It is most effective in the flaccid cauda equina lesion with pelvic-tilting muscles intact. It is most difficult to perform in a high spastic lesion.

The alternate two-point gait advances a crutch and the opposite foot at the same time and then the other crutch and foot (Fig. 14.16). This is less stable, allowing only two points to remain on the floor at one time. It is easier for the flaccid individual and usually permits a more rapid gait than the former.

The shuffle-to gait consists of advancing both crutches forward at the same time or alternately and then dragging the feet toward and even up to the crutches (Fig. 14.17). It is very stable and somewhat less tiring than the previous gaits, but it is impractical on a rough walking surface.

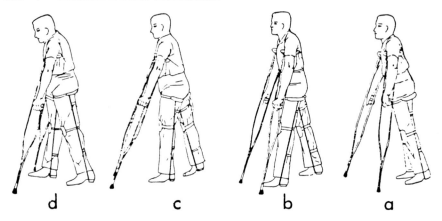

Fig. 14.15. Alternate four-point gait, from right to left: (a) right crutch forward, (b) left foot forward, (c) left crutch forward, (d) right foot forward.

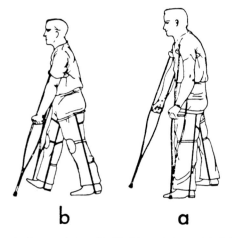

Fig. 14.16. Alternate two-point gait. Right crutch and left leg moved forward simultaneously, then left crutch and right leg.

The swing-to gait is the same as the shuffle-to gait previously described, except that the trunk is elevated, permitting the feet to hop toward the crutches. As the feet strike, the crutches are raised either together or alternately and placed forward and the same cycle is repeated. The work done in lifting the body is probably not much more than that done in dragging the feet forward against friction. It is slightly less stable than the shuffle-to gait. Both the shuffle-to and the swing-to gaits are more practical for the spastic since inadvertent flexion due to spasticity will not throw the patient off balance, as the crutches are well ahead of the hips.

The fastest, most graceful but most difficult crutch gait is the swing-through in which the crutches are placed forward, the body raised, and

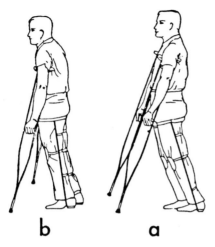

Fig. 14.17. Swing to gait in which feet hop to crutches by elevation.

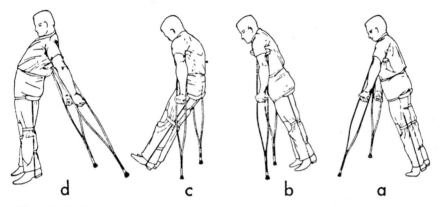

Fig. 14.18. Swing-through gait, from right to left: (a) crutches forward, (b) feet leave floor to swing forward, (c) feet completing swing through crutches, (d) feet have completed swing and crutches are ready to be lifted forward.

the legs swung forward, striking the heels in front of the crutches and throwing the hips in extension; the crutches are then carried in front of the feet again (Fig. 14.18). This is an effective gait for the flaccid individual but is a more difficult gait for the spastic since the shoulders and crutches must be back of the pelvis when the legs are forward. With sudden spasticity resulting in hip flexion, this may be difficult as the patient may lose balance and fall backward.

Conclusions

Functional improvement from bed to ambulation has been described in three stages. This progression can be a smooth flow from total helplessness to as completely an independent state as is possible within the individual's remaining reserves. The way from one state to another must be paved by specific exercises.

Function in the paraplegic is costly in terms of energy requirements. Despite the most positively directed motivation, activities such as ambulation should be limited if their toll is excessive. Thus rehabilitation goals must not be set beyond mechanical and metabolic capacities.

REFERENCES

1. ABRAMSON, A. S. Atrophy of disuse; definition. *Arch. Phys. Med., 29:* 562, 1948.
2. DEITRICK, J. E., WHEDON, G. D., AND SHORR, E. Effects of immobilization on various metabolic and physiologic functions of normal men. *Am. J. Med., 4:* 3, 1948.
3. ALBRIGHT, F., AND REIFENSTEIN, E. C. *The Parathyroid Glands and Metabolic Bone Diseases. Selected Studies.* Baltimore, 1948.
4. ABRAMSON, A. S., AND DELAGI, E. F. The contribution of physical activity to rehabilitation. *Res. Q., 31:* 2, 365, 1960.
5. ABRAMSON, A. S. Bone disturbances in injuries to the spinal cord. *J. Bone Joint Surg., 30A:* 982, 1948.
6. ABRAMSON, A. S. Modern concepts of management of the patient with spinal cord injury. *Arch. Phys. Med. Rehabil., 48:* 113, 1967.
7. GUTTMANN, L., AND FRANKEL, H. The value of intermittent catheterization in the early management of traumatic paraplegia and tetraplegia. *Paraplegia, 4:* 63, 1966.
8. ABRAMSON, A. S., AND EBEL, A. Rehabilitation in the management of prolonged illness. *Med. Clin. North Am., 37:* 915, 1953.
9. ROSE, D. L., RADZYMINSKI, S. F., AND BEATTY, R. R. Effect of brief maximal exercise on the strength of the quadriceps femoris. *Arch. Phys. Med., 38:* 157, 1957.
10. STOVER, S. L., HATHAWAY, C. J., AND ZEIGER, H. E.: Heterotopic ossification in spinal cord injured patients. *Arch. Phys. Med. Rehabil., 56:* 199, 1975.
11. FAY, T. Neurophysiologic aspects of therapy in cerebral palsy. *Arch. Phys. Med., 29:* 327, 1948.
12. GORDON, E. E., AND VANDERWALDE, H. Energy requirements in paraplegic ambulation. *Arch. Phys. Med., 37:* 276, 1956.
13. DUNNING, M. F., AND PLUM, M. Hypercalciuria following poliomyelits; its relationship to site and degree of paralysis. *Arch. Intern. Med., 99:* 716, 1957.
14. ABRAMSON, A. S. Principles of bracing in the rehabilitation of the paraplegic. *Bull. Hosp. Joint Dis., 10:* 175, 1949.
15. ABRAMSON, A. S., AND HIRSCHBERG, G. G. Studies on spasticity. The role of the contraction of certain muscle groups and the effect of its elimination on the over-all spasticity in patients with transverse spinal cord lesion. *Bull. Hosp. Joint Dis., 13:* 164, 1952.
16. DEAVER, G., AND BRITTIS, A. L. Monograph V., Institute of Physical Medicine and Rehabilitation, New York, 1953.
17. ABRAMSON, A. S. Principles of bracing in the rehabilitation of the paraplegic. *Orthop. Prosthet. Appl. J., 28,* 1955.

15

Therapeutic Exercise in Hemiplegia

────────────────── JAMES R. SWENSON

To comprehend the therapeutic exercise treatment of hemiplegia fully one must have a thorough knowledge of the whole range of therapeutic exercise and an appreciation of the pathophysiology of stroke and its evolution. Hemiplegia is characterized by a variable collection of neurological impairments only one of which is motor paralysis. This suggests that a variety of therapeutic techniques will be required to effectively treat the specific mosaic of impairments seen in each individual patient. This makes the establishment and strict adherence to a specific stroke exercise protocol illogical and at times ineffective.

The careful evaluation of each stroke patient is the first priority of treatment and the careful formulation of an appropriate exercise program is the second priority item. The initial evaluation of the patient rarely gives all the information needed concerning that patient's deficits. More often the therapeutic team needs to carefully observe the patient for several days or weeks before all of the impairments are detected and understood. Changes in impairments occur as a result of the evolution of hemiplegia and in response to the treatment program. This makes continuing evaluation of the patient and modification of the exercise program essential. The most effective ongoing patient evaluation and program modification is accomplished by a team effort between physician and therapists.

The severity of stroke depends upon five factors.

1. The *cause* of the stroke and its permanence. Is the initial stroke lesion reversible with time or does cell death occur so that no spontaneous recovery can be expected?

2. The *location* of the stroke. Which tracts and cell nuclei are involved? The location and extent of brain damage determine the symptoms and physical findings in the patient.

3. The *quantity* of brain tissue involved. In some locations a large quantity of brain tissue damage will cause only minimal functional impairment. In other locations, such as the brainstem, a small amount of tissue destruction can cause severe neurological and functional impairment. The degree of organic brain damage and impairment of higher intellectual functions is often of more significance than the degree of motor paralysis.

4. The *health status* of the patient before the stroke. One would expect a better prognosis in a young cardiac patient with an embolic stroke than in a 68-year-old patient with diffuse cerebrovascular disease resulting in occlusion of the middle cerebral artery.

5. The number and type of *complications* which occur after the onset of stroke. This is related to the level of care provided the patient which is related to the skill and sophistication of the therapeutic team.

The neurological picture is determined by the site of brain damage. The clinical features (14) found in occlusion of the internal carotid, middle cerebral, anterior cerebral, posterior cerebral, and the vertebral arteries are well known and useful in diagnosis.

Patient Evaluation

Before an appropriate therapeutic exercise program can be prescribed for the hemiplegic stroke patient, the physician must make a complete evaluation of the patient. In addition to the general physical examination, this should include state of consciousness, mental function, speech and language, cranial nerves, sensation, perceptual ability, motor function, joint range of motion, reflexes, and functional level.

The booklet, "A Classification and Outline of Cerebrovascular Disease — Part II" (14) lists the important information to be collected by the physician from the patient's history, physical examination, and laboratory examination to assist in the management of the patient. A standard description of *state of consciousness* (14) includes 1) normal, 2) semistupor (lethargy with slow response), 3) stupor (appropriate response to verbal stimulus), 4) deep stupor (purposeful response to noxious stimulus), 5) semicoma (nonspecific response to pain), 6) coma (no response to pain with present DTR's, pupillary reactions, and corneal reflexes), and 7) deep coma (no response to pain with absent DTR's, pupillary reactions, and corneal reflexes).

Mental function includes intellect (memory, recall, calculation, judgment, orientation), speech and language, emotion, and thought content. Traditional mental function tests should give answers to the following kinds of questions. Is the patient orientated to time, place, person? What kinds of psychic defenses does the patient have? How much rigidity of personality exists that will interfere with therapy? Is the patient aware of his surroundings? Since exercise therapy is a learning situation, is the patient capable of understanding objectives, following directions, and learning new skills? Does the patient have continence of bowel and bladder? Is the patient able to feed himself? Does the patient track with his eyes when others come into the room?

Speech and language evaluation should determine if the patient has dysarthria or aphasia. If aphasia is present, is it expressive, receptive, or combined? Do not confuse organic mental syndrome with aphasia. The aphasic patient will remain alert. He will be a good learner and will have a better prognosis for independence in ambulation and self-care activities. The patient with organic mental syndrome will have a difficult time learning transfer activities, dressing skills, and other complex motor acts. The severely global aphasic patient may initially be difficult to distinguish from the patient with organic mental syndrome. This distinction has clinical importance.

The *cranial nerves* are evaluated traditionally. Attention must be paid to the absence or presence of a visual field defect. Homonymous hemianopsia greatly interferes with the perception of visual cues from the environment on the affected side. This causes the patient to lean to the affected side and have a distorted perception of verticality. Rod and frame tests have clearly shown that left hemiplegic patients have a greater disturbance of verticality than right hemiplegic patients. Limited occular movements, nystagmus, loss of corneal sensation, vestibular dysfunction, paralysis of pharngeal and laryngeal muscles, and paresis of tongue muscles all complicate exercise therapy. Bulbar symptoms with inability to chew, swallow, or speak must be evaluated in these patients.

Sensory testing includes evaluation of vibration, two-point discrimination, position sense, pain, light touch, temperature, stereognosis, deep pressure, double simultaneous stimulation, graphesthesia, localization of touch, texture, and appreciation of weight. The standard neurological texts describe the techniques of sensory testing. Impaired sensation complicates and prolongs exercise therapy and may ultimately impair total function.

Perceptual defects also complicate the management of stroke patients. Perception is defined as the ability to integrate and interpret internal and external sensory information. Common perceptual problems in stroke patients include denial of the hemiplegic side, lack of visual awareness of objects or activities past the midline, astereognosis, visual neglect, disturbance of body image, constructional apraxia, defective right-left discrimination, topographic memory loss, altered vertical perception, and figure-ground problems.

Cohen (16) outlines the perceptual problems found in hemiplegic patients. For a stimulus to effect a given response, it must first be perceived. Basically two types of sensation are involved in normal reception, one at the primary thalamic level involving touch and pain, and the other at the cortical level involving discriminatory interpretations of sensory impulses by which the nature of trace figures and proprioceptive determinations are made. In general it seems the parietal lobes are concerned with sensory interpretation. Disturbances of body image, spatial judgment, and sensory interpretation are associated with damage to the nondominant parietal lobe of the brain.

Constructional apraxia is a perceptual deficit which occurs in the hemiplegic patient. The patient is unable to copy simple geometric designs. Apraxia can complicate dressing in the hemiplegic patient. The patient may have difficulty in putting on his clothes and may put them on back to front or upside down. Defective right-left side discrimination is another form of perceptual loss. Some patients suffer from topographic memory loss and have the inability to describe familiar routes.

One of the commonest but least investigated behavioral changes associated with brain injury in adults is visual-spatial neglect. The patient ignores objects, people, and activities in one half of the world around him. The lesion producing visual spatial neglect usually occurs in the posterioparietal or the occipitoparietal area of the nondominant cerebral hemisphere. The lesion frequently will extend beyond the cortex to involve the optic radiations.

Albert (1) presents a simple test of visual neglect consisting of having the patient cross out 40 randomly placed short lines on a paper. He found bilateral neglect both in patients with right and with left brain damage which was more severe in patients with right brain damage. Visual neglect can occur without a visual field defect. Visual neglect can be caused by disturbance of any of the following factors: attention, reception of visual stimuli, modality specific attention, perception, sensory motor integration, oculomotor function, cerebral dominance for visual-spacial organization, immediate recall and recent memory.

DeCencio et al. (19) found that persons having left hemiplegia were inferior to those having right hemiplegia in their perception of verticality within both the frontal and midsagittal planes. Right hemiplegic persons are deficient in the visual perception of verticality within the frontal plane only. This is explained on the basis of a bilaterally asymmetrical proprioceptive input. Left hemiplegic persons incorrectly perceive verticality both within the frontal and midsagittal planes. This is considered to be caused by asymmetrical proprioceptive input, combined with spatial perceptual dysfunction associated with a lesion of the right hemisphere.

Birch et al. (7) studied perception in hemiplegic patients and found three features of the visual perception of vertical and horizontal that are altered in the hemiplegic patient; namely, accuracy, directional shift, and variability. In all three of these aspects of visual functioning the hemiplegic patients perform more poorly than do control subjects. In their perception of the vertical, the left hemiplegics made errors which were preponderantly counterclockwise in direction. No such problem is apparent in the right hemiplegic patient.

Many perceptual tests have been published. A number of poorly defined perceptual terms are being used and creating confusion. The clinical correlation of these tests and these terms remains to be determined by careful, controlled experiments. The relationship of many perceptual terms to the traditional neurological sensory modalities is confusing and unclear.

Thus it can be appreciated that perceptual functions are complex. Future research is badly needed to standardize perceptual terminology for the adult hemiplegic patient, determine the best tests for perceptual functions, correlate perceptual test abnormalities with barriers to successful rehabilitation and clarify the best therapeutic exercise technique for a given perceptual defect.

Motor function testing includes evaluation of gait, strength, coordination, and muscle tone. Motor control is evaluated in terms of a background of knowledge of patterned movements. Traditional manual muscle testing is not applicable. The nonapplicability of traditional manual muscle testing terminology is evident to all with any experience in the field, but for some reason many persist in using inappropriate terminology. Many new muscle test forms have been developed which are based on the motor recovery characteristics in hemiplegics; such tests are those by LaVigne (33), Caldwell et al. (12), Brunnstrom (10), and Zankel (76).

Brunnstrom (10) has categorized the recovery from adult hemiplegia in six steps. Stage 1 describes the period immediately following the acute episode, when flaccidity is present and no limb movements can be initiated. As recovery begins, the basic limb synergies or some of their components may appear as associated reactions or minimal voluntary movement responses may be present. This is stage 2 and spasticity begins to develop. In stage 3 the patient gains voluntary control of the movement synergies, although full range of all synergy components does not necessarily develop. Spasticity has further increased and may become severe. Stage 4 is characterized by the ability to initiate movement combinations that do not follow the paths of either synergy and spasticity begins to decline. If progress continues in stage 5 more difficult movement combinations are learned as the basic limb synergies lose their dominance over motor acts. With the disappearance of spasticity individual joint movements become possible and coordination approaches normal.

Thus at first there is a period of flaccidity which usually lasts from 7 to 10 days. During the second week spasticity usually develops. This varies according to the severity of the lesion and the location of involvement.

Motor evaluation of the hemiplegic arm should compare the patient to the six recovery stages: Is the arm flaccid or spastic? Are the DTR's hyperactive? Is a withdrawal reflex present? Is there a complete or partial motor paralysis? Are weak synergistic motor patterns present? Can the patient perform isolated movement?

During the increasing spasticity phase, pattern movements can usually be evoked using the facilitation techniques. After pattern movements return and can be evoked, then voluntary initiation of pattern movements occur. Following this comes the period of voluntary control of isolated movements. In the evaluation of the upper extremity it is important to determine how much recovery has occurred.

Motor evaluation of the hemiplegic leg is similar. What is the tone? Are the reflexes hyperactive? Is there withdrawal on stimulation of the foot? What degree of motor paralysis exists? Can the patient voluntarily dorsiflex or plantarflex the ankle? Is the knee stable with standing?

Joint range of motion is evaluated using well known established techniques. Contracture formation can definitely limit function and needs to be assessed and recorded. Typical upper extremity contractures consist of adduction and internal rotation of the shoulder and flexion of the elbow, wrist, and fingers. In the lower extremity there may be flexion of the hip, flexion of the knee, and combined inversion and plantar flexion of the foot and ankle.

Testing the performance of the *activities of daily living* and determining *functional level* complete the evaluation. Activities of daily living evaluation should include the areas of eating, personal hygiene, dressing, and homemaking. Functional level evaluation should include the patient's ability to sit, stand, transfer, walk, and use a wheelchair.

The evaluation responsibilities should be multidisciplinary. Team evaluations with sharing of results will give the best data base to use for treatment. Rarely will a single team member be proficient in all needed evaluation areas.

A summary of any general health problems such as hypertension or congestive heart failure, or medical contraindications which will effect the rehabilitation program should be conveyed by the physician to all health team members.

Traditional Therapeutic Exercise

The first goal of therapeutic exercise in the hemiplegic is directed toward the prevention of the joint contractures. Choice of a proper bed and bed positioning early can help prevent contractures. A foot board helps prevent tightness of the heel cord. Intermittent prone positioning will help prevent hip flexion contractures. Daily range of motion exercises will also help prevent contractures. However, if contractures occur, reduction can be accomplished by a combination of muscle relaxation and pain relief by the use of heat or ice, stretching, positioning, and active exercise. Ultrasound is an effective modality for moderately severe contractures. Prolonged stretching is much more effective than brief stretching. Range of motion exercises can be the joint responsibility of nursing, physical therapy, and occupational therapy.

There are many published range-of-motion exercise programs for stroke patients. *Strike Back at Stroke* (69), currently distributed by the American

Heart Association, is a readily available source of range of motion exercises for families.

Prolonged use of bed positioning and range of motion exercises is limiting. The patient should be up and out of bed as soon as possible since early mobilization is an excellent form of range of motion exercises and also promotes neurological reintegration. The best way to stretch the heel cord is to stand and walk the patient early. If he is unable to stand, a tilt table can be used to stretch the heel cords. When muscle tone is flaccid, the maintenance of range of motion is simple. Later, very spastic muscles may require splints or braces to prevent contracture. As therapy progresses the patient should be taught self range-of-motion exercises to the involved upper extremity using the good extremity, pulleys, or a wooden stick.

After range-of-motion exercises come sitting activities with feet on the floor. Patients often have poor sitting balance when sitting on a high bed with their feet dangling, but have good sitting balance once the bed is lowered and the feet are placed on the floor.

The use of a tilt table prior to standing is useful to recondition patients who tend to develop orthostatic hypotension. Usually if the stroke patient is mobilized early, within the first 3 or 4 days, the tilt table will not be required.

Sitting in the wheelchair early is also useful to prevent deconditioning of the acute hemiplegic patient. Progressive wheelchair sitting helps maintain or restore cardiovascular function, builds endurance, and provides sensory stimulation to the patient.

The uncomplicated patient with stroke secondary to thrombosis or emboli should be mobilized at 2–3 days. Patients with stroke secondary to subarachnoid hemorrhage should stabilize for 10–14 days before mobilization.

The question of how early to mobilize the acute stroke patient with associated myocardial infarction is controversial. Some would claim a 21-day period of bed rest is indicated. However, if the patient stabilizes quickly, if there are no arrhythmias, and if the cardiologist agrees, careful mobilization should be started at 10 days.

Standing activities are important and come next in the scheme of treatment. Standing exercise can begin at the bedside and later in the parallel bars when the patient can go to the gymnasium. Early standing helps preserve body image, spacial relationships, and promotes early restoration of physical function.

Hirschberg (25) describes a simple preambulation program which can be done at bedside. If the patient can stand on his uninvolved leg, and if he is motivated, he has the potential to walk. His leg, trunk, and pelvis can be strengthened by a program of several sessions daily of 10 stand-ups from a chair holding on to a stable object for balance. In about 2 weeks, the patient proceeds to a progressive step up exercise program utilizing stairs and a hand rail.

Formal ambulation training starts with standing activities in the parallel bars. The patient is first taught to bend on each knee alternately and return to the extended position. This is followed by balancing first on the normal and then the hemiplegic side.

The common tendency of these patients to walk stiff kneed with a circumducted gait should be guarded against. If the ankle is unstable a temporary plastic short leg brace can be used. They are commercially available in several different sizes and are excellent for evaluation of ambulation ability in patients without the delay of waiting for a customized orthotic device.

As soon as knee stability is determined a permanent short leg brace may be ordered. If the knee is stable, a polypropylene foot ankle orthosis is usually satisfactory. If the knee is unstable, the double adjustable ankle joint brace with the ankle locked in slight plantar flexion will increase knee stability. A disadvantage of the double adjustable ankle brace is the inadvertent change of the ankle position by the patient's family because they feel the screws are loose and ought to be tightened. This can produce dragging of the toe or genu recurvatum with knee pain depending on the ankle position in a patient who at discharge had an acceptable gait.

Concomitant with ambulation training should be an applied exercise program aimed at developing 1) transfer skills, 2) stand-sit skills, 3) movement of body about on the bed and mats, and 4) the use of wheelchairs. As ambulation improves, stair climbing, curbs, and ramps are added.

Part of the traditional therapeutic exercise program includes training in the activities of daily living. This is an applied type of therapeutic exercise. An activity of daily living reference readily available for families is *Up and Around, A Booklet to Aid the Stroke Patient in Activities of Daily Living* (70), currently available from the American Heart Association.

Evaluation for assistive equipment is part of the overall physical restoration program, though not specifically related to exercise therapy.

The history of traditional exercise programs for hemiplegic patients has been reviewed by Westcott (74). Clayton (15) outlined in 1924 a basic hemiplegic exercise program consisting of active movements in a single joint, holding one joint corrected while moving another, teaching control of the entire limb, two-handed stick activities, pulley exercises, ball exercises for grasp and release, ball catching, exercises to train the use of individual fingers, exercises to music to teach rhythmic movements, and teaching normal use of limbs in functional activities (ADL's).

Later Coulter (17) outlined a walking education program consisting of bedside sitting with active leg movements, standing between two chairs and swinging affected leg, rocking back and forth while standing, first supported and then unsupported, and later progressing to walking.

Many of the muscle reeducation techniques designed for poliomyelitis patients have been used widely in hemiplegia; namely, passive motion, reciprocal motions, active assistive motions with attempted bilateral movements, and use of some basic reflex facilitation.

Group exercises have been used often in the treatment of hemiplegia to teach rolling, crawling, sitting balance, trunk balance, and self-range of motion. Bullock and Lupton (11) found that working in groups is an effective and economical way of treating hemiplegic patients provided progress is monitored regularly and groups are carefully graded.

Deaver (18) in 1951 outlined the goals of the traditional hemiplegic exercise program as preventing deformities, treating deformities if they occur, retraining the patient in ambulation and elevation activities, teaching the patient to perform the activities of daily living and working with the unaffected arm and hand, retraining the affected arm and hand to its maximum capacity and treating facial and speech disability if they are present.

The goals of stroke rehabilitation as outlined in 1972 in the Report of the Joint Committee for Stroke Facilities (59) restated Deaver's original physical goals and added as additional goals compensation for sensory loss, full social participation, achievement of maximum patient motivation, establishment of independent living post discharge, and in some cases vocational placement. These latter goals require a comprehensive team effort and adequate representation on the treatment team by the phychosocial therapists. Achievement in these areas produces life satisfaction and gives meaning to physical restoration.

Neuromuscular Facilitation Exercises

Over the past 20 years a number of muscle reeducation programs based on neuromuscular facilitation have been developed and widely used.

Fay (22) suggested the use of pathological and unlocking reflexes as a form of exercise in spastic children. He stated that the twice daily induction of these reflexes will improve spastic muscle function and decrease the level of spasticity. His reflex therapy stimulated further development.

The Bobaths (8, 56) developed a neurodevelopmental treatment program initially for cerebral palsied children and then later applied it to stroke patients. They feel the factors which interfere with normal motor performance in the adult hemiplegic are sensory disturbances of varying degrees, spasticity, a disorder of normal posture reflex mechanism, and a loss of selective movement patterns. The normal posture reflex mechanism is the basis for normal voluntary skilled movements. Their evaluation of patients assesses postural reactions, the ability to perform voluntary movement and the state of balance, and other automatic protective reactions. The techniques of therapy employed depend upon the stage of recovery the patient has achieved. The general aims of the exercise program are to either decrease, increase or stabilize postural tone (depending upon its effect upon movement), inhibit interfering patterns or movement reactions, and facilitate patterns leading to selective motor control and functional skills.

Brunnstrom (10, 50) developed a technique of muscle reeducation utilizing reflex training for hemiplegic patient. She described the basic flexion and extension synergies of the upper and lower extremity along with the associated reactions of hemiplegia evoked by yawning, sneezing, and coughing. Brunnstrom defines the associated reactions of hemiplegia as the involuntary limb movements and the reflex tensing of muscles which occur. Her treatment technique consists of using the associated reactions of hemiplegia, the synergistic patterns, and the pathological tonic neck and labyrinthine reflexes. Resistance to the normal limb, sensory input by tapping, and relaxation techniques are also used. The actual program techniques depend upon the stage of motor recovery in the individual patient. The goal of the Brunnstrom technique is selective motor control and then utilization of more advanced orthodox muscle reeducation techniques.

Proprioceptive neuromuscular facilitation is another neurophysiologic therapeutic exercise program developed by Kabat and Knott (31, 72). This system of therapeutic exercise uses basic neurophysiological mechanisms to increase central nervous system excitation and hence movement. These include maximum resistance, traction and approximation of joint structures, quick stretch, cutaneous pressure with holds and grips, reinforcement of weak movement with synergistic stronger movements, the use of simple verbal commands, and the utilization of the basic spiral diagonal patterns of movement.

The Rood technique of neuromuscular facilitation therapy stresses the concept that sensory input determines motor output (58). Her technique involves utilization of the skin receptors with brushing and icing to facilitate agonists and inhibit antagonists as a basis for exercise. She also uses proprioceptive techniques with stretching to facilitate agonists and both active and resistive contraction to facilitate antagonists. She uses pressure techniques of tapping, pressure, and joint compression along with a sequence of development activity program.

Thus a number of different neuromuscular facilitation exercise programs have been developed. They are described fully in Chapter 4. Initially the systems seemed to be contradictory, but in later years they seemed to be complementary. An analysis of the similarities of these various systems reveals that they are more alike than unlike. These different techniques for muscle reeducation all utilize proprioceptive techniques, sensory input (using commands, touching, tapping, and stretching), techniques of reciprocal inhibition, and utilization of various reflex activity which is released in the hemiplegic patient. There is no inherent advantage of one system over the other and the results of neuromuscular facilitation muscle reeducation depends more upon the skills of the therapist in any technique or given combination of techniques than in the specific technique itself.

Flanagan (23) lists come common denominators of the various systems of facilitation exercise. Sensation and motion are intimately related in the normal functioning of the human nervous system and sensory input to facilitate or inhibit movement is one of the basic concepts of these methods. Each method recognizes and utilizes the sequence of normal human motor development in the exercise program. Early motor behavior is vastly influenced by reflex activity and in treatment these reflex mechanisms are used to facilitate or inhibit voluntary effort. All methods employ the important concepts of motor learning such as repetition of activity, frequency of stimulation, and the employment of sensory cues to facilitate learning. All approaches center on the interaction of the body and its segments as a whole; in other words, the whole patient rather than one of his parts. A close, personal interaction between therapist and patient is critical for success.

Although the various techniques of neuromuscular facilitation exercise have been practiced widely for 20 years now, their real value and effectiveness has not been subject to sufficient controlled experimentation. Most physiatrists and therapists concerned with the rehabilitation of hemiplegic patients are convinced of the value of facilitation exercises in the individual patient, but usually prescribe a program combining the traditional methods with facilitation techniques.

Stern et al. (57) studied the value of facilitation exercise versus a traditional type exercise program. A group of randomly selected patients with hemiplegia from stroke were exposed to a specific therapeutic exercise program utilizing neuromuscular reeducation techniques based on neurophysiological and/or developmental theories. Results were compared with those in a control group of persons who had received a similar type program which did not contain these exercises. Patients in both groups were alike in the major clinical characteristics and were evaluated using objective, quantitative test measurements. In addition a numerical self-care scoring system (Kenny Rehabilitation Institutes Self-Care Evaluation) was used to assess functional improvement. Both groups showed comparable improvement. Thus, neuromuscular reeducation exercises added to a traditional exercise program were not more effective in improving patient motility and strength than traditional exercises alone.

Caldwell et al. (12) outlines an upper extremity exercise program for hemiplegic patients consisting of individual and group instruction on self-range of motion, self-care, and activities of daily living; along with the use of static splints, dynamic splints, and other orthotic devices as appropriate. Obtaining and maintaining a functional pain-free range of motion in the upper extremities is an important goal. A variety of therapeutic exercise techniques in the proprioceptive neuromuscular facilitation area are employed to develop better voluntary control using a combination of techniques described by Kabat, Bobath, Brunnstrom, and others.

Most current hemiplegic exercise programs tend to be a combination of traditional methods, facilitation methods, and, in some areas, biofeedback techniques.

Electromyographic Biofeedback Exercises

Since 1960 evidence has been accumulating of the value of electromyographic (EMG) biofeedback as a therapeutic exercise technique (Chapter 9).

Marinacci and Horande (42) first observed that during treatment of patients with stroke and peripheral nerve injuries, the presentation of an auditory EMG feedback was often followed by some return of voluntary movement. Andrews (3) in 1964 noted similar results in 20 patients with hemiplegia. In 1973 Johnson and Garton (29) reported on muscle reeducation in 10 hemiplegic patients with disability lasting more than 1 year with variable results. In addition to the EMG biofeedback they used any other techniques of facilitation or operant conditioning that would work. They suggested this technique of muscle reeducation would prove helpful in muscle reeducation about the shoulder, elbow, wrist, knee, and ankle soon after onset of hemiplegia. The reverse application of the technique could also be used to obtain relaxation of spastic, undesirable, antagonistic muscle groups.

Swaan (60) used auditory EMG biofeedback therapy to inhibit undesired motor activity of the peroneus longus muscle while contracting the quadriceps muscle in seven patients, four of whom had hemiplegia. Each patient was treated with a conventional physical therapeutic technique and then his biofeedback program. The data indicate that the feedback technique resulted in better inhibition of unwanted muscle activity.

In 1975 Basmajian et al. (5) reported twice as much improvement in a group of patients with foot drop after stroke who were placed on a program of therapeutic exercise and EMG biofeedback when compared with a control group on the therapeutic exercise program alone. They later reported no significant change in peroneal nerve conduction velocity or spasticity level in this group of patients (62).

Brudny et al. (9) reported varying degrees of improvement in upper extremity movement patterns in hemiplegic patients following an 8–12-week exercise program using EMG biofeedback. They noted that patients with a greater degree of sensory loss usually responded in a more rapid manner. Two patients showed good improvement in pattern movements which did not have carry-over into functional gains. This groups feels that the audiovisual sensory feedback from integrated EMG should be considered as an external feedback loop in the disrupted system which substitutes for the internal proprioceptive loop. They feel this external loop augments or helps restore the normal sensory motor interaction. The fact that retention persists after withdrawal of the feedback suggests that new sensory motor integration is taking place as a result of such therapy. In their opinion whenever a patient with a disorder of voluntary movement from a central nervous system insult fails to respond adequately to conventional rehabilitation procedures, a trial of biofeedback therapy is warranted.

Lee et al. (34) compared the short-term effects of brief EMG biofeedback with the effects of placebo feedback and with the effects of training with therapist encouragement but without feedback in 18 patients. Each patient was subjected to each different training strategy. There was no statistical differences between the myoelectric output of the three training techniques.

Basmajian (6) is currently treating subluxation of the hemiplegic shoulder with EMG biofeedback therapy to the deltoid muscle with promising results. He feels that weakness of the supraspinatus, which normally locks the shoulder in position and prevents downward disloca-tion, is responsible for hemiplegic shoulder subluxation. However, he has found that biofeedback exercise to the deltoid will strengthen both muscles and is therefore an effective means of exercise therapy.

Those engaged in biofeedback exercise systems use them to gain voluntary control and increase strength in weak muscles and also to relax overactive spastic muscles. Often the achievement of relaxation of the overactive muscles will produce more improvement of gait than increasing the control of weak muscles.

Thus, as the 1950s and 1960s were the years to explore the use of neuromuscular facilitation exercise therapy for hemiplegia, it looks as though the 1970s and 1980s will be the years to explore the use of biofeedback exercise therapy for hemiplegia. Results are encouraging, but much remains to be learned about the real value and indications for EMG biofeedback therapy. The wise clinician will avoid the noncritical total acceptance of biofeedback as a form of therapy, but instead will add it cautiously to his current system of hemiplegic therapeutic exercise for those patients who seem to respond. It is an excellent focusing device for hemiplegic patients.

Johnson et al. (28) reported on the sequence of fibrillations and positive waves on EMG in stroke syndrome and suggests that the muscle fibers have an abnormal irritability, perhaps as a consequence of the loss of neurotropic influence on the muscle fiber after the stroke. The release from central nervous system influences in hemiplegia occurs by 7–14 days in most instances. One wonders if the early use of biofeedback exercise therapy will hasten the sensory-motor reintegration of the central nervous system.

Other Methods of Exercise Therapy

Liberson et al. (37) in 1961 reported on the use of electric stimulation of the peroneal nerve for gait training in hemiplegic patients. More recently, Takebe et al. (63) reported on peroneal nerve stimulation in nine hemiplegic patients with foot drop using the Philips functional stimulator with only fair results. They later (61) used both EMG biofeedback and peroneal nerve stimulation for hemiplegic drop foot and found improvement from both techniques.

Teng et al. (66) studied the carry-over effect of gait synchronized stimulation of the peroneal nerve on voluntary ankle dorsiflexion and found that success was correlated with performance feedback, not peroneal stimulation. Thus, the feedback aspect of nerve stimulation techniques may be the most important factor in retraining.

Lee and Johnston (35) reported on the use of a train of electric impulses to the foot skin surface to evoke a flexion reflex as a means of gait training in six hemiplegic patients. On the basis of this preliminary report, he feels that this is a practical means of facilitating the swing phase of gait, thereby permitting earlier and more effective ambulation training.

In 1956, taking an entirely different approach, Psaki and Treanor (55) emphasized the control of afferent impulses in the management of spastic paralysis. They inhibit such afferent impulses by restriction of standing and ambulation before voluntary knee flexion was possible, selective reeducation of the extensors of the upper extremity and flexors of the lower extremity, early curtailment of sensory stimuli to the palm, and interruption of conduction of the afferent impulses by nerve blocks and even by surgery. Phenol nerve blocks and surgical control of spasticity are still used.

Licht (38) in his historical review of stroke rehabilitation techniques reported a technique being developed by Adams in Belfast. Patients are restrained on their functional side to treat denial, apraxia, or neglect of the hemiplegic side. Adams feels there are patients in whom recovery of the paralyzed side can be assisted with this technique, which appears worthy of being explored and developed in the future.

Zankel (77) reported a technique of neuromuscular reeducation which employs intensive repetitive sinusoidal stimulation over the muscle belly of the paralyzed muscle assisted by the patient's own exercise effort. He claims significant benefit from this technique, but clearly states that (74) no adequate controlled investigations have been accomplished.

Thistle et al. (67) studied isokinetic exercises, a type of exercise where the speed of motion is held constant by a special device and the resistance varies with the effort of the patient. From this preliminary study, they felt the method was more efficient than traditional resistive exercises to increase the strength of the quadriceps muscle in hemiplegic patients.

Inaba et al. (26) compared the effectiveness of progressive resistive exercises, simple active exercise, and training in the activities of daily living in attaining functional independence in patients with hemiplegia. A 1-month inpatient program of progressive resistive exercises and training in activities of daily living is more effective than a program of activities of daily living alone or when combined with simple active exercise. Following 2 months of treatment, however, no difference was evident between the two groups in levels of function.

A whole new area of therapeutic exercises developed by Ayres (4) and Frostig (24) for the perceptual-motor retraining of brain-damaged children is now being applied to adult hemiplegic patients by various occupational therapists such as Taylor (65), Okoye (48), Farber (21), Llorens and Seig (39), and others. These programs use a wide variety of sensory stimulation techniques aimed at promoting reintegration of the sensory-motor system. These systems are based on the concept that normally the sensory, perceptual, cognitive, and motor systems become integrated in consecutive order. The choice of stimulation technique depends on the developmental level. Some initial experiences are promising, but the real value of these programs needs to be determined in controlled clinical studies.

Ambulation

Using telemetered EMG activity, Peat et al (49) showed that the hemiplegic gait disturbances were characterized by a loss of the usual phasic pattern associated with the gait cycle. The anterior tibial, gastrocnemius, medial hamstrings, and quadriceps all have peak activity at midstance and lack the usual phasic variation related to the gait cycle.

In a study by Norton et al. (47) to correlate gait speed and spasticity in thigh musculature in hemiplegic patients, no statistically significant correlation appeared. Gait speed may have been affected by other variables, specifically, proprioceptive defect, intensive duration of gait training prior to study, or specific muscle weakness. Also gait speed was not correlated with spasticity in the anterior tibial or gastroc-soleus muscles.

Montgomery and Inaba (44) list the common gait problems in the hemiplegic patient. During stance phase these include inability to shift trunk laterally over the involved leg, inadequate control of pelvic rotation, pelvic drop on uninvolved side, trunk flexion at hips, unstable knee, equinus, and varus. During swing phase these include inadequate hip flexion, inadequate knee flexion, inadequate dorsiflexion of ankle, and scissoring.

According to Perry (52), during each step three fundamental tasks are performed: forward progression, single limb balance, and limb length adjustment. At heel strike the hemiplegic patient lacks the initial controlled plantar flexion that provides the shock absorber mechanism. The unvarying ankle plantar flexion from heel strike to midstance is obstructive to the maintaining of trunk balance in the midstance phase. Lack of activity in the gastroc-soleus at push off is inadequate and greatly interferes with normal gait. Controlled knee flexion with ankle extension is not possible at the end of push off in the hemiplegic patient when only patterned movement is available. At the early swing phase, simultaneous hip, knee, and ankle flexion is usually adequate, but during the late swing phase the pattern is obstructive since isolated knee extension with hip and ankle flexion is defective.

Peszczynski (54) described a certain walking pattern in hemiplegic patients which he called the intermittent double step gait. There are two variations of this extremely useful gait. In the first type the patient tends to lose balance abnormally during the stance phase of the hemiplegic leg. In the second type the patient loses balance abnormally during the swing phase of the paralyzed limb. In either case, in order to regain his balance the patient will pause after each complete step. Some patients with persistently poor balance can be deliberately taught the intermittent double step gait in order to assist them in walking safely.

Bracing

Bracing is a form of therapeutic exercise. Short leg braces may be required in the hemiplegic patient to control ankle and knee instability, varus from excessive spasticity, excessive pattern motions, contractures, or proprioceptive loss. Good hip stability and balance determine the ambulation level achieved. The patient's hip and trunk control determine the ability of the patient to initiate a stepping motion and to achieve enough hip and knee flexion to allow a good swing phase.

A short leg brace with a dorsiflexion stop may be needed to help stabilize the knee. If the hemiplegic patient is able to hike the pelvis and flex the knee, usually the patient can learn to walk with a short leg brace. Perry (51) has noted that the patient with adequate hip response to stabilize his trunk is assured good quadriceps action at the knee.

Perry (51) points out the value of the double adjustable ankle short leg brace in hemiplegic patients. The locked ankle joint is more effective in controlling spasticity and excessive patterned responses than braces which allow limited ranges with spring assists. A fixed ankle position avoids the difficulty of trying to stop an unwanted action after it has already been stimulated by a short range of free motion. The preferred position for the fixed ankle is approximately 90°. A few degrees one way or the other markedly influences the patient's ability to stand erect. The adjustability of the brace allows determination of the most effective position of the ankle joint for each individual patient. Uncontrolled varus may require the use of a T strap to the double upright brace or in some cases surgery. Holding the ankle in slight dorsiflexion through bracing will control hyperextension of the knee.

All but the most severe deformities of the foot and ankle can be improved with an appropriate orthosis, according to Waters and Montgomery (73). Management of the knee generally is restricted to problems which can be controlled by stabilizing the ankle. There is no effective bracing for the hip other than lateral support which can be provided with a cane. The three most common ankle braces used are the double adjustable rigid ankle joint brace, the limited ankle motion brace and the light weight toe pick up plastic orthosis. The basic rigid orthosis is a double adjustable ankle locking device which can be adjusted in both dorsi and plantar flexion. The limited ankle joint braces include the conventional double upright single adjustable ankle joint with the dorsiflexion spring assist. The toe pick up orthosis is helpful if there is no troublesome varus.

Exercise Treatment of Specific Conditions and Complications

Subluxation of the shoulder is a common problem in hemiplegics. Taketomi (64) stresses the importance of using an active exercise program to correct subluxation of the shoulder instead of the sling. Biofeedback exercises have been advocated by Basmajian (6) as a way to retrain the scapular-positioning and supraspinatus muscles which he feels are responsible for preventing subluxation of the shoulder.

Clumsiness of the nonhemiplegic hand is common. Jebsen et al. (27) found that the normal hand in 27 hemiplegic stroke patients had slower function when compared to normals. This was true for both right and left hemiplegic patients. This decrement in hand function may be related to loss of uncrossed ipsilateral motor or sensory fibers or to a disturbance of interhemisphere integration. Traditional ADL functional training usually is all that is needed to increase the skill of the nonhemiplegic hand.

Thrombophlebitis is another complication of stroke. The early use of foot boards, elastic stockings, and active foot exercises of the nonhemiplegic leg while in bed will help to minimize the incidence of thrombophlebitis. Early mobilization is also important in prevention of thrombophlebitis.

Troublesome, persistent spasticity is better treated with phenol blocks, surgical lengthening of tendons, tenotomy, or neurectomies than with an exercise program.

Genu recurvatum can be caused by weakness of the hamstrings or quadriceps muscles, impaired proprioception, or a spastic or contracted Achilles tendon. Genu recurvatum secondary to weakness of hamstrings or quadriceps muscles can be treated by exercises to build strength. The use of a double adjustable short leg brace fixed in slight dorsiflexion may control genu recurvatum. Occasionally a knee cage is required to prevent severe genu recurvatum.

Some ambulatory patients will later develop a spastic, tight Achilles tendon which causes late genu recurvatum and produces pain in the knee. Whenever a patient is seen in follow-up, heel cord length should be evaluated. If the heel cord is tight, then a vigorous range of motion program with self-stretching at home is indicated. If this is unsuccessful, lengthening of the Achilles tendon may be required. The technique of percutaneous heel cord lengthening allows mobilization of the patient at 14 days in a brace as opposed to 4 weeks of immobilization using older surgical techniques. Medications to control spasticity may decrease genu recurvatum secondary to a spastic gastrocnemius.

Shoulder hand syndrome or reflex sympathetic dystrophy is a common complication of hemiplegia. There is puffy nonpitting edema of the hand with loss of skin lines. The hand becomes painful in flexion. The shoulder is painful. Exercise therapy to the hand and shoulder should include vigorous range of motion exercises as well as modalities to decrease the pain. There is a wide variety of medical and surgical treatments for shoulder-hand syndrome which will not be reviewed.

Frozen shoulder secondary to untreated shoulder-hand syndrome or immobilization by a sling can be treated with ultrasound followed by manual range of motion with the scapula immobilized by the therapist. Later, broomstick exercises and pulley exercises can be added.

Impaired swallowing requires specialized programs. Larsen (32) outlines a swallowing exercise program consisting of leaning forward with neck flexed when swallowing, holding breath when swallowing, using voluntary initiation of swallowing instead of reflex swallowing, eating slowly, and using various techniques to stimulate swallowing such as placement of good-tasting, moist food in oral cavity, manual elevation of larynx, or tapping of lips.

Outcome and Prognostic Factors

Cassvan et al. (13) studied the relationship of laterality of stroke as a factor in ambulation and found that the right hemiplegics progressed more rapidly in all stages of ambulation (standing in parallel bars, ambulation in parallel bars, ambulation outside of parallel bars, and stair climbing) and achieved higher levels of ambulation.

An association exists between urinary incontinence and the ability to regain ambulatory status in hemiplegic patients, according to Lorenze et al (41). A study of 254 patients showed that persistent urinary incontinence was associated with delay or failure of the recovery process with respect to ambulation, but the causal relation was complicated. The functions of ambulation and urination are both impaired by the loss of cortical control. In their patients the overwhelming cause of urinary incontinence was the loss of cortical inhibition. Persistence of urinary incontinence is a poor prognostic sign. Recovery from loss of cortical inhibition usually followed the following phases: bowel and bladder incontinence, bladder incontinence, nocturnal urinary incontinence, and normal bladder control. In most situations where independent ambulation was not achieved, the patient not only had a bladder incontinence, but bowel incontinence as well.

Moskowitz et al. (45) in a long term follow-up of 518 post-stroke patients found that recovery of motor function occurs within 6 months. Return of function was not always consistent with motor recovery. Rehabilitation beyond the 6-month period can occur when superimposed complications have caused a functional deterioration in the patient. Recovery of function in upper and lower extremities varies inversely with the degree of late spasticity. The prognosis for ambulation in patients with hemisensory loss is only 47% and is equally poor in patients with a right or left involvement. The prognosis for ambulation without sensory loss was over 85% The incidence of post-stroke seizures was 5% at 2 years and increases with longer survival times. Clinical observations indicate that maximal functional improvement tends to occur within the first 6 months.

Lorenze et al. (40) also searched for the causes of failure in independent ambulation in their 200 cases of hemiplegia. Despite the presence of many complicating factors, by far the commonest cause of failure in ambulation in all groups was muscular weakness, atonicity, or severe spasticity. Poor motivation was the next most common factor followed by balance problems and cerebellar symptoms. Instances of failure due to anosognosia, poor vision, multiple complications, general weakness, poor endurance, and mental defects occurred, but were infrequent.

Van Buskirk and Webster (71) studied the prognostic value of sensory defect in the rehabilitation of hemiplegic patients. Serial examinations of pain, two-point discrimination and vibratory sense were made weekly for periods varying from 2 to 17 weeks on 35 male subjects. They found that patients with intact sensation had an average hospital stay of 68 days. Those who exhibited recovery of sensation had an average hospital stay of 76 days and achieved a satisfactory result in rehabilitation. Patients who failed to recover one or more of the sensory modalities had an average hospital stay of 236 days. The majority of these patients achieved a poor functional result. The degree of functional independence depends both upon the degree of motor and sensory activity of the hemiplegic side. The length of hospitalization can be correlated with the degree of sensory impairment present. This series suggests that the prognosis is worse if a disturbance of two-point discrimination persists.

Williams (75) studied the relationship of dressing ability in hemiplegic patients and the ability to copy three figures: a house, clock, and flower. She found patients who produce normal drawings are more likely to be independent in upper extremity dressing skills on admission and have higher capacity to achieve these skills than do patients who produce abnormal drawings.

Newman (46) documented the process of recovery after hemiplegia in 39 cases followed from onset for at least 20 weeks. Some neurological recovery occured in 34 patients. Recovery is usually best in the lower limb, but upper limb movement, sensation, body image, mental ability, and speech may also recover to some extent. Recovery may begin as early as the 1st week or as late as the 7th. Little neurological improvement took place after the 14th week and the average interval from onset to 80% final recovery was 6 weeks. Functional recovery closely follows neurological recovery. It is suggested that much of the early recovery and that of the upper limb could be due to return of circulation to ischemic areas. Transfer of function to undamaged neurons is suggested as a mechanism of late recovery, especially of the lower limbs and speech.

Peszczynski (53) reports on various clinical prognostic factors in stroke. He feels that prolonged bowel incontinence is the most important prognostic symptom in a stroke patient. If bowel incontinence persists for 3–4 weeks after onset, then achievement of a self-care functional level is doubtful. He does not feel that urinary incontinence has major predictive value. Flexion contracture of the hemiplegic knee is the second most important prognostic factor for rehabilitation. Prolonged flaccidity of lower extremity usually prolongs the period of gait training, although these patients usually always learn to ambulate. Sensory involvement in hemiplegia has a definite influence on the prognosis in that more time is needed to teach ambulation and ADL activities. Hemianopsia presents additional complications and risks because of the disturbed visual field. A painful shoulder in hemiplegia can be very disturbing if untreated and may interfere with dressing activities. Aphasia does not basically interfere with the hemiplegic patient's ability to walk, dress, or feed himself. Mental derangements, such as confusion, can be very disturbing.

Anderson et al. (2) studied 233 patients with completed stroke over a 4-year period of time to determine predictive factors in stroke rehabilitation. Initially there were 652 admission variables, 347 discharge variables, and 214 follow-up variables collected by a whole team of health workers. The important variables emerging were perceptual loss, low motivation, confusion and disorientated thinking, withdrawn and apathetic behavior, extended time since onset, previous cerebral vascular accident, nystagmus, low blood pressure, and extended period of unconsciousness at the time of stroke.

Unfortunately, Anderson's predictors are useful as group indicators, but less helpful in predicting individual patient achievement. This was the same conclusion reached by Lehmann et al. (36) who listed as negative group predictors congestive heart failure, gross perceptual deficit, lower level of education, and older age. However, individual prediction was not possible and all hemiplegic patients should be given a therapeutic trial unless they are so ill that they cannot take part in the therapeutic program.

How Long Should Treatment Persist?

Inpatient stroke rehabilitation programs vary in length of stay from 6 to 12 weeks with 8 weeks perhaps being an average. Mildly involved hemiplegic patients often return home after 1-2 weeks of therapy. Patients with dense perceptual problems are often discharged to nursing homes as not rehabilitatable after 10-12 weeks of intense therapy.

Miglietta et al. (43) reported on the fate of 25 elderly hemiplegic patients discharged as failures from a rehabilitation program after a nonproductive program which averaged 11 weeks in duration. All were placed on a continuing rehabilitation program and improvement in function and performance occurred in 10 patients, 8 of whom became ambulatory and independent in the activities of daily living after a program lasting 7 months on the average.

DiBenedetto (20) reported on 75 stroke patients with severe mental, motor, and sensory impairment who were considered not to have rehabilitation potential and were placed in a long term care facility with a less intense program. Over 6-10 months many of these patients did achieve enough functional independence to walk and return home. She stresses the potential of these patients if they are subjected to an ongoing less intense program instead of being abandonded.

It is difficult to provide the treatment needs for the severely disabled hemiplegic patient. The high cost of medical care and pressures by third-party carriers and by peer review tend to force denial of services to the hemiplegic patient whose deficits exceed the average.

Conclusion

The many conflicting claims in the medical and allied health literature concerning exercise therapy for the hemiplegic patient confuses the experienced and inexperienced physicians alike. In the search for improved treatment techniques, proven systems and principles are often disregarded for the latest new technique even when that technique has not be subjected to controlled experimentation. The wise physician will insist on documentation of effectiveness of new exercise techniques before he incorporates them into the clinical care of his hemiplegic patients.

Four factors are significant for any type of hemiplegic treatment program (68). As reorganization of the central nervous system occurs this facilitates the regaining or relearning of lost function. Rehabilitation is a learning process and if a patient is capable of receiving and interpreting the sensory input by the various modalities, then certain motor skills can be relearned. The acquisition of a motor skill requires repetition. The optimum conditions in which the person with brain injury may learn is a sympathetic and well structured environment and the attention and skill of the therapist seem to be more or at least as important as the technique being used.

Thus to fully comprehend the therapeutic exercise treatment of hemiplegia one must have a comprehensive knowledge of the whole range of therapeutic exercise and an appreciation of the pathophysiology of stroke and its evolution.

REFERENCES

1. ALBERT, M. L. A simple test of visual neglect. *Neurology, 23:* 658–664, 1973.
2. ANDERSON, T. P., BOURESTOM, N., AND GREENBERG, F. R. Predictive factors in stroke rehabilitation. *Arch. Phys. Med. Rehabil., 55:* 545–552, 1974.
3. ANDREWS, J. M. Neuromuscular re-education of hemiplegia with aid of electromyograph. *Arch. Phys. Med. Rehabil. 45:* 530–532, 1964.
4. AYRES, A. J. *Sensory Integration and Learning Disorders.* Western Psychological Services, Los Angeles, 1973.
5. BASMAJIAN, J. V., KUKULKA, C. G., AND NARAYAN, M. G. Biofeedback treatment of foot-drop after stroke compared with standard rehabilitation technique; effects on voluntary control and strength. *Arch. Phys. Med. Rehabil., 56:* 231–236, 1975.
6. BASMAJIAN, J. V., Personal communication.
7. BIRCH, H. G., PROCTOR, F., AND BORTNER, M. Perception in hemiplegia; I. Judgement of vertical and horizontal by hemiplegic patients. *Arch. Phys. Med. Rehabil., 41:* 19–27, 1960.
8. BOBATH, B. *Adult Hemiplegia: Evaluation and Treatment.* William Heinemann Medical Books Ltd., London, 1970.
9. BRUDNY, J., KOREIN, J., AND GRYNBAUM, B. B. EMG feedback therapy; review of treatment of 114 patients. *Arch. Phys. Med. Rehabil., 57:* 55–61, 1976.
10. BRUNNSTROM, S. *Movement Therapy in Hemiplegia.* Harper & Row, New York, 1970.
11. BULLOCK, E. A., AND LUPTON, D. Later states of rehabilitation in hemiplegia. *Physiotherapy, 60:* 370–374, 1974.
12. CALDWELL, C. B., WILSON, D. J., AND BRAUN, R. M. Evaluation and treatment of the upper extremity in the hemiplegic stroke patient. *Clin. Orthop., 63:* 69–93, 1969.
13. CASSVAN, A., ROSS, P. L., AND DYER, P. R. Lateralization in stroke syndromes as a factor in ambulation. *Arch. Phys. Med. Rehabil., 57:* 583–587, 1976.
14. Classification and Outline of Cerebrovascular Disease II. National Institute of Neurological and Communicative Disorders and Stroke, an ad hoc committee. *Stroke, 6:* 565–616, 1975.
15. CLAYTON, E. B. *Physiotherapy in General Practice*, pp. 106–115, William Wood Co., New York, 1924.
16. COHEN, C. A. Perceptual problems in hemiplegics *South. Med. J., 67:* 1329–1332, 1974.
17. COULTER, J. S. *The Use of Therapeutic Exercise in Internal Medicine and in Neurology*, pp. 46–50. W. F. Prior Co., Inc., Maryland, 1939.
18. DEAVER, G. C. The rehabilitation of the hemiplegia. *R. I. Med. J., 34:* 421–424, 1951.
19. DeCENCIO, D. V., LESHNER, M., AND VORON, D. Verticality perception and ambulation in hemiplegia. *Arch. Phys. Med. Rehabil., 51:* 105–110, 1970.
20. DiBENEDETTO, M. Optimal care for the severely involved stroke patient. *Rehabilitation (Br.), 91:* 27–35, 1974.
21. FARBER, S. D. Sensorimotor Evaluation and Treatment Procedures. Indiana, Indiana University-Purdue University at Indianapolis Medical Center, 1974.
22. FAY, T. The use of pathological and unlocking reflexes in the rehabilitation of spastics. *Am. J. Phys. Med., 33:* 347–352, 1954.
23. FLANAGAN, E. M. Methods for facilitation and inhibition of motor activity. *Am. J. Phys. Med., 46:* 1006–1011, 1967.
24. FROSTIG, M. *Movement Education: Theory and Practice.* Follett Publishing Co., Chicago, 1970.
25. HIRSCHBERG, G. G. The use of stand-up and step-up exercises in rehabilitation. *Clin. Orthop., 12:* 30–46, 1958.
26. INABA, M., EDBERG, E., AND MONTGOMERY, J. Effectiveness of functional training, active exercise, and resistive exercise for patients with hemiplegia. *Phys. Ther., 53:* 28–35, 1973.
27. JEBSEN, R. H., GRIFFITH, E. R., AND LONG, E. W. Function of "normal" hand in stroke patients. *Arch. Phys. Med. Rehabil., 52:* 170–174, 1971.

28. JOHNSON, E. W., DENNY, S. T., AND KELLEY, J. P. Sequence of electromyographic abnormalities in stroke syndrome. *Arch. Phys. Med. Rehabil., 56:* 468–473, 1975.
29. JOHNSON, H. E., AND GARTON, W. H. Muscle re-education in hemiplegia by use of electromyographic device. *Arch. Phys. Med. Rehabil., 54:* 320–322, 1973.
30. KNAPP, M. E. Problems in rehabilitation of the hemiplegic patient. *J.A.M.A., 169:* 224–229, 1959.
31. KNOTT, M., AND VOSS, D. E. *Propreoceptive Neuromuscular Facilitation.* Harper & Row, New York, 1968.
32. LARSEN, G. L. Conservative management for incomplete dysphagia paralytica. *Arch. Phys. Med. Rehabil., 54:* 180–185, 1973.
33. LAVIGNE, J. M. Hemiplegia sensorimotor assessment form. *Phys. Ther. 54:* 128–134, 1974.
34. LEE, K. H., HILL, E., JOHNSTON, R., et al. Myofeedback for muscle retraining in hemiplegic patients. *Arch. Phys. Med. Rehabil., 57:* 588–591, 1976.
35. LEE, K. H., AND JOHNSTON, R. Electrically induced flexion in gait training of hemiplegic patients; induction of the reflex. *Arch. Phys. Med. Rehabil., 57:* 311–314, 1976.
36. LEHMANN, J. F., DELATEUR, B. J., AND FOWLER, R. S. Stroke rehabilitation; outcome and prediction. *Arch. Phys. Med. Rehabil., 56:* 383–389, 1975.
37. LIBERSON, W. T., HOLMQUEST, H. J., AND SCOT, D. Functional electrotherapy; stimulation of the peroneal nerve synchronized with the swing phase of the gait of hemiplegic patients. *Arch Phys. Med. Rehabil., 42:* 101–105, 1961.
38. LICHT, S. Stroke; a history of its rehabilitation. *Arch. Phys. Med. Rehabil., 54:* 10–18, 1973.
39. LLORENS, L. A., AND SIEG, K. W. A profile for managing sensory integrative test data. *Am. J. Occup. Ther., 29:* 205–208, 1975.
40. LORENZE, E. J., DE ROSA, A. J., AND KEENAN, E. L. Ambulation problems in hemiplegia. *Arch. Phys. Med. Rehabil., 39:* 366–370, 1958.
41. LORENZE, E. J., SIMON, H. B., AND LINDEN, J. L. Urologic problems in rehabilitation of hemiplegic patients. *J.A.M.A., 169:* 1042–1046, 1959.
42. MARINACCI, A. A. AND HORANDE, M. Electromyogram in neuromuscular re-education *Bull. Los Angeles Neurol. Soc., 25:* 55–71, 1960.
43. MIGLIETTA, O., CHUNG, T. S., AND RAJESWARAMMA, V. Fate of stroke patients transferred to a long-term rehabilitation hospital. *Stroke, 7:* 76–77, 1976.
44. MONTGOMERY, J., AND INABA, M. Physical therapy technics in stroke rehabilitation. *Clin. Orthop., 63:* 54–68, 1969.
45. MOSKOWITZ, E., LIGHTBODY, F. E. H., AND FREITAG, N. S. Long-term follow-up of the poststroke patient. *Arch. Phys. Med. Rehabil., 53:* 167–172, 1972.
46. NEWMAN, M. The process of recovery after hemiplegia. *Stroke, 3:* 702–710, 1972.
47. NORTON, B. J., BOMZE, H. A., AND SAHRMANN, S. A. Correlation between gait speed and spasticity at the knee. *Phys. Ther., 55:* 355–359, 1975.
48. OKOYE, R. Functional Evaluation of the Adult with CNS Dysfunction. Long Island District New York Occupational Therapy Association, New York, 1976.
49. PEAT, M., DUBO, H. I. C., AND WINTER, D. A. Electromyographic temporal analysis of gait; hemiplegic locomotion. *Arch. Phys. Med. Rehabil., 57:* 421–425, 1976.
50. PERRY, C. E. Principles and techniques of the brunnstrom approach to the treatment of hemiplegia. *Am. J. Phys. Med., 46:* 789–812, 1967.
51. PERRY, J. Lower-extremity bracing in hemiplegia. *Clin. Orthop., 63:* 32–38, 1969.
52. PERRY, J. The mechanics of walking in hemiplegia. *Clin. Orthop., 63:* 23–31, 1969.
53. PESZCZYNSKI, M. Prognosis for rehabilitation of the older adult and the aged hemiplegic patient. *Am. J. Cardiol., 42:* 365–369, 1961.
54. PESZCZYNSKI, M. The intermittent double step gait. *Arch. Phys. Med. Rehabil., 39:* 494–496, 1958.
55. PSAKI, R. C., AND TREANOR, W. J. Afferent influences in the management of spastic paresis. *Arch. Phys. Med. Rehabil., 37:* 214–218, 1956.

56. SEMANS, S. The Bobath concept in treatment of neurological disorders. *Am. J. Phys. Med.*, *46:* 732-785, 1967.
57. STERN, P. H., McDOWELL, F., AND MILLER, J. M. Effects of facilitation exercise techniques in stroke rehabilitation. *Arch. Phys. Med. Rehabil.*, *51:* 526-531, 1970.
58. STOCKMEYER, S. A. An interpretation of the approach of Rood to the treatment of neuromuscular dysfunction. *Am. J. Phys. Med.*, *46:* 900-956, 1967.
59. Stroke Rehabilitation. Joint Committee for Stroke Facilities. *Stroke, 3:* 373-407, 1972.
60. SWAAN, D., VAN WIERINGEN, P. C. W., AND FOKKEMA, S. D. Auditory electromyographic feedback therapy to inhibit undesired motor activity. *Arch. Phys. Med. Rehab.*, *55:* 251-254, 1974.
61. TAKEBE, K., AND BASMAJIAN, J. V. Gait Analysis in stroke patients to assess treatments of foot-drop. *Arch. Phys. Med. Rehabil.*, *57:* 305-310, 1976.
62. TAKEBE, K., KUKULKA, C. G., NARAYAN, M. G., AND BASMAJIAN, J. V. Biofeedback treatment of foot-drop after stroke compared with standard rehabilitation technique (Part 2); effects on nerve conduction velocity and spasticity. *Arch. Phys. Med. Rehabil.*, *57:* 9-11, 1976.
63. TAKEBE, K., KUKULKA, C., NARAYAN, M. G., AND BASMAJIAN, J. V. Peroneal nerve stimulator in rehabilitation of hemiplegic patients. *Arch. Phys. Med. Rehabil.*, *56:* 237-240, 1975.
64. TAKETOMI, Y. Observations on subluxation of the shoulder joint in hemiplegia. *Phys. Ther.*, *55:* 39-40, 1975.
65. TAYLOR, M. M. Adaptive Learning Among Adults with Acquired Cerebral Dysfunction: Problems and Treatment. Minnesota Occupational Therapy Association Retreat Workship, 1971.
66. TENG, E. L., McNEAL, D. R., AND KRALJ, A. Electrical stimulation and feedback training; effects on the voluntary control of paretic muscles. *Arch. Phys. Med. Rehabil.*, *57:* 228-233, 1976.
67. THISTLE, H. G., HISLOP, H. J., AND MOFFROID, M. Isokinetic contraction; a new concept of resistive exercise. *Arch. Phys. Med. Rehabil.*, *48:* 279-282, 1967.
68. TOBIS, J. S. Re-evaluating the Management of the Stroke Patient. In *Neurophysiologic Aspects of Rehabilitation Medicine*, pp. 319-330, edited by A. A. Buerger and J. S. Tobias. Charles C Thomas, Springfield, Ill., 1974.
69. U.S. Department of Health, Education, and Welfare: Strike Back at Stroke. United States Government Printing Office, Washington D.C., 1969.
70. U.S. Department of Health, Education, and Welfare: Up and Around. United States Government Printing Office, Washington D.C., 1964.
71. VAN BUSKIRK, C., AND WEBSTER, D. Prognostic value of sensory defect in rehabilitation of hemiplegics. *Neurology, 5:* 407-411, 1955.
72. VOSS, D. E. Propreoceptive neuromuscular facilitation. *Am. J. Phys. Med.*, *46:* 838-898, 1967.
73. WATERS, R., AND MONTGOMERY, J. Lower extremity management of hemiparesis. *Clin. Orthop., 102:* 133-143, 1974.
74. WESTCOTT, E. J. Traditional exercise regimens for the hemiplegic patient. *Am. J. Phys. Med.*, *46:* 1012-1023, 1967.
75. WILLIAMS, N. Correlation between copying ability and dressing activities in hemiplegia. *Am. J. Phys. Med.*, *46:* 1332-1340, 1967.
76. ZANKEL, H. T. *Stroke Rehabilitation: A Guide to the Rehabilitation of an Adult Patient Following a Stroke.* Charles C Thomas, Springfield, Ill., 1971.
77. ZANKEL, H. T. Stimulation assistive exercise in hemiplegia. *Geriatrics, 15:* 616-622, 1960.

16

Exercises for Lower Motor Neuron Lesions

MILAND E. KNAPP

Lower motor neuron lesions damage or destroy the anterior horn cell, its axon, or the myoneural junction. Some classifications include primary muscle disease such as muscular dystrophy with motor neuron disease. In muscular dystrophy, however, while prevention and treatment of contracture is usually necessary, exercise to increase strength is contraindicated since it is more likely to produce weakness than strength. Therefore this presentation will not include exercise for muscular dystrophy.

Lower motor neuron lesions may be classified according to the pathologic course of the disease.

1. Those that progress in severity in spite of treatment. Examples include amyotrophic lateral sclerosis and Charcot-Marie-Tooth disease.

2. Those that begin acutely but reach a stable level. Examples include acute anterior poliomyelitis and avulsion of the brachial plexus without nerve regeneration.

3. Those that tend to improve after the original nerve involvement is completed. Examples are Guillain-Barré syndrome, peripheral nerve injury with regeneration and some toxic neuropathies.

Diseases in group 1 do not respond to treatment. Therefore therapeutic exercise should be limited to efforts to maintain range of motion and preserve useful function as long as possible. Increase of strength is not a practical goal. Groups 2 and 3 do respond to exercise. Therefore persistent treatment usually produces results that justify the effort expended.

Sensory loss makes treatment more difficult and recovery slower.

Basically, the exercise phase of treatment of lower motor neuron lesions may be divided into three parts:

1. Prevention or correction of factors limiting range of motion. These

349

factors are: (a) muscle spasm (nearly always present in poliomyelitis and Guillain-Barré syndrome), (b) pain produced by motion, and (c) contractures.

2. Reeducation of the afferent side of the motor pattern or engram to produce coordinated function. Sister Kenny called this "restoration of mental awareness." Its modern name is "biofeedback."

3. Reeducation of the motor portion of the motor pattern including exercise to increase strength.

Prevention or Correction of Factors Limiting Range of Motion

In poliomyelitis, Guillain-Barré syndrome, and irritative nerve lesions, hot packs of the Kenny type (4, 5, 8) are most effective, although other methods, especially whirlpool, may also relieve muscle spasm and pain. Gentle range of motion exercises, avoiding pain production but gradually increasing the arc of motion must accompany or follow the heat. Solidly developed contractures require prolonged stretch in addition to heat usually accompanied by massage.

It is generally believed that muscle imbalance causes muscle contractures due to differentials in muscle strength. Such imbalance, therefore, must be at a lower motor neuron level.

Therapeutic exercise as a treatment for lower motor neuron lesions under this concept becomes very simple. It consists merely of determining which muscles are weak and which are strong, analyzing the muscle balance between the involved muscles and then using strengthening exercises for the weak muscles while avoiding exercise of the strong, thereby restoring muscle balance. Technically, this is carried out by having the therapist perform passive motion of the strong muscle while the patient performs active motion of the weak muscle. This procedure has been called "muscle reeducation," but it does not seem to resemble "education" in any form and probably should be entitled "localized differential exercise." If muscle balance is restored, contractures should be prevented.

This explanation for development of contractures has several defects. In the first place, there is no location in the body, with the possible exception of the extraocular muscles, where agonists and antagonists are exactly equal to each other in strength. The extensors of the neck are much stronger than the flexors; the extensor of the knee is twice as strong as the flexor; the plantar flexors of the feet are more than 5 times stronger than the dorsiflexors in a normal person. This has been demonstrated quantitatively by Beasley, using very accurate tensiometer measurements.

Instrumentation and methods employed by Beasley (1, 2) in conducting quantitative muscle tests have been described in two published papers. Specific procedures used in testing the 12 actions, for which data are given in Table 16.1, were described by him in 1958 (3). Two significant

TABLE 16.1. *Maximum Average Strength for Six Antagonistic Pairs of Muscular Actions: 386 Children, Ages 10 to 12 Years*
(Data from Beasley*)

Muscular Action	Mean† (lb) $\bar{x}$	Standard Deviation s	Relative Dispersion $V\%$	Ratio of Antagonists Stronger/ Weaker
Neck				2.30:1
Flexion	22.42	3.474	15.50	
Extension	51.59	6.944	13.46	
Elbow				1.20:1
Flexion	46.92	9.010	19.20	
Extension	39.20	6.708	17.11	
Wrist				1.41:1
Ulnar flexion	46.54	8.570	18.41	
Radial extension	33.12	6.038	18.23	
Hip				1.66:1
Flexion	68.95	7.574	10.98	
Extension	114.18	21.892	19.17	
Knee				2.00:1
Flexion	57.79	8.512	14.73	
Extension	115.50	21.125	18.29	
Ankle				5.25:1
Dorsal flexion	51.92	10.758	20.72	
Plantar flexion	272.48	53.200	19.52	

* Data in this table were presented by Dr. Willis C. Beasley in a scientific exhibit and paper at the twenty-third Annual Scientific and Clinical Session, American Congress of Physical Medicine and Rehabilitation, Detroit, Michigan, August 28–September 2, 1955. This information is reproduced here with his permission.

† Mean values include correction for opposing gravitational component force of the body segment.

points to observe, according to Beasley, are: 1) these measurements were made with the most favorable positioning and angulation for each particular muscular action; 2) the lever length of the body segment is the same for each antagonist action of a particular pair. The ratio of stronger to weaker action in each antagonist pair, therefore, gives a fair representation of the relative maximum strength of each muscular action.

We are especially interested in the significance of the ratios between stronger and weaker aspects of antagonistic pairs of muscle systems as applied to the question, "Do muscular contractures arise from differences in the maximum strength of antagonistic muscles?" In normal children, who had no contractures at the time of the tests, the ratios between the average maximum normal strength of these six antagonistic pairs varied widely from a minimum of 1.20:1 for the elbow to a maximum of 5.25:1 for the ankle. Within this range of strength difference, therefore, we are not justified in explaining the contractures on the basis of imbalances in the potential voluntary strength of antagonistic pairs of muscles. It is apparent that muscle balance is located not in the motor unit, but in the higher regulating centers in the spinal cord or brain.

Secondly, contractures frequently develop in muscles of zero power, and, in fact, these are some of the most difficult contractures to overcome. These are most likely to develop in muscles which have been immobilized in splints or casts to prevent overstretching, whether the opposing muscle has strength or not.

Thirdly, contractures may develop in strong muscles that are opposed by strong muscles. In studying many thousands of post-poliomyelitic paralyses we have found no consistent correlation between strength and contracture formation.

It is true that fibrous tissue shortens to fit the space allowed for movement. A contracture may develop because a weak muscle is unable to move the joint through a full range, but this is not muscle imbalance. Some other means must be employed to perform the motion and prevent the contracture. Certainly immobilization promotes rather than prevents contracture. It may change the angle of the contracture but frequent motion through an adequate range is the only way to prevent it.

In treatment, some contractures may be removed by heat, massage, and motion, but some persistent, disabling ones require surgical release.

Reeducation of the Afferent Motor Pattern

Reeducation of the afferent side of the motor pattern will vary according to the level of sensation. If sensation is normal as in poliomyelitis and many Guillain Barré paralyses, the techniques developed by Sister Kenny are very effective. If sensation, especially proprioception, is impaired or lost, visual and auditory feed-back techniques may be used, but tactile and proprioceptive techniques must be modified. Electromyographic bio-feedback methods (9) which make motor contractions visible or audible may be of value.

Reeducation of the Motor Portion of the Motor Pattern

Before the widespread use of anti-poliomyelitis vaccines, acute anterior poliomyelitis was the lower motor neuron disease most frequently requiring treatment. Sister Elizabeth Kenny developed a method of muscle reeducation for that disease which, in my opinion, is logical and effective for the majority of lower motor neuron diseases if modifications are made for whatever sensory deficits may be present. Reeducation of motor function closely parallels the Kenny method although interrupted negative direct current stimulation of denervated muscles may be added in peripheral nerve injuries to maintain muscle contractility, to reduce contracture and to minimize muscle atrophy and fibrosis while the nerve is regenerating. Therefore I will describe her method in detail as the basis for exercise in the treatment of lower motor neuron disease. Modification must necessarily be made in the presence of sensory deficits.

According to her concept of poliomyelitis, muscle spasm occurs during the acute stage and is the major cause for contractures. The spasm is relieved by the use of hot foments and motion. The hot foments are of a special type which are extremely hot but do not contain droplets of water. The preparation and application of the packs have been described adequately elsewhere (4, 5, 8). Weakness is caused by denervation as in the conventional concept or by what Sister Kenny designated as mental alienation. Mental alienation is a physiologic interruption of function rather than a pathologic one. It can be corrected by proper therapeutic techniques. In addition to these factors, some of the poor function is caused by incoordination. This incoordination is not resident alone in the cerebellum but is the result of disturbances throughout the central nervous system, including the internuncial cells as well as the lower motor neurons (6).

The neuromuscular system is highly specialized. Although each muscle has a definite primary action (a direct pull upon its insertion), it rarely acts alone because of the integration and cooperation of the adjacent muscles. When a joint is moved in a specific direction, a number of related muscles come into play. However, there is usually one muscle which is primarily responsible for any given motion. This muscle is usually known as the prime mover of the joint in that particular direction. For each motion performed by a muscle, there is an opposite motion performed by an antagonistic muscle; the effective function of a joint depends upon the orderly regulation of these opposing units by the controlling nervous system. When a flexor begins to contract, the extensor must simultaneously elongate in a graduated manner so that a smooth action of the joint results. The elongating muscle must retain, at all times, a certain amount of tonus so as to be able to contract immediately and reverse the joint motion. This harmonious motion, which allows smooth, orderly and effective functioning of muscle, is well referred to as coordination. The disappearance of a particular muscle action from the motor scheme, whether due to direct involvement of that muscle by the disease, to indirect involvement by alienation or to interference with function by muscle spasm, will result in attempts by the adjacent muscles to substitute for the lost motion with the development of incoordination. In starting muscle training, this substitution of muscle action must be completely removed and prevented. Every mental and physical effort of the patient must be guided to the movement which is being trained and to that alone; allowing and even encouraging a patient in the free choice of substitution of muscles for the mere satisfaction of haphazard motion of the joint invite disaster.

As soon as possible after the diagnosis is made, treatment should be begun to minimize the aftereffects of the disease; it may often be started while the patient is still febrile. In the acute period the treatment is directed toward relief of pain and muscle spasm and maintenance of normal reflex patterns. This is done by the frequent application of special hot packs, by the use of reeducation techniques, and by positioning the patient in bed with a foot board to maintain the "standing" reflexes. These procedures can be used even while there is a threat to the patient's life and can be carried on in the respirator, although with some difficulty and lessened efficiency. We believe they should not be ignored or eliminated even for a few weeks in the respirator.

The muscle reeducation technique is based upon the normal processes of learning and starts at a reflex level in an attempt to stimulate proprioceptive pathways by having the therapist move the part passively. There are several techniques for this, depending upon the range of motion present, the tenderness of the part, and the size of the limb. One is a shaking or vibrating motion; another is a rapidly alternating movement; but the most commonly used method is to carry the part through a normal motion rather rapidly. The purpose of this maneuver is to stimulate the proprioceptive sensory endings in the tendon, muscle, and joint so that they will send impulses to the cord that will in turn produce an efferent impulse in the large motor neurons and cause contraction of the muscle fibers. Because this contraction shows up as a prominence of the tendon, Sister Kenny called it "tendon stimulation." This may be accomplished in spite of the fact that no voluntary motion can be demonstrated. However, it obviously means that motor fibers are present and, therefore, that intensive efforts at reeducation are worthwhile. During this procedure, the patient is completely inactive and makes no attempt to assist.

When an efferent pathway has been demonstrated by "tendon stimulation," a process of reeducating the afferent side of the motor pattern is begun by using every means available to produce sensory stimuli to make the patient aware of the motion to be performed. Sister Kenny called this "restoration of mental awareness." The motion which is carried out passively as described under "tendon stimulation" produces proprioceptive stimuli. The motion and the action of the muscles producing the motion are described to the patient; this involves auditory stimuli. The patient watches the movement performed, and this provides visual stimuli. The therapist strokes the skin over the area upon which the patient's attention is to be centered, usually the point of insertion of the prime mover. This adds tactile stimuli. Thus, every available method of reinforcing sensory stimulation is used. Probably the most important point in this phase of reeducation is that the therapist must carry out the motion exactly as the patient is to perform it. Physiologically, if learning consists of breaking down the resistance at the synapse, repetition is undoubtedly the most effective means of accomplishing this. Not only must the efferent pathway for the agonist be developed, but, in addition, similar coordinated pathways for the antagonist to let out slack, the synergists to help the motion and the stabilizers to fix the parts in a functional position must be developed.

Care in producing a coordinated movement seems to us to be essential to the production of eventual coordinated function. Reinforcement or facilitation by diagonal and rotatory movements as advocated by Kabat may result in stronger contractions but also may result in incoordination which interferes with function, in our experience. In the Kenny technique reinforcement is accomplished by adding various types of stimuli rather than by adding multiple stimuli of an incoordinate nature.

Simultaneously with the reeducation of the afferent pathways, attempts are made to reeducate the efferent pathways. This is done by having the patient attempt to assist the motion being performed by the therapist. This was named "restoration of muscle function" by Sister Kenny. The usual technique is for the therapist to perform two passive movements while executing all the procedures described under "restoration of mental awareness" and then to have the patient attempt to assist the third motion. If he succeeds, the treatment is discontinued for that session in order that he may be left with a sense of accomplishment, which will serve as a psychological boost for him. At later sessions the amount of active participation is gradually increased as function improves until the entire treatment is active. However, great care must be taken to avoid incoordination. If it occurs it is usually necessary to go back to an earlier stage of the treatment and start from there, even sometimes to put the patient back to bed and start the whole process over again.

Since muscle balance (or coordination) does not reside in the lower motor neuron or motor unit, no particular attention is paid to strength. The purpose of the reeducation is to produce a coordinated motion regardless of strength. Both the strong and the weak muscles are exercised, but the attempt is made to train them to work together. When this is successful the incidence of late contractures is minimal.

When the reeducation has progressed well and good coordination is established so that the patient has developed a solid motor pattern, heavy resistance exercises may be added to develop maximal strength of the involved muscles. However, the increments of resistance must be small and gradual, and great care must be used to detect the onset of incoordination in order to correct it before faulty habits are firmly established. Of course, when muscles are so weak that they cannot overcome gravity or cannot lift the weight of the part, every motion of ordinary activity is a heavy resistance exercise and helps to develop strength in the muscle. Thus the everyday activities of walking and daily living substitute for resistance exercise if the movement is not hampered by braces.

Muscle reeducation should begin as soon as the part can be moved through a small range of motion without pain or incoordination, while the patient is still in bed and even while the patient is still febrile. However, if pain is produced or spasm is increased by the motion, the attempts at muscle reeducation should be discontinued until those undesirable effects are no longer produced. In general, the earlier the reeducation can be started, the better the results will be. The ideal procedure, whenever possible, is early therapy to prevent the patient from losing his motor pattern.

The patient should be comfortable and relaxed throughout the treatment session. When treating a small child it is often necessary to spend a good deal of time gaining his confidence before satisfactory reeducation can be performed, because a child who is crying cannot be reeducated, nor can an adult who is fearful of the production of pain. The patient is placed on a hard table or plinth in as normal a position as possible (simulating the usual standing position if the patient were erect). He lies with his arms at his sides, legs in line with the body, feet at right angles and knees straight. The patient lies quietly (without moving muscles other than those to be treated) in a separate room so that his attention will not be distracted by other patients or unusual noises, for the treatment requires a great deal of concentration on the part of the patient as well as the therapist. No attempt is made to reeducate individual muscles nor to carry out localized exercise for individual muscles. The unit of reeducation is a movement of the joint in as normal a manner as possible, and this requires the coordination of many muscles. The usual technique is to carry out two passive movements after tendon stimulation has been done and then to attempt an active motion. If any visible or palpable motion is accomplished, the amount of active motion is gradually increased until the patient carries out the entire motion actively, but usually with assistance in order to prevent incoordination. Great care is taken to prevent the development of incoordinated movements. If a wrong muscle becomes active it is controlled by finger pressure on the muscle or by telling the patient not to use that muscle. In this reeducation technique we try to produce a pure motion. Care must be taken, also, not to tire the patient in any way. If the patient shows any evidence of fatigue the treatment should be discontinued and resumed at a later time, either the same day or on another day. The same procedure is followed if the patient becomes uncooperative. Sufficient assistance is given for each motion so that the patient does not have to use every muscle available to put forth a maximal effort. If a maximal effort is used, it is usually accompanied by a great deal of incoordination.

Reeducation is achieved by the use of alternate motions in as normal a manner as possible. The motion takes place first in the direction of the pull of the muscle which normally contracts within its own resting length, usually the flexor. Then extension is carried out, since the extensors usually must be removed from their resting length before a normal contraction can occur. Since joint motion is necessary in reeducation techniques, muscle setting (quadriceps setting in particular) has no place in this type of reeducation.

The patient is first placed in the supine position, and all of the muscles that can be treated in that position are treated first; then the patient is placed in the prone position, and the remainder of the muscles are treated. In the prone position, the same fundamental alignment is still maintained; the feet are placed over the edge of the table with a small pad under the ankle to avoid pressure on the toes, the knees are extended, and the arms are at the sides.

A complete list of the areas to be treated and the motions to be carried out follows:

I. Supine Position

Neck

1. Anterior neck muscles

Arm and Forearm

2. Elevation of shoulder
3. Flexion of arm at shoulder
4. Extension to neutral position
5. Abduction of arm
6. Adduction of arm
7. Internal rotation
8. External rotation
9. Flexion of forearm in supination
10. Extension of forearm in supination
11. Flexion of forearm midway between supination and pronation
12. Extension of forearm midway between supination and pronation
13. Supination in the extended position
14. Pronation in the extended position
15. Supination in the flexed position
16. Pronation in the flexed position

Wrist and Hand

17. Volar flexion of wrist
18. Dorsiflexion of wrist
19. Radial deviation
20. Ulnar deviation
21. Flexion at the metacarpophalangeal joints
22. Extension at the metacarpophalangeal joints
23. Flexion at the interphalangeal joints
24. Extension at the interphalangeal joints
25. Abduction of the fingers
26. Adduction of the fingers
27. Hyperextension of the fingers
28. Opposition of the thumb
29. Opposition of the little finger
30. Abduction of the thumb
31. Adduction of the thumb
32. Flexion of the thumb
33. Extension of the thumb

Trunk

34. Breathing and abdominal exercise
35. Forward flexion of trunk

Thigh and Leg

36. Flexion of thigh
37. Extension of thigh to the neutral position
38. Abduction of the thigh
39. Adduction of the thigh
40. Internal rotation
41. External rotation
42. Extension of the leg at the knee

Ankle and Foot

43. Inversion in plantar flexion
44. Eversion in plantar flexion
45. Inversion in neutral position
46. Eversion in neutral position
47. Plantar flexion
48. Dorsal flexion
49. Flexion of toes
50. Extension of toes

II. Prone Position

51. Posterior neck muscles
52. Retraction of shoulder girdle
53. Retraction of both shoulder girdles
54. Hyperextension of arm
55. Extension of elbow
56. Spinal muscles
57. Quadratus lumborum
58. Pull buttocks together
59. Hyperextension of thigh
60. Flexion of leg at knee
61. Plantar flexion of foot

The Neck

Spasm is commonly present in the posterior neck muscles while weakness is more common in the anterior; however, there may be spasm in the sternocleidomastoids, which will cause a tilt of the head. The sternocleidomastoid muscles have a double action; when working together they flex the head and neck forward; when working individually they rotate the head toward the opposite side and the face upward.

The patient lies in the supine position, his shoulders at the edge of the table and his head supported by the hands of the therapist. The patient is first instructed in the motions to be performed. He is told that the action of the sternomastoid muscles is to bring the head forward and downward, acting from their insertion on the mastoid process. The insertion is stroked by the therapist, and the direction of pull of the muscle is pointed out. He is requested to think about the movement and follow it mentally but not to make any actual effort. The motion is then carried out 3 times in each treatment session. When it is thought that he can carry out the motion actively, the therapist first performs two passive movements in this manner; then the patient attempts an active movement. If active movement is obtained, the patient must be watched closely to be sure that coordination is good. The contraction should be equal from both points of attachment. The patient must not bring the platysma into action, as evidenced by a downward pull of the corners of the mouth. There should be no activity in the posterior neck muscles; both sternomastoids should contract equally, and there should be no elevation of the shoulders. If greater pressure is felt on one side of the head than on the other, efforts are made to concentrate the patient's attention upon the weaker side until the action is equalized. If spasm is present in the posterior neck or in either sternomastoid, the movement may be distorted and the treatment delayed until this spasm has been overcome, after which each sternomastoid is exercised individually. While this is being done the patient's attention is focused on the single insertion of the muscle into the mastoid process, and the head is rotated according to the action of the muscle.

The important points about reeducation of the anterior neck muscles are: 1) the pull must be even when both sternomastoids are acting; 2) care must be taken that both the sternal and clavicular heads of the sternomastoid function; 3) substitution of the platysma or the strap muscles of the neck must be avoided; and 4) the pull must be from the insertion and not the origin of the muscle.

Arm and Forearm

ELEVATION OF THE SHOULDER

The upper trapezius, the levator scapulae, and the rhomboideus minor carry out this motion. The patient is usually in the supine position, but this motion may be reeducated with the patient in the erect position. The upper arm is grasped below the attachment of the deltoid to support the weight of the limb. The insertion of the trapezius to the spine of the scapula is the point of indication, and the patient's attention is centered on this insertion. Incoordination is shown mainly by use of the anterior neck muscles. Spasm in the pectoralis major or minor and the latissimus dorsi may interfere with the action. If the patient tends to elevate the shoulder when flexion or abduction is being performed, it may be well to treat this area after reeducation of the flexors and abductors has been performed.

FLEXION AND EXTENSION OF THE SHOULDER

Flexion is carried out by the coracobrachialis and anterior deltoid; extension to the neutral position, by the latissimus dorsi and the posterior deltoid. The insertion of the coracobrachialis, just below the medial margin of the humerus, is the point of indication. The therapist strokes this area and directs the patient's attention to this point. The therapist grasps the extended elbow, with the patient's forearm resting against the therapist's forearm. The arm is then carried forward and upward and returned to the neutral position. The point of indication for the return to the neutral position is the point of insertion of the latissimus dorsi into the humerus. Incoordination is likely to occur in the pectoralis major, particularly in the form of substitution of that muscle for the flexors.

ABDUCTION AND ADDUCTION OF THE SHOULDER

Abduction is performed largely by the deltoid, and the insertion of the deltoid into the deltoid tuberosity of the humerus is used as the point of indication. Adduction is performed by the latissimus dorsi and pectoralis major. Here a double insertion is indicated into the upper humerus anteriorly and posteriorly. Spasm is likely to be present in the adductor muscles and must be completely relieved in order to obtain complete abduction. It is very important that the shoulder should not be elevated during the performance of abduction. It is often necessary to place one hand over the acromion process to keep the shoulder from elevating. This is particularly true if there is spasm or muscle shortening present in the pectoralis major and latissimus dorsi.

INTERNAL AND EXTERNAL ROTATION OF THE SHOULDER

Internal rotation is performed by the latissimus dorsi, pectoralis major and subscapularis; external rotation, by the supraspinatus, infraspinatus and teres minor. Reeducation of these motions is carried out with the forearm flexed to a right angle midway between pronation and supination and with the arm partially abducted in order to secure a good range of rotation. One hand is used to maintain the abduction while the other grasps the hand and wrist to stabilize the wrist. In this case, the indication is not at the insertion of the muscle but is just above the elbow on its medial surface. For internal rotation the indication is toward the body, and for external rotation the motion is indicated away from the body. Incoordination of the wrist and fingers is likely to occur and should be watched for. Also, pronation and supination of the forearm may be attempted to substitute for rotation. The patient, in addition, may attempt to flex or extend the elbow.

FLEXION AND EXTENSION OF THE ELBOW

Flexion is performed primarily by the biceps and brachialis. The insertion indicated is that of the brachialis into the tuberosity of the ulna, with the forearm supinated. Extension is carried out by the triceps and anconeus. The insertion of the triceps into the olecranon is the point of indication. The arm is flexed to a right angle only because the biceps reaches its maximum contraction at that level. If flexion is carried beyond the right angle, attempts to extend the elbow again may result in incoordination (particularly by attempts to use the shoulder girdle incoordinately), and the shoulder will be raised off the table.

The second position for flexion and extension of the forearm is with the arm in mid-position. The indicated insertion is the same, but the motion is to carry the thumb toward the mouth.

PRONATION AND SUPINATION OF THE FOREARM

This motion, also, is done in two positions, first with the elbow extended and then with it flexed. With the elbow extended the muscles functioning are primarily the pronator quadratus for pronation and the supinator longus or brachioradialis for supination. The attachment of the pronator quadratus to the volar surface of the forearm near the wrist is used as the point of indication for pronation, and the attachment of the supinator to the dorsal surface of the radius, for supination. At the 90° angle the insertion of the pronator teres into the lateral surface of the radius is used as the point of indication for pronation; the insertion of the biceps into the bicipital tuberosity of the radius is used for supination. The hand is grasped by the therapist as in shaking hands; the forearm is supported with the other hand. The motion is started from the mid-position and carried into supination and then past the mid-position to pronation. The muscles of the hand present the most common substitution problems.

Wrist and Hand

FLEXION AND EXTENSION OF THE WRIST

Flexion of the wrist is carried out by the flexor carpi radialis, flexor carpi ulnaris and the palmaris longus. The insertions of these flexors are used for the points of indication, and they are usually stroked simultaneously. The extensors are the extensor carpi radialis longus and brevis and the extensor carpi ulnaris. The insertions of these muscles are also indicated in the same manner with the forearm supinated, usually with the elbow flexed. The patient's hand is grasped between the thumb on the dorsal surface and the fingers on the volar surface. Incoordination is likely to be shown by action of other muscles of the hand and fingers, especially of the thumb. It is very important to prevent the finger flexors and extensors from substituting for the wrist flexors and extensors.

RADIAL AND ULNAR DEVIATION OF THE WRIST

This function is performed by the same muscles, but in this case the extensors and the flexor carpi radialis work together to produce radial deviation, while the extensor and flexor carpi ulnaris do the same to produce ulnar deviation. The same position is used as for the previous procedure. The insertions of the muscles are indicated in the usual manner; both are stroked at the same time.

FLEXION AND EXTENSION AT THE METACARPOPHALANGEAL JOINTS

For flexion, the muscles used are the flexor digitorum sublimis and the lumbricales; for extension, the extensor digitorum communis and the interossei. The fingers are grasped as a group, leaving the thumb free.

The action is to bend the metacarpophalangeal joint without flexing the interphalangeal joints, so that a table top is made. Then it is returned to the straight position. The indication is the metacarpophalangeal joints.

FLEXION AND EXTENSION OF THE FINGERS AT THE INTERPHALANGEAL JOINT

The muscles used here are the flexor digitorum profundus and sublimis and the extensor digitorum communis, extensor indicis proprius and the extensor digiti quinti. This is done with the hand raised from the bed; each finger is exercised individually. The tip of the finger is used as the point of indication, and the last two joints are indicated.

ABDUCTION AND ADDUCTION OF THE FINGERS

Abduction is performed by the dorsal interossei and the abductor digiti quinti. Adduction is performed by the palmar interossei and the adductor digiti quinti. With the hand lying flat on the table, each finger is exercised individually. The finger is first abducted and then adducted. The indication for abduction is the lateral side of the finger and for adduction, the medial side. The middle finger is not exercised.

HYPEREXTENSION OF THE FINGERS AND THE THUMB

This motion is performed by the extensor digitorum communis, extensor indicis proprius, extensor digiti quinti, extensor pollicis longus and brevis. The hand is held flat on the table and each finger is grasped in turn to raise it off the table. The dorsal surface of the finger is used as the point of indication.

OPPOSITION OF THE THUMB AND LITTLE FINGER

This is performed by the opponens pollicis and opponens digiti quinti. The therapist grasps the thumb of the patient between his thumb and index finger. The insertion of the opponens to the first metacarpal is pointed out, and the therapist moves the thumb toward the little finger in a rotary motion so that the palmar surface of the thumb faces toward the palm of the hand and reaches over to the little finger. At the same time the little finger is brought up to the thumb.

ABDUCTION AND ADDUCTION OF THE THUMB

Abduction is performed by the abductor pollicis longus and brevis, and adduction, by the adductor pollicis. The treatment is performed with the hand resting on the table on its ulnar side with the arm midway between pronation and supination. The therapist grasps the patient's thumb between his thumb and index finger. The lateral side of the thumb is indicated for abduction and the medial side for adduction, and the appropriate motions are carried out. Substitution of the extensor pollicis longus and brevis should be avoided.

FLEXION AND EXTENSION OF THE THUMB

The muscles used are the flexor pollicis longus and brevis and the extensor pollicis longus and brevis. The point of indication is the tip of the thumb.

The Trunk

THE MUSCLES OF RESPIRATION

Inhalation is performed by the external intercostals, the serratus anterior and the diaphragm. The patient is directed to inhale through his nose and to fill his chest with air, expanding it as far as possible. Exhalation is performed by the internal intercostals and abdominals. The patient is then directed to exhale through his mouth, pull in the ribs and, finally, contract the abdominal muscles. It is important to avoid using the sternocleidomastoid muscles during inhalation (a common substitution for the muscles of respiration). If the patient cannot breathe without using these muscles, a respirator may be indicated. Many of the post-respirator cases who have lost intercostal function will use the sternomastoids rather extensively for inhalation. The use of hissing, coughing and grunting is of value in those patients who have difficulty in exhaling. Spasm in the back muscles may interfere with respiration to a certain extent; spasm in the pectoralis major is a very common cause of interference with respiratory function. Shortening may occur in the intercostals as well, and it may be necessary to manually stretch adjacent ribs to improve respiration.

FLEXION OF THE TRUNK

The muscles used in this motion are the masseters, platysma, sternocleidomastoids, intercostals, all abdominals and iliopsoas. The normal motion of flexion of the trunk is a rolling motion (the patient rolls up like a rug) accomplished in this sequence: the masseter fixes the jaw, the platysma depresses the chin, the sternocleidomastoids flex the neck and the head rises off the bed. The internal intercostals contract to hold the rib cage together, and the abdominals contract to bring the rib cage toward the pelvis. Finally, the iliopsoas flexes the pelvis on the thigh and brings the patient to a sitting position. It is obviously impossible for the patient to perform this sequence of events if there is any tightness in the back. Since muscle spasm is almost constantly present in the back muscles in the acute stage of the disease, it is extremely important that back tightness be relieved as early and as completely as possible. We feel that the ultimate goal is to get the patient to touch forehead to knees in the long sitting position with the knees absolutely straight. If this can be accomplished we can be sure tightness is relieved in the back. It is important that the patient touch the forehead to the knees rather than the chin or the mouth because, if the chin or mouth is used, a certain amount of tightness may remain in the posterior neck. If tightness remains in the back, the patient comes up abdomen first, using the psoas to pull himself foreward, even though his thorax and head may lag behind the lower trunk.

If one leg seems to become shorter in the long sitting position, there is tightness in the back muscles on that side. If an apparently short leg regains its full length on sitting, the tightness is in the abdominals.

Evenness of pull in all areas of the abdominal muscles is an important objective because weakness of the abdominals is a very common cause of scoliosis at a later date. Residual tightness is also a common cause of scoliosis and should be relieved if possible.

To achieve flexion of the trunk the therapist places his right hand under the patient's head and tells him to help bring his forehead toward his chest, to pull his ribs down and his stomach in and then to sit up. The indications are the forehead, chest and abdomen in turn.

Thigh and Leg

FLEXION AND EXTENSION OF THE THIGH

The prime mover for flexion of the thigh is the iliopsoas, which inserts into the lesser trochanter of the femur. The rectus femoris, sartorius and adductors (longus, brevis and minimus) also help to flex the thigh, as does the tensor fasciae femoris. However, the latter muscles, less likely to be nonfunctioning than the psoas, are less powerful and usually do not produce an even, coordinated movement. Therefore, we attempt to encourage the action of the iliopsoas as much as possible while discouraging substitution by these accessory muscles. In poliomyelitis the lower extremities are usually weak, and, since a satisfactory walking gait is one of the primary objectives of treatment, accurate reeducation of the thighs is very important. With the patient in the supine position, the therapist stands at the side of the bed and grasps the knee (or that region) with one hand while supporting the foot with the other hand. The motion is carried out by flexing the thigh with the knee flexed, keeping the leg parallel to the table. The point of indication is the insertion of the psoas into the lesser trochanter, a point about an inch below the inguinal ligament just medial to the bellies of the sartorius and rectus femoris. This spot can be palpated when the patient is relaxed. The arc of movement to be used depends upon the experience and judgment of the therapist. It should not be continued if the patient's physical effort disappears in any particular arc of the movement. If the psoas is very weak, the origin of the muscle may be stimulated and facilitation thus obtained by having the patient hold his head off the table while flexion of the thigh is carried out (reinforcement of psoas activity). Incoordination is likely to be present because of contraction of the sartorius, the adductors and, frequently, the hamstrings. Since spasm is commonly present in the hamstrings, it is important that the motion does not elicit pain. It may be argued that it is not necessary to be so insistent about reeducation of the psoas since flexion can be carried out by the other muscles mentioned. However, the substitution of these muscles for the psoas may prevent its reeducation and eventually cause its complete elimination from the motor pattern.

Extension of the thigh is performed by the gluteus maximus and long head of the biceps, with some assistance from the semimembranosus and semitendinosus. In the supine position the thigh and leg are returned to the table, with the leg held continuously parallel to the table. The point of indication for extension is just distal to the ischial tuberosity.

ABDUCTION AND ADDUCTION OF THE THIGH

There are two abductors of the thigh. The tensor fasciae femoris, together with the insertion of the gluteus maximus into the fascia, acts as a stabilizer in abduction and will abduct to the straight line but not much beyond because of lack of leverage. The gluteus medius is the abductor which carries the motion beyond the straight line because it inserts into the greater trochanter near its apex, which projects from the femur and offers adequate leverage. The point of indication for this motion is the insertion of the gluteus medius into the greater trochanter.

Adduction is performed by the adductors longus, brevis, minimus and magnus, the gracilis and the pectineus, all of which lie on the inner surface of the thigh. The inner surface of the thigh near the knee is used as the point of indication.

The patient lies in the supine position and the thigh is moved in abduction first, then back in adduction to the straight line. The knee is in a position of extension with the heel held in the therapist's cupped hand. It is important that the pelvis should not elevate during abduction, in order to get a true motion of abduction. Spasm is frequently present in the adductors as well as in the hamstrings, and these should be watched carefully to be sure spasm is relieved. External rotation of the thigh should be avoided as should any action in the quadriceps.

INTERNAL AND EXTERNAL ROTATION OF THE THIGH

Internal rotation is produced by the gluteus minimus; external rotation, by the quadratus femoris, obturators, gemelli and piriformis. Indication of the direction of motion is made on the anterior surface of the thigh near the knee rather than at the insertion of the muscles. The knee is placed in line with the lower extremity, which rests on the table. After indicating the areas, the motion is carried out by rotating the entire lower extremity internally and externally. The lower extremity should not be abducted when these motions are being carried out. The adductors aid in internal rotation but should be kept from working while this motion is being reeducated. Inversion and eversion of the foot is a common incoordinate act that accompanies this motion.

EXTENSION AND FLEXION OF THE KNEE

Extension of the knee is achieved by the quadriceps femoris. This group of four muscles inserts into the tibial tuberosity through a common tendon, the patellar tendon. To reeducate this muscle the patient lies supine with the thigh and knee flexed. The therapist stands at the side of the table, supporting the knee with one hand and the leg with the other. The insertion of the patellar tendon into the tibial tuberosity is indicated, and the knee is then extended from the flexed position. Contraction of the hamstrings and movements of the trunk should be avoided; it is especially important to keep the iliotibial band from performing this action. A very common substitution is hip extension, and this should be avoided while carrying out reeducation of the quadriceps. Muscle setting is condemned because it does not produce a motion and, therefore, tends to produce incoordination. It is not uncommon for the patellar tendon to be so stretched that the patella rests above the level of the condyles of the femur, if muscle setting has been practiced vigorously over a long period of time.

Flexion of the knee is performed by the hamstrings. While only three hamstrings are listed in anatomy books, we recognize five: the biceps femoris, the semimembranosus, the semitendinosus, the gracilis, and the sartorius. The insertions of the biceps femoris into the head of the fibula and the medial hamstrings into the medial tuberosity of the tibia are used as the point of indication. A more detailed description of the technique for flexion of the knee will be given when discussing the prone position. It is important that both the lateral and medial hamstrings should contract with equal strength in order that the motion may be well coordinated. Since there is more muscle on the medial than the lateral side, the medial side is usually stronger.

Foot And Ankle

INVERSION AND EVERSION OF THE FOOT

In the neutral position, inversion is produced by the anterior tibial and eversion by the peroneus tertius and brevis. The point of indication is the insertion of the tibialis anterior for inversion and the tuberosity of the fifth metatarsal for eversion. The most common incoordination is the use of the extensor hallucis longus to substitute for the anterior tibial and of the toe extensors for the peroneals.

In the plantar flexed position, inversion is performed primarily by the posterior tibial and eversion by the peroneus longus. The insertion of the tibialis posterior into the center of the arch of the foot is used for indication; the tuberosity of the fifth metatarsal, for the peroneal indication. When carrying out inversion and eversion of the foot in plantar flexion it is important that the anterior tibial does not substitute for the posterior tibial and that the peroneus tertius does not assist during eversion.

EXTENSION AND FLEXION OF THE ANKLE

Extension (plantar flexion) is carried out by the gastrocnemius and soleus, which insert into the tip of the calcaneus. Treatment is conducted with the patient in the supine position; the hand is placed over the sole of the foot and even pressure is applied over the heads of the metatarsals. The index and middle fingers are placed on either side of the calcaneus. The motion of plantar flexion is then carried out, and reeducation proceeds in the usual manner. To work primarily with the gastrocnemius, the knee is kept extended; to work primarily with the soleus, the knee is flexed. The point of indication is the insertion of the tendon into the calcaneus. The peculiar method of holding the foot is used so that variations in pressure against the heel of the hand can be felt. If it is found that the medial or lateral side of the foot is exerting unusual pressure, the patient is told to try to maintain even pressure. This is very important if good function is to be obtained. It is important to relieve all spasm in the gastrocnemius-soleus because its presence in either head interferes with even function.

Extension of the foot by the flexor digitorum longus or brevis, peroneus longus, tibialis posterior or the quadratus planti should be studiously avoided because this tends to allow shortening of the plantar fascia, which will result in a high arch and a peg heel. If the gastrocnemius-soleus is weak, it cannot give enough support to stretch these muscles satisfactorily, so that the end result of use of these muscles to substitute for the calf muscles accentuates the calcaneus deformity.

Flexion (dorsiflexion) is performed by the combined efforts of the tibialis anterior and peroneus tertius. The insertion of the tibialis anterior and peroneus tertius is used for indication; the foot is brought up into a slightly dorsiflexed position. It is important in retraining dorsiflexion that the toe extensors should not be used because they will often tend to completely overshadow the anterior tibial and peroneus tertius and to produce hammer toes.

FLEXION AND EXTENSION OF THE TOES

The flexor digitorum longus and brevis, lumbricales and flexor hallus longus and brevis carry out flexion. Extension is produced by the extensor digitorum longus and brevis and extensor hallucis longus and brevis. These are usually reeducated in a group by holding all the toes in the hand with the thumb on the dorsal surface and the index and middle fingers along the plantar surface. The tip of the toe is used as the point of indication for both directions. If total paralysis is present, the toes may be moved individually in the same manner as for the fingers. Flexion is always performed first.

Prone Position

After reeducation of the muscles in the supine position has been performed, the patient is turned to the prone position with the toes over the edge of the bed, and the posterior muscles are given special attention.

POSTERIOR NECK

Hyperextension of the head is produced by the rectus capitis posterior major and minor, while extension of the head is executed primarily by the trapezii (in addition to the paravertebral muscles). For this training the head is taken beyond the end of the table and supported with the hand. The point of indication is the base of the skull. It is very important that both sides of the neck contract evenly.

RETRACTION OF THE SHOULDERS

This motion is performed by the rhomboids, major and minor. The point of indication is the vertebral border of the scapula. The shoulder is raised a little off the table with the hand under it, after which the shoulder blade is brought back toward the midline. This may be done with each shoulder individually and then with both shoulders together. It is important that the upper trapezius does not elevate the shoulder; the inferior angle of the scapula must be anchored by the latissimus dorsi.

HYPEREXTENSION OF THE UPPER EXTREMITY

The muscles involved in hyperextension are the teres major and the posterior deltoid. Usually, the shoulder is first fixed in a position of retraction and then the arm is extended. The arm is grasped at the wrist in midsupination, holding the shoulder off the table. The point of indication is the insertion of the teres major into the upper end of the humerus. Common incoordinations occur in the latissimus dorsi, which result in adduction of the arm. The upper trapezius must not elevate the shoulder, and the patient must not try to pull the shoulder forward. The motion should be carried out with a directly posterior motion.

ELBOW EXTENSION

Extension of the elbow may be exercised in this position also with the triceps and anconeus. The patient may be placed near the edge of the table with a pad under the shoulder and the elbow flexed over the edge of the table. The point of indication is the olecranon, and the arm is extended from the flexed position.

EXTENSION OF THE SPINE

This action is performed by the erector spinae muscles. If the patient is small, one therapist can carry out this motion by placing his arm across the chest, being careful not to press on the neck. If the patient is an adult or a large child, it is often necessary to have two people perform the reeducation technique so that one can help lift the shoulders and upper trunk while the other stabilizes the pelvis. The erector spinae muscles consist of a great number of small muscles extending only a few segments vertically and divided into several groups laterally, but fused and overlapping so that they appear to be one large muscle. However, this motion is not performed by one muscle. If it is noticed that certain areas are not functioning, then special attention should be given to those areas. If the patient is very weak the upper portion of the back may be treated first, then the middle and then the lower. An additional stimulus can be given to the lower back by lifting both legs off the table simultaneously, with the head kept in good alignment. If weakness is greater on one side than the other, that side of the trunk and the corresponding leg can be raised to increase the amount of stimulus to the desired area.

QUADRATUS LUMBORUM

The quadratus lumborum is an extremely important muscle which is often neglected in reeducation. Complete paralysis of both quadrati makes walking impossible even with braces. The quadratus is a triangularly acting muscle which produces stabilization between the lumbar spine and the pelvis; it should not be thought of as an elevator of the pelvis. Reeducation of the longitudinal fibers may be performed by bringing the pelvis toward the ribs. However, reeducation of the oblique fibers is best carried on by having the therapist pull down on the leg on the strong side while pushing up on the weak side and asking the patient to push toward the therapist with the weak quadratus. The best strengthening exercise for the quadratus is walking in the erect position, best done between parallel bars.

HYPEREXTENSION OF THE THIGH

Hyperextension of the thigh is performed by the long head of the biceps, assisted by the semimembranosus and semitendinosus. The quadriceps stabilizes the knee in extension; the gluteus maximus stabilizes the thigh on the pelvis; and the iliocostalis lumborum stabilizes the pelvis on the trunk. The extended leg is grasped with the hand under the knee, as the leg rests on the forearm of the therapist. The point of indication is the origin of the long head of the biceps at the ischial tuberosity. Hyperextension is performed, and the insertion of the gluteus maximus is indicated as a stabilizer; the attachment of the iliocostalis to the pelvis is also indicated as a stabilizer. It is important that the contraction start in the long head of the biceps rather than in the gluteus maximus or medius. The biceps femoris has a double function: the long head extends the hip, while the combination of long and short head flexes the knee. However, it seems to us that it is better to think of this muscle as arising from the linea aspera at about the middle of the femur. The proximal insertion into the ischial tuberosity performs the function of extension of the hip; the distal insertion into the head of the fibula performs the function of flexion of the knee. This muscle is important because it figures prominently in maintaining the erect position. In order to walk without a brace there must be some way of stabilizing the thigh on the pelvis. This is not done by the quadriceps, which merely extends the knee. The flexors of the hip, which are often present when the extensors are nonfunctioning, interfere with the motion. The hamstrings, however, which arise from the ischial tuberosity, help to extend the thigh. Those muscles which arise from the pubis, on the other hand, only adduct the thigh and do not extend it, and the sartorius, which arises from the antérior superior spine of the ilium, flexes the hip instead of extending it. Therefore, in an examination of the patient we should determine which of the hamstrings are present in order to determine how useful they will be in walking.

The gluteus maximus can be exercised individually in the prone-lying position by having the patient approximate his buttocks. The indication is the insertion of the gluteus maximus into the fascia femoris. The pull must come from the inferolateral region and must extend upward and medially in order to have a useful function. Confusion may arise from other movements in this area, particularly those of the sphincter ani, which may produce enough movement to make it appear that the gluteus maximus is functioning.

KNEE FLEXION IN THE PRONE POSITION

The muscles involved in this action are the semimembranosus, semitendinosus, and short head of the biceps. The lower leg is grasped at the anterior surface of the ankle. The point of indication is the attachment of the lateral and medial hamstrings. The knee is flexed through a moderate range; the return of motion is extension by the quadriceps, and the tibial tuberosity is indicated. It is important that the pull come from the insertion and not the origin of these muscles; the long head of the biceps should not function. Both the inner and outer hamstrings should function evenly; however, the inner hamstrings are always more prominent than the outer. Added stimulation can be given to the inner or outer hamstrings individually. For the outer hamstrings, the leg is slightly externally rotated, and with the hand of the therapist placed on the dorsal surface of the patient's foot a combined flexion movement of toes, ankle and knee is carried out. For the inner hamstrings, the same procedure is performed except that the leg is internally rotated and the great toe is flexed with the index finger. We should try to avoid substitution of the gracilis and sartorius in this motion.

EXTENSION (PLANTAR FLEXION) OF THE ANKLE

The muscle performing this function is primarily the soleus, although the gastrocnemius cannot be completely excluded. The knee is flexed to a right angle, and the foot is grasped as in the supine position; then the indication is given to the Achilles tendon at its insertion into the calcaneus, and the motion is performed. The patient is instructed to relax, and the foot is returned passively to the starting position. As in the gastrocnemius, it is important that an even pressure across the ball of the foot be present.

Scoliosis

The prevention of scoliosis is of paramount importance because its presence constitutes a severely deforming, as well as a sometimes disabling, condition. Scoliosis is produced by a combination of muscle tightness and weakness. We do not believe that leg shortening produces a fixed curve except in the presence of weakness or tightness of the back or abdominal muscles. We have seen many patients with 2 inches or more of leg length difference continue for many years without scoliosis, provided that neither back nor abdominal tightness or weakness was present. However, the direction of scoliosis may be determined by leg length. This is true, also, of tightness in the tensor fasciae femoris. Generalized weakness of severe degree is almost certain to result in some degree of scoliosis in a child. We have followed children for 5 or 6 years in whom, in the erect position, x-ray films showed a curve first in one direction, then in another, before actual fixation occurred. Unfortunately, fixation does eventually take place, and a fixed scoliosis develops.

In treating scoliosis, all tightness is first removed from the back and associated areas with packs and stretching; the stretch must sometimes be localized to the involved area. We do not believe that tightness should be left in the back to gain support because it does not give support if the muscles are weak. On the other hand, forcible stretching should not be started late in the course of the disease because a tear in the fascia may develop which progresses in the same area on further stretch and thus tends to increase rather than correct scoliosis. The cause of scoliosis is difficult to determine because so many factors operate in varying degrees.

These factors include muscle tightness in the sacrospinalis, quadratus lumborum, hamstrings, abdominals, tensors or scapular muscles; weakness of abdominals, quadratus or thoracic muscles; and incoordinate action of any of these muscles. If these factors are sufficiently prominent it is virtually impossible to prevent some degree of scoliosis.

In order to delay the development of scoliosis for as long as possible, tightness should be overcome and flexibility maintained. To this end, the parents are taught to carry out the stretches at home and are impressed with the fact that this must be done very conscientiously and over many years or until the child has attained full growth. In addition, suspension at home by head traction is often useful. Coordinated muscle function is of utmost importance in those cases with weakness. It is much more common for scoliosis to follow weakness of the abdominal muscles than weakness of the back muscles. It is desirable to delay its development as long as possible because it seems that surgical fusion, if that becomes necessary, is more effective in older patients. If it can be postponed until the child has grown to adulthood, surgery may not be necessary. In our experience corsets and jackets have not been effective in preventing the development of scoliosis; their greatest function is to hide the curve from the doctor and the parents and, therefore, to make them all feel a little happier while the curve continues to increase.

Gait Training

The ultimate objective of muscle reeducation of the lower extremities is the production of a satisfactory gait for locomotion. In the order of their value for walking, the most important muscles are those of the trunk followed by those of the upper extremities (needed for crutch walking with braces on the lower extremities). In the lower extremities the most important muscles are the hip extensors (to stabilize the thigh on the pelvis), the other thigh muscles (except the quadriceps), the ankle muscles (for stabilization) and last of all the quadriceps. The quadriceps is not necessary for walking on one level. In going up and down stairs one quadriceps is all that is required; we have seen a few patients go up and down without a railing, without braces, without crutches, and without either quadriceps.

The normal gait consists of the following progression of events: the hip flexes and the knee bends; the lower extremity is brought forward, the knee extends, the foot dorsiflexes and the patient comes down on the heel with the toes off the floor and the knee extended (or hyperextended); the weight of the body is then brought forward over that leg; then, when the center of gravity passes the center of the foot, the patient rises on his toes and flexes the knee and hip and starts the same process over again. It has been shown that in the normal gait the foot is raised only a quarter of an inch or so off the floor; even a slight amount of foot drop may interfere with walking. However, the goal of training should be to barely clear the floor without elevating the pelvis abnormally. A high stepping gait is undesirable.

At the beginning of gait training the patient should stand with his weight evenly distributed on both legs, then bend each knee slightly in an alternating manner, returning each to complete extension before the other knee is flexed. The range of this motion is gradually increased until it is decided that forward progression is possible. The first step is performed by placing the body weight securely on the weaker leg and bringing the stronger leg forward first. This is necessary for stability on the step-off and to start the momentum of the gait. The succeeding steps are always easier than the first one because the inertia of the body weight has been overcome.

The essentials of a normal gait should be simulated as closely as possible in spite of the fact that many of the muscles are weak or perhaps entirely devoid of power. Momentum can be used to substitute for some of the motions, and the knee can be used in slight hyperextension to bear weight in the absence of quadriceps. Absence of quadriceps does not cause a back-knee; it is caused by absent hamstrings. Another cause of back-knee is persistent tightness of the soleus. This may give stability to the knee but tends to force hyperextension when the body is brought forward with the ankle partially but rigidly plantar flexed. Stretching of the posterior ligaments of the knee results, and it may even produce bony changes. This may happen while the patient is wearing a long leg brace. Many patients who have hamstring but no quadriceps function can be taught to walk very successfully without a brace and with no evidence of difficulty due to back-knee after many years. The problem of back-knee is much overemphasized; it is not likely to cause trouble in adults. In children who cannot be taught to walk with a slightly bent knee but who throw their full weight back against the posterior ligaments (if the hamstrings are weak), it may be necessary to use a brace to prevent the knee from going back too far. This is especially important because the developing bones will respond to such forces and may become deformed out of proportion to the actual force being placed upon them.

Momentum can be substituted for the function of the dorsiflexors of the foot, and a reasonably normal gait can often be obtained without a foot-drop brace and without a foot drop.

Tightness in the hip flexors, particularly in the tensor fasciae latae, is an important cause of gait problems. If there is the slightest degree of hip flexion contracture the patient with severe weakness cannot get his weight distributed over his lower extremity and, therefore, cannot walk without a brace. In fact, in many instances, he cannot walk with a brace, except in a very ungainly, quadruped type of gait with his crutches placed far ahead of his lower extremities.

General Comments

It should be emphasized that the reeducation process must extend over a long period of time; there is no miraculous fast method. Repetition of each motion many times daily is the only way to achieve success. Treatments once or twice a week are wasteful of time and money. Our experience has shown that follow-up treatment after the patient is discharged from the hospital is usually best done by the patient or his relatives or friends after specific training by the therapist. In this way exercises may be performed frequently enough to be of value.

When muscle reeducation has developed a sound, well established motor pattern which is not likely to be disturbed or lost by intense effort, heavy resistance exercise may be used to develop maximal strength (seeChapter 7). In our experience, it is of doubtful value since the duration of the increased strength may not be great and the development of incoordination is a very real danger.

Braces should be used when they increase the functional ability of the patient or when they prevent or retard the development of deformities. They should not be used merely because the muscle test shows weakness of a certain grade.

Follow-up examination by the physiatrist must continue at intervals for many years and, in some patients, for life. New problems may arise at any time. It is far better to detect them in the early stages and prevent their further development than to attempt to correct them after they have been firmly established.

REFERENCES

1. BEASLEY, W. C. Influence of method on estimates of normal knee extensor force among normal and postpolio children. *Phys. Ther. Rev., 36:* 21, 1956.
2. BEASLEY, W. C. Instrumentation and equipment for quantitative clinical muscle testing. *Arch. Phys. Med., 37:* 604, 1956.

3. BEASLEY, W. C. Quantitative estimates for the percentage level of fair muscular actions. *Arch. Phys. Med., 39:* 104, 1958.
4. COLE, W. H., AND KNAPP, M. E. The Kenny treatment of infantile paralysis. *J.A.M.A., 116:* 2577, 1941.
5. KENNY, E. *The Treatment of Infantile Paralysis in the Acute Stage.* St. Paul, 1941.
6. KNAPP, M. E. A hypothesis to explain the muscular after-effects of poliomyelitis. *Arch. Phys. Med., 29:* 334, 1948.
7. KNAPP, M. E. Function of the quadratus lumborum. *Arch. Phys. Med., 32:* 505, 1951.
8. POHL, J. F., AND KENNY, E. *The Kenny Concept of Infantile Paralysis and Its Treatment.* St. Paul, 1943.
9. SIMARD, T. G., AND BASMAJIAN, J. V. Methods in training the conscious control of motor units. *Arch. Phys. Med. 48:* 12, 1967.

17

Exercise in
Multiple Sclerosis

_____ RENE CAILLIET

Multiple sclerosis is one of the group of diseases of the central nervous system classified as a demyelinating disease, so called because the pathology is a focal or diffuse disturbance of the myelin sheaths (white matter) of nerve fibers in various regions of the central nervous system. Its etiology is unknown.

At first there is destruction of the myelin sheaths with varying sizes and locations of patches and a tendency toward fluctuation, remissions and exacerbation. The micropathology of multiple sclerosis is that of fatty swelling, followed by fenestration and vacuolization and ultimate degeneration of the myelin sheaths, gradually replaced by scarring (sclerosis) or proliferation of microglial glitter cells and astrocytes. Throughout the central nervous system can be seen numerous areas of demyelinization of varying sizes and in various stages of development and degeneration. Though old (so-called healed) plaques can be seen, many nerve fibers traverse the area. Edema and perivascular infiltrations may interfere with the conductivity of the axis cylinder. The presence of this edema and infiltration (1), which is reversible, accounts undoubtedly for the exacerbation and remissions of the disease.

The characteristic pathological alteration consists of myelin loss with relative preservation of axis cylinder. The presence of a demyelinating lesion in the nerve fiber greatly impairs the ability of the fiber to conduct repetitive impulses and to fatigue rapidly (2). The temperature at which conduction block occurs is directly proportional to the degree of demyelinization (3). A small degree of temperature elevation blocks an increasing number of conducting fibers. Conversely, increasing the pH by decreasing serum calcium or increasing phosphate improves the conduction velocity of the demyelinated nerves (4). These and many other, as yet unproven factors, influence the course of the disease and its reaction to a therapeutic regime.

There is no classical syndrome of neurological findings which establishes the diagnosis of multiple sclerosis. The diagnosis is suggested by the (young) age, history of previous mild transitory symptoms, tendency toward remission and exacerbation, the frequent presence of early visual disturbance associated with mild pyramidal tract symptoms or ataxia and the presence of neurological signs and symptoms not attributable to a single focal tract or level lesion. Laboratory diagnosis is of no assistance.

Four clinical classifications are recognized: 1) alternating type with recurrences and remissions (recurrences being frequent and of variable severity and duration; recovery of each attack being complete or partial); 2) gradual insidious type with no appreciable recovery phases and a continuing downhill course; 3) acute fulminating type with massive involvement in one episode leading to early marked disability or death; 4) stationary type with initial onset, a residual defect and no further exacerbation, and partial remission becoming static.

According to Grinker (5), this disease ranks third in frequency among neurological disorders. Wilson (6) ranked it as the most prevalent of all neurological diseases between 1908 and 1925.

The treatment of multiple sclerosis is empiric. Schumacher (7) in his excellent review concludes, "It may be said that the outlook for cure of the disease by drugs is unpromising and that the outlook for symptomatic relief by drugs is less optimistic. . . . " The consensus indicates that physical medicine and rehabilitation techniques have most to offer multiple sclerosis patients (8).

The use of physical medicine in the treatment of multiple sclerosis refers to the total rehabilitation of the patient in which exercise plays a vital role. Exercise, however, must relate to the specific neurological deficit exhibited by the patient. As any single or combination of central nervous system tracts may be involved, an exercise regime must be directed to that specific deficit.

Mortality and Morbidity

In a statistical study of 284 outpatients followed for 10 years, the survival rate 5 years after the initial clinic visit was 96.4%; at the end of 10 years, 88.3%. The percentage of patients walking and working after 5 years of initial clinic evaluation was 64.4%; at the end of 10 years, 42.0% (9). In a small (40) group of patients followed for 20 years, 12 patients (30%) survived 20 years, at the end of which time 4 had no or slight disability; 4, moderate disability; and 4, severe disability (10). The previously discouraging mortality and morbidity statistics must therefore be reviewed. Some indication of prognosis worthy of consideration was done by Mueller (11) for 810 patients. Approximately half the patients with multiple sclerosis become ill before the age of 25, and less than 10% at 40 or over. When the age at the onset is advanced, patches give rise to clinical symptoms more frequently. In this age group, there is a greater tendency for the disease to become progressive earlier. The disease is seldom disabling before it enters a steadily progressive stage. Spastic paresis is found more often at an advanced age, whereas cerebellar disturbances are more frequent at an early age and are relatively uncommon at an advanced age. Thygesen (12) found that 13% were virtually or completely free from symptoms after 8–15 years, with 12% of the cases characterized by long remissions, the disease having become stationary at an early stage. It has recently been stated, however, that spontaneous improvement cannot be expected after 2 years following the onset of an exacerbation (13).

Evaluation of benefits of treatment is difficult to ascertain clinically. A working scale has been devised which stresses disability as the standard (14):

0 – Normal neurological examination.
1 – No dysfunction, minimal signs (Babinski positive, minimal finger to nose ataxia, diminished vibration sense).
2 – Minimal dysfunction (slight weakness or stiffness, mild disturbance of gait, awkwardness, mild visuomotor disturbance).
3 – Moderate dysfunction (monoparesis, mild hemiplegia, moderate urinary or eye symptoms, a combination of lesser dysfunctions).
4 – Relatively severe dysfunction not preventing ability to work or carry on normal activities of living, including sexual functions.
5 – Dysfunction severe enough to preclude working, with maximal motor function (walking unaided up to several blocks).
6 – Assistance required for walking (canes, crutches, braces).
7 – Restricted to wheel chair (able to wheel self and enter and leave chair alone).
8 – Restricted to bed, but with effective use of arms.
9 – Totally helpless bed patient.
10 – Death due to multiple sclerosis.

Secondary related disability and pathogenetic factors may be pictured as in Figure 17.1.

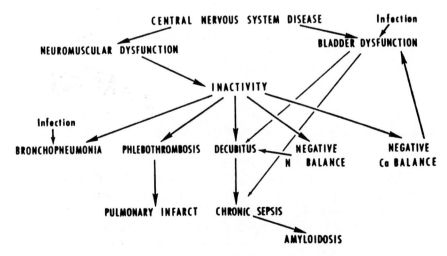

Fig. 17.1. Effects of inactivity in multiple sclerosis.

Since many neurological functional pathways may be involved, either isolated or in combination, consideration of the type of neuromuscular involvement must be considered in exercise prescription. Some generalities encountered in this illness must also be kept in mind. Multiple sclerotics exhibit a characteristic fatigue pattern almost diagnostic of the disease. A kind of fatigue is often seen; the patient awakens reasonably rested, reaches a peak of fatigue and excessive weakness by mid-afternoon and recovers energy and strength by early evening. This consistent diurnal cycle must guide us in prescribing the optimum time for therapeutic exercise.

Fatigue of muscular contraction noted generally in patients with multiple sclerosis, especially in repetitive contractions (endurance exercises), demands individualized exercise prescription. Clinical experience has failed to demonstrate any adverse effect on the patient from the repeated production of fatigue even during exacerbations of the disease.

External heat, whether originating in the weather or other forms of heat, is fatiguing to these patients; in some, to the point of complete exhaustion. This reaction is sufficiently common to be diagnostic. Thus the best time for exercise is in the cool of morning or of evening; hot tub baths should not precede exercise. It is of interest that ice baths in the summer, although they may temporarily increase spasticity, may, on the other hand, increase strength and endurance and, in some cases, increase tolerance to hot weather.

Corticospinal Dysfunction

Voluntary movement is an interaction between sensory and motor neurons and their internuncial connection interrelated at the spinal, supraspinal, and cortical levels. The lower levels control limited stereotyped reflexes. The supraspinal reflexes are more complex and more extensively represented with the cortical centers the most complex controlling larger segments of the body and integrating the sensory and motor function. The higher centers both increase and decrease the function of the lower centers (Fig. 17.2).

Damage to the central nervous system loses the control of the higher centers which permit the emergence of the uncontrolled or partially controlled middle or lower centers. The lower and middle patterns are always present and are *not* pathological; they merely become uncontrolled and thus have always been considered pathological.

Although many concepts of etiology, neuropathology and evaluation of therapeutic approaches have been applied to the adult "stroke" (cerebrovascular accident) or the neonatal central nervous impairment (cerebral palsy) similar aspects are related to multiple sclerosis. Similar techniques are thus applicable with certain basic differences.

The impairment of the central nervous system is spotty and not specifically localized in the central nervous system as they are in the

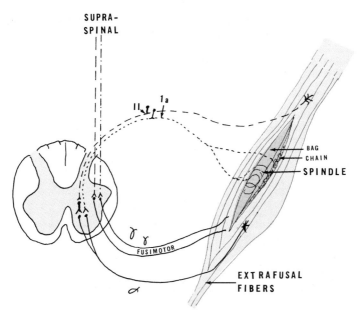

Fig. 17.2. Alpha-gamma ($\alpha\gamma$) linkage. The group II and Ia afferents are sensory from the nuclear bag and chain of the muscle spindle. They connect to the fusimotor nerves α to the extrafusal fibers to complete the cord level reflex arc. The supraspinal centers descend the cord to connect to the γ motor neurones to innervate the spindle.

stroke. The lesions are usually incomplete and often may be progressive and thus not consistent in their response to treatment. Numerous other systems of the supraspinal and cortical level may be simultaneously involved. Sensory loss is probably more extensively lost than in stroke. Extraneous factors such as metabolic or thermal influences modify the expected responses. Regardless, several neurophysiological principles apply to impairment of the pyramidal tracts.

Kabat (15) postulated that new pathways could be created through extrapyramidal pathways. Fay (16) claimed that the basic physiological reflexes that remained could be gradually controlled by the uninvolved higher centers. Bobath (17) felt that it is impossible to impose normal patterns upon abnormal ones and thus the abnormal patterns must be suppressed. She stressed that spontaneous recovery or the extent of recovery from therapy depended largely upon the degree of sensory involvement.

Birch (18) expressed the opinion that central nervous system damage is irrevocable and rehabilitation (of the hemiplegic) patient resides in training the utilization of residual motor abilities. In multiple sclerosis what is irreversible and what is reversible is not always immediately discernible.

Treatment of Multiple Sclerosis Impairment Based upon Neurophysiological Principles

Dependent upon the type of paresis present after the patient is evaluated the form of treatment can be considered. This may be divided into various stages.

1. Induction of voluntary motor activity.
2. Restoring or improving sensory feedback.
3. Inhibiting unwanted motor patterns.
4. Improving coordination.
5. Preventing or overcoming myostatic or articular constraints.

INDUCTION OF VOLUNTARY MOTOR ACTIVITY

In multiple sclerosis, paresis may exist very similar to the early flaccid stage of stroke in which the patient cannot initiate a voluntary movement. Spasticity of the antagonist may not be the principal disability at this stage. With no significant motor activity there can be no sensory feedback and no coordination.

To activate a nonresponsive muscle, various facilitation principles and

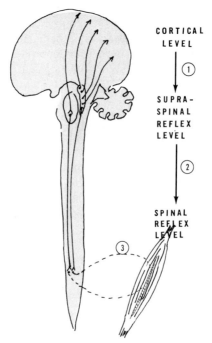

Fig. 17.3. Hierarchic organization (Jackson concept). The cortical level modifies all lower function. Contains the programmed organization of complex functions. The supraspinal reflexes facilitate or inhibit the spinal reflexes and maintain control for the cortical function. The spinal reflex is stereotyped and dependent in part on the gamma (γ) (spindle) system.

techniques may be utilized. These techniques are based upon neurophysiological concepts that are becoming increasingly clarified in the literature. Voluntary movement originally considered to be a function of alpha (α) motor control under direct control of the higher centers is no longer accepted (19). The accepted concept postulates motor function primarily a function of the gamma system via the spindle cell system. The gamma (γ) system maintains reflex motor tone and posture, but also initiates movement and facilitates coordination by adding sensation to the neuromuscular mechanism.

The proposal expounded by Hughling Jackson (20) of the central nervous system being organized in three motor levels is increasingly more accepted and implemented in therapeutic regimes. The Jackson concept "a hierarchy of centers according to the doctrine of evolution" formulates 1) lowest centers rigidly organized in stereotyped reflexes through limited pathways, 2) the middle center is more complex with greater representation that facilitate or inhibit the spinal reflex, and 3) the higher centers most complex where there occurs sensory motor integration that modify the lower centers (Fig. 17.3). In essence, motor action is produced by the higher centers modifying the lower centers in their reflex activities by enhancing (facilitating) or decreasing (inhibiting). The higher centers develop complex patterns.

Damage to the central nervous system impairs the control of the higher centers which allows emergence of reflex activities of the lower centers that are not under volitional control and not specific in their activities. These basic reflexes that have been considered *pathological* are not: they are physiological and only become pathologically significant when their higher center control is lost. This is the impairment in multiple sclerosis and the basis of exercises in its treatment.

The spinal reflexes form the basis of all motor function. At this level there is continuous sensorimotor interaction. The supraspinal level maintains the spinal reflex level in the controlled threshhold to permit the cortical levels to initiate coordinated movement.

Therapy must thus be concerned with modification of spinal reflex activity by influencing the facilitation or inhibition from the middle supraspinal level.

Activation of an unresponsive muscle may be by local excitation from electrical stimulation of the muscle or motor nerve when no significant voluntary control is evident.

Local facilitation using basic spinal reflexes may initiate movement. The most common of these reflexes is the stretch reflex by either manually stretching the muscle, tapping the tendon or local cutaneous stimulation over the muscle area such as brushing, stroking, ice. Any of these modalities may supply the necessary initiation of muscle contraction.

As some contraction eventually is elicited, movement can be hampered by the antagonistic spasm. Decreasing or eliminating antagonistic spasm may permit voluntary contraction of the agonist. As spasticity is not confined to any one muscle or muscle group, but rather to synergistic patterns, the entire pattern must be supressed. This can be accomplished by proper careful handling that does not initiate spastic antagonistic contraction. Application of ice to the antagonist may be effective. In severe cases selective denervation of spastic antagonist by phenol neurolysis may be needed (21).

Mass patterns or synergies can be employed to elicit the desired movement (22). Resisting any aspect of this reflex pattern may elicit excitation of the nonfunctioning muscle(s) in that pattern. This is the basis of proprioceptive facilitation. Resisting distal motions may initiate proximal movements. This is exmplified in utilizing of the tonic neck reflexes, the Marie Foix maneuver (23), or co-contraction of homologous muscles of the opposite extremity.

The position of the body as related to gravity influences the reaction of the extremities. This is allegedly due to labyrinthine reflexes. In the supine position the lower extremities have an increased extensor tone and the upper extremities an increased flexor tone. In the upright or sitting posture these reflexes are even more accentuated and may make it difficult to initiate upper extremity extension or lower extremity flexion.

In treatment of a patient this position must be altered to accomplish the desired result or desired patterns of movement.

As an example of the above, the "spastic" lower extremity is usually that of an extensor pattern with weakness of the flexor pattern. The erect stance enhances the lower extremity extensor tonus thus the patient is best exercised in the supine position or side lying. If the stronger flexor muscles are the hip flexors, these are manually resisted to have irradiation to the distal ankle dorsiflexors. Lesser resistance to the ankle flexors can thus reinforce this particular component of the flexor synergy. Simultaneously resisting the opposite normal extremity in flexion pattern will also reinforce the desired movement of the impaired ankle dorsiflexion.

RESTORING OR IMPROVING SENSORY FEEDBACK

Sensory feedback reinforces control and coordination (24, 25). Sensory awareness is relatively simple if proprioception is not impaired, but proprioception is frequently impaired or lost in multiple sclerosis. Visualization of the motion is a sensory feedback. Verbal reinforcement by the therapist's command or electromyographic (EMG) amplification is also auditory reinforcement.

INHIBITING UNWANTED MOTOR PATTERNS

Purposeless motions must be eliminated. In corticospinal tract involvement intense effort on the part of the patient may cause irradiation to other muscles in the similar pattern or in contralateral patterns. It is desirable to decrease the effort so that movement occurs mostly in the prime mover. Associated and unwanted movements can be manually suppressed by the therapist, but this is cumbersome and may reinforce abnormal patterns.

Bobath advocates the employment of "key points of control" to reduce spasticity. The therapist attempts to change part of the abnormal pattern of these which are usually proximal (neck, shoulders, and pelvis) in treating the distal motions as are distal "key points" (toes, ankles, and fingers) in reducing proximal spasticity.

Reduction of flexor spasticity in the trunk and arm is possible by utilizing neck extension and external rotation of the arm at the shoulder. Flexor spasticity can be further reduced by the therapist by extending the wrist and abducting the thumb. Extensor spasticity of the lower extremity can be reduced by initiating flexion of the big toe and ankle. While abnormal patterns are decreased with these techniques, normal activity is encouraged (26). The specific exercises and techniques are well illustrated in Bobath's text, *Adult Hemiplegia* (17).

IMPROVING COORDINATION

Coordination is considered to be programmed in the extrapyramidal tracts. Repetition of the specific movements reinforce and facilitate coordination while simultaneously inhibiting undesired motions. As certain pathways are enhanced, other unwanted patterns must be inhibited.

Coordination via the extrapyramidal tracts combine patterns that are smooth and require increasing less conscious monitoring.

Coordination requires continuation of voluntary activity with sensory feedback that is both conscious or subconscious and that is programmed in precise patterns. When resistance is applied, greater effort of the patient causes spread of activity to extraneous muscles both of the ipsilateral and contralateral side. By accurate and frequent repetition this spread to contiguous muscles is diminished and potentially abolished. Greater spread, greater strength and more complex activities gradually evolve (27).

Inactivity will rapidly cause a loss of coordination. This is true of normal individuals, but is even more true in patients with neurophysiological impairment. It is therefore desirable that treatment sessions be scheduled frequently on a daily basis and be continued for prolonged periods. In multiple sclerosis where fatigue and adverse reaction to temperature variations are prevalent, careful scheduling of exercise is necessary.

PREVENTING OR OVERCOMING MYOSTATIC OR ARTICULAR CONSTRAINTS

The restoration of neurophysiological patterns with volitional control is of limited value if the musculoskeletal system impairs function.

Joint contracture and myostatic contracture can restrict adequate joint range of motion. Balance and posture are impaired and the extremities limited.

Hip and knee flexion contracture occur early in neurologically impaired patients. Bed rest in flexed positions is largely responsible and even the extensor pattern of the corticospinal tract involvement does not prevent the contracture. In the reclining position the sensory stimulus of bed sheets, pillows, and handling initiates flexion patterns which can lead to contracture.

In the total extensor synergy of the lower extremity equinovarus deformity of the foot-ankle can occur which makes dorsiflexion during gait difficult even if the dorsiflexor muscles function in the gait pattern.

In the upper extremity internal rotation of the arm and elbow, and hand and wrist flexors as well as finger contractures may occur that will inhibit contrary movements.

Bracing, splinting, and positioning must be specifically utilized to prevent or decrease contracture. These are well documented in the literature. During the exercise regime all contractures may be minimized by insuring full range of motion of all involved muscle groups. Passive stretching must be done very gently to avoid stretch reactions which could initiate reflex synergies. Judicious use of phenol nerve blocks to the contracting muscles is of value, as is the use of ice during active exercise.

Cerebellar Dysfunction

Cerebellar dysfunction has been defined clinically as the presence of ataxia, dysmetria, intention tremor, dysdiadokinesis, and rebound phenomenon due to impairment of the cerebellum and its coordination with the remainder of the motor central nervous system. The mechanism of cerebellar dysfunction was attributed by Luciani (28) to weakness, hypotonia and incoordination. It is now mostly attributed to the weakness of hypotonia. Hughlings Jackson (29) wrote, "It will not suffice to speak of coordination as a separate faculty; coordination is the function of the whole and every part of the nervous system. . . . " Asynergia is due principally to asynchronous action of the fixation muscles and the prime movers; that is, loss of synergy between agonistic, antagonistic relaxation, synergistic and fixation muscles. Rebound phenomenon is due to deficient reciprocal inhibition which leaves residual tonus in the antagonists that govern the action of the agonists. Efficient proprioceptive pathways must obviously be impaired, for, as Sherrington taught, "The cerebellum is the head ganglion of the proprioceptive system. . . . "

In the management of cerebellar dysfunction, these clinical factors must be considered. Weakness of muscle implies weakness of innervation, and, consequently, resistance exercises utilizing pattern movements will tend to enforce prime movers. Resistance to antagonistic pattern groups applies here.

The cerebellum acts as a *comparator,* i.e., compares the sensory input of actual limb position and movement to the *intended* position and movement. Upon minute detection of deviation, correction is made via the cerebellar pyramidal system or to the cortex via the thalamic nucleus ventralis lateralis (VL).

Thalamotomy performed in alleviating tremor has been based on the assumption that the VL *generates* tremor. Tremor probably occurs because the sensory input from the periphery is defective and thus impairs the computer-like correction of the cerebellar pathways.

Improvement in ataxia could therefore explain the rationale of an exercise regime. By stabilizing supporting or restricting movement of all the body parts unrelated can permit attention on the prime mover(s). Sensory information can be enhanced by performing before a mirror for visual feedback and exercises can be performed by placing a weight upon the extremity. A wristlet or anklet with a weight of 1–3 lb secured by velcro permits proprioceptive feedback. Strengthening of fixation muscle groups may be effected by the technique of rhythmic stabilization (30). Resistance is applied to muscles in a rhythmic alternating manner, rendering a joint rigid as the muscles contract isometrically. Alternating isometric contraction of agonists and antagonists which prevents movement of the joint and the rapidity of alternation and the amount of resistance are dependent on the ease of reciprocation and the strength of contraction possible in the individual patient. This technique is time consuming, requires exceptional skill of the therapist and, unfortunately, in many cases fails to adequately improve the patient; but the technique has offered confirmation regarding the mechanism of cerebellar dysfunction.

The use of Frenkel exercises has a time-honored past in the treatment of ataxia. His exercises were devised principally for locomotor ataxis in which ataxis is due to loss of proprioception. They are useful in cerebellar ataxia (31). Frenkel exercises are begun from one of four positions: lying, sitting, standing or walking. Concentration of attention on each movement is mandatory. Each movement is done slowly and with repetition. The exercises are as follows:

1. Lying position: Flexion and extension of each leg at the knee and hip joints. Abduction and adduction with the knee bent; later, abduction and adduction with the knee extended.
2. Flexion and extension of one knee at a time with the heel raised from the bed.
3. Knee flexed and heel placed upon some definite part of the other leg; for example, on the patella, the middle of the leg, ankle and toes. These exercises may be given by changing the heel from one position to another or else by calling for extension between different placings (really the neurological heel-to-knee test).
4. Knee flexed, heel placed on knee of other leg, heel to flexed leg gliding down the tibia to the ankle joint and back to knee.
5. Flexion and extension of both legs, together with knees and ankles held close together.
6. Flexion of one leg during extension of the other (reciprocal movement).

7. Flexion or extension of one leg during adduction and abduction of the other. When the performance of these exercises becomes easy, the patient should repeat them with the eyes closed.

8. From the sitting position the patient tries to place his foot definitely in the hand of the operator while the operator constantly changes the position of the hand. Exercises may be given by means of special apparatus, consisting of a board with holes in which to place the heels and a bar which may be placed across the bottom of the bed at different heights and varying distances. The patient is encouraged to place his heels in the holes. The position of the board is changed after each attempt.

9. The patient maintains the fundamental sitting position for a few minutes at a time.

10. Raising each knee alternately and placing the foot firmly on the ground upon a traced footprint.

11. The patient is taught to rise from a chair and sit again with knees held together.

12. Foot placings forward and backward on a straight line. These exercises should be followed by walking maneuvers; e.g., walking along a zigzag strip following markings.

13. Walking between two parallel lines.[1]

14. Walking, placing each foot on tracing on floor which should be marked in fairly close adduction position, straight line walking (not toe out).

The physiological basis for these exercises is the attempt to regain coordination by utilization of other senses (for example, visual in locomotor ataxia and proprioceptive-visual in cerebellar dysfunction), by voluntary relearning of functions lost by repetition of neurological deficiencies and by retraining of functional patterns. Gravity adds some resistance but not enough to permit full strength and endurance development. Thus, it is desirable to employ proprioceptive facilitation pathways and to avoid substitution patterns (32). These exercises are physiologically sound in so far as they utilize total patterns, utilize righting reflexes, employ stabilization mechanisms while stressing prime movements and, in the later exercises, stress daily functional activities. Only in the more recent verification of the advantages of resistive techniques do the original Frenkel exercises become inadequate. Their chief value resides in their usefulness when loss of proprioception (impairment of muscle joint and tendon sense) needs to be compensated by visual sensation.

Summary

Total care in multiple sclerosis lacks any specific form of treatment which can prevent exacerbation, hasten remissions or insure completeness

---

[1] *Editorial note.* Many patients are anxious to stand, even if standing can be accomplished only with assistance. If the upper extremities are strong enough to handle canes and crutches, balancing and gait training exercises may be started between parallel or walking bars. Braces may be required to control equinus position resulting from gastrocnemius spasticity. In the ataxic patient weighted crutches are often helpful as are sometimes weighted shoes. Crutches may be weighted by wrapping lead foil around the lower end or, in the case of the hollow upright, by filling with shot.

of remission. Exercise remains foremost in making the patient more comfortable, self-sufficient and economically more independent. Exercise aims at regaining function where neurological deficit results in permanent residual disability and at preventing further disuse loss where the neurological deficit is considered partially or wholly remissive. Thus, the exercises reviewed are aimed at the neurological defect, in this disease a demyelinization of central nervous system pathways. Any nervous tract or combination of pathways may be involved; these are most often the pyramidal and, next most common, the cerebellar. Since disease progress has a good statistical possibility of becoming stationary and mortality figures favor longevity, much of the disability follows from disuse and secondary factors. Thus, treatment must employ every aid toward more functional recovery. The exercise based on neurophysiology offers an important approach to the treatment of this neurologic defect.

REFERENCES

1. LICHSTENSTEIN, B. W. *A Textbook of Neuropathology*. Philadelphia, 1949.
2. NAMEROW, N. S. The Pathophysiology of Multiple Sclerosis. In *Multiple Sclerosis: Immunology, Virology and Ultrastructure,* pp. 143–181, edited by F. Wolfgram et al. Academic Press, New York, 1972.
3. SCHAUF, C. L., AND DAVIS, F. A. Impulse conduction in multiple sclerosis: a theoretical basis for modification by temperature and pharmacological agents. *J. Neurol. Neurosurg. Psychiatry, 37:* 152–161, 1974.
4. BECKER, F. W., MICHAEL, J. A., AND DAVIS, F. A. Acute effects of oral phosphate on visual function in multiple sclerosis. *Neurology, 24:* 601-7, 1974.
5. GRINKER, R. R. *Neurology*. Springfield, 1943.
6. WILSON, S. A. K. *Neurology*. Baltimore, 1941.
7. SCHUMACHER, G. A. Treatment of multiple sclerosis. *J.A.M.A., 143:* 1241–50, 1950.
8. GORDON, E. E., AND CARLSON, K. E. Changing attitude toward multiple sclerosis. *J.A.M.A., 147:* 720–723, 1951.
9. MacLEAN, A. R., AND BERKSON, J. Mortality and disability in multiple sclerosis. *J.A.M.A., 146:* 1367–1369, 1951.
10. ALLISON, R. S. Survival in disseminated sclerosis; a clinical study of a series of cases first seen 20 years ago. *Brain, 73:* 103–120, 1950.
11. MUELLER, R. Course and prognosis of disseminated sclerosis in relation to age of onset. *Arch. Neurol. Psychiatry, 66:* 561–570, 1951.
12. THYGESEN, P. Prognosis in initial stage of disseminated primary demyelinating disease of central nervous system. *Arch. Neurol. Psychiatry., 61:* 339–351, 1949.
13. KURTZE, J. F. Course of exacerbations of multiple sclerosis in hospitalized patients. *Arch. Neurol. Psychiatry, 76:* 175–184, 1956.
14. KURTZE, J. F. A new scale for evaluating disability in multiple sclerosis. *Neurology, 5:* 580–583, 1955.
15. KABAT, H. Studies of neuromuscular dysfunction. XI. New principles of neuromuscular re-education. *Permanente Found. Med. Bull., 5:* 3, 1947.
16. FAY, T. Basic considerations regarding neuromuscular and reflex therapy. *Spastics Q., 3:* 1, 1954.
17. BOBATH, B. *Adult Hemiplegia: Evaluation and Treatment*. William Heinemann Medical Books, London, 1972.
18. BIRCH, H. G., PROCTOR, F., BORTNER, M., AND LOWENTHAL, M. Perception in hemiplegia; I. Judgment of vertical and horizontal by hemiplegic patients. *Arch. Phys. Med., 41:* 19–27, 1960.

19. WALSHE, F. M. R. On the role of the pyramida system in willed movements. *Brain, 70:* 329, 1947.

20. JACKSON, J. H. Croonian lectures on the evolution and dissolution of the nervous system. *Lancet, 1:* 555, 1884.

21. LANDAU, W. M., WEAVER, R. A., AND HORNBEIN, T. F. Fusimotor nerve function in man. *Arch. Neurol., 3:* 32–45, 1960.

22. KNOTT, M., AND VOSS, D. E. *Proprioceptive Neuromuscular Facilitation: Patterns and Techniques.* New York, 1956.

23. MARIE, P., AND FOIX, C. Les reflexes d'automatisme dits de defense. *Rev. Neurol., 28:* 225, 1915.

24. LOOFBOURROW, G. N., AND GELLHORN, E. Proprioceptive modification of reflex patterns. *J. Neurophysiol., 12:* 435–446, 1949.

25. GELLHORN, E. Proprioception and the motor cortex. *Brain, 72:* 35–62, 1949.

26. BRUNNSTROM, S. *Movement Therapy in Hemiplegia. A Neurophysiological Approach.* New York, 1970.

27. KOTTKE, F. J. Neurophysiologic Therapy for Stroke. In *Stroke and Its Rehabilitation* Ch. 11, edited by S. Licht. Elizabeth Licht Publisher, New Haven, 1975.

28. LUCIANI, L. *Human Physiology.* London, 1915.

29. JACKSON, J. H. *Collected Writings.* London, 1932.

30. KABAT, H. Studies on neuromuscular dysfunction. XIII. Rhythmic stabilization; a new and more effective technique for treatment of paralysis through a cerebellar mechanism. *Permanente Foundation Med. Bull., 8:* 1, 1950.

31. FRENKEL, H. S. in *Physical Therapeutic Technique,* edited by F. B. Granger. Philadelphia, 1929.

32. HELLEBRANDT, F. A., AND HOUTZ, S. J. Mechanisms of muscle training in man. *Phys. Ther. Rev., 36:* 118, 1956.

18

Exercises for Amputees

_____ ALLEN S. RUSSEK

"The literature woven around the subject of amputation is indeed voluminous: the story of surgical dismemberment goes back to the days of Hippocrates and Celsus and even beyond. John Woodall . . . said that 'It is no small presumption to dismember the image of God.'" So said Sir Gordon Gordon-Taylor in his Presidential Address to the Medical Society of London in 1942 (1).

A major amputation is defined as an amputation in the lower extremity through or proximal to the tarsometarsal joints or in the upper extremity, through or proximal to the carpometacarpal joints. It is estimated that 1 of each 250 persons in the United States has had a major amputation and that of these about 700,000 are in the lower extremities. Additional amputations are being performed at the rate of 35–40 thousand annually. These occur at a ratio of 5 in the upper extremities for each 20 in the lower extremities. The continuing supervision of these new and old amputees constitutes an appreciable medical responsibility in which the medical profession as a whole has only recently developed a special interest.

Causes and Indications for Amputation

A variety of clinical pathologic states terminate in amputation with its characteristic disability. This disability is rather a clinical paradox since it is the end result of the treatment, the pathology having been removed; in most other disabilities the pathology or its residuals persist. The amputee may be an otherwise healthy individual (particularly the traumatic amputee) with an isolated physical defect.

The indications for amputation fall into several groups (2):

Peripheral Vascular Insufficiency. In peace time, this is the largest group and accounts for about 80% of all amputations in adults in the

389

lower extremities. A variety of causes for circulatory failure lead to amputation. The most common are related to diabetes, Buerger's disease, arteriosclerosis, emboli, massive arterial thrombosis, arteriovenous aneurysm and others, all of which have failed to respond to medical or lesser surgical procedures. Improved vascular surgery is progressively reducing this number.

Trauma. Severe injuries with massive loss of tissue and destruction of blood supply may require immediate amputation. Most surgeons debride such wounds and wait until specific indications present themselves to the point where surgical or orthopedic reconstruction can no longer offer hope for viability or function.

Malignant Tumors. Benign tumors may occassionally require amputation if removal of the tumor is not possible without serious impairment of blood and nerve supply. When malignancy has been positively diagnosed, amputation should be accomplished high enough to prevent recurrence whether metastasis is present or not. Most of the high proximal amputations such as hip disarticulation, hemipelvectomy, shoulder disarticulation and interscapulothoracic are performed for malignant tumors.

Nerve Injuries. An anesthetic limb, over which a patient has little or no control, frequently develops pressure or friction phenomena of which he is not aware for some time. Amputation of such limbs is indicated when repeated ulceration and infection have developed beyond medical control and constitute a threat to the patient's health and function.

Infections. Amputation and a well fitted prosthesis are superior functionally, cosmetically, and physiologically to a painful, functionless member.

Thermal Damage. Amputations for burns may be performed early or late depending upon the extent of initial destruction or subsequent deformities and loss of function. Cold injuries are insidious in nature and usually require amputation for interference with blood supply.

Congenital Malformations. Congenital malformations are not uncommon, such as absence of the femur or tibia or a rudimentary limb at the end of which there is an apparently normal foot. Unfortunately even after successful, repeated surgery in childhood the growth discrepancy in time between the two lower extremities may be considerable. The reconstructed, deformed limb may be 8–30 cm shorter than the other side, necessitating the use of a cumbersome brace and foot extension or a prosthesis. In most instances the knee levels do not correspond and the device carries a locked knee for walking. The principle of prophylactic amputation in infancy, depending on the nature and extent of the deformity, should be considered in many cases.

Congenital Absence of Limbs. Some persons are destined to be amputees throughout their lifetime. Many congenital amputees have rudimentary structures at the terminal portions of their stumps. If these serve no useful purpose, or interfere with the fitting of a prosthesis, they should be removed and the stump reshaped.

Cosmetic Amputation. Many children grow into adult life with damaged or deformed limbs which have been sufficiently functional during childhood and adolescence. When they face the realities of life and become aware of their variations from the normal, they often seek amputation. The remarkable cosmetic, aesthetic, social, vocational, emotional, and personality improvement after amputation and prosthetic restoration in many cases justifies cosmetic amputation.

Levels of Amputation

The classical "sites of election" are only guide lines to indicate an "ideal" site in the segment of an extremity which satisfies the functional requirement and physical characteristics best adapted to the simplest available conventional prosthesis. Modern prosthetic techniques can fit any amputation at any level. There are some specific levels where surgical judgment may choose to sacrifice tissue and length for increased function:

1. *Partial foot amputations other than transmetatarsal*—these have outlived their usefulness. The results are not efficient weight-bearing members and require a bulky, cosmetically poor prosthesis with which the ultimate function is not as good as it is with a more proximal amputation.

2. *The lower third of the leg*—the long lever contributes nothing to stability, inteferes with standard methods of fitting, and the circulation in this area, already depressed, may be further impaired in a prosthesis. The formation of a shapely ankle is not possible with a very long, below-the-knee stump.

3. *The proximal 5 cm of the tibia*—this results in a short, broad, squared-off stump which cannot be adequately fitted. The lever is too short to preserve the knee functions and it is difficult to keep the stump from coming out of the socket.

4. *The distal 10 cm of the femur unless an end-weight-bearing stump is desired.* End-weight-bearing is a great advantage and should be accomplished whenever possible and feasible. Those long stumps in the supracondylar area, which have exposed the medullary cavity of the bone and cannot be used for end-weight-bearing are a source of difficulty. They are hard to fit, require outside knee joints which cannot be adjusted for friction, disturb the symmetry of the levels of knee motion, and interfere with gait.

In summary the most acceptable and convenient levels for best function in the lower extremity are (Fig. 18.1):

1. *Partial foot* (transmetatarsal only)—if it becomes infected, it is not worth trying to salvage.

2. *Symes*—this is the best below-knee level if it is done properly. It is not advisable in women or diabetics.

3. *Below-the-knee*—the ideal level is in the middle third of the leg.

4. *End-weight-bearing*—above the knee, including disarticulation, when specifically indicated.

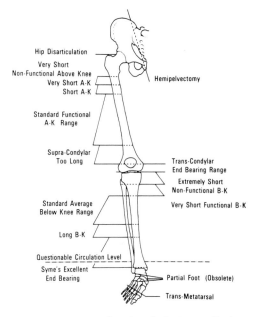

Hip Disarticulation

Very Short

Non-Functional Above Knee

Very Short A-K

Short A-K

Hemipelvectomy

Standard Functional
A-K Range

Supra-Condylar
Too Long

Trans-Condylar
End Bearing Range

Extremely Short
Non-Functional B-K

Standard Average
Below Knee Range

Very Short Functional B-K

Long B-K

Questionable Circulation Level

Syme's Excellent
End Bearing

Partial Foot (Obsolete)

Trans-Metatarsal

Fig. 18.1 Amputation levels in lower limb.

5. *Above-the-knee*—from 4 inches above at any level, preferably mid-thigh.

Similar surgical judgmental choices exist inthe upper extremity (Fig. 18.2). Most experienced surgeons will avoid:

1. *Partial hand amputations in which there is no possibility of function.* When in doubt, everything viable is saved, with the understanding that later revision may be necessary. Any active pinching or prehension with sensation is better than any prosthesis. Even an amputation through the carpometacarpal joints, with good wrist function, can result in acceptable function against an opposition post or plate and can be alternately used with a prosthetic hand.

2. *The proximal 5 cm of the forearm*—the extremely short below elbow stump, if it functions at all, does so at a very low level even with the specially modified prosthesis necessary.

3. *The elbow disarticulation and the distal 8 cm of the humerus.* These require outside elbow joints and disturb the symmetry of elbow centers.

The Role of the Physiatrist in Amputee Management

The physiatrist plays a major role in prescribing for and directing the performance of those activities, before and after amputation surgery, which contributes to restoration of maximal function. It is therefore essential that the physiatrist have insight into the background and techniques of modern amputation surgery and the physiological alterations associated with it. This permits participation in preoperative confer-

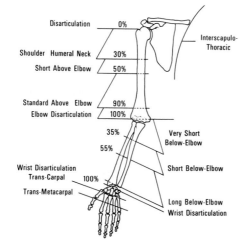

Fig. 18.2 Amputation levels in upper limb.

ences and discussions as well as in the postoperative management and the rehabilitation process. The responsibilities of the rehabilitation team have changed since the advent of immediate postsurgical fitting and training and the practice of early ambulation. Whereas previous concentration was on preprosthetic activities, stump shrinking, crutch ambulation, and gait training, it is now primarily judgmental in an integrated and continuous program with the surgeon, prosthetist, physiatrist, therapist, and patient, before and after the amputation.

Postoperatively, whether or not the patient ambulates as soon as possible, starting even on the first postoperative day he should be instructed and supervised in an exercise program. This starts in bed for body alignment, posture, preservation of muscle power and range of motion. Special attention is given to the upper trunk, shoulder depressors and elbow extensors in anticipation of using crutches. Evaluation of the capability of the remaining lower extremity must be made and an appropriate program set up to keep it functional. These exercises and others play a major part of the management of the patient who goes through months of waiting for a prosthesis. Fortunately, present-day management leaves little time for the new amputee to deteriorate. Every uncomplicated lower extremity amputee can be made ambulatory with some type of temporary prosthesis within a month of surgery.

Immediate Post Surgical Prosthetic Fitting and Early Ambulation

GENERAL CONSIDERATIONS

From World War II until the mid-1960s, great progress and improvements had been made in the design, quality, and function of artificial limbs. But progress in amputation surgery was needed to make it possible for amputees to get the most out of these new designs and devices. The relatively modern practice of early mobilization, as applied to the management of many other surgical conditions, did not filter down to amputees. As a group, lower extremity amputees benefited from this principle only to the extent of achieving earlier use of the remaining leg (3). There still remained a long pre-prosthetic program of exercises, wrapping the amputation stump for shrinkage, shaping, and conditioning, all of which took a great deal of time even with good management. The postamputation period resulted in excessive loss of time and productivity and the deteriorating emotional and physical effects of inactivity and disuse.

Although it had long been known that the amputee could be made ambulatory in a much shorter time than was customary, the implementation of this knowledge was very limited. Isolated efforts on the part of individual doctors to eliminate wasted time were made in military hospitals, and with some success. These included the use of plaster of Paris sockets, pylons, temporary prostheses, and other improvisations with which the amputee could function until he was ready to be fitted with a permanent prosthesis.

In principle, these devices were based upon protecting the amputation stump by concentrating weight on proximal parts. The stump itself was a passive member and often, when not sufficiently protected, showed signs of stress from early use. These devices served a useful purpose by demonstrating that amputees could become ambulatory shortly after surgery, but were restricted to military hospitals and other institutions where a resident prosthetist was available. There was no carry-over to civilian amputees, since civilian hospitals were not equipped with specialized facilities or personnel who had sufficient interest to conduct those early efforts at reducing disability time. Moreover, it was customary for commercial prosthetists to take 6–8 weeks to deliver a prosthesis. The idea of getting amputees up and walking with double support in a short time remained a challenging dilemma for those interested in the rehabilitation of the amputee.

SPECIAL CONSIDERATIONS

Every major amputation in the lower extremity involves loss of the foot. Not much attention has been paid to the foot as a functioning organ, and its loss has not until recently been considered a major problem since it can be replaced by an artificial foot (4). The reality of this situation, however, is not that simple. The foot is a highly compound and complex organ which is controlled by an elaborate signaling system from the surface, the muscles, and the tendons. The efficiency of the foot is dependent upon the sum of its afferent sensations and stimuli in relation to its weight-bearing factors and its contact with the ground. It is intimately bound up in proprioception of the entire extremity and coordination of the proximal joints and muscles through its connection with the central nervous system and the spinal cord reflexes.

The proprioceptive functions of the foot are derived from integrated sensations and impulses conveyed proximally to provide information as to the immediate conditions at the ground. It conveys information whether it is hard or soft, level or slanted, rough or smooth. It also evokes an immediate spinal cord reflex reaction to any displacement of the center of gravity upon loss of equilibrium or upon encountering an unexpected depression or obstacle in the process of walking. It not only conveys this information to the same side but it also alerts the opposite side to take over in the event that an immediate correction is not possible on the affected side. This defensive system of communication originates in the central nervous system organs in the skin, in the muscles, and in the tendons. It therefore also communicates information proximally with regard to the tension of muscles and the amount of weight on the limb and alerts antagonistic muscles to create a system of balance in relation to the positive efforts which are made. It is a highly defensive and compensating system of protection and coordination.

Amputation seriously disturbs this chain of events from the level of the sectioned muscles to the neurologic silence below it. Electromyographic studies have indicated that shortly after amputation even sectioned muscles contract in the phase of gait in which they normally participated before the amputation (5). When these muscles are not reattached to bone they eventually atrophy and become fibrotic, losing all of the proprioceptive functions and afferent signaling. It is also interesting to note that pairs of muscles, agonists and antagonists, which have been coordinated prior to amputation may accidentally work together; but most often after amputation both muscles either may be simultaneously stimulated and contract together, (throwing off the coordination) or else neither will be stimulated at all. As a consequence, after a below-knee amputation the knee-stabilizing muscles that prevent the knee from buckling do not get the information they need; thus, after above-knee amputations the hip and lower back do not receive the necessary information for their participation in the kinetic chain for balance and coordination. This is the reason many amputees never lose their sense of insecurity and instability when using a prosthesis.

It has also been demonstrated electromyographically that if muscles are sutured to bone to create a new insertion under slight tension they will continue to contract in the phase of gait in which they normally participated and will not atrophy or lose this function by disuse and fibrosis. This isometric contraction is capable of generating the signaling necessary for the proximal muscles to take over their responsibility for both stabilization of the proximal joints and for appreciation of the tension of the muscles below in relationship to the degree of weight borne and of the support line (relative to the position of the center of gravity of the superincumbent body mass). Moreover, retracted muscles which have lost their capability of contracting have also lost the venous pump factor which contributes to healing of the severed tissues. It has also been determined that time is an important factor; the longer the individual is separated from a weight-bearing situation on the amputated side, the less liklihood there is for his developing an adequate signaling system for sufficient coordination to feel secure in placing weight on that limb with a prosthesis.

The two-joint muscles are most efficient in providing a new system of communication and balance with antagonistic muscles after amputation. These are the rectus femoris and the hamstrings in the above-knee amputation and the gastrocnemius in the below-knee amputation. The first is to reestablish physiologic and neuromuscular conditions as close to the pre-amputation state as possible by reattaching the key muscles to the bone in order to make it possible for them to contract in the normal phase of gait in which they participate. The second factor is to reduce the time during which there is a disturbance in weight bearing and in interpretation of signals from the ground in the weight-bearing position.

BACKGROUND AND PROCEDURES

In 1963, Dr. Marion A. Weiss (6), Director of the Rehabilitation Institute of Konstancin, Poland, reported on his procedure of immediate postsurgical fitting and ambulation. On the basis of his convincing evidence, which became well known after he had visited the United States and lectured at numerous medical centers, activity in this procedure spread like brush fire in many countries. Within a year, numerous grants, primarily federal, were made to support serious investigation of this procedure. The Veterans Administration contracted to conduct a full-time research effort at the University of Washington in Seattle, directed by Dr. Ernest M. Burgess (7) and major research programs were organized at New York University, the University of California, Northwestern University, Duke University, and the United States Naval Hospital at Oakland, California. All of these research projects were closely monitored by the National Research Council and numerous meetings were held with the project directors, who exchanged information on their procedures. Commercial devices became available to meet the need and commercial prosthetists were brought into the program to provide services in the operating room and to deliver prostheses rapidly. From this extensive research, there has emerged a body of knowledge which was sound, practical, and teachable, to the extent that it could be carried out in any well equipped hospital.

SURGICAL ADAPTATIONS FOR IMMEDIATE POSTSURGICAL FITTING

Above-knee and below-knee amputations are performed with modification of standard technique to form and shape the stump as a plastic or reconstruction procedure with tension myoplasty. This is the best amputation technique at present whether or not a rigid dressing is applied.

The essential feature of myoplasty in constructing a functional amputation stump is anchoring the muscles that cross two joints. They are used to shape the stump and preserve a significant part of the feed-in mechanism for communication to proximal parts. Above the knee they are the rectus femoris and hamstrings. Below the knee the gastrocnemius is the major muscle. Stabilization and shaping of the stump, by trimming and suturing down other muscles as well, establish a new proprioceptive system of integrated impulses which the nervous system can understand by training and reassociation. This has been demonstrated by electromyographic studies.

The specific procedure above the knee is to suture the rectus femoris and hamstrings to the periosteum and to each other in balance, avoiding a pulley action over the end of the bone. In addition, depending upon the length of the stump, the adductor magnus medially and fascia lata laterally are anchored. This is done with the amputation stump in the neutral extended position, rather than in an acutely flexed position, to avoid flexion or adduction contracture at the hip.

Below the knee the tendon of the gastrocnemius-soleus is trimmed and tapered to fit and match the blended thin anterior fascia and periosteum of the tibia and fibula. Devitalized muscle, particularly in the soleus, and excessive muscle bulk should be removed to avoid necrosis and for proper shaping of the stump. With the muscles under slight tension in myoplasty the bone is stable and does not move within the muscles.

In immediate postsurgical fitting, it is deliberately intended to perform a tension myoplasty amputation and cover this with a contoured surgical dressing, over which a sterile stump sock is applied. On the stump sock, shaped and skived felt pads are glued to protect the patella, the medial flare of the tibia, and the anterior tibial crest in below-knee cases. Thereafter, a plaster cast is applied with the knee in 10° of flexion. The cast extends halfway up the thigh. It is applied at first with the use of elastic plaster of Paris. When this has set, it is reinforced with regular plaster of Paris bandages. The elastic plaster of Paris is so applied that there is proximal pressure (from below upward) at the end of the amputation stump and the method of applying it is such that there is no circular compression of the stump or the thigh. This is extremely important, since it simulates the position of the amputation stump in a total contract prosthetic socket. This is known as the rigid dressing, which is applied whether it is intended to have the patient walk in this socket or not. The rigid dressing is compressive while the plaster is wet, but when it sets, it is no longer compressive but is simply firm, and the circulation is not embarrassed by a properly applied rigid dressing.

When it is intended for the patient to walk in this socket, a coupling device with steel straps is placed over this cast and with further plaster of Paris bandages is incorporated in the cast. Because the patient has been previously measured for length and alignment, a pylon device can be attached to the coupler. This pylon device terminates in a foot and can be removed for sleeping. If all goes well, it is possible to stand the patient the next day and in the ensuing period, progressively have him shift weight onto this amputated side and gradually ambulate with partial weight-bearing until he develops stability and confidence. The temporary prosthesis is adjustable for rotation, mediolateral angulation, and length, so that a satisfactory weight-bearing line can be achieved without placing undue stress on the tissues and having the patient distribute weight through every surface of the amputation stump and onto the thigh as well.

Early ambulation is basically the same procedure, with the application of the rigid dressing but without applying the walking device. This does not interfere with the usual procedure of getting the patient up on his unamputated leg, bearing weight and walking between parallel bars or using crutches, in order to preserve and maintain function in that extremity. In 10–20 days, the cast and sutures are removed and a temporary prosthesis is applied for ambulation.

In amputations above the knee, several methods of performing the tension myoplasty are available. In mid-thigh amputations, the method used at the New York University Medical Center has been to preserve a long tongue of the adductor magnus medially, bringing this over the cut end of the femur and suturing it to the bone. The anterior compartment, consisting of the severed quadriceps muscles, is sutured to the front portion of the adductor magnus and the hamstrings posteriorly. This is all covered by a flap of fascia lata from the lateral side, making a closed envelope for the stump, all being under slight tension and stabilizing the bone in the center of the amputation stump so that it does not move from side to side within the soft tissues. In above-knee amputations nearer to the knee, particularly in the supracondylar region, the long flap is made from the quadriceps group and sutured posteriorly over the entire stump after anchoring the other muscles to the bone.

A rigid dressing is then applied as after below-knee amputation. If immediate ambulation is planned, an extension wood block is used to equalize the knee centers and an ambulating device with adjustable knee and alignment controls is added. This pylon terminates in a SACH foot.

Some prosthetists prefer to apply the above-knee rigid dressing in a manner similar to the formation of a quadrilateral, ischialgluteal weight-bearing socket. This can be done with casting devices in the operating room, but an experienced prosthetist can also do it by hand. Suspension of this socket to prevent it from coming off when the patient sits up is still a problem not yet solved. Many methods have been employed, and all have resulted in both successes and failures. This is an individual problem resting with the prosthetist who assists the surgeon in the operating room. If the cast becomes loose and begins to slide, it must be removed and another cast applied. This is sometimes carried out 3–4 times before a removable prosthesis is used.

POSTOPERATIVE MANAGEMENT AND TRAINING

Training procedures are somewhat different from what they would be for a patient who has waited out his period of conditioning and shrinking.

It was common to have amputees use elastic bandages for shaping and conditioning the amputation stump and, at the same time, do various exercises to preserve the range of motion, to prevent contractures, and also to relieve pain, which sometimes has been severe in the early postoperative period. This preprosthetic activity has been entirely by-passed with the use of the rigid dressing, whether or not early ambulation is instituted. There is much less postoperative edema to overcome with the use of the rigid dressing and pain has not been a prominent factor.

The use of a prosthesis alleviates excessive stresses on the remaining leg, if the patient has the capability of walking. Walking is far better than abstract exercise, since there is no exercise that the patient can do lying in bed which is comparable to what happens when the patient stands on the leg, even if he does not walk on it. The kind of shoes the patient wears is extremely important, because the shoes as well as the walking and other therapy must not be traumatic to the remaining leg. Even if the patient is not able to wear a shoe, a large foam rubber boot can be used to allow the patient to put weight on the limb. The purpose of doing this is not so much to affect walking, but to preserve the remaining limb. The ground reaction and proprioception of weight-bearing has a satisfactory effect on circulation. The metabolic demand is not tremendously increased by weight-bearing alone, and partial weight-bearing in parallel bars or with the use of crutches appears to provide the greatest amount of circulation which the patient can derive from his vascular tree.

The postoperative course and training constitute an integrated continuous team effort. It varies with individual patients but in general with the rigid dressing there is less pain and fewer complaints of phantom discomfort. Some patients have no pain at all but most patients complain of pain of varying intensity for 3 or 4 days. The pain is usually accompanied by a feeling of general constriction of the amputation stump. This is no indication to do anything about the cast. If the patient complains about focal pain over a subcutaneous bony area, it should be relieved if its persists. Relief is usually created by splitting the cast and taping it together wherever it separates. Persistent local pain over a bony point may require complete removal of the cast socket and reapplication with protection of the bony points. The reapplication must be done immediately since the stump will swell rapidly if the cast is removed within the first 2 weeks.

On the first postoperative day the surgeon meets with the patient, the physiatrist, the prothestist, and the physical therapist for aligning the prosthesis properly and working out a schedule of training. A walker is placed in the patient's room so that he may stand beside the bed. The pylon is attached to the rigid dressing in bed and the patient is helped to sit up. If there are no orthostatic problems he is allowed to stand with the support of the walker and to touch down with the prosthesis so that it can be adjusted. Five minutes of standing with contact of the prosthetic foot against the floor is all that is necessary. There is no advantage in placing any considerable weight into the prosthesis at that time. If the patient is not medically well or has a great deal of pain, it is advisable to postpone the initial standing for a few days.

Training with this type of postoperative prosthesis is not designed to achieve any great gait characteristics. The real objective is to reestablish proprioception and feedback by contact with the floor, which alerts the muscles and reestablishes the signaling system. Pain is also relieved by distal pressure on the stump by contact with the floor.

It is inadvisable at this early stage to attempt to train the patient with a three-point gait either between parallel bars or with crutches and the unamputated leg because the prosthesis has a tendency to fall off and will lose its compressive value. The patient is encouraged to place more weight on the prosthesis progressively but never more than 15–20 lb (or about 8–9 kg). This can be judged by having the patient stand on two scales each time he gets up to get the feeling of which 15 lb (about 6 kg) of weight on the prosthesis is like. Walking in the prosthesis is achieved progressively between parallel bars in the physical therapy department twice daily so that the patient does not have any long sessions of walking. It is never necessary for the patient to have his full weight on the prosthesis. This has been done by many patients without damage but there is no real purpose in doing so until the definitive prosthesis is obtained.

Concomitant with the standing, balance, and limited ambulation the patient continues his exercises for the turnk and upper extremities to maintain a satisfactory degree of muscle power in the upper extremities and to ensure that he can sustain proper postural attitudes while standing and walking.

Daily supervised exercises and training are carried out in the below-knee cases for 14 days. If all goes well and there are no complications, the initial cast socket may be left on for 21 days. When it is removed in 14 days, it may be possible to take out all of the sutures, or at least those from healed areas in the scar. At that time another cast or cast socket and pylon are applied as soon as possible. If healing is delayed or prolonged, it is still possible to keep the patient ambulatory with the cast socket and pylon if there is no infection. The vertical position is one of the most effective means of improving the healing qualities of an amputation wound, particularly in the case of vascular impairment since the isometric contraction of the muscles creates the so called "venous pump" which becomes much more efficient in the verticle than in the horizontal position.

In above-knee cases it may be necessary to remove the cast socket in 1 week and reapply another because of displacement of the amputation stump within the socket. It is difficult to maintain an undisturbed relationship between the stump and a cast socket in the above-knee case since the socket may fall off and usually is loose within a week.

A new cast is then applied just as it was in the operating room but it is somewhat easier with the patient awake. This is left on for 1 to 2 additional weeks while the patient is given balancing and ambulation training. After 2 or 3 more weeks of comfortable use of the second cast the prosthetist is asked to split the cast and apply and remove another cast for the purpose of making the socket of a permanent prosthesis. The split cast is taped back and used until the prosthesis is delivered and fitted. This should not take more than a few days so that the ambulating process is not interrupted for any length of time if the split cast does not function well. The permanent prosthesis is removable so that it is essential to wrap the stump or use a properly fitted elastic stump shrinking sock at all times when the prosthesis is off.

When a rigid postsurgical dressing is not used, the stump may tend to swell for many weeks unless a compressive bandage is used when the prosthesis is off. The training process is supervised to check the posture and tolerance of the patient. Full weight should not be permitted during the first 6 weeks after surgery because it takes that long for the tissues to heal and to withstand the tensions and pressures of full weight.

During this entire period the patient is seen daily by the physical therapist who reports to the surgeon, physiatrist, or prosthetist any variations in function, fit, and alignment or the development of pain. In general, with good surgery and management designed to accomplish early ambulation the uncomplicated amputation patient should be able to leave the hospital ambulatory with a walkerette or crutches using a temporary or permanent prosthesis within a month after amputation. The preprosthetic preparation period which used to take up so much time now consists of using ambulation for shrinkage and strengthening instead of wrapping and bed exercises.

In many cases a walking pylon is not applied to the cast socket because of the general condition of the patient or other contraindication. The rigid dressing, however, still retains its value in enhancing healing and diminishing the postoperative phantom. In such cases, the cast is removed in 2–3 weeks for removal of sutures and measurement for a temporary removable prosthesis which should be delivered in just a few days. The temporary prosthesis then serves a useful purpose for 8–10 weeks until a permanent one is fitted. This applies in both above- and below-knee amputations. With immediate fitting and early ambulation, many older patients who previously would have been considered poor candidates for a prosthesis, do rather well and become surprisingly active with their prostheses. This is attributable to the preservation of maximal residual proprioception after proper myoplastic surgery and shaping of the stump with little time to deteriorate. When the permanent prosthesis is fitted, the gait characteristics of the patient must be seriously considered.

Gait training is now concerned with the manner of ambulating and leads to a more advanced series of exercises. At this point attention is directed toward equal length of steps. There is a tendency to take a long step with the prosthesis and a short step with the other leg. *This should be corrected early in the training.* It is helpful to have lines or foot prints painted on the floor and a full length mirror. The subject is to be instructed to look straight ahead and stop watching his feet. Knee flexion and heel rise are now concentrated on. When training is started the knee friction may be released or made tight, according to the ability of the patient to handle the prosthesis. It must now be adjusted to the speed of the gait which is developing. Increased friction and tight extension aids lead to circumduction of the prosthesis or vaulting on the other foot. Patients using the polycentric knee or positive friction locking knee must be taught to break the knee by first taking weight off the prosthesis. When the prosthesis is comfortable there should be little difficulty in practicing an even cadence. This corrects the sudden, rapid, short step with the normal leg.

These exercises should be done repeatedly and deliberately until safety and confidence are certain. As progress is made there may occur gait impairments which can only be corrected in the prosthesis, such as rotation at heel contact, foot slapping, whips, knee buckling, etc. Prosthetic adjustments are made to prevent habitual defects.

This is the general way gait is supervised. There are other methods and many supplementary exercises with and without the prosthesis which are contributory to good training and good performance. Each patient will progress at his own pace so that there is no time-table to follow. Patients who lag in progress are those who are known in advance to have lower potentials. The patients who do best require much less time than those who struggle for their low-level potential function. The slow and older amputees should not be forced to endure long practice periods in an effort to achieve the ability to put full weight on the prosthesis. The physician and therapist will recognize that these patients are failing and resort to the use of crutches. Most of these patients can learn stable three-point or four-point crutch gait as they may need. The patients who will walk well may advance from the parallel bars to independent gait without using crutches or canes. For these individuals there are a number of additional activities to be learned. These consist of stepping up and down a curb, stair climbing and descending, walking sideways, walking up and down an incline, bending and kneeling, stepping over obstacles, walking in a circle, sitting down and rising from chairs, and getting up from the floor. All of these are taught with techniques, which ensure stability of the prosthesis.

When a definite objective has been set and achieved, training should be discontinued. For those amputees who, at best, are functioning at a low level, time and experience can provide the necessary loss of fear and ultimate sense of stability.

During the training period and in follow-up contacts with amputees, an attitude of encouragement and praise will sustain the motivation to continue especially the slow patient for whom even small skills may be a long and arduous experience. Where a vocational objective depends upon function with the prosthesis, training in special activities may be necessary, such as driving a car.

Upper Extremity Amputees

The indications for amputation in the upper extremity are predominantly for traumatic accidents, industrial and thermal. They occur in a much younger average age group in the population than do accidents involving the lower extremity.

There are standard elective levels, as there are in the lower extremity but, in general, the amputation site will be dictated by the degree and extent of injury. There are, however, many more adaptive prosthetic components to serve the nonstandard upper extremity amputee than the lower.

The myoplastic stump closure is almost universally used and very early improvised functional use is common practice. Rigid dressings can be applied postoperatively as in the lower extremity. Many types of clips, clasps, or other fittings have been devised to hold a pencil, spoon, hook, or other device for early functional use since there are not special components available.

Functional devices are readily improvised by occupational therapists in training amputees in activities of daily living. The myoplastic closure preserves the proprioceptive qualities of the amputation stump as it does in the lower extremity. It also is followed by less swelling and shrinkage, diminishing the atrophy from disuse.

The specific exercise program is directed toward preserving the strength, range of motion and coordination of the shoulder girdle (scapulothoracic), shoulder (scapulohumeral) and elbow joints for the operation of the harness and prosthesis, depending upon the level of amputation. Trunk and postural exercises become part of the supervised program immediately following surgery to compensate for the discrepancy in weight across the shoulder girdles by loss of part or all of the upper extremity. Scoliosis and deviations of the head are not uncommon secondary developments. The objectives of training are functional use of the prosthesis in proper body alignment.

STANDARD ABOVE-ELBOW AMPUTEES

Normal range of all scapulohumeral motions as well as scapulothoracic motion is essential for control of the above-elbow prosthesis. Early active or passive exercises to maintain range of motion are necessary. If contractures develop (usually of the shoulder adductors and rotators), passive stretching in addition to the active exercises should be instituted immediately. Although bilateral shoulder motion is still required, major control of the prosthesis in standard above-elbow amputees is by flexion of the arm at the scapulohumeral joint. Consequently, powerful arm flexion must be developed. Control of the prosthesis elbow lock is by extension of the arm. Therefore, the extensor muscles of the arm must likewise be well developed.

STANDARD BELOW-ELBOW AMPUTEES

Forearm and wrist amputees require normal shoulder mobility and strength of the shoulder and arm muscles for activation and control of the prosthesis.

Every effort should be made to obtain the maximum range of pronation and supination, since at best it is difficult to incorporate this function in the use of the prosthesis. In addition to the active or passive exercises to maintain or increase elblow flexion and extension, active or passive exercises to maintain or increase the range of forearm rotation are essential. If limitation of this motion develops, passive stretching by the physical therapist should be performed in addition to the active exercises.

PROSTHETIC CONTROLS TRAINING

There are four basic body control motions used to operate upper extremity prostheses (8). Depending upon the prosthesis, a single basic motion or a combination of the basic motions may be required.

Arm-Flexion Control Motion

Shoulder flexion is used as the major power source in upper extremity amputees who retain this function. The motion is flexion at the scapulohumeral joint with the arm or arm stump kept in the saggital plane. Only the humerus should be moved, with minimal or no motion of the shoulder girdle taking place.

Shrug-Control Motion

Control is accomplished by protraction of the normal shoulder plus some protraction of the shoulder on the amputated side.

Pronation-Supination Control Motion

Pronation-supination motion is used as a power source for step-up rotation units used in some below-elbow prostheses.

Training in prosthetic controls consists of first training the amputee to perform singly and independently the major control motions indicated for his prosthesis. Practice will be necessary and should be continued until proficiency is attained.

Manually operated accessories for the prosthesis, such as the arm turntable unit, wrist rotation unit, and wrist flexion unit, are not operated by a control system but are pre-positioned prior to the movement of the prosthesis (9). Training in their use is taught before teaching coordination of the basic motions and consists primarily in learning the proper settings of the particular device for different activities.

Depending upon the type of harness system used, combinations of the basic motions will usually be required for activation and control of a prosthesis. When proficiency in performing each basic body motion singly is attained, the amputee can then be trained to coordinate these individual motions for efficient, smooth operation of his prosthesis.

The type of harness control system used will depend upon the level of amputation.

BELOW-ELBOW SINGLE-CONTROL SYSTEM

Patients with a forearm amputation or wrist disarticulation use the below-elbow single-control system to operate the prosthesis (10). Arm flexion is used to provide the force necessary for actuation of the terminal device.

In training the below-elbow amputee in the control motion, he first flexes the elbow to 90° and then flexes the shoulder without movement of the shoulder girdle until the terminal device operates. The amputee should be directed to concentrate on learning the feel of the shoulder harness as he operates the terminal device and to use this "feel" as a guide in developing control. The control motion should be practiced until the terminal device can be opened and closed partially, rapidly and slowly with the arm and forearm in various positions.

ABOVE-ELBOW DUAL-CONTROL SYSTEM

Elbow disarticulation and standard above-elbow amputees use the dual-control system. In this system the arm-flexion control motion is used to perform two prosthetic operations. With the prosthetic elbow unlocked, flexion at the shoulder causes flexion at the elbow of the prosthesis. With the prosthetic elbow locked, flexion at the shoulder operates the terminal device. The elbow lock is controlled by the arm-extension control motion, using a separate cable.

The elbow lock and its control, and the means by which shoulder flexion controls both elbow flexion and operation of the terminal device, are explained to the amputee. Then the amputee is taught to control the elbow lock, first, by hyperextension of the shoulder, while holding the shoulder girdle steady, and, then, by a combined motion of should extension and protraction of the shoulder girdle. Unlocking the elbow is by the same motion. When mastery and smooth operation of the elbow lock control are attained, the amputee is trained to flex the prosthetic elbow by shoulder flexion. With the elbow unlocked and the forearm positioned at 90° elbow flexion, the amputee flexes the shoulder without shoulder girdle motion to hold the forearm at 90° elbow flexion; then the arm stump is slowly relaxed, allowing the elbow to extend and the prosthetic forearm to drop. Next, the amputee learns to slowly flex the elbow to 90° by flexion of the shoulder and then to flex the elbow completely.

With mastery of flexion of the elbow and the ability to smoothly position the forearm at any degree of elbow flexion, the amputee is next trained in the combined operation of elbow flexion and elbow locking. The sequence of motions is flexion of the shoulder to flex the elbow and then (while maintaining the forearm in position) protraction of the shoulder girdle, with either a backward motion or a pushing down motion of the arm stump, to lock the elbow. It may be necessary to abduct the shoulder slightly to maintain tension on the elbow flexion cable. When mastery of these combined motions is attained, the amputee is trained to operate the terminal device. The forearm is positioned by flexing and locking the elbow; then, by flexion of the shoulder, the terminal device is operated. Practice is continued until all the combined control motions can be performed efficiently and smoothly. Body motion should be minimal and all shoulder and arm motions should be limited on the amputated side. The amputee should practice control of the prosthesis, not only in the sitting and standing positions, but also in all the other positions which normal daily activities may require.

ABOVE-ELBOW TRIPLE-CONTROL SYSTEM

In the triple-control system for standard above-elbow amputees, elbow flexion is produced by the arm-flexion control motion, elbow locking by the arm-extension control motion and operation of the terminal device by the shrug-control motion, utilizing protraction of both shoulders.

The amputee is first trained in control of the elbow lock and flexion of the elbow as described for the dual-control system. When mastery of these combined motions is attained, the amputee is trained to operate the terminal device. The elbow is flexed to 90° and the forearm position is maintained without locking the elbow. Then the terminal device is operated primarily by protraction of the shoulder on the normal side. Practice in performing all the control motions simultaneously with a coordinated and smooth operation is carried out, not only in the standing and sitting positions, but also in all other positions which may be required in the activities of daily living.

For shoulder disarticulation and interscapulothoracic amputations it is possible to derive some minimal function from conventional fitting and harnessing in a small number of cases. The development of myoelectric functional prostheses offers more hope for the very high single or double amputee.

The INAIL-CECA myoelectrically controlled prosthesis, developed by Hannes Schmidl of Budrio, Italy, is being used and has been improved at the Institute of Rehabilitation Medicine of the New York University Medical Center. In this prosthesis two sensitive contacts pick up the myopotentials generated by muscle contraction within the socket. The electrical potentials (microvolts) are amplified by microcircuitry and power a servomechanism by operating a switch, turning it on and off. The motion power is derived from compact batteries. No harness is needed except where suspension is critical. The pick-up electrodes are placed over flexors for flexion and extensors for extension so that wherever possible, depending on the level of amputation, the thought of flexion and contraction of the flexor will switch on the flexion or grasping motion of the special hand; similar action taking place for extension. These prostheses cost about 2½ times as much as conventional ones but provide more function for the very high above-elbow, shoulder-disarticulation and bilateral above-elbow cases.

Training for use requires intensive exercise of the muscles which will be monitored by the built-in electordes until they generate the minimal or more number of microvolts needed to operate the mechanisms. The patient is trained with a mock-up arm on a console and can observe his progress objectively as he is trained. The battery power pack and electronic components are miniaturized and are incorporated within the prosthesis.

Summary

Lower Extremity. The concept of training the lower extremity amputee in recent years has changed drastically. The principles of immediate fitting, the rigid dressing and early ambulation have made it unnecessary to perform the pre-prosthetic activities of wrapping, shrinking, crutch walking, intensive general body conditioning and difficult specific exercises which used to part of amputee rehabilitation. This has been replaced by cooperative planning with the surgeon, prosthetist and physical therapist to have the patient ambulate:

1. With an immediate prosthesis consisting of an adjustable pylon coupled to a rigid cast socket, within a few days after surgery.

2. With a walking pylon on a removable socket when the sutures are removed (14–21 days).

3. With a temporary ambulator or pylon for stump conditioning and shaping when the operative scar is healed (3–4 weeks).

The ambulating devices and partial weight bearing provide essentially all of the conditioning and strengthening and range of motion which the patient needs.

Upper Extremity. On an individual basis, each patient can be practicing functional activities with an improvised temporary prosthesis while performing the exercises necessary for achieving maximal use and skill with the prosthesis in a much shorter time than was previously expected.

REFERENCES

1. Cited by PACK, G. T., AND ARIEL, I. M. *Treatment of Cancer and Allied Diseases, Vol. VIII,* Ed. 2. Harper & Row, New York, 1964.
2. RUSSEK, A. S. Management of lower extremity amputees. *Arch. Phys. Med. Rehabil., 42:* 687–703, 1961.

3. Russek, A. S. Immediate postsurgical fitting of the lower extremity amputee. *Med. Clin. North Am., 53:* 665–676, 1969.

4. Russek, A. S. Amputations: Immediate postoperative fitting and early ambulation. In *Vascular Surgery, Principles and Techniques,* edited by H. Haimovici. McGraw-Hill, New York, 1976.

5. Russek, A. S., Thompson, W. A. L., Clauss, R. H., and Truchly, G. *Investigation of Immediate Prosthetic Fitting and Early Ambulation Following Amputation in the Lower Extremity;* Rehabilitation Monograph No. XLI, Institute of Rehab. Med., N.Y. Univ. Med. Center; Final Report, Project HEW-RD-1958, 1969.

6. Weiss, M. *The Prosthesis on the Operating Table from the Neurophysiological Point of View;* Report of the Workshop Panel on Lower Extremity Fitting, National Academy of Sciences, Committee on Prosthetics Research and Development, Feb., 1966.

7. Burgess, E. M., Romano, R. L., and Zettl, J. H., *The Management of Lower Extremity Amputations; Prosthetics Research Study,* Seattle, Wash., prepared for the Prosthetics and Sensory Aids Service, Veterans Administration Control No. V5261P-438, Tr 10-6, August 1969.

8. Aylesworth, R. D. (Ed.) U.C.L.A. Dept. of Engineering, *Manual of Upper Extremity Prosthetics,* 1952.

9. Fletcher, M. J. The upper extremity armamentarium. *Artif. Limbs, 1:* 15, 1954.

10. Taylor, C. L. The biomechanics of control in upper extremity prostheses. *Artif. Limbs, 2:* 4, 1955.

19

Therapeutic
Exercise for Back Pain

JOHN E. SARNO

Rational, effective therapeutics follow from accurate diagnosis. Therapeutic eclecticism is usually an indication of diagnostic incompetence. But success in treatment does not automatically indicate accuracy of diagnosis since factors unrelated to the therapeutic modality may supervene and bring about a resolution of symptoms and/or pathology. In the human organism, either self-restorative processes (which we share with other animals) or the psychic apparatus contribute to the end result of therapeutic intervention and are sometimes primary. Before the advent of modern medical techniques they were solely responsible for sickness or health, life or death.

There is no more controversial subject in medicine today than the diagnosis and treatment of back pain. The mainstream of current medical thinking on the etiology of low back pain revolves around disorders of the last two lumbar intervertebral discs, disease of the apophyseal joints of the lower lumbar spine, postural aberrations in this area, and certain structural abnormalities of the lumbosacral skeletal structures, most of which are thought to be congenital in origin. Consideration of the value of therapeutic exercise in the treatment of low back pain depends upon whether or not the current assessment of etiology is accurate for if certain structural abnormalities are the causes of this pain syndrome then there is no rational basis for the use of therapeutic exercise for it is difficult to see how the conditioning or strengthening of trunk and/or limb musculature can alter the pathological aberrations which are the concomitants of herniated disc, spondylolisthesis, osteoarthritis, scoliosis, etc. And yet there is clinical evidence that therapeutic exercise frequently plays a role in the elimination of low back pain (1, 2).

If true objectivity is to be employed one must also admit that the methods of chiropractors, osteopaths, and a host of lesser known healers are also often effective. Distasteful as it may be, an assessment of the efficacy of therapeutic exercise in the treatment of low back pain must somehow account for the occasional success of these disciplines, some of which are clearly unscientific. If one is not prepared to engage this question the validity of all claims for therapeutic efficacy must be suspect.

We shall advance the thesis in this chapter that the majority of low back pain, and indeed upper back pain as well, is the result of a nonstructural disorder, as a consequence of which therapeutic exercise may be a rational, effective treatment modality. As the problem is analyzed an attempt will be made to identify the factors upon which this efficacy is based. Unfortunately there is no objective data to substantiate such assertions at this point in time. However, we share this dilemma with all who claim merit for the variety of treatment methods which have been advanced in the treatment of back pain; to our knowledge none enjoys the virtue of scientific validation except perhaps the debridement of disc material in a clear-cut case of herniation.

The diagnostic situation has not changed since a writer for the *British Medical Journal* editorialized in 1971 that in most cases of back pain a specific abnormality is not found and that in those cases in which congenital abnormalities or deformities are demonstrated radiographically, their significance in the production of pain is doubtful (3). How, then, can treatment success be verified if the etiology of a process is so much in doubt? What claim can one make for the value of bed rest, a lumbar corset, traction, medication, transcutaneous coagulation of the nerves of Luschka, chemonucleolysis, etc., when the pathologic process being treated is so poorly understood? To be sure an assertion by a writer for the *British Medical Journal* does not establish something as fact but this is a generally accepted view. Nowhere in the literature is there to be found convincing evidence to demonstrate that the writer was in error or that the treatment modalities enumerated above are of dependable value. Conjecture is rampant, some of it cogent and logical but none supported by unequivocal data. Let us review some of the more commonly presented diagnoses in clinical practice.

Common Diagnoses in Low Back Pain

Statistically most patients with persistent low back pain syndromes are told that the problem is due to "a disc," "a degenerated disc," or "a slipped disc." If there is leg pain associated with lumbar, lumbosacral, or gluteal pain the figure approaches 100%. In a series of 65 consecutive patients with back and/or limb pain seen in consultation, 37% came with this diagnosis (Tables 19.1 and 19.2). The demonstration in 1932 that a lumbar intervertebral disc may herniate, producing a radiculopathy, has been very much a mixed blessing. No one doubts that this pathology exists but its true incidence is probably far below the frequency of diagnosis. Dillane et al. (4) noted an incidence of 7.6% in males and 5.6% in females in a

TABLE 19.1. *Admitting Diagnoses in 65 Consecutive Patients with Skeletal Pain*

Diagnosis	Patients	
	no.	*%*
Lumbar disc disease	24	37
Lumbar osteoarthritis or sprain	9	14
Lumbar muscle spasm	3	05
Congenital lumbar abnormality	1	02
Fracture lumbar vertebral body	1	02
Cervical sprain, strain trauma, osteoarthritis, radiculopathy	17	26
Cervical disc disease	1	02
Overstretched neck ligament	1	02
Thoracic outlet syndrome	1	02
Frozen shoulder	1	02
Tendonitis, thigh or knee	2	03
Dislocating knee	1	02
Arthritis, knee	1	02
Muscular problem, thigh	1	02
No admitting diagnosis	3	05

TABLE 19.2. *Diagnosis and Site of Pathology in 65 Consecutive Patients with Skeletal Pain*

Diagnosis	Total		Low Back		Upper Back and Cervical		Both Lower and Upper Back		Other	
	no.	*%*	*no.*	*%*	*no.*	*%*	*no.*	*%*	*no.*	*%*
Tension myositis	52	80	36	82	23	96	8	100	1	20
Psychogenic regional pain ("conversion")	12	18	8	18	1	4	0		3	60
Somatic process	1	2	0	0	0	0	0		1	20
Total	65	100	44	100	24	100	8	100	5	100

group of 470 patients who suffered 605 attacks of low back pain over a period of four years. Based upon our work this incidence may be high.

The diagnosis is usually prompted by coexistent low back and leg pain, the presumption being that a posterolaterally bulging or herniated disc impinges on the ipsilateral root at L.4–5 or L.5–S.1. It is frequently made without benefit of myelography or electromyography but is often buttressed by radiologic evidence of a narrow disc space at the appropriate level. Indeed, x-ray evidence of a narrowed disc space often prompts the diagnosis in the absence of leg pain. But Nachemson, one of the most knowledgeable and ardent advocates of lumbar disc pathology as the basis for most low back pain, has stated categorically that radiologic evidence of a single narrowed intervertebral disc cannot be correlated with low back pain (5). Splithoff (6) and others have also indicated the lack of diagnostic specificity of radiologic abnormalities of the lumbosacral area. And yet the diagnosis continues to be made with astonishing regularity despite the additional facts that the leg pain often involves areas that do not correspond to the appropriate spinal segment and is sometimes bilateral. The reason seems clear: there has been no satisfactory alternative explanation. Nachemson has reviewed what is known about the lumbar disc and wistfully concludes that the answer to the question of how it causes back pain still eludes us, that the etiology of most back pain is unknown (5).

When a patient presents with the complaint of low back pain without leg pain he may receive one of a number of diagnoses, depending on his age and the appearance of his lumbar spine films. If the patient is young and the x-rays are normal he or she may be told that the problem is "postural"; if x-rays demonstrate a narrowed disc space, facet tropism, spondylolisthesis, scoliosis of any degree, either lumbar or thoracic, a transitional vertebra, spina bifida occulta, defects of the pars interarticularis, an exaggerated lumbar lordosis or a lumbosacral tilt, these will be cited as the cause of the pain despite a number of substantial reports invalidating this conclusion (5–10). Patients in the older age group with back pain unassociated with leg pain are at even greater risk since in addition to the statistical possibility that they will have one of the above abnormalities, they are almost certain to have some evidence of osteoarthritic change in the articulating elements of the lumbosacral structures, to which the pain is attributed. Back pain with leg pain at any age usually calls forth the diagnosis of radiculopathy based on disc herniation regardless of the findings of plain x-rays, myelography, or electromyography.

Another common diagnosis is that of instability in the lumbosacral area. It is usually based upon presumptive evidence of abnormal mobility in low back skeletal structures, radiologically determined, and common after surgical fusion. The assertion that an "unstable" back produces pain has never been objectively verified.

In cases where laminectomy has been performed with recurrence of pain frequent diagnoses are "scar tissue" or "arachnoiditis." It is difficult to escape the conclusion that these diagnoses are often made in an attempt to explain recurrent pain that is otherwise highly enigmatic.

What pervades the entire spectrum of diagnostic possibilities in low back pain is the concept that the pain must be attributed to a structural disorder of the lumbosacral elements. It is a bias which is deeply ingrained in medical practice and teaching but, unfortunately, largely unsupported by objective data.

There is no alternative to these diagnoses which currently enjoys serious consideration; it is our view that they are in error in most cases and that there are other processes responsible for back pain in well over 95% of those who present with the syndrome. It would appear that the majority suffer from a benign, reversible, psychosomatic process involving the musculature of the back which we have suggested calling *tension myositis.* Though there is at present meager hard data supporting the existence of this entity, clinical studies are highly suggestive.

Tension Myositis

In 1946 Sargent reported a series of cases in which 96% of the subjects were diagnosed as having psychosomatic backache (11). These patients were carefully studied at an Air Force convalescent hospital and it was concluded that the majority suffered from a disorder which was painful and related to the patient's psychic state. To our knowledge no one has specifically confirmed or contradicted Sargent's findings and the paper has remained hidden in the literature.

Table 19.1 details the clinical diagnoses in a series of 65 consecutive patients seen in consultation for skeletal pain syndromes. The majority were subsequently diagnosed as having tension myositis (Table 19.2). This muscle disorder appears to be pathologically analogous to other psychosomatic processes such as peptic ulcer, spastic colitis, bronchial asthma, and migraine headache, to name the most prominent. One can hypothesize that all of these disorders originate in limbic nuclei and are mediated through the autonomic nervous system. Conversion pain is psychogenic in origin as well and has been well described by Walters (12). Patients with the latter variety of psychogenic pain generally have more complicated psychological problems than those with tension myositis.

The close relationship of tension myositis and other psychosomatic disorders is illustrated in Table 19.3. Clearly there is a valid correlation among these pathological entities.

Like much of medical nomenclature the term tension myositis only

TABLE 19.3. *Associated Psychosomatic Disorders in 108 Patients with Tension Myositis*

Disorders	Patients	
	no.	%
Total number with some related disorder	78	72
Peptic ulcer and related disorders	41	38
Allergic rhinitis and/or asthma	31	29
Colitis, spastic colon or diverticulitis	24	22
Tension headache	18	17
Migraine headache	10	09
Idiopathic cardiac palpitations	4	04
Angeoneurotic edema	5	05
Neurodermatitis, eczema or psoriasis	7	06
Four of above	3	03
Three of above	17	16
Two of above	37	34
One of above	21	19

approximates the actual disorder; the word tension is meant to represent the psychic component of the process, which will be dealt with in greater detail later; the muscle pathology is probably not purely an inflammatory one although there may be secondary inflammatory changes (13). We suspect it is a local disorder of the contractile state of muscle and the location and degree of pain are functions of the actual muscle tissue involved. On occasion it is sufficiently widespread to be perceived by the patient as spasm. More often the patient is only aware of an aching or burning pain in a well circumscribed area.

Clinical Description of Tension Myositis

In the majority of cases the pain is sudden in onset and related to a minor injury or "back strain." Commonly the syndrome is precipitated by a minor automobile accident in which the patient's car is struck from behind. Typically he has little or no pain immediately after the accident but will experience the gradual onset of low back and/or neck and shoulder pain during the next 1–5 days. Often the patient needs no acute medical treatment or leaves the hospital to which he is taken without having had x-rays. The pain generally comes on gradually and, once established, tends to become increasingly severe. At this point medical advice is sought, x-rays are taken, and one of the following diagnoses are made: if the pain is in the neck, shoulder and/or arm—cervical sprain, cervical spondylosis or osteoarthritis with cervical radiculopathy ("pinched nerve" to the patient); for low back and/or leg pain—lumbosacral sprain, herniated disc or osteoarthritis with lumbar radiculopathy. Treatment is invariable: rest, "muscle relaxants," tranquilizers, analgesics, cervical collar, and cervical traction for the neck pain patient. (So pervasive is the prescription of a cervical collar that patients are occasionally given them in anticipation of the development of pain, a practice which has a most damaging psychological effect.) For the patient with a low back syndrome, rest in bed is the major treatment modality; if the pain persists or worsens the next step is admission to the hospital for "traction" and the patient is frequently discharged with a lumbar corset. All too frequently these measures are without benefit, the pain continues and the patient becomes increasingly anxious and depressed.

More common than a minor auto accident is a history of sudden, acute pain precipitated by lifting, bending, twisting, or stretching. The patient usually has the perception of having suffered some acute structural derangement and describes the moment of onset with such phrases as, "my back went out" or "something snapped." (Thereafter, if he has recurrent episodes he will use the same phrase to describe onset.) In the majority of cases there is a marked disproportion between the severity of the pain and the violence of the precipitating movement. More often than not it is an innocent twist or bend of the trunk. It is difficult to conceive that we are of such fragile construction that a minor twist can result in a catastrophic structural aberration. In fact, we believe that no such thing occurs but that the physical movement or activity serves to trigger an acute, focal muscle spasm, very much as a turn or stretch in bed will precipitate a "cramp" in the gastrosoleus in people who are subject to them. The sudden, excruciating nature of the pain at the moment of onset suggests to the patient that something catastrophic has occurred. The pain most often is located in the lower lumbar, lumbosacral or gluteal musculature, usually unilateral but often bilateral. Once the syndrome has become established the pain tends to predominate on one side or the other but occasionally shifts to the other side. This is a fact of great significance, particularly if there is leg pain associated with back pain, and it is often ignored. The shifting locus of pain casts doubt on the diagnosis of a radiculopathy of spinal origin.

Shoulder and neck pain due to tension myositis is more apt to be insidious in onset though occasionally it is precipitated by a sudden head movement. Characteristically, the muscle most often involved in the upper back is the upper trapezius; there will almost always be pain in the paracervical muscles on the same side, often occipital pain as well and less frequent but by no means rare there is pain in the middle and lower trapezii, rhomboids or latissimus dorsi. Pain may involve any part of the arm but is commonest in the deltoid-biceps-triceps regions, though we do not believe the pathology involves these muscles but that the pain is secondary to a mild neuropathy, to which we shall return later.

In a small but significant proportion of cases in both the lower and upper back the pain comes on without an obvious precipitant. Often the patient is aware of its presence on awakening in the morning. Regardless of mode of onset once the pain has occurred it tends to remain and get worse in a significant proportion of cases.

The simultaneous occurrence of upper and low back pain, which is not infrequent, reflects our hypothesis that tension myositis is a single pathologic entity which may involve any of the postural muscles. Twenty-seven percent of a group of 108 patients with tension myositis had involvement of muscles in both the lower and upper back. Though it is often associated with an incident which implies structural damage, the history and physical findings together with certain personality or psychologic factors suggest that the pathologic process is psychosomatic in origin.

With the persistence of pain each patient tends to develop a characteristic pattern of factors which either aggravate or relieve the pain. With a low back syndrome, for example, most patients complain that sitting, prolonged standing or lifting even light objects increases or brings on the pain. Many patients find that walking a short distance relieves the pain, sometimes completely, but prolonged walking tends to bring it back again. About one-third of patients find that the recumbent position relieves the pain while the majority find that the pain is not relieved and in some cases is aggravated when they are in bed.

Upper back pain is almost always aggravated by use of the arms or head movement. Many of these patients complain of the onset of numbness and paresthesias in the fingers during the night, relieved by getting up for awhile or exercising the arm and hand vigorously.

Not infrequently patients claim some relief with a cervical collar or lumbar corset and there are undoubtedly some who obtain complete relief and do not seek further consultation. In view of the inability of either of these devices to immobilize the segment of spine for which they are designed one is strongly inclined to believe that relief is obtained through the mechanism of suggestion. We have rarely failed to wean these patients from their collars or corsets within a matter of a few weeks.

The persistence of symptoms for months and years usually tends to produce increasing disability. Older patients who have been told that the problem stems from degeneration of spinal structures are often extremely anxious when first seen in fear that they will eventually be totally incapacitated.

A common history in patients within the third, fourth, and fifth decades is that they have episodes 1–4 times a year, usually increasing in frequency as they get older, each of which may last for 2 or 3 weeks. Between incidents they are free of pain but tend to restrict their activities sharply, avoiding sports or anything that requires physical exertion. Parents often decry their inability to pick up or play with their children. Sexual activity may be curtailed because of fear of precipitating an episode. Because of great variability in the location and severity of the pain it is difficult to escape the conclusion that the pathology is not structural.

The coexistence of leg or arm pain represents an important aspect of these syndromes for it is upon these symptoms that the diagnosis of a herniated disc or radiculopathy most often depends. Pain in the leg generally involves the posterior or lateral aspect of the thigh and leg and the lateral and dorsal foot. The patient rarely describes lancinating pain; it is usually aching and occasionally burning in character. It is frequently but not consistently associated in the patient's mind with pain in the buttock or just above the posterior pelvis. Arm pain most often involves the extensor surface of the arm and the fourth and fifth fingers of the hand but is not restricted to these areas.

It is usually presumed, with and without benefit of x-rays, that these limb symptoms are due to embarrassment of a nerve root at the spinal level, lumbar or cervical. There is good reason to hypothesize that there is, indeed, a mild neuropathy, but that it is distal to the spine; we suspect that spasm in the vicinity of the sciatic nerve as it emerges from its foramen is responsible for the leg symptoms and that spasm in the upper trapezius muscle somehow compromises a nerve root or roots after they emerge from their intervertebral foramina. We base these suppositions, 1) upon our ability to eliminate the entire syndrome by conservative means that could not possibly change the structure of the spine, 2) because of the intermittent and shifting character of the clinical picture, and 3) assertions by several workers that one cannot correlate structural aberrations in the cervical and lumbar spine with pain syndromes (5–10).

Indeed, the last of these reports asserts that cervical myelography lacks diagnostic specificity in the evaluation of cervical disc or spondylotic root compression and that "large defects of any shape with or without adjacent dural compression may be totally asymptomatic." In addition we have accumulated a small series of patients referred with the diagnosis of "lumbar disc disease" in whom electromyograms demonstrated mild denervation in the leg but none in the paravertebral musculature, strongly suggesting that the compression of nerve tissue was distal to the spine.

The physical examination in patients with tension myositis is remarkably consistent. Even in patients with prolonged symptomatology, that is months or years, there is usually a paucity of objective findings. In low back syndromes, a reduction in motor power in the legs is rarely seen and an occasional patient will have a diminished or absent ankle reflex. This may occur following a severe episode of spasm in the gluteal musculature and is usually temporary, though it may persist for a number of months. A reflex change of this kind is always attributed to a herniated disc. The various tests designed to identify spinal nerve compression must be interpreted with care for they are frequently positive in patients with tension myositis. Pain in the posterior thigh on straight leg raising will certainly reflect root pathology but it will also result from compromise of the sciatic nerve itself. Patients with tension myositis in the gluteal musculature always have buttock pain with straight leg raising and it often radiates down the leg. Similarly, if there is lumbosacral or gluteal pain with forward bending one may conclude that this too results from stretching of the muscles in spasm. The sensory examination is usually negative but may be positive if there is sciatic irritation. Characteristically, it is rarely restricted to one segment, throwing doubt on the root as the source of the deficit. Most often there is minimal hypesthesia and patients report that they sometimes experience paresthesias in the same distribution. The most constant and dependable finding on examination is tenderness on palpation, strongly suggesting soft tissue pathology. The area of tenderness correlates with the reported locus of pain and in virtually all patients who report leg pain the tenderness is in the buttock musculature. These areas of tenderness are undoubtedly synonymous with the trigger points of Travell (14) and Kraus (15).

In the upper back and shoulders there are analogous findings on examination. Reflex, motor, and sensory testing are usually negative. As in the low back there is a rare reduction in reflex amplitude. Head motions generally result in pain in the posterior cervical or upper trapezius muscles but not in the arms. Head extension in a case of bona fide foraminal root encroachment will produce arm pain with good consistency;

it does not occur in patients with tension myositis. As in the low back, tenderness in the upper trapezii and less commonly in the lower scapular musculature is a consistent finding.

The Psychosomatic Basis for Tension Myositis

Psychosomatic illness is not a new concept, thanks to the insights of such workers as Alexander (16), Dunbar (17), and Grinker (18). What is of great interest, however, is the fact that this knowledge is rarely used in clinical practice. No one denies that peptic ulcer is a psychosomatic disorder but few patients report that they have been counselled by their physicians or sent for psychotherapy after the diagnosis has been established. All report in detail on the antacid and anticholinergic drugs prescribed. The term "psychosomatic" is assiduously avoided as though it implied inferiority, weakness, or mental illness. Indeed patients will often state when the subject is introduced that they fear these implications. It is of great interest that this reaction appears to be culturally determined for it has been observed, though not systematically recorded, that patients from Latin America, parts of the Middle East, and some European cultures are not threatened by the diagnosis. Except for rare exceptions North Americans are disturbed by and will initially reject a psychosomatic diagnosis. Naturally this orientation exists in physicians as well, which probably accounts for their reluctance to confront their patients with the diagnosis and may be the key reason why they are slow to recognize the psychic etiology of pathologies.

Kraus (15) has suggested that "tension" plays a role in backache but has not identified the problem as psychosomatic, nor do his treatment methods reflect such a view. The term "psychological overlay" is often used inside and outside of the literature, sometimes accurately to reflect intensification of a somatically caused pain syndrome by psychic factors, but more often as a vague reference to the fact that the pain syndrome cannot adequately be explained by objective phenomena in a patient who appears to be neurotic.

It has been our observation that patients with tension myositis almost uniformly possess one or more of the following personality characteristics: a highly developed sense of responsibility or duty, a strong desire to achieve or accomplish, compulsiveness, perfectionism, conscientiousness, a tendency to worry. Their inner motivation is strong and they are "solid citizens," good family men and women, often very active in community and religious activities. Clearly these characteristics are very common in North Americans, but so is tension myositis. In addition, as indicated earlier, tension myositis is only one of a repertoire of possible psychosomatic reactions including gastric hyperacid states, hiatus hernia, colitis, spastic colon, migraine headache, allergic states, idiopathic cardiac palpitations, angioneurotic edema, and others. Most patients with tension myositis have a history of one or more of these related disorders. Table

19.3 details the incidence of these associated psychosomatic processes. The high incidence of peptic ulcer and related disorders is highly suggestive.

These assertions to not prove the point. Clinical experience demonstrates, however, that patients who are made aware of and accept the diagnosis do well with a simple program of physical therapy; those who reject the diagnosis generally do not improve. There is a small group of patients whose symptoms disappear upon learning of the diagnosis, without benefit of physical therapy. Finally, patients with severe, prolonged tension myositis of the incapacitating variety usually respond favorably when treated with intensive psychotherapy in a rehabilitation setting. That program will be described in greater detail below.

As stated previously the onset of tension myositis is frequently associated with situations of external stress but not always. One has the impression in many patients that there has been an accumulation of tension, sometimes over many years, which may manifest itself as tension myositis insidiously or be precipitated by a more or less dramatic incident. In the latter, as noted above, the syndrome is frequently precipitated by a minor automobile accident in which a so-called "whiplash" injury occurs. It is well known in clinical medicine that these injuries are frequently persistent and resistant to all forms of treatment. When they occur in young people, who do not have significant spondylotic or osteoarthritic changes in the cervical or lumbar spine, it is particularly difficult to attribute the continuing pain to a structural problem. The presence of tension myositis is logical and consistent. Once having been apprised of the proper diagnosis, and so reassured that there is nothing to fear from permanent disability, the majority of patients do well. The therapeutic approach will be elaborated below.

One can only speculate on the intracerebral process which transforms psychic into somatic phenomena, if "transform" is the proper word. We have the impression that the postural muscles of "susceptible" individuals are "sensitized," much as the nasal tissues of a person with allergic rhinitis. In the latter case the offending allergen precipitates the symptomatic manifestation of the disorder; in tension myositis some physical maneuver or occurrence triggers the acute "spasm," which is painful. The process of "sensitization" will surely remain a mystery for a long time since it will require knowledge of brain processes about which we now have only the most primitive understanding.

Case Reports

Following are two case reports illustrating typical histories and findings in patients with tension myositis.

Case 1. The patient is a 28-year-old housewife, mother of two young children, who was a passenger in the back seat of an automobile which was struck from behind while at a stop light. She was thrown about in the car but did not strike her head or lose consciousness. She experienced no immediate pain and elected not to go to a hospital or to her own physician. However, on the following day she began to feel pain in the posterior cervical area. Over the next week the pain became increasingly severe, and spread to involve the top of both shoulders, the lateral aspect of both arms (triceps area), the parascapular region on both sides of the midline, and eventually lumbar and lumbosacral areas. The pain was described as aching, burning, and occasionally sharp. She consulted her physician, films of the cervical and lumbar spine were done and read as normal. She was told she had suffered a severe "strain" in the cervical, thoracic, and lumbar areas. A cervical collar and a muscle relaxant were prescribed and she was advised to rest. For a few days after seeing her doctor she improved but then found that even at bed rest she was having significant pain. After 3 weeks of almost complete rest she began to move around and attempted to do some chores, with marked aggravation of the pain. She was then referred to another physician who changed her medication and suggested a lumbar corset. Her mother was summoned to come and help with the care of the home and children. At 3 months post-onset there was no change so she consulted a chiropracter. With daily treatment she improved somewhat but after 3 weeks when she attempted to do some housework there was a marked recrudescence of pain. Over the next 5 months she became increasingly anxious and depressed while her husband and mother struggled to maintain a normal family life.

When seen in consultation it was noted that the patient had a history of allergic rhinitis (grass pollens and molds) since the age of 19; she had suffered from hives for 9 months during her senior year in high school and since the age of 23 had experienced from three to five classical migraine headaches a year. She had been married 6 months prior to the first migraine episode.

Physical examination failed to reveal any evidence of a neural deficit or limitation in range of motion of the trunk, neck, or limbs. On palpation, marked tenderness was found over the upper trapezii bilaterally, the medial parascapular muscles on both sides of the midline, and the paravertebral lumbar musculature. The diagnosis was tension myositis. The patient appeared to comprehend the nature of the process, recognized that she had a basically anxious personality, and became pain-free after 4 weeks of physical therapy.

Case 2. The patient was a 38-year-old policeman who developed low back pain after helping lift a stretcher. He was treated conservatively for 6 months and then had a laminectomy and foraminotomy at L.4–5 bilaterally and L.5–S.1 on the left. He was better postsurgically but his symptoms continued and after a few months began to increase in severity. Thirteen months after the surgery a repeat myelogram was normal. At this point he was having recurrent attacks of severe low back pain which necessitated bed rest for a few days, doing light desk duty between attacks. He had multiple courses of physical therapy over the next 2 years. Thirty-nine months post-onset percutaneous rhizotomies of the nerves of Luschka were performed at L.3–4, L.4–5, and L.5–S.1 bilaterally resulting in temporary reduction in symptom severity once more. About 3 months later, however, the attacks of severe pain resumed, now occasionally requiring hospitalization. During one of these, a repeat electrodiagnostic study was negative except for the paravertebral changes described above.

When first seen 7 months after the last surgical procedure he described pain involving the entire lumbosacral region, without radiation into either leg, but with feelings of "heaviness" in the entire left and posterior aspect of the right leg. He required Demerol for pain control and was severely restricted in all aspects of his life. He was emotionally distraught since he feared for his ability to work, to be a good husband and father.

His past medical history was benign except for an episode of "viral meningitis" 2 years before the onset of his present problem.

On examination he presented as a healthy male who looked his stated age. He had no gait abnormality, the trunk was not tilted laterally but was rigid, and the lumbar area was flat. He could bend forward to 75° without discomfort but straight leg raising was limited to 45° bilaterally. The reflex, motor, and sensory examination of the legs was normal. There was a midline scar in the lumbar region. Marked tenderness was noted on palpation of the entire lumbar area from L.1 to the sacrum and over the upper buttocks.

The admitting diagnosis was severe, chronic tension myositis.

Admission laboratory studies were normal. Plain films of the lumbar spine showed straightening of the lumbar spine and posterior narrowing of the lumbosacral joint.

Psychological investigation revealed that he had an extremely low self-image. He thought himself to be stupid and uneducated and felt inferior to others socially and intellectually, usually causing him to avoid or withdraw from social situations. He doubted his ability to be a good husband, father, and provider but resented and then felt guilty about his resentment of the demands made on him by his family. Throughout he was unable to discuss these matters with his wife or anyone else.

The treatment program consisted of physical therapy for 3 hours each day, occupational therapy, and individual and group psychotherapy. During his early psychotherapeutic sessions he was skeptical about working with a psychologist and expressed great doubt that his symptoms could be psychologically engendered. He met with the attending physician daily at which time the details of the psychosomatic process were carefully and repeatedly explained. By the end of the third week after admission he became more receptive to the idea and started to work very well with the psychologist. He began to develop many insights into his behavior, often dealing with painful emotions. As this occurred his pain began to decrease in severity and frequency. Before his discharge he had also begun to discuss sexual problems with his wife and for the first time in many years felt that the deteriorating situation might be reversed. By discharge 7 weeks after admission he was free of pain and planning to continue psychotherapy at home. He had made some major insights into his behavior and feelings. As of this writing, 8 months post-discharge, he is leading a normal life and remains pain-free.

Treatment of Back Pain

This is the subject to which the entire exposition thus far has been directed for, as stated earlier, if most back pain syndromes are structural in origin there seems little theoretical value in an exercise program. And yet most experienced workers in rehabilitation medicine have often observed improvement in patients with low back and/or leg pain treated primarily with exercise. The most dramatic are those with a "sciatic" syndrome in whom it is ordinarily presumed there is disc protrusion or herniation. Nachemson and Elfstrom (19) have pointed out that contraction of the iliopsoas muscle increases the intradiscal pressure at L.4–5 and L.5–S.1; how then explain successful treatment of a patient with a presumed herniated disc when the exercise program includes difficult sit-ups, and exercise which includes powerful contraction of the iliopsoas, particularly if the legs are in extension? If this is the case sit-ups are contraindicated in a patient with a herniated disc. However, in the period before we recognized tension myositis as an entity, large numbers of patients with presumed "discs" were treated in our clinic with this type of exercise and many were relieved of symptoms. It was a result that was accepted gratefully though it could not be explained.

Similarly, on the basis of practical observation, one of the basic tenets of exercise therapy for low back pain was violated many years ago at our institution; back extension exercises were incorporated into the therapeutic regimen for low back pain patients. They continue to be used to this day. In the case of both of these exercises, their use or interdiction has been based upon certain theoretical principles both as to etiology and therapy for low back pain. It has been presumed that all back pain syndromes are structural in origin, involving primarily posterior elements, i.e., the posterior aspect of the annulus fibrosis and the articulating elements; therefore, back extension exercises are forbidden, flexion exercises are recommended.

If, however, the etiology of most back pain is tension myositis, the inconsistencies disappear. There is no need to be concerned about intradiscal pressure and, for reasons to be discussed below, abdominal strengthening exercise is often valuable in patients with sciatica. Similarly, there is no reason to avoid back extension exercise if the pathology is muscular; indeed, exercising the muscles in spasm may be beneficial.

Logic suggests that a psychosomatic disorder should be treated by psychotherapy. In fact, of 52 patients in whom the diagnosis of tension myositis was made, only 3 required psychotherapy (6%); of 12 patients in whom a diagnosis of "conversion" pain was made, 5 had psychotherapy (42%).

Though psychotherapy is prescribed for only a small proportion of the patient population, experience strongly suggests that patients with tension myositis must both understand and accept the psychosomatic diagnosis before they can hope to be free of pain, regardless of the physical therapy program. This understanding and acceptance may be at a fairly superficial level, in which case suggestion may play a salutory role. But recovery seems to be heavily dependent on this factor since patients who will not or cannot accept the diagnosis generally do not do well.

There appears to be a powerful role for the non-psychiatrist physician in the diagnosis and treatment of physical disorders of psychic etiology. The patient is more inclined to listen to and believe such a physician precisely because he is not a psychiatrist and because, therefore, his diagnosis does not bear the stigma of "mental illness." If the psychic aspect of the problem is presented as related to personality characteristics rather than psychopathology, though still undesirable, it is more acceptable to the patient. The attending physician then assumes the additional role of educator; he explains the mechanism by which psychic phenomena are translated into physical disorders and makes it possible for the patient to accept the diagnosis. Having established this clinical bridgehead it is then possible to introduce the psychiatrist or psychologist into the therapeutic process when necessary.

A physical treatment program for tension myositis must of necessity be empirically derived, based upon experience, logic, and conjecture. If the pathology is a psychosomatic muscle disorder it is reasonable to believe that it is benign and reversible. Further, the disorder has the clinical appearance of a painful change in the contractile state of muscle, a "spasm," despite the fact that the pain often involves only a small, well localized area. Once more, the experiences of Travell (14) and Kraus (15), appear to coincide. Based upon this formulation the following therapeutic regimen is suggested:

1. The use of a local modality for the purpose of heating the muscle tissue involved, based upon the hypothesis that heat is often efficacious in relieving muscle "spasm." Any penetrating modality can be used such as diathermy or ultrasound.

2. Mild electrical stimulation, alone or in combination with ultrasound, appears to have value in the reduction of "spasm." (A specific device is not suggested since this is not the focus of this presentation.)

3. Massage may be helpful in reducing or even eliminating the pain during a treatment session. It is presumed that the process is capable of relaxing the abnormal contractile state, but how this is accomplished is in question. Direct pressure may induce reflex relaxation of the muscle; the soothing effect of massage may produce a centrally induced relaxation

or the effect may be mediated by suggestion. The improvement is usually temporary but has value for it demonstrates to the patient that his pain is remediable, that he does not suffer from an irreversible structural disorder.

4. Therapeutic exercise, the focus of this chapter, is presented as the cornerstone of the physical treatment program. When used for low back tension myositis it is primarily a strengthening program, with the emphasis on the abdominal musculature. For tension myositis involving the neck and shoulders, or in less frequent cases, the posterior thorax, active, resistive and relaxation exercises are prescribed.

The skill of the physical therapist is employed in the ability to teach the patient to perform the exercises properly and overcome his fear or resistance, particularly if there is discomfort or pain with performance of particular exercises. This is not uncommon, for the contraction or stretching of muscles that are the focus of tension myositis may produce pain. The therapist must be trained to understand the nature of the pathology as well as the personality configuration which underlies it in order to treat the patient more effectively, which means to allay fear and encourage increasing activity. The therapist must also decide when to have the patient progress to more advanced exercises.

Following is a suggested exercise program for low back pain syndromes:

General Instructions:
A. Do all exercises on the floor or a hard surface.
B. Do each exercise twice a day, 5 times each, increasing the number as strength increases.
C. Do not rush; always allow adequate time.
D. Do not hold your breath.
E. Consult your therapist if an exercise increases pain.
  1. Pelvic tilt (lumbar isometric flexion exercise) (2)
     Position: Supine with knees bent (hooklying)
     Purpose: A preliminary exercise to strengthen abdominals and relax the muscles in "spasm"
     Instructions:
     a. Contract abdominal muscles strongly, forcing low back into the floor; then relax
     b. Contract glutei strongly; then relax
     c. Combine abdominal and gluteal contractions, then relax
  2. Sit-up I (first in a series of six)
     Position: Supine—arms extended forward
     Purpose: Strengthen abdominals
     Instructions:
     a. Chin on chest, lift head and shoulders and sit up slowly
     b. Lower body slowly, keeping chin on chest
     c. Relax
  3. Sit-up II
     Position: Supine—arms folded across chest
     Purpose and Instructions: Same as Sit-up I
  4. Sit-up III
     Position: Supine—hands behind head

Purpose and Instructions: Same as Sit-up I
5. Sit-up IV
   Position: Hooklying (supine with knees bent), arms extended
   Purpose and Instructions: Same as Sit-up I
6. Sit-up V
   Position: Hooklying, arms folded across chest
   Purpose and Instructions: Same as Sit-up I
7. Sit-up VI
   Position: Hooklying, hands behind head
   Purpose and Instructions: Same as Sit-up I

Exercises 2 through 7 (Sit-up I through VI) are designed to be used progressively, that is, as abdominal strength increases the patient progresses to the next in the series. In general, only one of these should be used at a given point in the treatment program though the therapist may choose to introduce a hooklying exercise sooner because of good progress.

8. Lateral Sit-up
   Position: Supine
   Purpose: Strengthen lateral abdominals
   Instructions:
   a. Bend both knees and lift them toward the left shoulder
   b. Simultaneously, tuck in the chin and roll up reaching both hands toward the right hip
   c. Hold for count of 3, slowly relax to starting position
   d. Repeat to the opposite side
9. Bridging—I
   Position: Hooklying
   Purpose: Strengthen back muscles
   Instructions:
   a. Tighten the glutei
   b. Lift hips off the floor keeping trunk straight
   c. Maintain for count of 3 without arching back
   d. Relax to starting position
10. Bridging—II
    Position: Hooklying, hands behind head
    Purpose: Strengthen back and hip muscles
    Instructions:
    a. Tighten glutei, lift hips off floor
    b. Extend left leg; do not flex hip
    c. Return left foot to floor after count of 3
    d. Lower hips and relax
    e. Repeat with right leg
11. Bridging—III
    Position: Hooklying, hands behind head
    Purpose: Strengthen back and hip muscles
    Instructions:
    a. Tighten glutei, lift hips off floor
    b. Extend left leg; do not flex hip
    c. Abduct left leg slowly
    d. Adduct left leg and return foot to floor
    e. Lower hip to floor slowly
    f. Repeat with right leg

A low back program should consist of at least four exercises: a pelvic tilt, good as a warm up, one of the sit-up series, the lateral sit-up (exercise 8) and one of the bridging series.

Despite traditional views to the contrary, as noted earlier, neither the sit-up exercise with the legs extended or back strengthening exercises have proven to be deleterious in our patients, many of whom have had leg as well as back pain.

Since it would appear that the majority of neck and shoulder pain syndromes are examples of tension myositis following is a group of suggested exercises for that area:

General Instructions:

A. Perform exercises sitting in front of mirror
B. Do each exercise twice daily; the number of repititions prescribed by therapist
C. Do not rush; allow adequate time
1. Move head in a circle: chin to chest first, then to right with chin in line with right shoulder, continue back and look at ceiling, then to left with chin in line with left shoulder and back to chin on chest. Relax. Repeat circle in opposite direction
2. Tilt head to right; try to touch ear to right shoulder, eyes straight ahead. Repeat to left
3. Pull chin back into "West Point" posture
4. Elevate both shoulders (shrug);
   Depress both shoulders;
   Bring shoulders forward;
   Bring shoulders back; approximate scapulae
5. Clasp hands above head and reach for ceiling; hold for count of 3 and relax.
6. Clasp hands in front of chest, reach forward; hold for count of 3 and relax.
7. Clasp hands behind low back, approximate scapulae; hold for count of 3 and relax.
8. Isometric resistance group; patient manually resists following movements:
   a. head and neck flexion
   b. lateral rotation to right and left
   c. head and neck extension
   d. lateral tilt to right and left

Empirical Rationale for Therapeutic Exercise

At this moment it is not possible to identify the precise reason or reasons for the value of exercise in these disorders. One can hypothesize that well conditioned muscles are less susceptible to the postulated state of "spasm" or that, like massage and ultrasound, exercise has the capacity to relax "spasm."

There is reason to believe that strong abdominal muscles are important for the integrity of the intervertebral disc by providing visceral support for the lumbar spine (20). Though it is probably less frequent than generally thought, lumbar discs do herniate. It is theoretically possible that strong abdominal muscles may protect the low lumbar discs. Once having ruptured, however, it is difficult to imagine how strengthening the abdominals could remedy the situation. Nevertheless strengthening the abdominal muscles is considered an exercise in preventive medicine and is presented to the patient as one of the important reasons for its inclusion in the therapeutic regimen.

It must also be considered, as with every other facet of the therapeutic program, that it works through suggestion. It is a common experience that even after patients have been apprised of the diagnosis and accepted the psychosomatic explanation, they tend to focus heavily on the physical treatment. They generally perform their home exercise routines very faithfully. The exercise program may provide an important facesaving device for those patients (the majority) who are ashamed of the diagnosis.

Because of the occasional success of other types of practitioners (chiropractors, osteopaths, etc.), one is obliged to give serious consideration to the hypothesis that the efficacy of the entire treatment program, including exercise, is a function of suggestion. If, as we believe, tension myositis is a psychosomatic disorder, it is eminently susceptible to the power of suggestion. Not all scientific observations are made in the laboratory. Some of the most important medical advances have been the result of acute observation and intellectual power. Suggestion as a therapeutic tool has been poorly understood and inadequately utilized. It can explain many of the enigmatic phenomena associated with the treatment of back pain.

Disabling Back Pain Syndromes

The use of therapeutic exercise extends beyond the treatment of ambulatory patients with back pain. There is a large population of "incorrigibles," i.e., patients with severe, disabling syndromes of many years duration, often operated upon many times, who are more disabled than most paraplegics and many quadriplegics. Experience with a population of these patients, treated with intensive physical and psychotherapy, attests to the value of therapeutic exercise (21). In the series of 28 patients reported in this study, 64% were rendered free of pain or sufficiently so to resume a normal existence; this statistic is based upon a follow-up of from 6 to 24 months.

In each of these patients the continuing pain syndrome was the result of significant psychic conflict which had resulted in the production of either severe tension myositis (20%) or a "conversion" pain syndrome, usually accompanied by paresis and hypesthesia (80%).

The physical therapy program consisted of at least 3 hours of treatment daily including exercise in a warm pool, mat exercises, ambulation, and the trunk exercise regimen described earlier. Manual projects to increase endurance were carried out in the occupational therapy section. Though psychotherapy was mandatory and intensive with each patient, and probably of crucial importance, one cannot estimate with certainty the relative value of each treatment component. Therapeutic exercise was clearly an important part of the program described in that study but a final determination of the value of the various treatment modalities must await a controlled study.

Reference has been made to "conversion" pain syndromes; the term is qualified by quotation marks to indicate that patients with such symptomatology are not all hysterics, as pointed out by Walters (12). We have adopted Walters terminology and call this psychogenic regional pain. What these patients have in common is a syndrome of neural symptoms which cannot be explained on the basis of structural pathology, of which pain is the most prominent, and a variety of non-psychotic behavioral disorders, of which hysteria is the most common. Physical findings are usually bizarre; e.g. in a case of suspected disc herniation hypesthesia is noted in multiple segments, often including L.2, L.3, L.4 and S.2, in addition to the commonly involved L.5 and S.1. The pattern of sensory loss is often bizarre and usually accompanied by extensive paresis in the involved limb. Another common finding is exquisite tenderness on light palpation over wide areas of the back and legs, not explainable on the basis of either neural or muscle pathology. In a series of 65 ambulatory patients who presented with pain syndromes, 18% had psychogenic regional pain and 82% had tension myositis (Table 19.2). As stated above, 80% of the group of severely disabled back pain patients had psychogenic regional pain.

In general, the psychopathology in "conversion" patients is more severe than in patients with tension myositis. Endogenous depression is not uncommon and serious psychic conflict is frequently seen, based on a variety of character disorders, hysterical personality patterns and occasionally borderline schizophrenia. While it is not expected that the non-psychiatrist will identify the precise psychopathology, he has a crucial role in distinguishing psychogenic (psychosomatic or "conversion") from somatic syndromes on purely physical grounds. His willingness and ability to do this induces patient confidence in the diagnosis which cannot be achieved by a psychiatrist.

The necessity of adopting the role of quasi-psychiatrist may be burdensome to the practicing physician for he is generally not prepared by traditional training to do so. But surely this is a deplorable deficit in medical education for human beings are not merely complex mechanical structures. There is no mind-body dualism; function of the spiritual-psychic apparatus is inextricably intertwined with that of the physical being and they cannot be treated separately. Pain is a symptom which may indicate somatic pathology or, just as frequently, a disorder of the psyche. To be unaware of the latter is to miss the diagnosis in a significant proportion of patients, particularly when back pain is the symptom.

Therapeutic exercise is a powerful force for good health and is increasingly being recognized as such. Though the hypotheses must be validated, it may have a unique role in the treatment of back pain syndromes in that it can contribute to the support of lumbar spine structures and help reverse a benign muscle pathology both physically and through the mechanism of suggestion. It has been the thesis of this chapter that exercise can fulfill this role only if back pain is not structural in origin; it is hypothesized that the majority of such syndromes are not structural.

REFERENCES

1. LIDSTROM, A., AND ZACHRISSON, M. Physical therapy on low back pain and sciatica. *Scand. J. Rehabil. Med.*, 2: 37, 1970.
2. KENDALL, P. H., AND JENKINS, J. M. Exercises for backache; a double-blind controlled trial. *Physiotherapy*, 54: 154, 1968.

3. Study of back pain. Editorial in *Br. Med. J., 4:* 4, 1971.

4. DILLANE, J. B., FRY, J. AND KALTON, G. Acute back syndrome; a study from general practice. *Br. Med. J., 2:* 82, 1966.

5. NACHEMSON, A. F. The lumbar spine an orthopedic challenge. *Spine, 1:* 59, 1976.

6. SPLITHOFF, C. A. Roentgenographic comparison of patients with and without backache *J.A.M.A., 152:* 1610, 1953.

7. HULT, L. The Munk Fors investigation. *Acta Orthop. Scand.,* Supp. 16, 1954.

8. HORAL, J. The clinical appearance of low back disorders in the City of Gothenberg, Sweden. *Acta Orthop. Scand.,* Supp. 118, 1969.

9. COLLIS, D. K., AND PONSETI, I. V. Long term follow up of patients with idiopathic scoliosis not treated surgically. *J. Bone Joint Surg., 51A:* 425, 1969.

10. FOX, A. J., LIN, J. P., et al. Myelographic cervical nerve root deformities. *Radiology, 116:* 355, 1975.

11. SARGENT, M. Psychosomatic backache. *N. Eng. J. Med., 234:* 427, 1946.

12. WALTERS, A. Psychogenic regional pain alias hysterical pain. *Brain, 84:* 1, 1961.

13. KRAFT, G. H., JOHNSON, E. W., AND LaBAU, M. M. The fibrositis syndrome. *Arch. Phys. Med. Rehabil., 49:* 155, 1968.

14. TRAVELL, J. Basis for multiple uses of local block of somatic trigger areas. *Miss. Valley Med. J., 71:* 13, 1949.

15. KRAUS, H. "Pseudo-disc." *South. Med. J., 60:* 416, 1967.

16. ALEXANDER, F. *Psychosomatic Medicine.* New York, 1950.

17. DUNBAR, F. *Mind and Body: Psychosomatic Medicine.* New York, 1947.

18. GRINKER, R. R., AND ROBBINS, F. P. *Psychosomatic Case Book.* New York, 1954.

19. NACHEMSON, A. L., AND ELFSTROM, G. Intravital dynamic pressure measurements in lumbar discs. A study of common movements, maneuvers and exercises. *Scand. J. Rehabil. Med., 2* (Supp 1): 1, 1970.

20. BARTELINK, D. L. The role of abdominal pressure in relieving the pressure on the lumbar intervertebral discs. *J. Bone Joint Surg., 39B:* 718, 1957.

21. SARNO, J. E. Chronic back pain and psychic conflict. *Scand. J. Rehabil. Med., 8:* 143–153, 1976.

20

Exercises
for Scoliosis

_____ RENE CAILLIET

Scoliosis may be *functional* or *structural* with the latter type being considered potentially symptomatic (1). Functional scoliosis is usually reversible and attributed to a mechanical basis. Structural change of the vertebral bodies or the intervertebral discs are usually not implicated as causative nor are they considered to result from functional scoliosis. Functional scoliosis decreases or disappears when gravity is eliminated or when the causative factor is removed. An implicated factor such as a short leg or faulty habit may cause a functional scoliosis and can be remedied. Lateral bending corrects a functional curve, but does not significantly alter a structural curve except in the very young patient with minimal early and flexible scoliosis.

Structural scoliosis has many etiologies, but the true causative factors remain unknown. Spinal curvatures progress in a lateral direction and are usually accompanied by rotatory deformities. Scoliosis is potentially progressive in all children with remaining epiphyseal growth (2) and progresses insignificantly in curves of less than 40° upon completion of apophyseal closure. Epiphyseal closure is approximately 15 years of age in girls and 17 years in males. Progression of curvature in adult scoliosis occurs in curves exceeding 50° and is attributed to asymmetrical disc changes in which there is compression on the concave side (3).

Scoliosis is specified by its anatomical level and extent in the vertebral column (Fig. 20.1). Viewing the vertebral column laterally reveals the physiological curves: the cervical and lumbar lordodis: the thoracic and sacral kyphosis (Fig. 20.2). Only an increase in the thoracic kyphosis: the "round back" is concerned in discussion of scoliosis. Scoliosis implies a lateral curving of the usual straight vertebral column and can be viewed from the anterior-posterior aspect.

Curves are classified as major or compensatory. The major curve is the

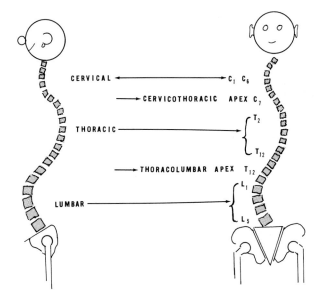

Fig. 20.1. Spinal level of scoliotic curvatures. Scoliosis is specified at the level of the spine and includes a specified number of vertebrae in the curve. The cervicothoracic and thoracolumbar curves are so designated by the site of the apex of the curve.

largest curve with the greatest angulation. The compensatory or "secondary" curve develops above or below the major curve (4) in an attempt to maintain bodily alignment with its center of gravity (Fig. 20.3).

Proper spinal alignment, without scoliosis or in a "compensated" scoliosis, has the occiput directly over the sacrum. A plumb line dropped from the seventh cervical spine (C7) process falls directly in line with the intergluteal fold (Fig. 20.4).

Curves are also differentiated according to the patient's age. A curvature during the first 3 years of life is termed *infantile*: between age 4 and 12 is termed *juvenile*: after age 12 in girls and 14 in boys (before maturity) is considered *adolescent*. Curves that exist after skeletal maturity are considered *adult* scoliosis.

Curves must be objectively measured on the x-rays. As standardized by the Scoliosis Research Society, curves are universally measured and reported by the Cobb method (Fig. 20.5). The *apical* vertebra is considered to be the most rotated vertebra in a curve. There is no current standard method of measuring the degree of rotation and various techniques differ in various clinics. Whatever is considered the accepted method of reporting rotation enables the specific clinic to evaluate progression or amelioration of the scoliosis.

The concurrent rotation of the spine with lateral curving presents the

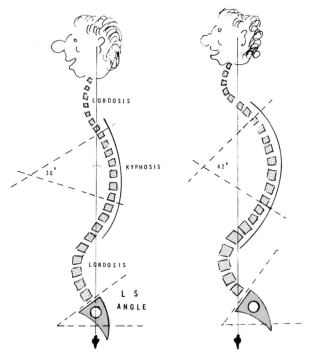

Fig. 20.2. Physiological curves of the spine. The four curves: cervical and lumbar lordosis and the dorsal-sacral kyphosis must transect the center of gravity. Increase of the lumbosacral angle increases all superincombent curves; 30–35° dorsal kyphosis is considered within "normal" range.

most deforming aspect of the scoliosis and, in the thoracic spine, the most responsible for cardiopulmonary difficulty.

As scoliosis is best treated by early recognition and prevention of lateral and rotatory changes, proper examination is mandatory. The child is examined from behind while adequately undressed and in the upright position. Both knees must be extended and the legs facing forward to reveal the true pelvic level. A short leg for any reason can cause pelvic obliquity with a superincumbent *functional* scoliosis. The cause of the leg length discrepancy can be revealed by thorough clinical and x-ray investigation (Fig. 20.6). Proper balance is discernible by suspending a plumb line from the spinous process of the seventh cervical vertebra and measuring the lateral deviation from the intergluteal fold.

With the patient bending forward to a right angle and viewed from behind, minor curves with or without early rotation can be readily discovered (Figs. 20.7 and 20.8). X-rays taken confirm the presence of the curve, the vertebral level of the curve and the measured degree of curving.

Treatment consists of early recognition, correction of existing curves and prevention of further progression. Upon discovering a curvature, treatment must be immediately considered. With current concepts of

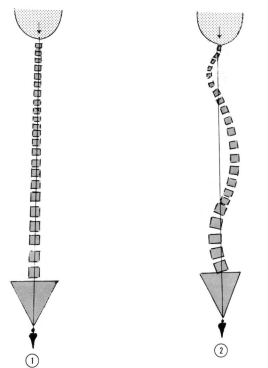

Fig. 20.3. Center of gravity: balanced curves. Normally (1) the occiput should be directly over the sacrum. In scoliosis (2) if all curves permit this alignment the curves are considered "balanced."

treatment, bracing and exercise is considered for any curve of 20° or more. A lesser degree of curving may suggest bracing if a rotatory component of any significance is present, as the thoracic rotational deformity of scoliosis is the most symptomatic. Surgical intervention is considered in a curve that exceeds 50°, is of a congenital etiology such as hemivertebrae, or is progressing in spite of adequate conservative nonsurgical treatment.

The details of bracing and the surgical intervention are well documented in the literature and not the concern of this presentation. Exercise with regard to scoliosis will be the basis of this presentation (5). It has been claimed that in the treatment of scoliosis exercises are an "exercise in futility." Exercises alone have not been considered to significantly alter the progression of scoliosis. Blount and Bolinske in 1967 stated the current thinking by stating: "Most orthopedic surgeons 'watched' the patients while the curves became tragically worse. For lack of any really effective program, some actually waited until the deformity became 'bad enough' to justify surgery. Many prescribed exercises during this watching period because they knew of nothing else to do. Physical therapists were frustrated by the lack of improvement. Eager patients became neurotic for the same reason and then completely bored by the ineffectual routine" (6).

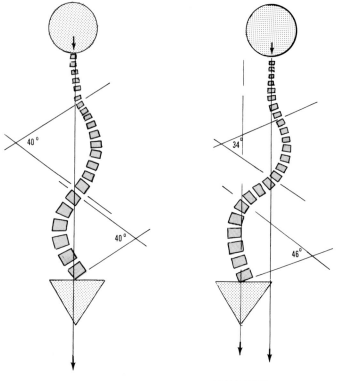

DOUBLE MAJOR
BALANCED

UNBALANCED

Fig. 20.4. Double major curves. Equal thoracic and lumbar curves with occiput remaining above the sacrum are "balanced" and less deforming. The right side curve is "unbalanced" and tends to progress more and are more difficult to treat.

Risser states: "It was customary at the scoliosis clinic at New York Orthopedic Hospital, as late as 1920 to 1930 to send the new patients with scoliosis to the gymnasium for exercises. Invariably the patients who were 12 to 13 years of age showed an increase of the scoliosis . . . it was therefore assumed that exercises and spinal motion made the curve increase" (7).

The early and most complete system of exercises for scoliosis were the creeping exercises devised by Klapp (8) in 1905. These exercises are still in vogue and are still considered effective so long as gravity is avoided. Unfortunately maintaining the prone or quadruped position throughout the remaining spinal growth is not feasible; thus concurrent bracing with exercises has remained necessary.

LeGrand-Lambling in the previous edition of this volume wrote an extensive review of exercises for scoliosis (9) and divided his program between exercises for functional and structural scoliosis. He also alluded to the detrimental effects of gravity by stating " . . . the aim of exercise

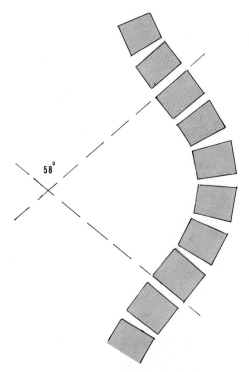

Fig. 20.5. Cobb method of measuring curves. A line is drawn perpendicular to the upper margin of the vertebra which inclines most toward the concavity. A line is also drawn on the inferior border of the lower vertebra that has the greatest angulation toward the concavity. The angle of these transecting lines constitutes the recorded degree of curvature.

therapy (in functional scoliosis) will not be to develop muscular forces to straighten curves, but to select an initial position to make them disappear. The object will be to avoid the reappearance of the deviation in the *standing position* (italics mine) by progressive reeducation of automatic and reflex mechanisms . . . ." LeGrand-Lambling expressed the concern that osteoarticular lesions tend to fix the lateral deviations and the associated rotation " . . . that is, to render them more or less reducible by passive maneuvers or the active motion . . . ."

In spite of the limited benefits attributed to exercises in scoliosis, the question of their value does not completely negate their being properly prescribed and utilized. Their greatest value is to—

1. Improve posture;
2. Increase flexibility (elongate the concave aspect of the spine and elongate soft tissue contractures);
3. Increase strength of abdominal muscles for posture;
4. Correct muscular imbalance; and
5. Improve respiration.

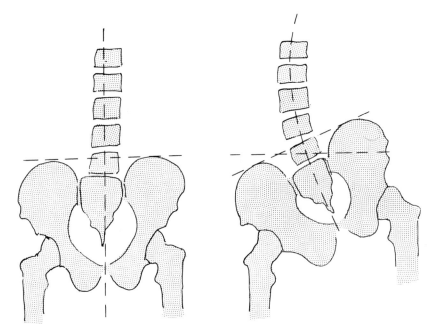

Fig. 20.6. Pelvic obliquity and functional scoliosis. The left sided figure pictures a balanced pelvis. The right figure depicts a short left leg with pelvic obliquity and a superimcumbent functional scoliosis.

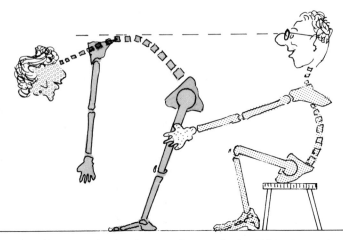

Fig. 20.7. Method of examination for scoliosis. With the patient standing and flexed forward 90°; legs extended and arms dangling the spine is examined by viewing directly from behind. This method frequently diagnoses curves not noted in the erect position.

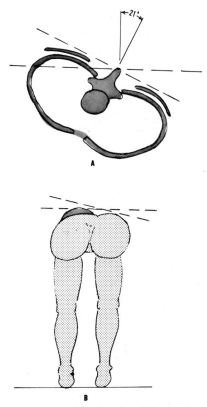

Fig. 20.8. Scoliosis noted by examination. Viewed from behind, the scoliosis is revealed as elevation of the rib on the convex side of the curve. This rotation may not be as noticeable as the erect posture.

Muscular imbalance has long been recognized as an etiological factor in idiopathic scoliosis and interest has recently been revived. Although no histological differences have been confirmed between the muscles on opposite sides of the scoliotic spine (10) there are histochemical (11), and neurophysiological differences (12). Histochemical studies have revealed a greater proportion of "slow twitch" muscular fibers as compared to "fast twitch" fibers on the convex side at the apex. These studies were done of the multifidus muscle which was found to be shorter on the convex than on the concave side. This paradoxical situation arises from the rotation of the vertebrae with lateral curving (Fig. 20.9).

"Slow twitch" muscle fibers are the dark (red) fibers that predominate in the dark muscles of many vertebrates except man whose muscles are mixed. They are used during sustained tonic activity such as postural functions, contract slowly, contain myoglobin, and, due to their metabolism, are resistant to fatigue. The "fast twitch" are light or "white",

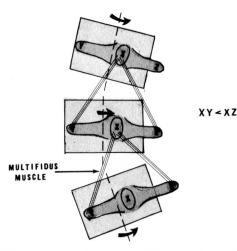

XY < XZ

MULTIFIDUS
MUSCLE

Fig. 20.9. Multifidus muscle shortening. The paradoxical shortening of the multifidus muscle on the convex side *XY* occurs because of the rotation of the vertebrae. The transverse process (*Y*) lies more posteriorly on the convex side and spinous process (*X*) deviates toward the convexity. The other erector spine muscles are *longer* on the convex side.

depend upon anaerobic metabolism, and therefore tire quickly during strenuous activity. They are used for short-term phasic activity.

"Slow twitch" muscles by virture of their physiology should shorten on the concave side of a curve to adapt to the shorter length. Recent studies have revealed a preponderance of slow fibers of shorter length on the *convex* side of the curve. These changes imply that the muscle changes are *not secondary* to the scoliosis but actually may be a primary causative factor.

Electromyographic studies have recently revealed hypersensitivity of the muscle spindle system on the concave side suggesting muscle imbalance as a possible causative factor in idiopathic scoliosis. As postural tone depends largely on stretch reflex in the extensor muscles this would be further implication of muscular etiology of scoliosis (12).

Although with current technique scoliosis cannot be controlled or improved with exercises alone, there is physiological basis for the belief that exercises have value in addition to other orthopedic measures of which the Milwaukee brace principle is an example.

Posture Exercise

Posture exercises are aimed at elongating the spine by decreasing the lumbar and cervical lordosis. In the growing child before the epiphyses close, the thoracic kyphosis can also be decreased.

The base of the spine that influences all superincumbant curves is the lumbosacral angle. The greater the angle the greater the lumbar lordosis;

and the converse is also true. To decrease the lumbar lordosis the lumbosacral angle must be decreased. To decrease the lumbosacral angle the anterior portion of the pelvis must be elevated and the posterior aspect depressed. The former is accomplished by the abdominal muscles and the latter by the gluteal and posterior thigh muscles.

The proprioceptive concept of pelvic motion, however, requires a sensory function secondary to muscular contraction. The "feeling" of "pelvic tilting" is far more valuable than merely strengthening the participating muscles. This function is trained by a supine exercise. With the patient lying supine, hips and knees flexed, the (1) low back is pressed to the floor (or treatment table) (2) is held there while the (3) buttocks is smoothly and rhythmically elevated from the floor (Fig. 20.10). The buttocks must *not* be elevated to a degree that would cause the low back to arise from the floor.

As this pelvic tilting movement is learned it is continued with the legs becoming increasingly more extended until both the hips and knees are fully extended.

Then in the erect posture this exercise is done with the back against a wall simulating the surface of the floor (Fig. 20.11). As this exercise is

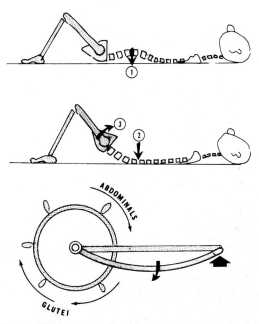

Fig. 20.10. "Pelvic tilting" exercise. Exercises to decrease the lumbar lordosis are done in sequence. With hips and knees flexed the low back (1) is pressed against the floor and held there (2). The pelvis (3) is then slowly raised. This action performed by the abdominal, hamstring and gluteal muscles decreases the lordosis and gives the patient the "feeling" of the pelvic motion.

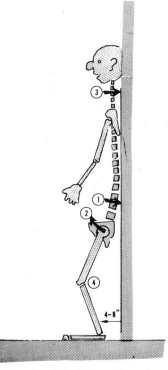

Fig. 20.11. Erect position of pelvic tilting. Leaning against a wall the low back (1) is pressed to the wall. The pelvis is "tilted" anteriorly (2) decreasing the lumbar lordosis. The neck is also pressed to the wall (3) decreasing the cervical lordosis and elongating the spine. The knees are flexed and the feet placed 4–8 inches from the wall. As this exercise becomes easier, the feet are placed closer to the wall and the knees are extended.

performed the neck is gradually added to the exercise along with the low back. The cervical lordosis is decreased by the neck being forced against the table or wall.

Should the concept of lumbar curve decrease be difficult for the patient to understand, a preliminary exercise in the prone quadriceps position can be performed (Fig. 20.12). With the patient on all fours, the low back is "arched" and rhythmically depressed. This undulating motion of the spine (lumbar kyphosis alternating with lumbar lordosis) can be reinforced by manual resistance or by the addition of a weight placed on the lumbar spine.

During all pelvic tilting exercises, either supine or erect, the chest must be repeatedly expanded in a deep breathing exercise.

As the abdominal muscles play a vital function in pelvic tilting they must be strengthened. The utilizable strength, however, is that of *isometric* contraction for sustained contraction and thus for endurance rather than phasic strength. Endurance gained by sustained isometric contraction is performed by the "sit up" position from the *flexed* posture to gradually lowering the trunk and holding the newly acquired position for varying periods of time (Fig. 20.13).

Decrease of the dorsal kyphosis is also desirable. This is an exercise performed in the prone position in which the upper back is hyperextended while the lumbar lordosis is kept at a minimum. With the pelvis "tilted" the head and shoulders are raised against resistance. "Push ups" performed while the pelvis is kept "tilted" are also prescribed.

"Distraction" has proven effective in elongating the spine, improving the erect posture by indoctrinating the patient in the "feeling of proper posture" with no concentration on the muscles involved. This is the concept of "standing tall" and can be done by manually pressing down on the patient's head while he or she attempts to push "up" against the hand. A weighted bag placed on the head and balanced can be used instead of the therapist's hand and permits the patient to walk, stand or sit in the sustained erect posture (Fig. 20.14).

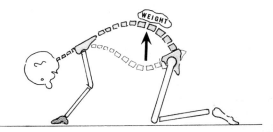

Fig. 20.12. Prone "pelvic tilting" exercise. In patients who experience difficulty in "tilting their pelvis" the quadriped position is assumed. The low back is arched and lowered—with or without a superimposed weight. Pelvic tilting is accomplished as is greater flexibility of the lumbar spine.

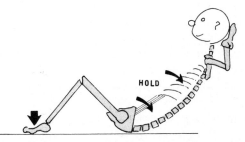

Fig. 20.13. Isometric abdominal exercise. To develop endurance and the "feeling" of abdominal contraction the patient goes from full sit-up position and leans back then sustains that position. Gradually the reclining degree is increased as is the duration of the sustained position.

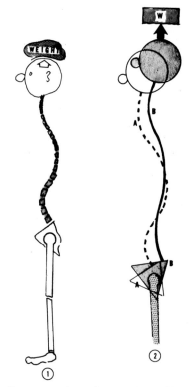

Fig. 20.14. Distraction exercises for posture. By attempting to elevate a weight placed on the head (1) all the curves of the vertebral column approach the center of gravity. (2) The cervical and lumbar lordoses (A) are decreased (B) as the pelvis "tilts" (A to B).

Increase Flexibility

These are exercises of "stretch" that can be considered to be related to "asymmetrical" exercises. The creeping exercises of Klapp stress stretching and elongation of the vertebral column. The EDF (elongation, derotation, and lateral flexion) technique of Cotrel relates to increasing flexibility and employment of exercises combined with traction (13).

General stretching exercises can be performed in the prone position. With the body in straight alignment with arms extended overhead and both legs fully extended, the back can be gradually arched fully, held there for a period of time then lowered to the floor (Fig. 20.15).

In the prone position, crawling can elongate the spine. Reaching forward (overhead) with one arm and simultaneously stretching the ipsilateral leg distally stretching that side of the spine. This can be termed "dry swimming." The same exercise can be performed in the four legged (quadriped position). With the patient on all fours the arm can reach forward in a horizontal direction and the opposite leg stretched toward the rear. Crawling exercises depicted in Figure 20.16 laterally flex the spine.

Merely standing erect and bending laterally as far as possible can stretch the spinal column in that direction.

As most scoliosis has segmental curving exercise that would elongate that segmental curve should be beneficial. Most exercises, however, are

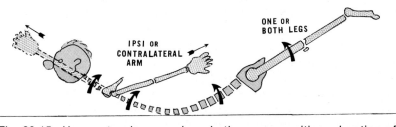

Fig. 20.15. Hyperextension exercises. In the prone position, elevation of the head and shoulders extend the upper spine. Elevating the legs extend the lumbar area. Elevation of one leg and the ipsilateral arm asymmetrically extend the spine and can correct lateral curving. The arm(s) can be held behind the body or overhead: as tolerated.

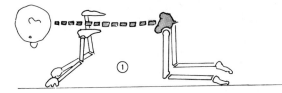

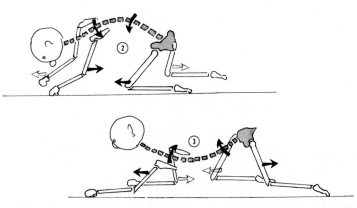

Fig. 20.16. Crawling exercises. The starting position (1) is the quadriped posture. As the right leg is extended with simultaneous overhead extension of the right arm, the spine is lateral flexed causing it to convex to the right. The opposite movement occurs (3) if the opposite arm and leg are extended.

more general and do not have specific segmental effect. Exercises performed in a brace about the restraining contact of a pad can be more specifically localized.

Lateral flexion and derotation of the thoracic spine can be accomplished in the following exercise. The patient kneels on the floor with buttocks on the heels then leaning forward until the abdomen rests on the thighs; this position immobilizes the lumbar spine (Fig. 20.17). The patient then stretches the arms overhead (horizontal to the floor) and places both hands on the floor. The head is now between the outstretched arms. In this position the hands are "walked" as far to one side as possible. This stretches and derotates the thoracic spine and can be performed to the right or the left as indicated.

In the prone position on a treatment table the patient can grasp the sides of the table which immobilizes the thoracic spine. A therapist or a trained member of the family can grasp both feet, bring both legs to one side then the other, and laterally stretch the spine by pulling the extended legs laterally as far as tolerated.

Within the Milwaukee brace, exercises are specifically performed to diminish the major curve by reducing the major posterior hump and forcing out the opposite anterior thoracic depression. With the pelvis tilted to decrease lumbar lordosis, the patient "pulls away" from the posterior pad applied against the apex of the hump (on the convex side of the curve). After deep inhalation the thoracic spine is pressed backward

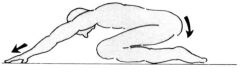

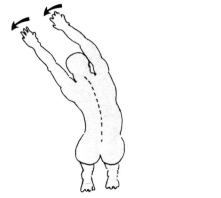

Fig. 20.17. EDF exercises. In the above position of the patient sitting on his feet the lumbar is immobilized. The overhead extended arms permit the fingers to "walk" to the left (or the right). This exercises lateral stretches and derotates the thoracic spine.

against the upright bars of the brace (Fig. 20.18). The rib hump on the convex side contacts the pad, resisting further movement and thus causing the spine to rotate. The forward shallow thoracic spine (on the side of the posterior hump) moves forward.

All exercises done within the brace must avoid an increase in lumbar lordosis and must be sustained to impart the sensation of the movement to the patient.

Cotrel advocates EDF exercises for the patient in treatment with his form of traction (13). The traction is applied actively by the patient. Within the traction, as the patient's legs are extended force is applied to the foot pads that exert traction upon the head halter. The spine is thus

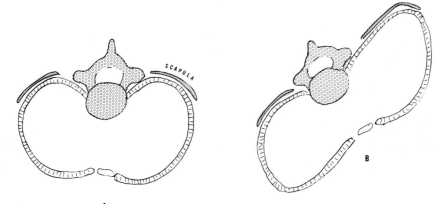

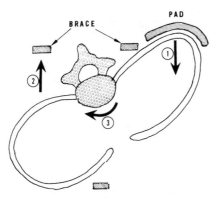

Fig. 20.18. Milwaukee brace exercises. The *upper figures* depict: (A) the normal rib contour in the straight spine; in scoliosis (B) lateral curving is compounded by vertebral rotation and rib deformity. In the brace (*lower figure*), the exercises are for the patient to "pull" his rib hump away from the pad (1) simultaneously press back against the opposite upright of the brace (2). These motions tend to derotate the spine (3) and decrease the rib cage deformity.

elongated (Fig. 20.19). The length of the rope must be carefully adjusted to assure that the patient receives maximal yet tolerable stretch. By extending the legs in a lateral direction, to the left or the right of the traction table, lateral spinal stretching can be achieved.

Improvement of Respiration

In thoracic curves of 50° or more and with significant rotation, respiratory difficulty is frequent. The decrease in vital capacity has been related proportionately to the degree of scoliosis (14). Treatment of scoliosis regardless of the method or technique must consider this aspect. Exercises for improving flexibility, posture and derotation of curves must include respiratory exercises.

Exercise usually prescribed for pulmonary disease emphasizes the conditions of asthma and emphysema with respect to teaching relaxation. This aspect of respiratory difficulty is not frequently noted in structural scoliosis so it will not be emphasized (15). Posture is also stressed in exercise for respiratory impairment. Rib cage immobility noted in older emphysema patients is also noted in scoliosis patients, but for different etiological reasons.

The rib cage excursion in scoliosis is limited due to angulation of the rib and the costovertebral articulation. Increased range of motion of the ribs must be attempted. The auxiliary muscles of respiration, the scalenes, may be shortened on the concave side of the neck and can be elongated by gradually and frequently forcing the head laterally with the hands away from the restricted side. This may be done by the patient or to the patient by a therapist. Cervical vertical traction also can elongate the neck and stretch these auxiliary respiratory muscles.

The scapulocostal articulation must be fully mobilized. Overhead arm elevation, clasping the hands together in the back and moving them away from the body, placing the hands behind the head and gradually bringing the elbows posteriorly, and full elevation and depression of the arms: all these exercises mobilize the scapulae.

Excursion of the lower rib cage must be increased. This can be accomplished by deep breathing exercise while manually resisting the rib cage excursion. Direct manual pressure can be applied to the lower rib cage bilaterally or unilaterally. If general rib cage excursion is desired, both sides of the rib cage can be restricted simultaneously. If the right rib cage requires expansion, the left side of the rib cage is restricted, causing the opposite side to expand further.

Resistance to the rib cage can be applied by placing a wide belt about the thoracic area crossing in front of the body and held by the patient's hands. By pulling the belt with both hands (Fig. 20.20), general restriction occurs; pulling the belt with the left hand applied pressure to the right side of the rib cage, and vice versa.

Patients have the tendency to develop thoracic breathing with little

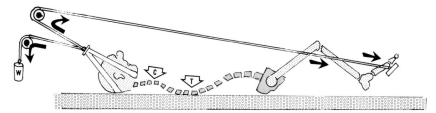

Fig. 20.19. Cotrel traction. As the traction is connected, gradual extension of the legs cause increased cervical traction and elongation of the spine. The force is applied by the patient who had supervised control.

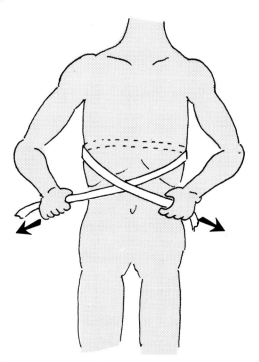

Fig. 20.20. Respiratory resistive exercise. A belt placed about the lower portion of the rib cage exerts corrective pressure upon the rib cage and segmentally resists respiration. By pulling with the right hand the left lower rib cage is prevented from expanding during deep inspiration and thus the right lower rib cage protrudes. The opposite action also can be performed.

diaphragmatic breathing. This often occurs in normal people, but it must not be permitted in scoliosis patients. Instruction in proper abdominothoracic breathing involves the following sequence:

1. Patient assumes the supine position with knees and hips flexed;
2. The rib cage is prevented from moving by concentration by the patient;
3. As the patient inspires, the abdomen should protrude. This can be witnessed

visually or manually and can be reinforced by placing a sand bag on the abdomen;

4. On deep expiration the abdomen retracts to its maximum;
5. Gradually the combination of abdominothoracic breathing is initiated; after a slow gradual abdominal inspiration (with protrusion of the abdomen) the rib cage is fully expanded; as the expiration follows, the abdomen retracts and the rib cage depresses;
6. Slow exercises of inspiration and expiration are practiced; the expiration phase is usually twice the length of inspiration; and
7. Abdominothoracic breathing practiced in the supine position is then attempted in sitting then the standing position.

Correction of Muscular Imbalance

Of the numerous etiologies of scoliosis there are some that are secondary to neuromuscular disease and are related to muscular imbalance. These include anterior poliomyelitis, spinocerebellar degenerative disease, muscular dystrophy, and other neuromuscular diseases. A careful muscle evaluation can detect the weakness or imbalance. Resistive exercises for the particular muscle group involved can be prescribed. Exercises of the extremities may be related, but usually are not significant. Trunk muscles are more involved.

The abdominal exercises have been discussed. If there is asymmetry in that the right obliques are weaker than the left, the flexion exercises can be performed by concommitant trunk rotation or lateral flexion with trunk flexion. The same position of the "sit up" exercise is assumed, but the trunk is rotated or flexed to strengthen the weaker side.

The extensor muscles must also be strengthened and, as for the flexors, if asymmetry occurs the strengthening of the weaker side must be

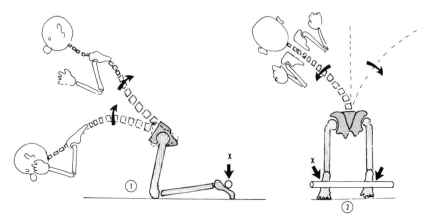

Fig. 20.21. Resistive extension exercise. In the kneeling position with the feet held down under a bar or furniture (1) the back can be straightened by slowly arising to a more erect posture. Asymmetrical strengthening can be accomplished (2) by incorporating lateral flexion as well as extension in the exercises.

stressed. Extension exercises may be performed by lying prone and raising the head and shoulders from the floor to strengthen the upper extensors. By raising the legs simultaneously, the lower extensors are strengthened. By raising one leg from the floor, the ipsilateral trunk extensors are strengthened. This asymmetrical extensor strengthening exercise can be further enhanced by elevating the overhead outstretched arm on the same side as the extended leg (see Fig. 20.15).

Resistance to extensor exercises can be added to the program by using the patient's body weight. In the kneeling position and the feet held to the floor by weights or by being placed under a piece of furniture, the patient can slowly arise from the fully flexed position to the full erect kneeling position (Fig. 20.21). Here, also, by simultaneous lateral flexion or rotation of the trunk asymmetrical stress of the weaker side can be accomplished.

REFERENCES

1. CAILLIET, R. *Scoliosis: Diagnosis and Management.* F. A. Davis Co., Philadelphia, 1975.
2. ROAF, R. Vertebral growth and its mechanical control. *J. Bone Joint Surg., 42B:* 40–59, 1960.
3. ENNEKING, W. F., AND HARRINGTON, P. Pathological changes in scoliosis. *J. Bone Joint Surg., 51A:* 165–184, 1969.
4. COBB, J. R. The problem of the primary curve. *J. Bone Joint Surg., 42A:* 1413–1425, 1960.
5. ARKIN, A. M. Correction of structural changes in scoliosis by corrective plaster jackets and prolonged recumbency. *J. Bone Joint Surg., 46A:* 32–52, 1964.
6. BLOUNT, W. P., AND BOLINSKE, J. Physical therapy in the nonoperative treatment of scoliosis. *Phys. Ther., 47:* 919–925, 1967.
7. RISSER, J. C. Scoliosis; past and present. *J. Bone Joint Surg., 46A:* 167–199, 1964.
8. KLAPP, B. *Das Klapp'sche Kriechverfahren.* Georg Thieme Verlag, Stuttgart, 1966.
9. LeGrand-Lambling, Y. Exercises for Scoliosis. In *Therapeutic Exercises,* Ch. 21, Ed. 2, edited by S. Licht. Elizabeth Licht, New Haven, 1965.
10. JAMES, J. I. P., LLOYD-ROBERTS, G. C., AND PILCHER, M. F. Infantile structural scoliosis. *J. Bone Joint Surg., 41B:* 719–735, 1959.
11. FIDLER, M. W., AND JOWETT, R. L. Muscle imbalance in the aetiology of scoliosis. *J. Bone Joint Surg., 58B:* 200–201, 1976.
12. HOOGMARTENS, M. J., AND BASMAJIAN, J. V. Postural tone in the deep spinal muscles of idiopathic scoliosis patients and their siblings. *Electromyogr. Clin. Neurophysiol., 16:* 93–114, 1976.
13. LaBRECHE, B. G., LEVANGIE, P. K., AND SHARBY, N. H. Cotrel traction; a new approach to the preoperative management of idiopathic scoliosis. *Phys. Ther., 54:* 837–842, 1974.
14. COLLIS, D. K., AND PONSETI, I. Long term follow up of patients with idiopathic scoliosis not treated surgically. *J. Bone Joint Surg., 51A:* 425–445, 1969.
15. SINCLAIR, J. D. Exercises in Pulmonary Disease. Chapt. 22, In *Therapeutic Exercise,* Ch. 22, Ed. 2, edited by S. Licht. Elizabeth Licht, New Haven, 1965.

21

Exercise in Sports Medicine

_____ FRED L. ALLMAN

Sports medicine is the study of problems and the application of solutions to them as they relate to the physiological, psychological, and pathological nature of the athlete. It involves sports, but it is not limited to organized athletics; it involves medicine, but it is not limited to injuries. Sports medicine concerns itself with the health implication of the organism in physical activity; thus, sports medicine spans the gamut from the highly trained athlete who is endowed with sufficient skill and physique to participate in modern competitive athletics with great intensity and diversity to the neophyte "little leaguer" who often lacks skill and physique and who might play in the vacant lot without any supervision.

The assumptions to which sports medicine subscribes require the interpretation and refinement that only competent research activity can offer. They also require application to the individual of the appropriate decisions that only a competent practitioner can make. Sports medicine thus has a task of linking research and practice.

Sports medicine requires a team: various professions, each with its own responsibilities, cooperate with mutual understanding and respect, while physicians, dentists, educators, athletic trainers, biological scientists, and behavioral scientists comprise most of sports medicine's professional reservoir.

Sports medicine differs from other forms of medicine in a number of ways. The attainment and maintenance of high levels of physical readiness required of top athletes produces significant effects on the working of the human organism. This high level of physical fitness or physical readiness often so alters the physiological makeup of the individual that his response to injury or disease actually differs from that of the non-athlete. The same process by which physical readiness is achieved may give rise to pathological conditions of one form or another which may fall outside the scope of "normal" clinical practice.

Practicing physicians often are so concerned with the grossly subnormal that the supernormal, when it is only slightly disabled, is apt to receive scant attention. Yet, to the athlete himself, even a slight disability might mean the difference between playing or sitting on the bench, or between winning and losing.

A sprained wrist would hardly incapacitate the banker but would be certain to alter the performance of a pole vaulter. Similarly, a businessman might be able to transact business nearly as usual with a strained hamstring muscle, while the hurdler, running back, or flanker would have his performance altered appreciably.

Also, it should be remembered that, in addition to his office, the doctor who treats athletic injuries must include observations of the athlete in the gymnasium or on the playing field as an integral part of the evaluation. It is there that function can best be determined and unless there is a complete return of function, performance is likely to be altered.

Another very important difference between sports medicine and other forms of medicine exists because injuries which are sustained during athletic participation are usually produced by circumstances inherent in respective athletic performance and they are therefore characterized by exposure to recurrent identical trauma, making reinjury likely. Therefore, in conditioning for athletic participation, and in rehabilitation following injury, the ultimate goal must be complete normal function to the greatest possible degree and in the shortest possible time.

Two Classifications of Exercise in Sports Medicine

Exercises that are utilized in sports medicine may be either *conditioning* or *rehabilitative*. Many of the exercises in each of these categories are the same – the biggest difference being in the intensity of the exercise. Conditioning exercise should be as intense as possible while rehabilitative exercises must necessarily be much less intense, especially in the early stages. Rehabilitative exercises must also consider the condition for which the rehabilitation has been prescribed, and therefore the exercise must be administered within the limits imposed by the existing status of the individual. The kinetic hazards imposed by the exercise must also be considered. Conditioning exercises are utilized to attain and maintain a high level of physical readiness which is required of top athletes in order that significant effect on the working of the human organism are affected. Rehabilitative exercises are designed to restore function to the greatest possible degree and in the shortest possible time and again, to attain and maintain high levels of physical readiness.

Conditioning Exercises for Sports Participation

THE PURPOSE OF CONDITIONING

Bilik (5) has stated that the primary objective of intensive conditioning is to "put the body with extreme and exceptional care under the influence of all the agents which promote its health and strength in order to enable it to meet extreme and exceptional demands upon it. Training aims to condition the muscles, the heart, the lungs, the joints, the nervous system, the mind, the whole body, every tissue and every cell, to function at maximum possible efficiency and to stand up under the most gruelling stress and strain." The primary purpose of conditioning, then, is to promote physical fitness and sports fitness.

Physical fitness, while important for every individual, is essential for the athlete. Physical fitness helps the athlete to enjoy physical activity. Physical fitness sustains learning skills. Physical fitness enhances excellence. Physical fitness decreases the chance of injury, and physical fitness helps to speed recovery following injury.

General Principles of Conditioning

A. ESTABLISH A GOAL

The goal of a conditioning program (1) should be to achieve optimum or near optimum fitness. The proper utilization of exercises is undoubtedly the single most important factor for the prevention of sports injuries. Proper exercise increase strength, cardiovascular endurance, and flexibility.

B. SELECT THE PROPER PROGRAM

Select a conditioning program that will develop all parts of the body with special emphasis on areas of greatest need based upon the demands of the sport. Do not overemphasize any one area or aspect. No single sport, no single exercise, and no single piece of apparatus provides total balanced development for all parts of the body. Optimum fitness requires balance.

C. WARM-UP PRINCIPLES

Always warm up. Calisthenics such as side straddle hop and running in place are good warm-up exercises. The warm-up not only prepares the body for the forthcoming increased activity, but also is a good way to detect areas of stiffness and discomfort prior to beginning the exercise program. Darling and Downey (8) have stated, "the temperature of the muscles rises during work in spite of the efficient circulation. This is probably advantageous to muscular function. The optimum for the speed of chemical reaction and metabolism is 102–103° F. There is some evidence that the speed, strength, and efficiency of contractions are enhanced by a rise in the temperature of muscle toward this range. The only efficient method of raising muscle temperature is by work of the muscle itself."

Recent studies seem to indicate that many people who engage in sudden severe exercise may have irregularities of the heart as opposed to exercise after a warm-up period. Scientists at the University of California at Los Angeles School of Medicine have demonstrated that warming up your heart before strenuous exercise increases your circulation to the heart muscle. Also, the blood pressure was found to increase abnormally when strenuous exercise was done without a warm-up period. Abnormal electrocardiograms were found after sudden exertion but in all cases the changes were less marked or did not occur at all if the subjects warmed up for 15–20 min prior to being exposed to severe exertion.

D. EXERCISE TOLERANCE

Each training should be adapted to the individual's tolerance level. Exercise tolerance is the level at which the body responds to exercise favorably. The exercise level should not be so high that the body has not fully recuperated in 24 hours or less. Alteration of work and rest is best and should be adapted to one's ability to recover. If the exercise is too easy it will fall short of the tolerance level; if too demanding it will exceed tolerance level and cause possible damage.

E. PROGRESSIVE OVERLOADS

The training plan must provide for progression until a high performance level or optimum fitness is achieved. In order to improve performance, overload is necessary. Overload is extending the work level beyond usual physical effort. This is achieved by exercising longer or with greater intensity than usual, or both. In the early stages of conditioning, a higher proportion of slow, long-continued endurance work is favored over speed work. Later as the physiological mechanisms adjust to the work load, the proportion of speed work to slow work is increased.

F. DOSAGE

In order to obtain a good cardiovascular response, the heart rate during the exercise period should reach a peak rate of at least 70% of its capable range. Cooper (7) has laid down two basic principles in this regard: 1) "If the exercise is vigorous enough to produce a sustained heart rate of 150 beats per minute or more, the training effect benefits begin about five minutes after the exercise starts and continue as long as the exercise is performed," and 2) If the exercise is not vigorous enough to produce or sustain a heart rate of 150 beats per minute but is still demanding oxygen, the exercise must be continued considerably longer than five minutes, the total period of time depending on the oxygen consumed." It therefore becomes obvious that the dosage necessary to produce a training effect will depend upon the state of the individual. The poorly conditioned individual may obtain a training benefit with relatively little intensity of exercise, whereas he increases the dosage and intensity as he becomes better conditioned in order to achieve the training benefit.

G. RECUPERATION

Following vigorous exercise, it is best to keep moving and not to sit down. Sitting or assuming the recumbent position allows for pooling of large amounts of blood in the lower extremity, thus depriving the heart of sufficient return of blood. This, in turn, can lead to syncope and other more serious disorders. It is much wiser to cool down slowly while continuing with some upright movement such as walking.

H. RECORDS

Records are essential if the individual is to progress optimally. Progress should be noted to be rising and rhythmic although time trials should not always indicate continued improvement. Even the gifted athlete cannot peak each week. It therefore becomes necessary to select certain key dates or events in which it is desirable to peak, and the conditioning should be directed toward those particular events.

I. MOTIVATION

Motivation is all-important. Ultimate success in any conditioning program depends to a large degree on motivation. Those individuals and teams who are able to maintain a high degree of motivation are likely to succeed. Those without motivation are almost certain to fail. The greatest motivation of all seems to be the desire for improvement, the desire to be better tomorrow than today, the desire to achieve competitive greatness.

General Principles of Basic Sports Fitness

Doherty (9) has noted the following basic sports fitness principles.

1. The hard core of basic sports fitness cannot be gained completely through the action of the event itself.

2. The hard core of basic sports fitness develops gradually over a period of years.

3. The basic fitness work should always be supplementary.

4. The basic fitness work should always include the practice of skills of many sports, even though they seem unrelated to one's special event. This is especially important during the early years of training and during the months of "active rest" from each year of training. Other sports are basic training in skill learning.

5. Basic sports training must be continuous.

6. The intensity of basic sports training must be varied (rising and rhythmic).

7. Basic sports training must be individualized. Broer (6) has stated, "The amount of daily exercise that is needed to reach and maintain physical efficiency at the highest attainable level is still determined mostly by observation or empirical methods. Experiments show that a daily amount of practice which is suitable for an individual is either too much or too little for others. They also demonstrate that regardless of the physical capacity of a given subject, there is a level of exercise which frequently repeated will lead to chronic fatigue 'staleness.'"

Specific Factors to Be Included in a Balanced Conditioning Program

Conditioning work is both general and special. General conditioning refers to total body development. Special conditioning concentrates on exercises and drills to develop the muscle groups for a special event in which the athlete wishes to concentrate. There are a number of specific factors that are necessary to include in a conditioning program if total fitness is to be achieved.

A. STRENGTH

Progressive Resistive Exercise

In 1945 scientific experimentation in clinical application by DeLorme proved that the best way to build muscular strength and endurance was a program of progressive resistive exercise. This has been confirmed many times in the last 30 years. More recently, Jones (13) has proved that with properly performed progressive resistive exercise an increased range of motion and improved flexibility is not only possible but also highly desirable. This is because injury is far less likely when flexibility has improved as much as possible in association with good strength.

Muscle Tension

Baer et al (3) concluded from a study they conducted that neither total work done nor power in the physical sense is a major factor in determining the improvement of muscular strength. They contended that the common denominator which explains strength improvement is the tension developed by the muscle during exercise. Earlier studies by others demonstrated that the tension which a muscle produces during contraction decreases as the speed of shortening increases. Thus, in isotonic exercise greatest tension is developed at a slower rate rather than a faster rate of contraction, thereby establishing a condition which is conducive to greater improvement in muscular strength. Muscles must be put under tension in order for them to develop strength. Strength is obtained by loading muscles and pressing activity to the threshholds of fatigue. This may be accomplished by the use of isometrics, isotonics, or isokinetic exercise. Isometric contractions are those in which no shortening takes place in the muscles. The joints do not move in the direction of the contraction and no actual work is done. Isotonic contractions are those in which the involved muscle shortens under load with the result of production of work. Isokinetic exercises are those in which joint motion occurs at a controlled rate. McCloy (15) writing on the mechanical analysis of motor skills has stated that the first prerequisite for the economical learning of a skill is sufficient strength to perform the task. Hellebrandt and Houtz (11), reporting on the overload principle, stated that the limits of performance must be persistently extended to improve muscle strength and that the rate of improving depends upon the willingness of the subject to overload.

Maximum Intensity of Contractions

The maximum intensity of contraction is produced when the highest possible percentage of the muscular mass is involved at a given moment, and certain factors are required to produce this situation. Good form, or the style of performance, is very important if maximum benefit is to be obtained with the progressive resistive exercise. Proper form includes the speed of movement, the range of movement, and beginning the movement from a pre-stretched position. Also the resistance should be moved in a smooth fashion and briefly stopped in the position of full muscular contraction. Jerking movements should be avoided.

1. The speed of movement must not be too fast or too slow. If it takes 2–3 sec to raise the weight, then it should take 4–5 sec to lower that same weight.

2. The range of movement must be great as possible. Prevention of injury is most likely when the muscles have been strengthened in every position and over full range of possible movement.

3. The movement must start from a pre-stretched position. Pre-stretching is involved when a relaxed muscle is pulled into position of increased tension prior to the start of contraction. Pre-stretching properly applied enables one to handle heavier weight and thus bring into action a greater percentage of the muscle mass during the repetition. For example, the weight should be lowered from the contracted position in a controlled manner until the bar or resistance arm is about one inch from the position of full stretch. At that point there should be a very quick "twitch" or "thrust." Immediately the quick "twitch," the movement should be slowed down in a controlled manner. The only rapid movement of the bar or the resistance arm should be during the first postion of the raising (positive) part of the repetition. The remaining portion of each repetition should always be smoothly performed.

4. The load must be heavy enough to require maximum intensity of contraction. High intensity exercise requires the repetitive performances of a resistive movement that is carried to the point of momentary muscular failure. When performing high intensity exercise, at least 8 repetitions should be performed and usually not more than 12–15. If 8 repetitions cannot be completed, then the resistance is too high and if one can perform more than 12–15, it is too light. Consider the set complete when it is momentarily impossible to perform another full repetition in good form. High intensity contraction must be practiced on an infrequent basis, with adequate allowance for total recovery between training sessions (must not work too long or too often). Total recovery from a high intensity training session may require as much as 48 hours. (During the early stages of rehabilitation, the intensity of the work is so low that training is possible on a daily basis. Later, as the intensity increases, the workouts are reduced to three times per week and during in-season training to only twice per week.)

5. The sequence of exercise in which the various muscle groups are to be worked should be such that the largest muscle group is worked first, proceeding down to the smallest group last. Working the large muscles first causes the greatest growth stimulus. Also, it is sometimes impossible

to reach the required condition of momentary muscular exhaustion while working large muscle groups if the system has been previously exhausted by exercises for other small muscle.

B. ENDURANCE

Systemic or general endurance involves the sustaining of activity in many of the large muscles of the body and is usually called cardiovascular respiratory endurance. Local endurance refers to the ability to sustain or repeat contraction in a single muscle or group of muscles. Cardiovascular endurance is the ability of the heart to perform more work than is usual more economically for prolonged periods and the heart's ability to recover quickly upon cessation of the activity. An efficient cardiovascular system is capable of adjusting the flow of blood in order to supply oxygen to the necessary tissues and to remove chemical by-products produced in muscle contraction. Exercise requires more oxygen to be delivered to the working muscle. The increased amount of oxygen is delivered by the circulation— this is a basic important concept. Unless the exercise requires a greater delivery of oxygen to the body, it will have little or no effect in maintaining the functional capacity of the heart and circulation. Aerobic exercises are those in which there is adequate oxygen intake. Anaerobic exercises are those in which there is inadequate oxygen intake or a gradual increase in oxygen intake or a gradually increasing oxygen debt. Only when you extend yourself is optimum effect from cardiovascular training achieved. Optimum effect is not readily achieved, in other words, if all training efforts are within the submaximal or aerobic capacity range. The body is capable of adapting specifically to imposed demands. In order to be of benefit in improving cardiovascular fitness, the organs need to be "stressed." Thus, anaerobic work becomes a part of the aerobic training, and this is the basis of a training which is known as "interval training" (alternately stress and nonstress work). Improving endurance is primarily a matter of building resistance to the many effects of fatigue (production of lactic acid, lowered oxygen supply to the muscles, decreased sensitivity of muscle fibers to stimuli, etc.). This is done by gradually increasing, as the training effect improves, the amount of work that is done during each exercise period. The upper limits of endurance training are still unknown. Bannister, because of the disappointment of defeat at the Helsinki Olympics in 1952, increased his work load severalfold and set a world record when he ran the first less than 4-min mile on May 6, 1954. Snell's training included approximately 5 times the amount of work that Bannister's training included and he soon lowered the record. Before training, Bannister's resting heart rate was over 70 beats per minute. At the time he broke the world record, his resting heart rate was below 40 beats per minute.

Balke (4) has reported on the seminomadic Tarahumara Indians in the northwestern region of Mexico. These people have not only adapted to the stresses of a relatively high elevation of their habitat, of rapid changes between hot and cold temperatures, and of their apparently inadequate nutrition, but have also accomplished unbelievable performances in running. Reports indicate that these people have run a distance of 600 miles in a 5-day period. Actual observations have shown that the winners of the typical kick ball races ran 125 miles, nearly continuously. The energy expenditure in such a race should amount to more than 15,000 kcal over a 24-hour period.

C. METABOLIC CONDITION

Metabolic condition is the ability to work at a high level of intensity for a prolonged period of time. In developing circulatory efficiency, Lamb (14) has pointed out that this is achieved through gradual conditioning of complex reflex mechanisms. The development of the nerve pathways that enable shutting down the arteries to one part of the body and opening those to others requires time and training, just as it requires time to train the nerve mechanism to be a sprinter. The fact that the legs are trained for circulatory efficiency does not mean that some other part of the body is trained for circulatory efficiency.

In order to obtain metabolic condition, every exercise must be continued to a point of momentary muscular failure within a limited number of repetitions, usually 8–12. The larger muscle groups are worked first. Very little in the way of rest can be permitted between exercises and the total elapsed training time during each workout should be no less than 15 min or no more than 45. These workouts must be conducted at a somewhat slower fashion initially, with brief rest intervals between each exercise.

However, as training continues from week to week, the pace of the training should be increased, so that after 4–6 weeks little or no rest is permitted between exercises. At that point in the training program the subject should move from one exercise to the next exercise as rapidly as possible with very little rest between exercises. Such training greatly improves both strength and cardiovascular endurance while being essential to promoting metabolic condition.

A recent study at the United States Military Academy at West Point, New York, indicates that such a training program does in fact induce metabolic changes that are capable of improving strength and cardiovascular endurance simultaneously and at levels which have seldom been produced in such a short period of time with any other previously known methods.

D. FLEXIBILITY

Flexibility is the ability to yield to passive stretch and to relax. Flexibility training is designed to increase the range of motion of the joints. This process requires the stretching of the tissues, especially connective tissue, beyond the normal limit and sometimes to the point of discomfort. Flexibility or suppleness is desirable to facilitate muscular action with minimal resistance to the tissues. When connective tissue is not actively stretched, it periodically shortens. Flexibility is necessary in order to obtain perfection of movement and perfection of movement is necessary to achieve peak performance.

In 1968 Holland (12) presented a review of the research literature pertaining to flexibility. Among the generalizations drawn from the studies were the following:

1. Little agreement was found with regard to the definition and limits of so-called normal flexibility and in what constitutes hypo- or hyperflexible range of motion.

2. General agreement existed that flexibility is a highly specific factor and that measurement of one of several body joints cannot be used to validly predict range of motion in other body parts.

3. In the intact joint, the connective tissues principally responsible for resistance to movement are, respectively, muscle, ligament, joint, capsule, and tendon. It is reasonable to assume that the myotatic stretch reflex significantly effects the role which muscle plays in relation to joint movements. Elastic connective tissue is more resilient during joint excursion than is collagenous tissue.

4. Insufficient data were evident comparing the efficacy of ballistic and static stretching in improving joint mobility, but probably less danger of connective tissue trauma may exist with static stretching.

5. Two kinds of flexibility may exist—one that is functionally dynamic and one that can only be measured in inactive positions of the body.

6. Participation in specialized forms of physical activity results in the development of specific patterns of flexibility. This generalization from research findings suggests that human patterns of joint mobility are modifiable.

Specificity Of Flexibility

Previously flexibility was commonly thought to be a general trait rather than a number of specifics related to the various joint movements. This concept has now been reversed by several investigators. Through correlation and factor analysis studies, joint flexibility has been shown to be highly specific throughout the body rather than existing as a general trait common to all joints. For boys, flexibility generally increases from age 6 to 10 years, then declines to age 16. For girls, a similar result has been found except the flexibility peak was at 12 years. Extensive and prolonged participation in the different physical activities or kinds of performances produces unique patterns of flexibility. When compared with 16-year-old boys, studies using 30 flexometer tests have shown that swimmers and baseball players have greater flexibility, exceeding the 16 year olds in 25 of the 30 tests. Basketball and track athlete, weight lifters, and gymnasts were superior in 14–15 of these tests. Wrestlers were the least flexible of groups listed, exceeding the boys on 8 tests only.

The concept that weight training causes a muscle bound condition has proven to be a myth. Habitual weight trainers and athletes who have achieved international recognition for best developed physique and for weightlifting generally have greater flexibility than normal groups including 16-year-old boys. Stretching exercises designed to produce greater range of movement in joints have resulted in pronounced improvements. The effects of these improvements have continued for at least 8 weeks after the cessation of exercises. Warm-up exercises substantially improve mobility, even a single preliminary trial results in a higher flexibility score for a given test.

Stretching exercises are especially important for the older athlete. Throughout life after age 25 there is a general steady loss of flexibility in the principle joints. This is probably related to many factors but most notedly to dehydration and disuse of the tissues. This decline is so parallel with aging that flexibility is one form of measurement of physiological aging.

Specific Training Programs

A. FARTLEK

Fartlek or marathon training is used early in the training program in an attempt to develop positive attitudes, confidence, and mental toughness while increasing endurance capabilities at a relatively leisurely pace.

B. CONTROLLED INTERVAL TRAINING

Controlled interval training consists of a repeated series of underdistance efforts at a controlled speed with a controlled period of rest between each effort. The rest interval is long enough to permit partial but not complete recovery of the heart rate to normal. The distance is never longer than the distance that the athlete is training for.

C. REPETITION TRAINING

Repetition training is used in the training program to develop quality. Fixed distances are repeated in exactly the same amount of time. The rest intervals, however, are long enough to permit more complete recovery of the heart rate than allowed in interval training.

D. OVERDISTANCE TRAINING

Overdistance training is that form of training that takes place at distances greater than the event being trained for, usually at a lower speed than that which will be possible in the event itself. This method of training is most often used in the early part of the season. This system helps to develop endurance that is more stable and longer lasting.

E. CIRCUIT TRAINING

Circuit training is the scientific arrangement of known and proven exercises designed to elicit maximum overall training effectiveness. Total balanced development for all parts of the body is the objective. Circuit training is based on sound, physiological principles and aims at providing various activities and a continuous challenge. A circuit utilizing proper exercise equipment will improve muscular strength and endurance, cardiovascular endurance and flexibility, apply the principle of "progressive overload," provide balanced development to the whole body, enable large numbers of performers to train at the same time, each according to his individual capacity, allow each individual to acquire a maximum workout in a short but adequate time, and inspire motivation through variety offered as well as by the application of new goals that become readily apparent almost daily.

F. SPEED TRAINING

The "speed principle" of training, as advocated by McGraw (personal communication) at the University of Texas, and others, can be utilized with many other types of training programs. Utilizing the "speed principle," an athlete performs the movements in a given exercise as rapidly as possible within a prescribed time. For each exercise, a proposed range of "sets" and a time interval are given. For example, the recommendation for push-ups is one to three sets of 10–30 sec each with a rest interval of 30 sec. The athlete performs one set of push-ups for 10 sec, rests for 30 sec, then repeats. The time of exercising is gradually increased while the rest period is gradually diminished. As fitness improves, the number of sets of each exercises may be increased. Thus, the effort-recovery cycle, referred to previously as interval training, is again utilized.

Rehabilitative Exercises in Sports Medicine

Rehabilitation following an athletic injury is a commonly neglected procedure. Few injuries sustained by athletes are so minor that some form of rehabilitation is not necessary. Any injury that necessitates removal of the athlete from practice or competition for as little as 3 or 4 days requires necessary evaluation to determine that function has not been impaired. Measurements of strength, flexibility, endurance, and coordination help to determine the ability of the athlete to return safely to competition.

These determinations must be quantitative and reliable and should not be based on "general clinical impression" alone. (See Appendices 1–3.)

The goal of rehabilitation is balanced bilateral muscular strength as well as antagonistic muscle balance. The goal of treatment must be restoration of function to the greatest possible degree and in the shortest possible time.

In rehabilitation for vigorous sports activity following injury, the SAID principle should be understood. The letters SAID stand for specific adaptation to imposed demands (Wallis and Logan (16)) and mean that the training program must attempt to adapt the individual to the demands that may be made upon him during athletic performance. Adaptation is specific and refers to the alteration of the structure or function of an organ or part as a result of an altered environment. Function increases with use, and that which we do not use we lose. The intensity, duration, and frequency of activity are all related to the functional capacity that is developed.

Rehabilitation of the athlete with an injury deals primarily with restoration of muscle function. The effectiveness of rehabilitation in the recovery period, either postinjury or postsurgically, will usually determine the degree and success of future athletic participation. The assurance given the athlete that his muscular strength and functional capacity are at a very high level of supportive quality is both a physiological as well as a psychological necessity in order for him to return to the field of competition. Haphazard, unproven methods of rehabilitation are usually ineffective and fall far short of the desired goal. Practice for the event itself does not make sufficient demands upon all of the physiological systems supporting the performance. The performer must therefore supplement his practice of the event with artificial exercise designed to develop supporting physiological mechanisms to the point that they can make a maximum contribution to the overall effort.

Rehabilitative exercise is defined as bodily movements prescribed to restore or alter favorably specific functions in an individual following an injury. They may be active or passive. Active exercise is purposeful voluntary motion that is performed by the injured individual himself, with or without resistance, and with or without the aid of gravity. Active exercise may be static, kinetic, or isokinetic. Static exercise is that which is performed without producing joint motion. The muscle being utilized maintains a fixed length, which is an isometric contraction. Kinetic exercise is that which is performed to produce joint movement. The contracting muscle shortens, producing the movement which is an isotonic exercise. Isokinetic exercises are those in which joint motion occurs at a controlled rate. Concentric contraction occurs when a muscle is contracted from the extended to the shortened position. Eccentric contraction occurs when the tensed muscle lengthens. An example of a concentric contraction would be flexion of the elbow in performing a pull-up. An example of an eccentric contraction is that of slowly lowering the body into the extended position from the flexed position after doing a pull-up since the muscle is maintaining tension while actually lengthening. Passive exercises are those performed for the injured athlete by another person or by a mechanical appliance. Passive exercise is carried out by the application of some external force with minimal participation of the muscle action by the injured athlete. It may be forced or nonforced. The nonforced exercises are those utilized to help maintain normal joint motion and are kept within a painless range of motion, for the most part, while forced passive exercises are those that usually produce movement beyond the limits of the free range of motion and are often associated with some discomfort to the individual.

The following factors should be considered in formulating the exercise prescription (Allman, (2)):

1. *The Exercise.* Three main factors must be considered in prescribing the exercise: the purpose of the exercise; how it is to be administered; and its relationship to other exercises that might be prescribed.

2. *Precautions.* The precautions should include concern for any existing conditions that might alter the response of the individual to the exercise program. It should be remembered that the exercise must be administered within the limits imposed by the existing status of the individual.

3. *Duration.* The duration of each exercise period and of the total amount of time required for the program must be considered.

4. *Intensity.* The intensity will vary according to the extent of the injury for which the exercise prescription is being ordered. For minor injuries, the intensity may be very great initially and of short duration, while in a more severely injured athlete, the intensity will be very low initially and then, over a period of months, will progress to that of high intensity prior to his being released for further competition.

5. *Nature of the Movement.* The nature of the movement is characterized by its speed, the method of loading as it effects joint dynamics, and whether or not it is performed unilaterally or bilaterally, either simultaneously or alternately. The length of the lever arm, the attachment points of muscles and tendons, and their angles of insertion are important in determining these characteristics.

6. *Range of the Movement.* The range of movement is determined by the distance the body part covers in exercise. Immediately following injury, or following surgery, an exercise might be prescribed without any movement of the involved joint, whereas as improvement takes place, the range of movement will be gradually increased. Toward the final stages of rehabilitation, and as soon as possible in the recovery period, the range of motion should be as complete as possible. The best results in restoring full muscle function are achieved when the muscles are contracted throughout the entire range of motion of the joints involved.

7. *Rhythm.* The rhythm relates not only to that which is carried out during each movement but also as it relates to different other movements. In the initial phases of the rehabilitation program, it is important to teach effort-relaxation cycles so that the muscle does not remain in a state of constant tension. As the exercise program progresses, less emphasis needs to be placed on effort-relaxation cycles as they become more or less subconscious.

8. *Timing.* Timing relates to exposure with a given exercise as well as the time allowed between each exercise. It relates to the coordination of muscle response, and also the stages of rehabilitation, whether immediately post-injury or late in the rehabilitation program.

9. *Progression.* Progression in a training program is essential. It relates to range of motion, load, speed, power, and energy expenditure in relationship to each exercise as well as to the total exercise program. An attempt should be made to produce some sign of progress in each exercise session. Muscles must be worked to the point of "momentary failure" or "exhaustion" if a high performance level is to be achieved.

10. *Neuromuscular Reeducation.* Neuromuscular reeducation primarily involves development of a proprioceptive awareness. Correction of posture and the use of passive, active, and resistive movements all seem to be essential to complete proprioceptive response.

Examples of Specific Rehabilitation Procedures*

A. REHABILITATION FOLLOWING SHOULDER INJURIES IN ATHLETES

Rotator Cuff Injuries

a. Early Rehabilitation

At this stage the rotator cuff is compromised by its subacute or postsurgical status. The shortness of the cuff muscles and the disproportionate strength of the other musculature of the pectoral girdle make conventional full range exercise inappropriate, even if active range of motion is possible. The following exercises are indicated:

i. Gripping Exercises. Gripping a hand dynamometer or tennis ball at several points along the arc from full (pain free) abduction-flexion-external rotation to full adduction-extension-internal rotation. This brings the rotator cuff into synergistic (fixative) contraction, as well as conditioning forearm muscles which have probably atrophied if inactivity has been of long duration.

ii. Codman (Pendulum) Exercises. This exercise increases the range of motion while stimulating contraction of the rotator cuff due to the gentle traction applied to the muscle systems.

iii. Bench Press Supports. Lie supine on the bench, holding the barbell in a "locked-out" position. A freely held barbell or dumbbells are preferable to a statically held weight machine since four-way control is stimulated by the free barbell and not by the weight machine. The weight should be only heavy enough to stimulate fixation of the cuff gently. Progression is accomplished by widening the grip gradually from about 20 to 30 inches (to pain tolerance). This increases the external rotation gradually. The weight is also increased gradually.

iv. Deadlift Supports. Hold the barbell or corresponding level of the multistation weight training apparatus with an overhand grip at the front of the thighs. The shoulders are held in a shrug position. Single efforts of 10 sec are performed. Progression is obtained by widening the grip and increasing weight.

v. Hanging from Chinning Bar. A bench or chair is used to elevate the body so that the bar can be grasped regardless of a deficient range of motion. The bar is gripped but no effort is made to support full or partial

---

* The program outlined is that used at the Sports Medicine Clinic in Atlanta, Georgia.

weight until the arms can be painlessly held over the head. The patient merely grips the bar and isometrically sets the latissimus group in a comfortable range. Once full weight bearing is possible, progression is obtained by widening the grip.

b. Intermediate Rehabilitation

At this stage the rotator cuff should be able to contract fully without pain, but full range is not present, and strength is not yet fully developed. The cuff is, however, adequate to take on conventional shoulder conditioning exercises that will develop strength and further increase range of motion. The following exercises are performed:

i. Light Dumbbell Circles. This is a progression of the pendulum exercises. Done while standing upright, the dumbbell is directed upward and outward in a rotary manner, and then upward and inward in the opposite manner. These circles progress by widening the excursion of the circle and increasing the weight.

ii. Bench Presses. Progressing from supports, the patient gradually adds bending to the movement until a full range bench press is possible. More weight is added. Once again, because of the need to support the weight in all directions, freely held weights are preferable to weight machines. Dumbbell bench exercises, or "flyes," while they may present a safety problem, will offer a wider range of motion.

iii. Upright Rowing. This is a progression of the deadlift supports, using the same grip, in which the weight is raised to a position high on the chest. Varying the width of hand grips is desirable.

iv. "Lat" Machine Pull-Downs to the Rear of Neck. A shoulder-width grip is used at first with later progression to a wider grip. Weight is added until the patient is able to progress to behind the neck pull-ups (only if a minimum of six can be performed).

c. Advanced Rehabilitation

The progress of the intermediate stage has probably left the athlete at near normal development. To develop extra strength of the structures in question, along with increased flexibility, the following program might be utilized:

i. Alternate Dumbbell Presses or Presses Behind the Neck.

ii. Dumbbell Benches, Incline Presses, Flyes, or Parallel Bar Dips.

iii. Bent-Arm Pull-overs.

iv. High Pulls with a Snatch Grip, or Repetition "Cleans." All of the above are done for strength at a level of weight, repetitions, and number of sets to assure maximum development in accordance with the individual's potential. The exercises are done to the extremes of motion so that flexibility is improved. If properly done in this manner, no specific flexibility exercise is needed. To supplement any deficiency, however, the following exercises can be performed:

v. Straight Arm Pull-overs Across the Width of a Bench, Using a

Progressively Wider Grip. The weight is kept at a permanently light poundage (30 lb).

vi. Light Dumbbell Flyes with a Medicine Ball between the Shoulder Blades, or Elastic Cable Stretching at Pulley Weights. In the latter, the cable is held in back of the shoulders with the palms facing forward at shoulder height and the cable is worked forward and backward, stretching the pectoral girdle and rib cage.

B. GLENOHUMERAL DISLOCATIONS AND SUBLUXATIONS

All stages of rehabilitation are similar to the rotator cuff with the following exceptions:

1. If the surgical intervention has not been instituted to correct the dislocations, no exercise should be done which places the shoulder in a compromised position (abducted and externally rotated). Thus, grips should never be wide, bench work should only be done in the top one-third of the movement, and presses are best performed in only the lower half of the range. To accomplish this, the use of a "power rack" is beneficial. If unavailable the barbell with the assistance of two spotters is used.

2. The extent of damage to the cuff and surrounding structures may be such that progress is slower, and there is greater atrophy and limitation of range.

3. Special emphasis is given to strengthening the internal rotator (subscapularis muscle).

C. ACROMIOCLAVICULAR INJURIES

1. Early Rehabilitation

At the subacute or postoperative stage, pain is often a limiting factor, with associated tightening of all the shoulder musculature (trapezius, pectoral, deltoid, latissimus, etc.) as well as the possibility of tightness and weakness in the adjacent arm muscles. For this reason, the following exercises are used:

a. Light, active range of motion for shoulder flexion, abduction, internal and external rotation, flexion and extension of the elbow, and supination and pronation of the forearm.

b. Light resistive exercise for the trapezius (shrug).

c. Light resistive exercise for the anterior deltoid (upright row).

d. Resistive exercise, to tolerance, for the forearm, biceps, and triceps muscles. All should be done in such a fashion that little or no downward pull is affected at the shoulder (lying or seated rather than standing).

e. Codman (pendulum) exercises are done to increase the tolerance of the shoulder to weight support with a limited range of motion.

2. Intermediate Rehabilitation

Pain should be absent and the range of motion nearly full. The main goal is strengthening the muscular attachments of the trapezius and deltoids in the area of the clavicle and acromion near the acromioclavicular joint. This is done by strengthening the entire deltoid-trapezius group. The following exercises should be done:

   a. Dumbbell presses done alternately (emphasis is on the anterior deltoid).

   b. Wide grip press behind the neck (emphasis on the lateral deltoid and trapezius).

   c. Shoulder shrug (emphasis on the trapezius).

   d. Upright row (emphasis on the anterior deltoid and trapezius).

3. Advanced Rehabilitation

Increasing the general muscle bulk in the anterior shoulder area should have a strengthening effect on the acromioclavicular joint. All of the above exercises are appropriate when done intensively with a heavy progression of weight. Also beneficial are all incline presses, all "cleans," snatches, and deadlifts, bench presses, and pull-overs.

D. INJURIES RELATED TO THE THROWING SPORTS

The key is prevention. Assuring general fitness of the musculature through adequate strength training is important. More important, however, is the establishment of fluid agonist-antagonist function for each associated movement at the shoulder and elbow. Development of appropriate flexibility and coordination of movement are extremely important, as well as of a proper kinesthetic sense by the athlete. The following general points are important:

   1. Full range strength training, mostly with dumbbells. Done to extremes of stretch and with "ballistic" movement to assure the maintenance of quick, fluid reaction in the muscles.

   2. Additional stretching movements for the entire shoulder-elbow area.

   3. Maintenance of flexibility and fluid motion in the thoracic and lumbar spine. This can have a beneficial effect on the general state of flexibility in the extremities.

   4. Thoughtful practice of the throwing skill to establish the most fluid and efficient pattern possible.

   5. Always practicing proper warm-up, and not abusing the endurance and recovery capabilities of the structures involved (not throwing too often or too much at one time, or too soon after a lay-off).

E. REHABILITATION FOLLOWING KNEE INJURIES IN ATHLETES*

1. Injury Classification

It is important to classify injuries by type and extent, since the course of rehabilitation will differ from one type to another. The injury classification and specified therapy routines should not be considered to be

---

* The program outlined is that used at the Sports Medicine Clinic in Atlanta, Georgia.

inflexible or to limit further detailing or specialization. See also Appendices 4 and 5.)

a. Single ligament or uncomplicated meniscus injury.

b. Multiple ligament injury or complicated single ligament and/or meniscus injury.

c. Multiple ligament injury associated with other complicating factors, such as a fracture.

d. Chondromalacia of the patella and/or femoral condyle erosion, either alone or in combination with any of the above types.

2. Stages of Rehabilitation

Rehabilitation following knee injury and/or surgery can be divided into five stages: presurgical, immediate postoperative, early intermediate, later intermediate, and advanced.

a. Presurgical Stage

The presurgical stage is usually significant only when elective surgery is to be performed. If a specific diagnosis has not been made, therapeutic exercise may be instituted for purposes of aiding in diagnosis as well as for functional benefits. Therapeutic exercise at this stage is designed to build or maintain strength, while at the same time not to aggravate the existing injury. Thus, the exercise must be, for the most part, not through a full range of motion. Isokinetic exercise is especially desirable during this stage because of its reasily controlled, noncompelling nature. The following exercises should be carried out:

i. Quadriceps setting—10-sec contractions for 5 min each hour while awake.

ii. Straight leg raising—15 nonstop repetitions with the maximum possible resistance each hour while awake.

iii. Isometric knee extension (at or near full extension)—15 repetitions each hour while awake.

iv. Isometric or isokinetic knee flexion—15 repetitions (optional).

v. Hip extension (wall pulley)—20-25 repetitions (optional).

vi. Hip flexion (wall pulley)—20-25 repetitions (optional).

vii. Hip abduction (wall pulley)—20-25 repetitions (optional).

viii. Hip adduction (wall pulley)—20-25 repetitions (optional).

The above routine should be performed daily for 10–14 days prior to surgery. In so doing, the preservation of muscle tone and the improved kinesthetic sense will help in preparation for the practice of similar exercises immediately postoperative. Instruction in three-point gait training should also be given during this stage. Touch weight bearing with the injured extremity is allowed; however, while the involved extremity is in the weight bearing phase of gait, the knee is fully extended and the quadriceps muscle is "set." Complicated or more serious injuries are usually treated by elective surgery and, therefore, are not included in this stage of therapy, since surgery is most often indicated immediately.

b. Immediate Postoperative or Postinjury Stage

The optimal time for commencement of therapeutic exercise is approximately 24 hours following surgery or injury. An earlier beginning is often met by an unreceptive and confused patient. Any beginning later than 24 hours must be considered a loss of valuable time. As soon as normal function ceases, atrophy and other debilitating mechanisms begin to occur and serve to delay further return of normal function. Exercises in this stage are similar to those in the presurgical stage, except for those movements that are precluded by the presence of a cast, dressing, or associated immobilization. The following exercises should be carried out:

i. Quadriceps setting – 10-sec contractions for 5 min each hour while awake.

ii. Straight leg raising – 10 repetitions each hour while awake with maximum possible resistance.

iii. Isometric hip extension – 10-sec "presses" onto the bed for 10 repetitions each hour while awake.

iv. Abduction and adduction of the hip – 10-sec presses against resistance for 10 repetitions each hour while awake.

v. Ankle plantar flexion – 10-sec presses against resistance for 10 repetitions each hour while awake.

vi. Ambulation. As soon as the patient is able voluntarily to elevate the involved extremity from the bed, he is allowed to ambulate on crutches, using a three-point gait, with touch weight bearing on the involved extremity. The touch weight bearing stimulates proprioceptive receptors that provide the central nervous system with an awareness of body segments (in the involved extremity). Proprioceptive awareness has been shown to be of primary importance in neuromuscular reeducation.

The goals during this stage of rehabilitation are maintenance of muscle mass, strength, and function during the period of time that immobilization is indicated. These exercises should be progressive and continuous during the entire immobilization period. It is important that exercises be prescribed for the entire extremity as well as other major body segments, since bed rest and immobilization deprives all of these segments of normal activity.

The above exercises are recommended for uncomplicated single ligament and meniscectomy cases. More complicated injuries introduce elements of increased instability, increased pain, increased potential for hemorrhage, and the need for more extensive tissue repair. These conditions are, therefore, indications for the most judicious choice of activity and dosage. In most cases, however, given time and proper supervision, the level of activity can approach that of less complicated cases. Careful control of the rate of exercise progression is the key to success, the following immediate postsurgery or postinjury routine is usually possible, even with very complicated cases:

vii. Quadriceps setting – 10-sec sets, for 5 min each hour while awake.

viii. Straight leg raising – to tolerance for 30 sec each hour while awake.

ix. Hip extension (isometric) – to tolerance for 30 sec each hour while awake.

c. Early Intermediate Rehabilitation

At the end of the immobilization period, the patient proceeds immediately into the early intermediate stage of rehabilitation. This stage is a continuation of the postsurgical stage and the exercises are similar but with added emphasis on progression. Exercises are also included to increase the active range of motion (ROM). Passive stretching is seldom used, as active ROM exercises usually provide full ROM within a reasonable period of time. In cases in which terminal extension is a problem, the patient is instructed in passive-active exercise to correct this deficit. The following exercises should be carried out:

i. Straight leg raising – using maximum possible resistance.

ii. Pulley exercises:

Hip extension – progressive to 15–20 repetitions.

Hip flexion – progressive to 15–20 repetitions.

Hip abduction – progressive to 15–20 repetitions.

Hip adduction – progressive to 15–20 repetitions.

iii. Knee extension – flexion utilizing isokinetic exercises, beginning with a relatively low speed and gradually increasing the speed.

iv. Ankle plantar flexion – progressive to 15–20 repetitions.

v. Terminal extension exercise ("hurdler's exercise") with the addition of a towel looped over the forefoot for additional stretching of the popliteal area.

The above exercises are done once in a circuit during the first session, two sets at the next, three sets at the next, and never more than three sets subsequently. Progression is consistent and judicious. As soon as a pain-free ROM in excess of 90° is present at the knee with no apparent swelling and no significant pain, the following changes are made:

vi. Leg raises are eliminated.

vii. Isotonic leg extension is added – one leg at a time, alternating legs. Resistance is added progressively, 15–20 repetitions.

viii. Isotonic knee flexion-resistance is added progressively, 15–20 repetitions.

ix. Terminal extension is continued if necessary.

x. Active stretching of the rectus femoris muscle, the hamstring muscles, and the Achilles tendon is initiated at the same time that isotonic exercises are introduced.

xi. Stationary bicycling is added to tolerance, usually 2–4 miles at one sitting, with a resistance based upon the capability of the individual.

xii. At this stage the leg press is added to tolerance. Resistance is progressive, 20–30 repetitions.

Each of these exercises is performed 2–3 times daily. The rationale at this stage is no longer one of maintenance of function, but is one of building (rebuilding) muscle mass and function. Still, aggressiveness should not gain the upper hand over judicious choice of exercise dosage. Of primary importance at this stage is mobilization and achievement of pain-free flexion and full extension. Secondarily, proper form in the performance of exercise is indicated. Of third importance is the actual amount of resistance used in the exercise, although once motion and proper form have been achieved, the resistance load becomes allimportant. More complicated or extensive injury may call for a slower beginning at this stage. By observing the signs of pain and swelling, however, as well as following basic precautions as far as the rate of progression is concerned, there is no reason to believe that most such cases cannot eventually progress to the same level of performance as less complicated ones. The difference is one of a slower rate of progress. In many cases of extensive erosion of the joing surfaces either on the patella or the femoral condyle, resistive ROM exercise may be permanently contraindicated. In these cases isokinetic types of exercise usually are helpful.

d. Late Intermediate Rehabilitation

The criteria for advancement to this stage are pain-free full range of motion of the involved joint, and a strength deficit in the quadriceps group of no more than 25%. The following exercises should be carried out:

i. Leg extension — both legs simultaneously, 15–20 repetitions.

ii. Leg flexion — both legs simultaneously, 15–20 repetitions.

iii. Leg press — 15–20 repetitions.

iv. Stationary bicycle — emphasize high speed and high resistance. Progress with distance up to 5 miles.

v. Running — preferably uphill or, if on the treadmill, with a grade of 5–10%. Progress in distance and speed.

At this stage of rehabilitation the rationale becomes less one of therapy and more one of sports conditioning. Sports conditioning centers about a concern for "functional power." Considerations must include resistance, speed of movement, range of movement, and repetitions. By this stage it has been determined whether or not intensive exercise is indicated. If not, then exercise is limited to nonresistive exercise of the isokinetic type, and to non-ROM exercises such as straight leg raises, isometrics at various angles, and full ROM hip and ankle movements.

e. Advanced Rehabilitation

The criteria for entry into this phase of rehabilitation are that the athlete be deemed able to participate in competitive sports, and have no more than 5–10% strength deficit in the quadriceps mechanism. The following exercises are to be carried out:

i. Warm-up using a stationary bicycle or jump rope. Maximum performance, 3–5 minutes duration.

ii. Leg press — to exhaustion, 20–30 repetitions.

iii. Leg extension — to exhaustion, 15–20 repetitions.

iv. Half knee bends — to exhaustion, 15–20 repetitions.

v. Leg curl—to exhaustion, 15–20 repetitions.

vi. Toe raise—to exhaustion, 25–30 repetitions.

vii. Stationary bicycle—taper off. Moderate resistance for 3–5-min duration.

The above exercises should be performed with absolutely no rest between exercises, and, with the exception of the stationary bicycle or jump rope, should be performed in approximately 5 min. The central focus of advanced rehabilitation is exactly the same as advanced sports conditioning. Done properly, sports conditioning should simultaneously provide maximum benefit in developing power, endurance, and flexibility.

F. REHABILITATION ROUTINES FOLLOWING SPRAINS AND STRAINS TO THE LUMBOSACRAL REGION OF THE BACK*

The purpose of these exercises is to improve the mechanics of the back through improved strength, coordination, and elasticity. This is accomplished by developing actively the flexor muscles of the lumbosacral spine and stretching passively the extensor muscles and fasciae. Faulty posture must be corrected, and once corrected, proper posture must be maintained at all times.

1. Acute Stage

This stage is marked by the presence of pain and muscle spasm, and requires bed rest. Back exercises should not be attempted during this stage. The following exercises should be carried out:

a. Muscle setting of major muscles of the extremities may be performed safely in order to maintain as much strength in the extremities as possible.

b. Deep breathing exercises may also be helpful.

2. Subacute Stage

This stage is marked by the relief of muscle spasm and the absence of significant pain. The following exercises should be carried out:

a. Gluteal muscle and abdominal muscle setting.

b. After 24 hours of the above two exercises, pelvic tilt exercises are initiated.

3. Intermediate Stage

The intermediate stage of rehabilitation for lumbosacral sprains usually starts about the fifth to seventh day following the acute episode. The following exercises should be carried out:

a. Abdominal Setting and Pelvic Tilt. The knees are bent. The back is flattened against the floor by pulling the abdominal muscles in and up, tilting the pelvis. The lower spine should be completely flat. This exercise must be performed on a rigid surface so that the back can be flattened with certainty. The abdominal and gluteal muscles should be "set" during

---

* The program outlined is that used at the Sports Medicine Clinic in Atlanta, Georgia.

this exercise. This exercise helps to strengthen the abdominal and gluteal muscles.

b. *Head-Shoulder Curl*. Sit-ups often aggravate existing back problems. Therefore, head-shoulder curls should permanently replace sit-ups. From the starting position, with the knees flexed and back flat on the floor, raise the head first, then the shoulders as far as possible, while keeping the small of the back flat. Hold this position in an isometric contraction with the abdominals.

c. *Knee-Chest*. From starting position of the head and shoulder curl, grasp the knees with outstretched hands and pull the knees toward the axilla as far as possible while attempting to push the head between the knees. This exercise passively stretches the erector spinae muscles and the contracted lumbar fasciae and ligaments posterior to the center of gravity at the lumbosacral level. Double leg raises are usually contraindicated in individuals with back problems and therefore should always be avoided.

d. *Trunk Flexion*. Sit on the edge of the chair, slowly drop head and shoulders, and then bend the back so as to attempt to touch the folded elbows to the floor between the feet. Relax. This exercise helps to overcome or prevent extension contractures of the lumbosacral spine.

e. *Hamstring Stretch*. Sit on the floor with the legs extended in front in a "V" position. Slowly bend the head, shoulders, and trunk forward while reaching for the toes of the left foot with the outstretched fingers. If unable to reach the toes, push the hands along the leg as far as possible. Slowly stretch. Repeat to the opposite side. This exercise stretches the erector spinae and hamstring muscles.

f. *Anterior Hip Stretch*. Assume the squat position, with both hands on the floor, the left foot placed flatly on the floor with the knee fully flexed and the right hip and knee fully extended behind the body with the weight on the ball of the foot and the ankle dorsiflexed. The forward knee is slightly extended and then flexed repeatedly, thus moving the pelvis up and down, and stretching the anterior portion of the extended hip. This exercise stretches the anterior thigh and hip structures (rectus femoris muscle, fascia lata, and iliofemoral ligament).

g. *Back Flattening Against Wall*. Stand with the back to the wall, and heels 6–8 inches from the wall. Flatten the spine against the wall by tilting the hips backward, with the abdomen pulled in and up, the chest up, and the chin in and down. Set the abdominal and gluteal muscles. This exercise helps to strengthen the abdominal and gluteal muscles.

4. Advanced Stage

This stage is not undertaken until the patient is totally asymptomatic. The goal of this stage is to restore sufficient strength so that the individual may safely participate in athletics, but the weight training program is modified so that it is not likely to aggravate the preexisting back condition. During this stage the exercises that were outlined for the intermediate stage are continued, and in addition endurance activities are progressively added to the program. These include cycling, jumping rope, and running.

REFERENCES

1. ALLMAN, F. L., JR. *Executive Fitness Desk Diary,* p. 11. MB Prod., Inc., Dallas, Tex., 1969.
2. ALLMAN, F. L., JR. *Sports Medicine.* Academic Press, New York, 1974.
3. BAER
4. BALKE, B. *Am. J. Phys. Anthropol., 23:* 293–301, 1965.
5. BILIK, S. E. *The Trainers Bible,* Ed. 9. Atsco Press, New York, 1941.
6. BROER, M. R. *Efficiency of Human Movement,* Ed. 2. W.B. Saunders, Philadelphia, 1966.
7. COOPER, K. H. *J. A. M. A., 203:* 201–204, 1968.
8. DARLING, R. C., AND DOWNEY, J. *Therapeutic Exercise,* Williams & Wilkins, Baltimore, 1971.
9. DOHERTY, J. K. *Modern Track and Field,* Ed. 2. Prentice-Hall, Englewood Cliffs, N. J., 1963.
10. Flexibility. In *Physical Fitness Research Digest,* Series 4, Oct. 1975.
11. HELLEBRANDT, F. A., AND HOUTZ, S. J. *Phys. Ther. Rev., 35:* 371–383, 1956.
12. HOLLAND, G. J. The Physiology of Flexibility. In *Kinesiology Review,* p. 49, 1962.
13. JONES, A. Flexibility and metabolic condition. *Athletic J., 56:* 2, 1975.
14. LAMB, E. *The Health Letter, 11,* 1973.
15. McCLOY, C. H. *Res. Quart., 11:* 28–39, 1940.
16. WALLIS, E. L., AND LOGAN, G. A. *Figure Improvement and Body Conditioning through Exercise.* Prentice-Hall, Englewood Cliffs, N. J., 1964.

Shoulder Evaluation Form

	Right	Left
Girth		
Arm	_____	_____
Forearm	_____	_____
Strength		
Hand	_____	_____
Shoulder		
Internal rotation	_____	_____
External rotation	_____	_____
Flexion	_____	_____
Extension	_____	_____
Abduction	_____	_____
Goniometric		
Abduction	_____	_____
Flexion	_____	_____
Internal rotation	_____	_____
External rotation	_____	_____
Extension	_____	_____

Comments:

Knee Evaluation Form

	Right	Left
Girth		
Quadriceps		
At ___ cm above patella		
Mid-patella		
Calf		
Strength		
Quadriceps		
Hamstrings		
Gastroc soleus		
Hip flexor		
Hip abductor		
Hip extensor		
Hip adductor		
Goniometric		
Extension		
Flexion		

Comments:

Ankle Evaluation Form

	Right	Left
Girth		
Foot	_____	_____
Ankle	_____	_____
Strength		
Plantar flexion..............	_____	_____
Dorsiflexion	_____	_____
Internal rotation	_____	_____
External rotation	_____	_____
Goniometric		
Plantar flexion..............	_____	_____
Dorsiflexion	_____	_____
Inversion	_____	_____
Eversion	_____	_____

Comments:

Protocol
for Testing
Quadriceps Strength

The key in this test is to arrive at a bilateral strength comparison—absolute accuracy is not needed. The following protocol should satisfy this need.

1. Test right knee first always (even if athlete is left handed, since most sports activities are right-foot oriented).
2. Have athlete tighten lap belt on Nautilus Knee Extensor Unit (or similar resistive exercise device).
3. Place right leg only under roller pad—do not allow other leg under as this could result in accidental help from the other leg.
4. Choose weight as follows: Estimate muscular body weight of athlete (discount fatty weight). Subtract 20 lb from this weight and use this to test.
5. If the athlete cannot actually complete one full repetition with the weight, this is satisfactory. Merely note the highest angle to which the weight can be lifted.
6. If the athlete can complete one or more full repetitions, count the number of repetitions, including the last incomplete repetition.
7. Retest left leg and compare results.
8. Strength differences can only be estimated in general terms. They may be calculated as follows: Same weight can be lifted with both legs, even though the height to which the weight can be lifted on the last (or only) repetition may not match—*equal strength*.

Ten or 20 lb difference, or one or two repetitions difference—10–20% difference, interpreted as *slight disparity*.

Greater discrepancy than above—*significant disparity*.

Example: Athlete weighs 200 lb, 10% body fat.
Muscular body weight = 180 lb.

Right Leg	Left Leg
180 lb × 1$\frac{3}{4}$ repetitions	180 lb × $\frac{1}{4}$ repetition only

10–20% strength disparity.

appendix
5
Prescriptions for Exercises

Home Knee Exercises

I. Lie on back. Keep knee absolutely straight as you lift it to 45°. Lower slowly. Do not relax the leg, but repeat 15 repetitions. As you get stronger, add weights by means of putting weight in a gym bag or "flight bag" and draping the handles over the ankles.

Straight leg raise

Gym bag for weights

II. Standing front leg raise is done exactly as above, only you stand to do the lift. Perform 15 repetitions. Add weight when you are able. Standing side raise is done exactly as above, only the weight is lifted to the side. Do 15 repetitions.

III. This "Quad-setting" exercise is performed seated on the floor. Place one or two rolled-up towels under the knee. While pushing the back of the knee down into the towel as

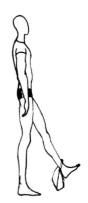

Standing front leg raise

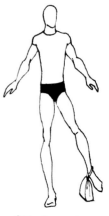

Side leg raise

hard as possible, attempt to keep the entire surface of your leg in contact with the floor. Hold 5 sec. Repeat 10 times.

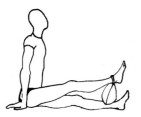

"Quad-setting" exercise

DO EACH EXERCISE
AS INSTRUCTED_____

TIMES DAILY
DAYS WEEKLY

SPECIAL NOTES: _____

IV. Sit on a high table, with the back of the knee just at the edge of the table. You may wish to use towels to pad the back of the knee. From the fully bent position, straighten the knee as much as possible. Hold for 3 sec at the top. Repeat 15 times. As you get stronger, add weight by means of a weighted bag. Continue using this exercise only as long as no increased pain or swelling is caused as a result of the exercise.

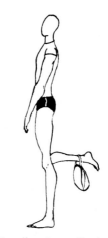

Standing knee-flexion

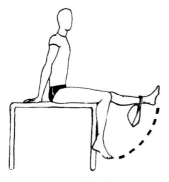

Seated leg extension

V. Stand erect and balance by holding onto a stable piece of furniture. Bend the exercising knee backward. Use the weighted bag as in the above exercises. Do 15 repetitions.

Stretching Exercises for Hips and Legs

NOTE: Before you do the following exercises, which are meant to be done intensely, you must warm up. This may include any light exercise and/or jogging, which does not cause pain. Allow 10 min for warm-ups.

ICE MASSAGE – You may wish to preceed your stretching with ice massage if you are in real pain or if your muscles are in spasm. If you do the massage, omit the warm-ups mentioned above.

Use a large piece of ice frozen in a 10- or 12-oz paper cup. Massage your injured muscle in firm, overlapping circles. Attempt to massage an area no greater than a softball, with the center being the point of most pain. Allow 15 min, then proceed directly to the stretching exercises below.

HURTLER'S STRETCH — assume a seated position on the ground with one leg stretched straight in front of you and the other bent under itself in back of you (see figure).

NOTE: In any stretching exericse, it is more beneficial to assume a slow, steadily increasing stretch, which builds to a peak (will be quite painful) after 15 sec; release slowly. Never jerk or fall into a stretched position.

This exercise is done in two parts — first the hamstring stretch; while keeping the knee straight, attempt to bring the chin as close to the knee as possible. If need be, loop a belt over the foot and pull. Do one hamstring stretch and then one thigh stretch, as shown below.

Second is the thigh stretch; while keeping the point of the knee on the floor, and the ankle directly under your hips, bend your entire body backwards until you are as far as you can get (full range should be with your elbows resting on the floor in back of you.

Now reverse your entire position and perform both exercises in the new position.

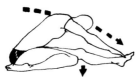

Hamstring stretch

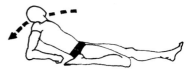

Thigh stretch

GROIN STRETCH — assume a stance with feet planted about double shoulder width and feet pointing forward and flat on the floor (keep them this way throughout). Now, lower your body to one side so that your finger tips support your balance by being placed on either side of your supporting leg. The opposite leg, will experience a stretch from the inside of the knee clear into the groin area. Release and do the other leg.

SPECIAL INSTRUCTIONS JUST FOR YOU!

DO EACH
 EXERCISE   TIMES DAILY
 _____
                              DAYS WEEKLY
 _____

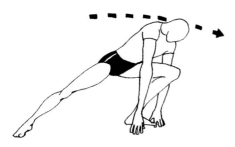

Groin stretch (side lunge)

William's Flexion Exercises

These exercises are designed to decrease low back pain by strengthening those muscles which flex the lumbosacral spine (especially the abdominal and gluteus maximus) and stretch the back extensors. But in order to do this, you must do these exercises *daily*. Do NOT exercise beyond the point of pain.

1. Lying on your back on a firm surface with your knees bent and your feet flat on the surface, flatten the small of your back against the bed, tightening your stomach and buttocks muscles. Hold 5 sec, relax. Repeat this exercise 10 times. (Place one hand under the small of your back to make sure your back flattens.) Do NOT arch your back when you relax.

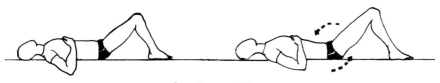

Starting position

2. Lying on your back as in Exercise 1, tighten your stomach muscles, fold your arms across your chest and pull your head forward so your chin touches your chest. Raise up until your shoulder blades are just off the floor and hold here for 5 sec. Relax. Begin by doing this exercise 10 times and work up to 25. Do NOT do regular sit-ups.

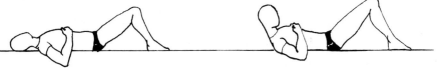

Starting position   Finished position

3. Lying on your back in the same manner as above, bring one knee up toward your chest as far as possible, then reach up with your arms and pull the knee on down to your chest. At the same time, raise your head and shoulders up off the floor as above. Hold for 5 sec. Now repeat with the other leg. Do this exercise 10 times. Do NOT do double straight leg raises as this may aggravate your back problem.

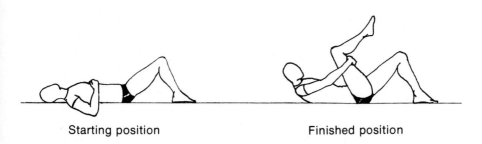

Starting position   Finished position

4. This exercise is the same as Exercise 3 except both knees are raised up and pulled to your chest. Raise your head and shoulders off the floor as you do this. Repeat 10 times holding each time for 5 sec.

Remember: it is important in both Exercises 3 and 4 to bring your knees up as far as you can *before* you use your arms to pull them to your chest.

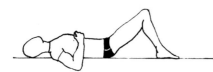

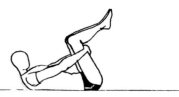

Starting position   Finished position

5. Begin in an exaggerated starter's position (one leg extended, the other forward, hands on floor). Press downward and forward several times, flexing front knee and bringing chest to thigh. Keep your forward foot flat on the floor and support weight on the ball of the back foot. After rocking several times, alternate legs. Repeat 10 times.

6. Stand against the wall with your heels 4 to 6 inches from the wall; flatten your back against the wall. Walk away from the wall maintaining this position. Hold for 10 sec. Gradually increase this time as you get stronger.

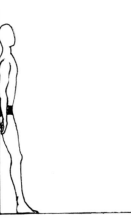

Exaggerated starter's position

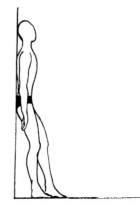

Exercise 6

22

Exercise in Foot Disabilities

JOSEPH H. KITE

Some foot disabilities, such as congenital clubfeet, are present at birth; others, such as congenital metatarsus varus, are noticed several months after birth; and others, like flat feet, still later. Some of the flat feet may have been present at birth but were not noticed until later. Other flat feet may be acquired from faulty sleeping and sitting habits.

Certain foot disabilities are associated with infancy, others with early childhood, and still others with the late childhood and adolescence. Some patients do not complain about their feet until they reach old age. Some foot disabilities may be caused by disease, as poliomyelitis, spastic paralysis, arthritis, gout, diabetes and arteriosclerosis, to mention a few.

Foot disabilities may follow poor posture, knock-knees and general relaxation. Obesity may tire the muscles and stretch the ligaments and cause the foot to pronate. A few children are born with an absence of some of the bones of the foot. A still rarer condition is a fusion of some of the bones in the foot, such as calcaneonavicular bar, which may cause a deformity of the foot.

The most common patterns seen in infants and early childhood are lateral rotation of the legs and flat feet and "medial torsion of the legs and pigeon-toes." Because of their frequency we shall present a detailed discussion of these.

Flat Feet

In times past our attention has been focused on the foot itself. We have talked about what has happened to the ankle, heel and forefoot, paying little attention to the entire leg. It is generally assumed that the deformity has been inherited from one of the parents. The parents frequently volunteer this information, and too often it is accepted as being true. Children do inherit the shape of the toes and of the foot but probably not the flat foot deformity itself, unless it is the congenital type. The parents probably acquired their flat foot deformity, so could not transmit it.

In order to have a better understanding of flat feet it is necessary to divide flat feet into two groups: the congenital and the acquired.

CONGENITAL FLAT FEET

Only a few children are born with flat feet. In these there may be a variation in the severity of the foot deformity. The foot may be only a little more flat than in the acquired deformity, or it may be so deformed that it might be called a reverse clubfoot. It may also be referred to as a "vertical talus." Only those feet with a severe deformity should be included under this congenital classification.

In a few cases the foot is folded up on the lateral side of the leg at birth in a calcaneovalgus position. If the foot is long and narrow and flexible the deformity may not be difficult to correct; in fact some of these deformities tend to correct themselves.

The more difficult cases to treat are those with rigid flat feet. The heel is fixed in a valgus position, and the forefoot is held in abduction. The longitudinal arch is completely obliterated, and there is bulging along the medial border of the foot (Fig. 22.1A). In these cases the anteroposterior roentgenogram shows, that the talus points medially toward the other foot at an angle of 60–75° instead of straight forward toward the great toe (Fig. 22.2A). In the lateral roentgenogram the talus points almost straight down toward the sole instead of forward, approximately parallel with the sole. In these cases, the navicular, instead of being in front of the head of the talus, rests on the superior surface of the neck of the talus.

It is very difficult in these cases to change the position of the talus by exerting force. These cases of congenital flat feet cannot be helped by

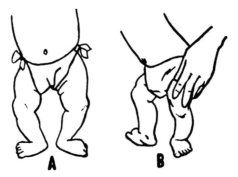

Fig. 22.1. Two-month-old baby with congenital flat feet. The forefoot is abducted, heel everted, and the foot dorsiflexed, resulting in a calcaneovalgus position. The longitudinal arch is obliterated, and there is bulging along the medial border of the foot. The toes on the lateral side of the foot do not touch the floor. These feet might be thought of as being reverse clubfeet. They are very difficult to correct.

exercises or corrective shoes. They should be referred to the orthopedist for correction by a series of cast applications similar to those used in the correction of clubfeet. In congenital flat feet the forefoot is turned inward as the cast is applied in just the opposite direction from that used in correcting a clubfoot. Figure 22.3 shows a patient with congenital flat feet and the result four years after treatment with casts.

ACQUIRED FLAT FEET

Most flat-footed patients belong to this group of "acquired" flat feet. The foot deformity is not as severe as it is in the congenital group. The

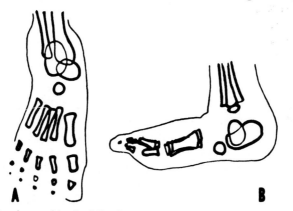

Fig. 22.2. Tracings of typical flat foot roentgenograms. In an anteroposterior view, the talus does not point straight forward toward the great toe but points medially toward the other foot. There is a wide separation of the shadows of the head of the talus and the anterior end of the calcaneus. In the lateral view the talus points straight down toward the sole of the foot and not forward in the normal manner. When the center of ossification for the navicular appears, it is not in front of the talus but is on the superior surface of the neck of the talus.

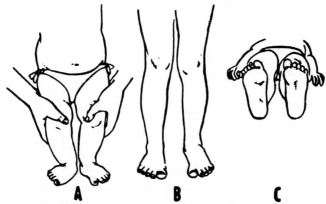

Fig. 22.3. Nine-month-old girl with congenital flat feet, corrected by a series of casts. The last two drawings show the correction 4 years later.

foot is more flexible, and when it is held in the hand it can be placed in an almost normal position. The arch may appear normal when the child is sitting, but when weight is borne the arch flattens out and the foot pronates. The forefoot is abducted and the heel turns out in a valgus position.

The first thing we notice in observing the flat-footed child walk is that his feet do not point straight forward in the direction in which he is walking, but, rather, they point laterally. If we examine the child more closely we see that his knees also point laterally, which means that there is a lateral or external rotation of the entire leg at the hip.

When we examine a child with foot trouble we should always do the "rotation test." This is done preferably with the child lying flat on his back. The legs are grasped at the ankles and rolled to determine the amount of rotation. If the legs can be rotated medially or laterally a great deal farther than normal, we speak of the patient as having either medial or lateral rotation of the legs.

When we do the rotation test in a flat-footed child and try to turn the legs medially at the hips, we find that the legs can be rotated medially only until the patellas point straight forward or a little medial to the midline (Fig. 22.4). When the legs are rotated laterally they may be turned outward at least 90°. The child in walking will naturally place his feet about halfway between these two positions. For this reason many children with flat feet walk with their feet abducted about 30–45°.

If the child was not born with the severe variety that we call congenital flat feet, he must have acquired the deformity, and we must look for its etiology. This is done by observing the sleeping and sitting habits of

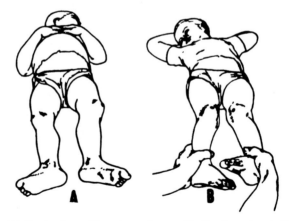

Fig. 22.4. (A) Typical position for a boy with "outward rotation of the legs and flat feet." The entire leg is rotated laterally at the hips, so that the patella and feet point outward or away from the midline. (B) When an attempt is made to rotate the legs medially at the hips, the legs can be rolled medially until the patella points straight forward, but the legs cannot be turned in much further.

infants and small children. Most of the deformity is produced during the first four months when the infant is too small to turn over. The position in which he is placed shortly after birth soon becomes his "position of comfort," and he objects to any other position.

The baby who has been floating in amniotic fluid before birth is placed on a firm mattress. A stiff, new diaper which is much too large for him is applied. His legs are held at right angles to the body in the frog or spread-eagle position. The knees must flex, and this makes the legs rotate laterally at the hips. He is in about the same position as a child would be placed in if he were wearing a Frejka pillow for correction of congenital dislocation of the hips. His legs are held in this same frog position when he is sleeping on his stomach or back. Most babies are kept on the abdomen during the first four months when they are not able to turn over. This is the safer position if they should regurgitate. This soon becomes their "position of comfort." They do not like to be placed in any other position and will cry until they are again placed on the abdomen (Fig. 22.5).

In this frog position the legs become fixed at the hips in outward rotation. The ligaments are stretched to this position. The medial rotators of the leg are stretched and weakened, while the lateral rotators are allowed to contract and are in the stronger position. The baby has more power in the outward rotation than in medial rotation. However, it is impossible for him to rotate his legs medially as long as the hips and knees are flexed in the frog position.

In addition to the fixed outward rotation of the legs in the hips, another deformity is occurring in the feet. As the baby lies on his abdomen, the

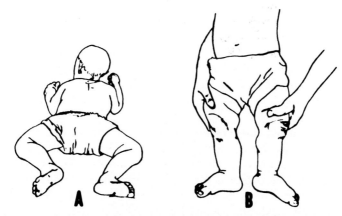

Fig. 22.5. (A) Nine-month-old boy who has always slept on his abdomen in the frog position, which forces the legs into an outward rotated position. The anterior surface of his thigh does not rest on the mattress as does the anterior surface of his body but is rolled outward 90°. (B) When he is placed on his feet, the entire leg rolls outward from the hips, so that the knees and feet both point outward about 45° or more.

great toe rests on the mattress and this pushes the foot around into a flat foot position. The foot is held in this position most of the day and night. The anterior and posterior tibial muscles are stretched, and the three peroneals, along with the extensor digitorum longus, are allowed to contract. According to a physiological principle, a stretched muscle is weakened and a contracted muscle gains in power. The stretched tibial muscles are weakened, and the contracted peroneal muscles gain in strength.

There is also a mechanical principle involved. The muscles which pull in a direct line work at an advantage, while those which pull from around the corner work at a disadvantage. The peroneals pull in a direct line and gain in power, while the tibial muscles have to pull from around the corner and work at a mechanical disadvantage. For this reason the foot is pulled out and up in a flat foot position.

This foot is somewhat like a foot after an attack of poliomyelitis. At first there is very little deformity, but as the months go by, we see more and more deformity if there is a muscle imbalance. We find that this flat foot is pulled out and up in a calcaneovalgus position more often than it is inverted, and it is held for a longer time in this flat foot position. As the infant grows older the flat foot deformity becomes more noticeable, and it becomes fixed by the contracted muscles. Bony changes now begin to take place. The calcaneus is rolled out from under the talus in a valgus position. The foot is also bent at the mid-tarsal joint, so that the forefoot is abducted on the posterior foot. The cuboid is pulled a little lateral to the normal position in front of the calcaneus, and the navicular is pulled around lateral to the head of the talus. The head of the talus and the tubercle of the navicular can now be seen and felt as a sharp bony prominence on the medial side of the foot (Fig. 22.6).

When the child is old enough to pull himself up and stand in the crib, he holds on to the side of the crib and stands with the feet wide apart to maintain his balance. This puts the feet in a pronated position. He now shows outward rotation of the legs and all the elements of a flat foot. The heels turn out in valgus, the longitudinal arch is obliterated, and there is bulging along the medial side of the foot, with a prominence about the tubercle of the navicular. When the baby is old enough to walk, the imprint will be that of a flat foot. We must remember that the infant who has not walked has a pad of fat in the sole of the foot. This will give a flat foot imprint when he is placed on his feet. However, we do not depend on the imprint of the sole to make a diagnosis of flat foot. The diagnosis is made on the previously mentioned findings.

Treatment of Flat Feet Before the Baby Begins to Walk

Obviously, the first step is to break the habit of sleeping always in the frog position. If the baby will sleep part of the time with the knees drawn up under him and part of the time in the frog position, he will have no fixed deformity in rotation. It is still better if we can teach the infant to

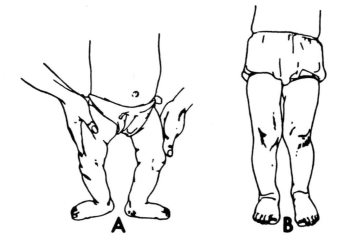

Fig 22.6. (A) Seven-month-old girl with outward rotation of the legs and flat feet. The tubercle of the navicular and the head of the talus can be seen pointing medially. Weight is born on the medial side of the foot. (B) Result 18 months after treatment with exercises, swung in shoes and a bar across the shoes at night to rotate the legs medially.

sleep on his side. This position is best begun when the baby comes home from the hospital. If he has not been placed on his side there, he can be taught to sleep on his side better at this time than he can later. This is done best by placing some support to his back to prevent him from turning over. A pillow may be used. A rolled blanket makes a firmer support (Fig. 22.7). When he is on his side the anterior surfaces of the thigh and abdomen are in the same plane, and the legs are in a neutral position. He is turned alternately on his right and left side after each feeding. If he should regurgitate when on his side he is safe, but, if placed on his back with a full stomach before he is old enough to turn over, he might regurgitate and drown, as has happened.

If the outward rotation and flat feet have already occurred, they must be corrected at the earliest possible time. With the baby on his back, the mother is taught to grasp the knees and to rotate the legs gently medially at the hips (Fig. 22.8). She may find it convenient to let the baby sit in her lap, facing forward, and to reach around the baby and grasp each knee and rotate the legs medially. (Some mothers do this while watching television.) She turns them in as far as she can without hurting the baby, and she holds them in this position for at least a half-minute. She is told that wiggling the legs or holding them for a few seconds will not stretch the contracted muscles and ligaments and capsule of the hip as effectively as a longer steady stretch. It is suggested that she hold the legs in medial rotation for half a minute. To appreciate how long half a minute is, she must count slowly to 30. Of course, there is no virtue in 30, but there is virtue in holding the legs in an overcorrected position for a long while.

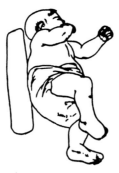

Fig 22.7. It is recommended that the baby be taught to sleep on his side. In this position the anterior surfaces of both legs are in the same plane with the anterior surface of the body. There is no torsion of the legs. The baby can be taught to sleep in this position by placing a support to his back. A pillow or rolled-up baby blanket is helpful.

She then relaxes for a few seconds to rest herself and the baby and repeats the exercise. If the baby objects and struggles she is told not to release the legs and reward the baby for struggling but that she should continue to hold the legs, even if the baby resents it, and that he will soon realize that it does not hurt and that he is not going to free himself. It is suggested that the mother stretch the legs medially for about 5 min each night and morning and that she make it a part of her routine either when she gives the baby his bath or when she puts him to bed.

If the flat foot deformity is not severe and the feet are fairly flexible, this is all that we teach the mother to do on the first visit. If the feet are quite flat she may be taught how to stretch the feet on the first visit, but it is confusing to the mother to try to teach her too much at one time.

If the flat foot deformity has been produced as described and the foot has been forced in the valgus position, the treatment is to stretch the foot back to the normal position. This is neither massage nor exercise but more like "stretching."

Various ways of holding the foot have been tried. We have found it best for the mother to place the baby on his back and for her to stand at his feet (Fig. 22.9, A–F). It is recommended that she begin with the right foot first, because it comes easier for her if she is right-handed. She places her index finger over the tubercle of the navicular. We explain to her that it is a pea-shaped bone on the medial side of the foot, about halfway between the base of the big toe and the heel. Usually by abducting the forefoot she can better see and feel this prominence. If she will move her finger back and forth a little toward the heel and toe, she can feel when she is off and on this bony prominence. The index finger should be straight and parallel with the foot. Some mothers like to flex the index finger, and when they do the nail presses into the skin and hurts the baby. The ball of the foot rests on the mother's flexed third finger, and her thumb rests on top of the big and second toes. This gives the mother a good grip on the front half of the foot.

The heel is then placed in the palm of the left hand, and a firm grip is taken on the posterior half of the foot. The heel which is in valgus is turned gently into varus. The fingers of the left hand surround the heel and the medial side of the foot. The middle finger of the left hand rests on top of the index finger of the right hand, so pressure can be made inward on the tubercle of the navicular more easily. The forefoot is carried in toward the midline of the body or toward the other foot. The forefoot is adducted, the heel is inverted and the foot is bent in the middle. The pressure is made straight in on the navicular and the head of the talus. It is not an upward thrust. We have found in treating the severe flat foot cases with casts that more improvement can be obtained by displacing the bones medially than can be obtained by trying to push up in this region. It is sometimes difficult to get the mothers to hold the heel. We try to explain to them that if they hold only the forefoot and twist the foot at the ankle, they accomplish nothing. They must hold the heel and bend the foot in the middle. It is like trying to straighten a wire. They cannot do it when they hold only one end. It is the same with the foot as with the wire; it must be held at both ends to bend it in the middle.

After doing this maneuver a few times, the foot seems to fit nicely in the hands. The mothers are instructed again to hold the foot for half a minute, release it and then repeat the operation. They often have a little more trouble learning to work on the left foot. Since 1950 we have taught more than a thousand mothers how to stretch flat feet. Most of them

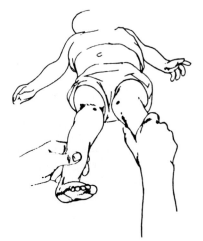

Fig. 22.8. To correct the outward rotation, the mother is taught how to grasp the legs and rotate the legs medially as far as they will go and to hold them in this position for about 30 sec, to release the legs for a few seconds, and to repeat the stretching.

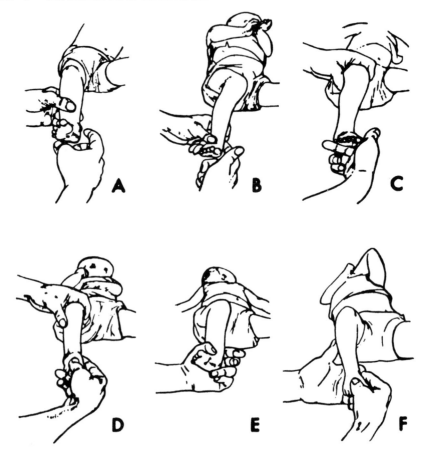

Fig. 22.9. (A) How to stretch a flat foot to form an arch. The tubercle or the navicular can be felt as a bony prominence on the medial side of the foot halfway between the base of the great toe and the heel. (B) The mother begins by placing her index finger on this pea-sized prominence. (C) The ball of the baby's foot rests on her flexed third finger. (D) Her thumb rests on top of the great and second toes, gives a good purchase on the forefoot. (E) The heel is placed in the palm of the left hand; the middle finger is placed on top of the right index finger, which is on the tubercle of the navicular as shown above. The two grips are then combined (F) If the baby's foot is small as shown in the drawings, the heel may be placed in the space between the index and middle fingers. This gives a firm grip on the heel. The two grips are then combined, the forefoot is carried inward toward the other foot, and the heel is inverted to correct the valgus deformity.

learned readily and have been rewarded by seeing their children develop arches in their feet.

The mother may give the child something to play with while doing the exercises or give him his bottle or make a game of it. The exercises do become monotonous, but the mothers are anxious to see an arch develop and are willing to suffer the tedium. The child begins to invert the foot after a few weeks, and the mother is encouraged to carry on.

This method will not correct every foot, but the percentage of success is high enough to make it well worth using. Success depends on the patience of the doctor and his ability to teach the mother the little details of the method.

Treatment of Flat Feet After the Child Begins to Walk

When the baby is old enough to begin walking, swung-in shoes are prescribed. There are many shoes on the market from which to select the proper shoe for the child. Some shoes are stiffer than others. For the first pair after the child is pulling up, we prefer the lightest swung-in shoes. The stiffer shoes which are often recommended delay walking. After the child has been walking a few months a heavier shoe may be used. We reserve the heaviest shoes for boys and overweight girls. All of these so-called corrective shoes have about the same features. The forefoot is swung inward into an adducted position, in some more severely than in others. In each there is a lift under the medial side of the heel. When the shoes have spring heels, a wedge of leather is inserted under the arch. When the shoe is large enough for heels, a Thomas heel is used. This carries the support a little farther forward under the arch than in the normal shoe and has $1/8$-inch lift on the medial side. In some shoes the counter is carried forward under the arch to give more support.

We are strongly opposed to a lift under the little toe side of the sole, since it elevates the lateral border of the foot and makes the foot assume more of a pronated position and does harm to the foot.

If the mother will not stretch the legs medially and the child still turns knees and feet outward, a bar may be placed across the shoes (to be worn at night) to turn the legs medially (Fig. 22.10). This is not seen by

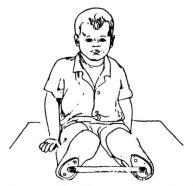

Fig. 22.10. If the mother is not willing to stretch the legs medially, or if the legs do not respond to her efforts, a bar to be worn at night may be placed across the shoes to rotate the legs medially.

friends, and the mothers do not object to the child wearing this. If the feet are flat, as they usually are, the bar is bent toward the body. This will invert the ankles and help correct the valgus deformity of the heels.

After the child begins to walk, if the flat foot deformity is so severe that he tends to break down the shoe on the medial border, he may have a support inside the shoe under the arch made of elastic or metal. The elastic supports may be made of sponge rubber, felt or leather; they are a stimulus to better foot posture. In heavy individuals a steel arch support may be used. These are made in our clinic to fit the shoe exactly with no flanges. The shoe holds the foot in the proper position on the metal support. Children never complain about these supports when they are properly made. In years past the physician had to make a plaster model of the foot and trim it before the brace-maker shaped the metal to fit the mold. Now our brace-maker has dies made for these foot plates, and all he needs is the shoe, which should be fitted without telling the shoe clerk that a foot plate is to go into it.

Treatment of Flat Feet in the Older Child

When the above recommendations have been carefully followed, most of the feet will have good arches and the child will walk with the feet straight by the time he is 2 or 3 years old. If the child has not been seen until he is several years old, he may be taught exercises in lieu of manual stretching by the mother.

In examining the older child we often find, in addition to the deformities mentioned above, a short heel cord. At first we may wonder why a child would have a short Achilles tendon (Fig. 22.11). If we watch the child

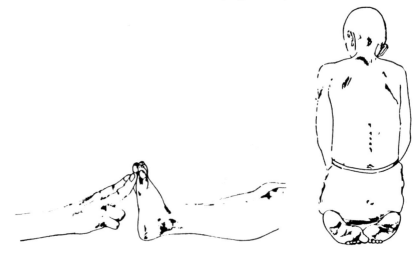

Fig. 22.11. (*Right*) Six-year-old boy sits on his feet much of the time; heel cords become contracted. (*Left*) When held in the midline the foot cannot be forced up in dorsiflexion above a right angle.

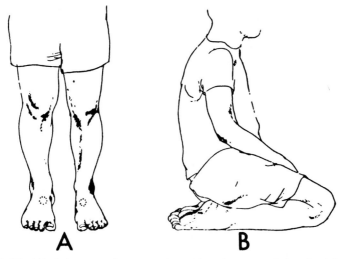

Fig. 22.12. (A) A bony enlargement on the dorsum of the foot has been called "over bone," once thought to result from lacing the shoe too tightly. (B) "Over bone" is produced by the child sitting on his feet. The pressure causes hypertrophy of the bones, just as the pressure of a tight shoe produces a bunion over the head of the first metatarsal.

play for a few minutes the answer becomes apparent. We see him on his knees sitting back on his feet, which are forced into an extreme equinus position. He sits this way a good part of the day at his play, in his chair at the table at meal time and on the floor watching television. The Achilles tendon becomes contracted in a manner similar to that in which his mother's develops from wearing high-heeled shoes constantly. Often he has "over bone" on the dorsum of the foot, from the irritation of the pressure on this part of the foot (Fig. 22.12). When he tries to walk with his feet straight in front of him, he cannot flex the ankle to a right angle. He has to let the foot turn out in a valgus position to relieve the strain on the tendon. The foot which cannot be brought up to a right angle, or 90°, when held in the midline can be dorsiflexed 15–20° above a right angle when allowed to turn out in a valgus position.

In order for this child to walk with his feet straight we must teach him exercises to stretch his heel cords. This may be done by someone holding his feet in the midline and manually stretching the foot in dorsiflexion. It is done better by teaching him an exercise in which he can use his body as the long arm of a lever and stretch the Achilles tendon. This exercise will be described below.

When a flat-footed child is requested to pull the foot up in dorsiflexion, he usually pulls it out and up, using the extensor hallucis longus, extensor digitorum longus, and the peroneals. The anterior tibial, which is the strongest dorsiflexor, is often not used at all in this action. The first exercise we like to teach the child is one to relax the other muscles and to strengthen the anterior tibial muscle.

Exercises. The exercises are done with the child barefooted. From the sitting position he is taught how to turn the foot "down in, and up." The foot is first carried through this motion manually. Then he is encouraged to follow a finger with his big toe, making a game of it. He plantar flexes the ankle as far as it will go and flexes his toes. This strengthens the short flexors of the toes. He then relaxes his toes and turns the foot in toward the other foot to invert the heel and get the foot in a position for the anterior tibial muscle to function. He continues to follow the finger with his big toe, pulling the foot up in dorsiflexion as far as possible. This causes a contraction of the anterior tibial muscle. At first it is easier to get him to pull the forefoot up against the resistance of a finger and to continue to pull as he slowly counts to ten. On the last count he is encouraged to give the foot an extra hard pull. This exercise strengthens the anterior tibial muscles and at the same time stretches the Achilles tendon. The child rests for a few seconds and repeats this exercise very slowly. Later he will learn to do it without the resistance of the examiner's finger. He will have to be taught to do one foot at a time for several days, and then he can do both at the same time. He is taught this exercise first because it is the most difficult for him to learn. His mother will have to work with him for a while to teach him how to do it correctly.

In the second exercise the child stands slightly pigeon-toed and raises himself on the lateral border of the feet, inverting the feet. This exercise again strengthens the tibial muscles. If the peroneal muscles are contracted, this exercise will stretch these muscles as did the first exercise. He does this exercise slowly and holds the position for a couple of seconds, relaxes, and comes back to the standing position. He may have to hold on to something at first to maintain his balance. He is to repeat this exercise a dozen times at first and then may gradually increase the number of times.

In the third exercise he stands slightly pigeon-toed and raises himself on the tips of the toes. He is to do this to the same count and in the same manner as the previous exercise.

The fourth exercise is designed to stretch the contracted Achilles tendon. This is done by standing about a foot and a half from the wall in a slightly pigeon-toed position. The heels must be kept flat on the floor. With his hands on the wall, he leans forward and touches his chest to the wall. If he cannot keep his heels on the floor he is too far from the wall. If he does not feel a pull of the muscles back of the knee he is too close to the wall and should move back an inch or two. He does this exercise slowly a dozen times and gradually increases the number of repetitions. These four exercises are performed for about 10 min each morning and night. The child is taught how to walk with his feet straight in front of him. This is probably the most important part of the training. He is taught to shift his weight, when standing, to the lateral border of the foot, away from the arch. This places the weight on the little toe side where there is no arch, thereby avoiding a strain on the muscles and ligaments of the arch.

Other exercises have been recommended which we seldom use. These include toe-curling and supination exercises and consist of picking up objects with the toes. The child is seated on a low chair, and a number of marbles are placed before him. He starts with his right foot and picks up one marble at a time and places it in a container to the left of the left foot. When he has finished, he repeats the process with the left foot. It is recommended that this be done for 10 min twice a day.

Toe-curling exercises can be performed by having the child stand on a large book or on the edge of a stair, trying to grasp the edge with his toes. He may also try grasping a chair rung.

The correction of flat feet is a slow process, and it should be explained to the parents at the beginning that it may take several years and that not all children so treated will develop a high arch, in fact, that a high arch is not necessarily a goal to be desired, since an arch of average height is better. They are also told that, if they will follow the instructions, the child probably will not run over his shoes or have pain in his feet.

There are a few foot disabilities which cannot be corrected by exercise. These are found in children whose joints are relaxed and hypermobile, whose feet turn either to a clubfoot position or to a flat foot position. Swung-in shoes and arch supports will keep these children from running over the shoes and should be used. A series of plaster casts may be needed in some cases. If these children suffer pain in later life, the foot can be made to assume the normal position by one of several operations to be performed by orthopedic surgeons with experience in this type of surgery.

Treatment of Flat Feet in Adults

In adults the findings are somewhat different. At one time the Army rejected recruits because of marked flat foot deformity even though many of them had earned a livelihood standing and walking without difficulty. It is only those adults who have discomfort who come for treatment; they seldom come for cosmetic reasons.

Often we find that the patients who are beginning to have pain have recently changed their occupations. We see individuals who had no trouble in an occupation which required walking develop trouble when they change to work which requires standing all day, especially in elevator operators, dentists, nurses, and surgeons. Others who walk most of the day may also have foot troubles, as postmen, policemen, waiters, and others who spend long hours on their feet.

Another frequent cause of foot trouble in the middle-aged is excessive weight. Often the feet have to carry 25–50 lb more than they did in the early years of life. The accumulation of this extra weight comes on gradually and is not noticed at first, but after a while a breaking point is reached. Frequently, these feet will cease to cause trouble if the patient will lose 10 to 15 lb.

Patients recovering from a long illness may complain of foot trouble when they begin walking again. The muscles and ligaments have become weak while they were in bed. In such patients walking should be resumed gradually, and shoes should be worn which give good support to the arches.

In an adult the position of the foot has become fixed, and the shape of the foot cannot be corrected simply by wearing a swung-in shoe as is possible in a child. Patients are sometimes seen who never had foot trouble but, after reading an advertisement, decide they should protect their feet by wearing some queer-shaped shoe recommended in the advertisement. They almost immediately develop pain in the feet because the feet cannot conform to the so-called corrective shoe. These corrective shoes should be used only by children whose feet are flexible. The adult who has changed to the abnormal shoe may get relief by going back to his original shoes.

The adult who is suffering from "foot strain" can get relief by being shown how to stand and walk and by being given some exercises to strengthen the weak, stretched muscles of the foot. We see more patients suffering with feet which are not really flat than we do those with extremely flat feet. They may still have about an average arch in the foot and an imprint between a normal and a flat foot. These are the feet which are beginning to collapse into a flat foot and might better be referred to as suffering from "foot strain." They can be helped by placing a wedge of leather $1/8$–$3/16$ inch thick in the medial border of the heel and by teaching them how to walk and stand with the toes pointing straight forward. They are taught to shift the weight to the outer borders of the feet when standing. The same exercises recommended for the older child should be carried out until the discomfort has been relieved. The correct walking and standing position should become a lifetime habit and not something to be followed for a few weeks.

Many older patients complain of pain in their feet from causes other than acquired flat feet. Probably the most common finding in them is a sprain of the ankle or a fracture of one of the small bones in the toe or foot. A rare finding occasionally has been tuberculosis of the foot. Nonmalignant and malignant tumors may force the foot out of balance and cause pain. One of the most common findings in middle-aged women with acute attacks of pain is a Morton's toe neuroma. This tumor causes excruciating attacks of pain between the third and fourth toes as a rule and can be relieved by removal of the small neuroma. Deformities following poliomyelitis, spastic paralysis, and spina bifida and congenital deformities offer no problem in diagnosis. These should be referred to the orthopedist for treatment.

SPASTIC FLAT FOOT OF ADOLESCENTS

One type of foot which should be described in some detail is the "spastic flat foot of adolescents." This is seen chiefly in young athletes who have overburdened their feet in their athletic endeavors, or who have injured the feet and have continued to strain them. It is seen in football players, often in the best players. One patient of ours who had earned all four letters in athletics in his preparatory school developed a very painful foot, and the muscles would go into spasm to help immobilize the foot or prevent motion. It is somewhat like arthritis. The extensor digitorum longus and the three peroneal muscles go into spasm and fix the foot until it is almost as rigid as a wooden foot. Any attempt at movement causes pain. The patient walks with the foot in an extreme flat foot position and avoids any motion in the foot or ankle. Even a jar may cause pain. It is more often unilateral, and the patient may come in walking on crutches.

Treatment. If the pain is due to arthritis, the treatment should begin with a search for the cause and treatment of the arthritis. Occasionally the foot can be helped by applying a cast, with the foot molded so as to correct as much of the flat foot deformity as possible. The foot is kept at rest in the cast for about a month. Often the foot is so sensitive it is necessary to give the patient an anesthetic and gently mold the foot into a more normal position and apply a cast for 4-6 weeks. This cast may have to be reapplied. When the cast is removed, a corrective shoe and foot plate may be necessary for some months. Heat, massage, and exercises are helpful at this stage, and care must be exercised to prevent recurrences. These patients are seldom able to return to college athletics.

CONGENITAL DEFORMITIES OF FEET

Another rare condition met with in youth is a congenital fusion of some of the bones in the foot, really a lack of segmentation of the bones. The foot may present the symptoms of a spastic flat foot or may give no symptoms for a long time. The most common finding in this condition is a calcaneonavicular bar or a talocalcaneal bridge. A bridge of bone crosses from one bone to the other, which serves as a checkrein to the motion between the bones and holds the foot in a slightly abnormal position. Patients suffering from this condition may do well if their feet are not subjected to abnormal strains. Often the foot is fixed in a flat foot position. When the discomfort cannot be relieved by rest and supports and exercise, it can be relieved by removal of the bar or by a triple arthrodesis.

An accessory tarsal navicular causes a prominence on the medial side of the foot along the arch. This may become sensitive from the pressure of the shoe. It causes an abnormal insertion for the posterior tibial tendon and changes its direction of pull. This may cause the foot to go into a pronated position. Occasionally the accessory navicular may require surgical removal for relief.

Medial Torsion of Legs, Pigeon-Toes

Medial rotation of the legs causes the child to walk pigeon-toed. This is one of the two patterns mentioned above: the first is that of the child who walks flat-footed, with the toes and knees pointing outward; the second is that of the child who turns his feet toward each other, and who looks bow-legged. He may trip on his feet and may fall frequently. This deformity is usually noticed shortly after he begins to walk.

Medial torsion varies in severity and in location. The deformity is not alike in all of these children, and for this reason the etiology differs. The torsion may occur at one, two or three locations, separately in each or in all three at the same time. We must study each of these three locations and the mechanics which produce the deformity in each in order to understand the problem and to successfully treat it.

MEDIAL TORSION AT THE HIPS

In children with this condition, the entire leg is rotated medially so that the toes and knees both point toward each other or toward the midline of the body. In examining these children we must first do the "rotation test" mentioned above. With the child sitting or preferably lying flat on his back, the legs are grasped above the ankles and the amount of rotation possible is judged by noticing the distance the patellas can be rotated medially and laterally. In medial torsion the legs can be rotated medially until the patellas face each other. The entire leg can be turned inward at the hip ninety degrees or more. The legs cannot be turned outward much past the mid-position. The muscles, ligaments and joint capsule at the hip have become stretched and fixed in this position of medial torsion. In order to understand the mechanics which have brought about this condition, we must watch how this child sits when he is on the floor playing and watching television (Fig. 22.13).

When the medial torsion is in the hips, the child sits with his knees flexed and his feet back on the side of the hips. He does not necessarily sit on his feet. He sits between his feet. The feet may be placed at varying distances from the hips. This gives him a broad base to balance himself better when he begins to sit alone. The anterior surfaces of the thigh are always rotated medially a full 90°. The anterior surfaces of the thighs face each other; this becomes the "position of comfort." When the child crawls about and goes back to a sitting position, he always returns to this same position.

While discussing inward torsion, we may pause to look at the feet. At times, the great toe rests on the floor and the foot is bent out in a flat foot position. The foot is held in eversion as shown under the description of flat feet above. This explains why the child may walk pigeon-toed and at the same time be flat-footed. The treatment for this combination is to use a normal or straight last shoe and insert a $1/8$-inch wedge in the medial side of the heel.

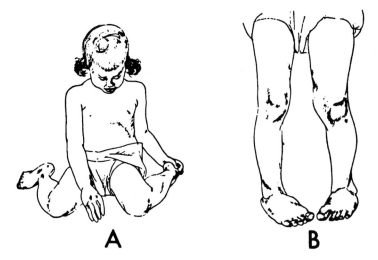

Fig. 22.13. (A) Medial torsion is produced in the hips by the child sitting with the knees flexed and the feet folded back opposite the hips. This rolls the anterior surfaces of the thighs medially about ninety degrees, so that the anterior surfaces face each other. (B) When the child stands she is pigeon-toed. It is more noticeable when she walks than when she is standing.

MEDIAL TORSION OF THE LEGS (BETWEEN KNEES AND ANKLES)

In this by far the largest group of children, the twist is between the ankles and the knees. A small segment of this group may be called "congenital" medial torsion of the legs, but most segments are called "acquired" medial torsion of the legs.

Congenital Medial Torsion

The deformity in these infants is frequently noticed when the baby is born. There is, in addition to the medial twist between the foot and the knee, a rather marked lateral convexity of the lower leg (Fig. 22.14). This deformity has been described by Nachlas, who says that it may be either an atavistic reversion or a developmental arrest. The orangutan, the gorilla and prehistoric man demonstrate medial torsion of the leg. The human fetus shows an inward torsion of the tibia, which disappears during the last few months before birth. The developmental-arrest theory is the more acceptable theory to the parents.

The chief complaint given by the mother is that the child is clumsy, pigeon-toed and bow-legged. When the deformity is noticed shortly after birth, there can be no doubt about its being congenital. However, it may be overlooked until the child begins to walk. It is then more difficult to tell whether the patient has a congenital or an acquired medial torsion. The deformity may be symmetrical and may occur in well nourished

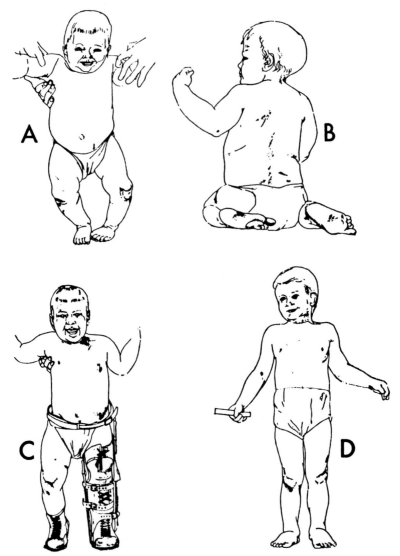

Fig. 22.14. (A) Congenital medial torsion of the left leg. Most of the deformity is in the lower leg between the knee and the foot. The knee points outward, and the foot turns in. There is lateral convexity of the leg. This is a 6-month-old boy, whose medial torsion was noticed by the pediatrician shortly after birth. (B) This boy sits on his left foot, which might make one think that the deformity was acquired. It is congenital because it was present before the child slept in the knee-chest position or sat on his feet. This deformity did not respond to stretching the foot in external rotation. (C) The deformity was corrected by wearing the bow-leg brace on the left leg. (D) Bow-leg deformity nicely corrected one year later.

children. In former times this deformity was called rickets and the child was treated with additional doses of vitamins.

The rotation test is helpful here. In the congenital medial torsion the knees can be rotated medially and laterally the normal amount. In the acquired type the knees can be rotated medially 90° or more.

The roentgenograms never show any cupping or fraying suggestive of rickets. The shaft of the tibia is straight, but the soft part shadow shows the lateral convexity of the leg (Fig. 22.15). The epiphyseal lines are not perpendicular to the shaft of the tibia as they normally are but are oblique. This is more noticeable at the distal end of the tibia. The epiphyseal line slants medially at each end, so that it gives the appearance of the shaft of the tibia being bowed. The metaphysis above and below the knee is expanded, and the epiphysis appears small. Children with congenital medial torsion show very little tendency to spontaneous improvement.

Acquired Medial Torsion

In acquired medial torsion the legs may be normal at birth, but the deformity is produced by the position in which the infant sleeps and, later, sits.

Etiology. These infants sleep on their stomach with their knees doubled up under them, their hips high and their feet turned in under them. They resemble a Moslem at prayer. The newborn may cry until he is placed in this fetal position, and then he will go to sleep. This soon becomes his "position of comfort." Pediatricians frequently recommend sleeping on the stomach, as it aids the expulsion of gas and is safe. There is no danger of the baby strangling on regurgitation. It the baby sleeps in this position

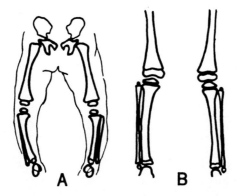

Fig. 22.15. (A) Tracings of roentgenograms of legs showing bowing of entire leg. The soft part shadow of the lower legs shows curving, but the shafts of the tibia are straight. There is tilting of the epiphyseal lines at each end, which causes the bowing; there is no suggestion of rickets. (B) Three years later, bow-leg deformity corrected by double bow-leg braces; epiphyseal lines now perpendicular to the shafts.

only occasionally, no harm is done. If he sleeps with his feet doubled up under him and turned in day and night for weeks until he is old enough to turn over, a twist will be produced between the ankle and the knee. The foot will also be bent in the midtarsal joint so that it will look like a congenital metatarsus varus deformity. In some cases the child continues to sleep in this knee-chest position for several years.

When the child who sleeps in the knee-chest position begins to sit, he will get on his flexed knees, put his feet behind him, turn his feet in toward each other and will sit back on his feet. This position forces a twist of 90° between the ankles and the knees (Fig. 22.16). This position does not produce a twist in the hips but only in the lower legs. However, it does cause a definite change in the feet, according to the two positions in which the feet are usually placed. If the feet are turned in toward each other, the weight will come on the head of the talus and the anterior lateral corner of the calcaneus; the child will develop a bony prominence over these two bones and the skin will later become brown and thick (Fig. 22.17). If he sits with the feet straight back behind him, he will develop "over bone" on the dorsum of the foot, and the Achilles tendon will become contracted (Fig. 22.12).

Signs and Symptoms. The child is also bow-legged and pigeon-toed as in the congenital group. The findings are similar to those of the congenital group but may not be as marked. In doing the rotation test, the legs may be rotated medially and laterally the normal amount, if the child sits on

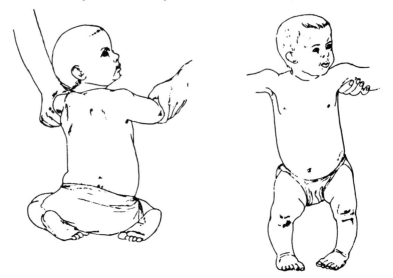

Fig. 22.16. (*Right*) Thirteen-month-old girl who stands and walks pigeon-toed. The twist here is between the feet and the knees. She slept in a knee-chest position. (*Left*) Her favorite way of sitting. Often the feet are more directly under her than shown in this drawing. This is an acquired medial torsion.

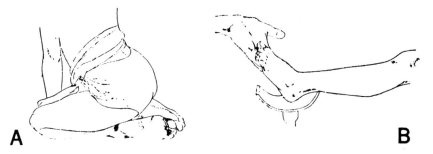

Fig. 22.17. (A) Eleven-year-old girl who sits on her feet, with the feet straight back in equinus at times, and at other times turned inward. (B) Her heel cord is contracted, and there is a prominence over the head of the talus and the anterior external corner of the calcaneus. The mother calls these "ugly knots."

his feet all of the time and not with his feet to the side of the hips. However, most of these children do sit part of the time with the feet by the side of the hips, and this position rolls the thighs medially as described above. In these cases the legs can be rotated medially 90° or more.

We also see children who always sit on one foot and will keep the other leg straight in front of them. This will give them a unilateral medial torsion and bow-legged deformity. They sit on the left leg much more frequently than they do on the right (Fig. 22.18)

The bow-legged deformity associated with this medial torsion is usually more apparent than real. When we bring the feet together with the toes pointing forward, the knees are rolled outward. This makes us look obliquely at the legs, and they look bowed (Fig. 22.19). When the feet are turned medially to make the knees point straight forward, the knees are closer together than the feet, and the legs are knock-kneed.

Treatment. The first thing to do in acquired medial torsion is to correct the sleeping and sitting habits of the infant, for prevention is most important. If our analysis of this condition is correct, we should teach the pediatricians, nurses, and mothers to insist that the baby sleep in all positions. It is not safe to place an infant on his back after a bottle until he can turn and take care of himself. Babies have regurgitated and have drowned when placed on their backs with a full stomach. The safest position is on the stomach, but this may cause torsion of the legs if the infant always sleeps in the same position. The recommended position is on his side. In this position the front of the legs and the front of the body are in the same plane (Fig. 22.7).

Exercises will vary according to the location of the torsion. If the torsion is in the hips, the mother is shown how to grasp the knees and roll the legs outward. The object is to untwist the deformity that has been put in the legs by the child sitting with his knees flexed and his feet opposite the hips. The mother should roll the legs laterally as far as they

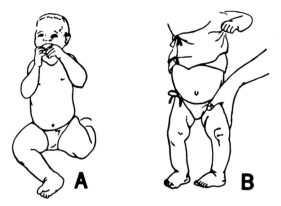

Fig. 22.18. (A) One-year-old boy who always sits with the right leg rotated laterally with the left knee flexed and the foot folded back by the hip or sitting on the left foot. (B) When he stands the right foot is placed in abduction and the entire leg is rotated laterally. There is marked medial torsion between the knee and the foot on the left. This is still more noticeable when he walks.

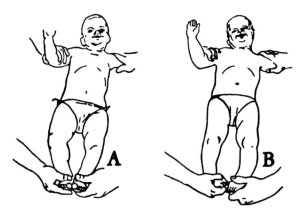

Fig. 22.19. (A) A year-old boy who is quite bow-legged when he stands. When the feet are brought together the knees are about three fingers' breadth apart. In this position, with the feet pointing straight forward, the knees are rotated laterally because of the torsion in the legs. This gives an oblique view of the legs, and an apparent bow-leg deformity. (B) When the feet are turned medially until the patellas point straight forward, in a true anterior position, the child is knock-kneed. The knees are closer together than the ankles, which is normal for this age.

will go without hurting the baby, and she should hold them in this position for half a minute, relax for a few seconds and repeat the outward rotation. This stretching exercise is done for 5 min twice a day.

If the medial torsion is between the feet and the knees, the mother should hold the leg with the knee extended and grasp the knee and hold it with the patella pointing straight forward. She grasps the ankle with her other hand and twists the foot outward, as far as it will go, and holds it so for half a minute (Fig. 22.20). The maneuver is easier if the hand is placed on the medial side of the ankle. The mother will have to change hands for each foot, twisting it outward, as though she were wringing clothes, for about three minutes.

The second maneuver is to correct the lateral convexity of the leg. The mother stands at the side of the child, grasps the knee with one hand and the ankle with the other, and puts pressure on the lateral side of the leg with her thumbs (Fig. 22.21). The thumbs are placed near the middle of

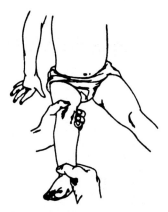

Fig. 22.20. To correct the medial torsion between the knee and ankle, the mother grasps the medial side of the ankle with one hand and the lateral side of the knee with the other and rotates the foot laterally. She twists the foot against the deformity.

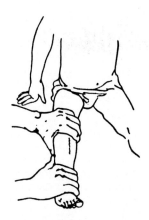

Fig. 22.21. The lateral convexity of the lower leg is corrected by the mother standing at the side of the patient and grasping the knee with one hand and the foot with the other. Pressure is made on the lateral side of the leg with the thumbs, as one would do in straightening a wire.

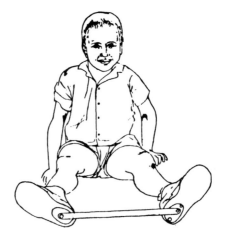

Fig. 22.22. A bar may be placed across the shoes to rotate the legs laterally. This is worn only at night.

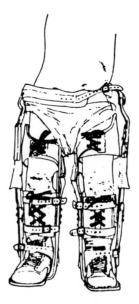

Fig. 22.23. A double leg brace is worn if the deformity cannot be corrected by the means described. The lateral bars of the braces are attached to a pelvic band so as to rotate the legs outward at the hips. There is also a rotation twist in the braces between the knees and the feet to rotate the feet out a little further. The lateral convexity is corrected by a pad at the medial side of the knee and a strap around the medial malleolus and the lateral bar. This holds both ends of the leg, while counterpressure is made on the lower leg by a strap around the lateral side of the leg and the medial bar.

the fibula, and the ankle and knee are drawn laterally, as in straightening a bent wire. This position is held for half a minute; the leg is released for a few seconds, and the exercise is repeated. About 10 min should be devoted to these two exercises morning and night.

If there is no improvement after 6–8 weeks, a metal bar may be placed across the shoes to rotate the feet and limbs laterally (Fig. 22.22). It may be worn only at night if the child is walking. This bar rotates the limbs outward at the hips. It has little effect on correcting the torsion between the knees and the ankle. The bar does more good in the acquired deformity than in the congenital group.

If the deformity has not been corrected by the time the child is 18–20 months old, double leg braces may be needed. Braces are seldom needed for the acquired group, but they may be needed for the congenital cases. Both groups should first be treated by the above stretching exercises. The brace recommended has bars on each side of the limb, with the lateral bars attached to the pelvic band (Fig. 22.23). There are freely moving joints at the hips, knees, and ankles. The lateral bars are set on the pelvic band so as to rotate the legs laterally. There is also a slight twist in the bars between the knees and ankles to turn the feet laterally even a little more. To correct the lateral convexity of the lower leg a pad is placed on the medial bar at the knee and a strap is placed around the medial malleolus and the lateral bar, thus fixing each end of the leg. There is another strap around the mid-portion of the leg, which is

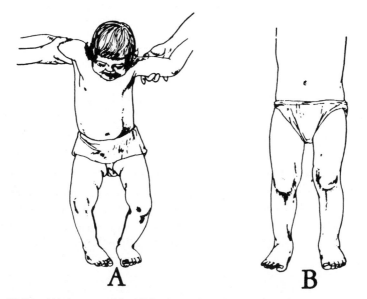

Fig. 22.24. (A) A year-old child whose bow-leg deformity was corrected by wearing a brace. (B) Appearance of the legs 8 months later after wearing a double bow-leg brace for 5 months.

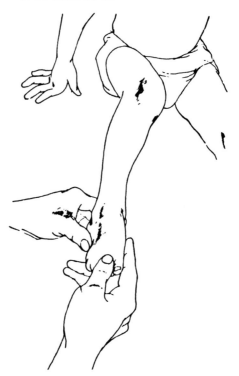

Fig. 22.25. Mild cases of congenital metatarsus varus may be corrected by the mother holding each end of the foot and pressing in on the middle. Pressure is made laterally on the medial side of the heel and the head of the first metatarsus. Counterpressure is made with the thumb on the base of the fifth metatarsal bone.

attached to the medial bar by buckles. This pulls in on the lateral side of the leg and corrects the lateral convexity. The deformity is usually corrected in from 3 to 9 months, depending on the age of the child and the severity of the deformity (Fig. 22.24).

Medial Torsion Between the Toes and Heel

The third place to find medial torsion is in the foot itself. The child who sits on his flexed knees with his feet turned in under him will develop forefoot adduction and inversion of the forefoot. Sometimes it is difficult at first glance to tell whether the forefoot adduction is the result of the child sitting on his feet, or whether it is a congenital metatarsal varus. If it is the result of sitting on the feet, the foot will be flexible and will feel normal when held in the hands. If this deformity is acquired, it will need no special treatment. We will accept a slight forefoot adduction as being desirable and indicating strong feet. If the child is flat-footed, sitting on his feet will help to produce an arch in the foot.

CONGENITAL METATARSUS VARUS

Congenital metatarsus varus is a fixed adduction of the forefoot. The correct term when we observe the child standing is "metatarsus adductus," but when he is sitting he will invert the foot as well as adduct it, so the term "metatarsus varus" is preferred. It is frequently called a "third of a clubfoot." In metatarsus varus not only is there forefoot adduction, but there is also a higher arch than normal and a prominence on the lateral side of the foot near the base of the fifth metatarsal. Muscle imbalance is present; the forefoot is always adducted and supinated and cannot be passively abducted to the midline. The foot is less flexible than normally.

Metatarsus varus deformity, which was a rarity 30 years ago, is now on the increase and is more common than clubfoot. Some cases are severe enough to be diagnosed at birth, but most are not recognized until the baby is 2 or 3 months old. The mild cases can be corrected by the mother stretching the foot. To do this she holds the toes and heel and presses in on the lateral border of the foot, on the prominence at the base of the fifth metatarsal (Fig. 22.25). If the deformity does not improve after a few weeks of stretching, it can always be corrected by the application of casts.

OTHER CONGENITAL DEFORMITIES OF THE FOOT

Clubfoot and other gross deformities cannot be corrected with exercises. These deformities require casts and operations for their correction. After casts are removed, the child may be taught exercises to strengthen the weak muscles. This will help the muscles to hold the foot in the corrected position. After operations children have to be taught to use crutches, how to walk to keep the feet straight and how to take steps of equal length. Heat, massage and exercises are helpful in removing the soreness and in strengthening the muscles and restoring a normal gait.

23

Exercise
for Arthritis

——————————————COLON H. WILSON, JR.

When discussing the problem of rheumatism with his students a century ago, Trousseau (27) said, "It behoves every practitioner to consider the form of treatment of each patient"; he advocated rest and exercise as the two main therapeutic pillars.

In the past two decades great advances have been made in the knowledge of the etiology and pathology of arthritis in its various forms. Newer drugs have been developed to complement salicylates, gold, and corticosteroids, including newer analgesic-anti-inflammatory drugs, penicillamine and cytotoxic-immunosuppressive drugs. Nevertheless rest and exercise continue to be fundamental parts of any basic management program (16, 23, 25).

To the practitioner, however, the prescription of rest and exercise for an arthritic presents a considerable problem. Special clinics are not universally available, and, even if they were, the number of arthritic patients is so large that the physician must prescribe treatment for the majority in their homes. A basic knowledge of the advantages and disadvantages of the forms of treatment and how they may be practiced is therefore a great asset.

Three main questions must be answered in relation to rest and exercise for the patient with arthritis: 1) In what forms of arthritis is exercise of value? 2) When are the afflicted joints to be rested and when are they to be exercised? 3) What forms of exercise should be prescribed?

It is the purpose of this chapter to discuss and answer these questions in so far as is possible and to consider the basic principles involved.

The modern conception of arthritis is very much simplified by a clinical classification in which three clear-cut types of arthritis are recognized, two chronic and one acute, each of which presents distinctive features: chronic inflammatory arthritis (e.g., rheumatoid arthritis and rheumatoid variants), degenerative joint disease (osteoarthritis), and specific infective arthritis. The chronic nonspecific inflammatory arthritides are generalized diseases usually affecting many joints. Osteoarthritis, on the other hand, is a slowly progressive disease in which the patient is not usually subject to acute exacerbations unless the affected joint has been subject to superimposed trauma, overuse or is in the stage of "active advance" as described by Fletcher (12).

In discussing the treatment of rheumatoid arthritis and osteoarthritis, it is easiest to consider them in three main phases: acute, subacute, and chronic. Rheumatoid arthritis may occur in any one of these three stages depending on whether or not an exacerbation is in progress. Osteoarthritis, on the other hand, is usually seen in a static form, and exercise therapy similar to that applied in the chronic stage of rheumatoid arthritis can be prescribed; it is only when the joint is subjected to trauma that osteoarthritis resembles the acute stage of rheumatoid arthritis and should be treated as such. The third form of arthritis we shall discuss in "specific infective arthritis" and includes acute suppurative arthritis, tuberculous arthritis, brucellosis, fungal arthritis, etc. The physical treatment of this group is the same as that of the acute stage of rheumatoid arthritis, provided the correct antibiotic therapy is exhibited. In the later stages when the suppuration has been controlled, the joint can be treated as though in the rheumatoid chronic stage.

Acute Stage

The aim of treatment in this phase of arthritis is twofold, namely, the relief of symptoms and the improvement of the patient's general health. The achievement of these objectives outweighs any consideration of the restoration of function, which therefore means waiting until the affected joint has become less inflamed. As there is usually a generalized constitutional disturbance which becomes worse if it is not treated, it is far more important to gain the patient's confidence by relieving pain and ensuring comfort than to concentrate on rehabilitation which at the time may seem to him to be a hopeless task.

This maintenance of a confident attitude and constant reassurance that the patient will eventually improve probably play a greater part in the reduction of pain and discomfort than has hitherto been recognized. Beecher (2), in a carefully conducted statistically controlled study, was often unable to demonstrate a greater effect on pain threshold from morphine than from placebos. In over 20% of patients receiving placebos, psychic modification of pain stimuli was considerable. The mere suggestion of relief appeared to reduce the thalamocortical spread of impulses. Patients did not claim that pain was absent; they were mentally divorced from painful experience, and the pain no longer bothered them.

In our experience we have found that a confident attitude, constant reassurance that the acute phase would soon pass and careful attention to the patient's comfort have done much to relieve pain. It is nevertheless vitally important to consider the advisability of the usual systemic measures associated with the acute stage of arthritis. Salicylates, the newer nonsteroidal anti-inflammatory drugs, synthetic adrenal cortico-steroids, penicillamine and the cytotoxic-immunosuppressive drugs all have a part to play in its treatment. No patient should be denied the careful assessment which the administration of these drugs requires.

It is impossible to lay down any hard and fast rules as to the local physical treatment of patients suffering from arthritis, as there are so many individual variations of the disease. In many, the pain appears to be a less prominent feature than joint swelling and restriction of motion; in others, pain appears to be more severe, though the local joint findings are less remarkable. The three factors important in treatment at this stage are rest, splinting, and gently joint movements.

REST

It is in the acute stage of arthritis that rest plays its greatest part. A patient suffering from an acutely inflamed joint which is painful at the slightest movement does not willingly move it. For this reason alone total bed rest has been used as a means of treatment for arthritis from time immemorial. One of the first publications concerning the use of rest came in the early nineteenth century when Sir Thomas Watson (29) cited the dictum of Warren, who, when asked what was good for rheumatism, replied, "Six weeks." At the same time Sir William Gull (14), in a well controlled trial, showed that patients who were treated with 16–30 days of bed rest alone fared better than those treated by the other methods which were then fashionable.

Too often in the past, however, the undesirable effects of bed rest were ignored, with a resulting high incidence of joint deformities. This presented a serious obstacle to subsequent rehabilitation, and bed rest fell into disrepute as a more active approach to the treatment of arthritis was advocated.

More recently, however, there has been a swing back toward total rest, and Duthie (9) has suggested that at least part of the systemic symptoms in rheumatoid arthritis may result from the inflammatory changes in the joint and that the greater the use of the joint in the inflamed stage, the greater is the generalized disturbance. Where the disease involves the joints of the upper limb exclusively it is usually not necessary to rest the body as a whole. In rheumatoid arthritis, however, generalized involvement of the joints is seen far more frequently, and in this type of patient. There is now general agreement that complete bed rest is essential (16, 23, 25).

When a patient suffering from an acute polyarthritis is put to bed, not only must the state of the affected joint and its surrounding muscles be considered but also the general posture of the body must receive attention.

GENERAL POSTURE

In emphasizing that it is essential that bed rest should not be allowed any longer than necessary, Fletcher (12) points out that most rheumatoid arthritis deformities result from inadequate attention to the postural position of the patient in bed. It may, however, be essential to prolong this period for a matter of weeks when detailed attention must be paid to posture in bed.

The bed should be firm and not sag in the middle. Sagging can be prevented by placing a board between the mattress and spring.

A cradle should be placed over the legs and the feet should be placed against a padded board at the foot of the bed to prevent the foot drop which may develop rapidly in the presence of the diminished muscle tone that accompanies disease of the ankle joint. Pillows behind the knees should be avoided, and at night only one pillow for the head should be allowed. During the day a firm back rest with a minimum number of pillows should be used as part of the attempt to maintain good posture of the spine.

In an attempt to avoid pain, the patient will tend to relax the joints of his upper extremities. The arms are held close to the sides with elbows flexed, the wrist drops and the fingers turn to the ulnar side. As a result the adductors and internal rotators of the shoulders become tight and flexion contractures may develop in the deviations mentioned. The position of the upper extremities should be changed frequently and supported at different times of the day by pillows or splints, particularly in the later subacute and chronic stages, in functional position.

SPLINTS

The inflamed joint is probably best safeguarded in the acute stage by the application of suitable splints. Dunlop (7) believes that the use of properly fitting splints is probably the most important advance yet made in the management of the joints in rheumatoid arthritis. With splints swelling can be reduced and pain relieved more effectively than by any other method. The function of the splint is to protect and immobilize the acutely inflamed tissues with the ultimate aim of preserving a movable and functionally useful joint. The possibility of ankylosis is, however, always present; thus, the affected joint should be maintained in the optimum position. Some form of light, comfortable apparatus should be used which is easily removable for physical treatment, since it is recommended that the splints be removed at least once daily for exercises. Duthie (9) asserts, however, that the splint can be maintained continuously in position for 2–3 weeks without subsequent diminution of the range of movement. This is not a universal practice, although in the author's experience it has much to recommend it in certain cases.

The splints may be made of wood, soft iron, steel alloys, duraluminum, molded leather, or plastic materials as well as plaster of Paris. Compound splints such as those described by Timbrell Fisher (26) for rheumatoid ailments and the Goldthwait brace (13) for spinal disease are effective except that they are costly and require time to manufacture. There is no place for the temporary or makeshift splint; it usually proves both uncomfortable and harmful.

The most useful materials available for splint making today are the newer lightweight heat mouldable plastics and plaster of Paris. If plaster of Paris is used the cast must be bivalved soon after its application so that no undue pressure is caused; in this way the joint is also made accessible for examination and exercise therapy. The splints used by the author and the joint position recommended for immobilization are shown in Table 23.1.

Good splinting should be comfortable and should allow for increased swelling of the joint yet prevent the slightest movement. Maximum comfort is the goal and this may necessitate the use of the newer light plastics instead of plaster.

GENTLE JOINT MOVEMENTS

When the patient is comfortable and the inflamed joint is adequately splinted, attention can be turned to the restoration of joint function. Function is maintained during the acute stage of the disease by gentle local joint movements for a short period once each day from the very onset of the disease regardless of how acute.

Opinion is divided as to whether these movements should be achieved by the patient's voluntary unaided effort or by passive movement. By passive movement we mean a gentle flexion and extension of the joint through as complete a range of movement as the pain and spasm will allow; the entire weight of the limb is supported in the therapist's hands throughout. No attempt at forcing should be made, for any passive stretching of a joint may aggravate the stiffness. That the elbow is particularly susceptible in this respect has been pointed out by Watson-Jones (30).

TABLE 23.1. *Recommended Splints and Joint Position for Immobilization*

Joint Involved	Position of Joint	Splint Recommended
Hand and fingers	Slight degree of flexion (25°) at metacarpophalangeal joint; curved to prevent ulnar deviation	Plastic
Wrist	30° to 45° extension	Plastic
Elbow	100° flexion, midway between pronation and supination	Plastic with reinforcement or plaster of Paris
Shoulder	Slightly flexed (30°), abduction 45°, external rotation 15°	Kramer wire or axillary cuff
Spine	Normal curves without attempt at correction	Flat bed as described
Hip	20° flexion, slight abduction, no rotation	
Knee	Almost complete extension	Plaster of Paris
Ankle	Flexed to 90°	Plaster of Paris
Foot	Normal position with slight flexion of the metatarsophalangeal joint and extension of the interphalangeal joint	Plaster of Paris

In our opinion the most effective approach to daily joint range movements is the "active assisted" exercise. The therapist learns to grip the extremity in such a way that it will not cause pain and so that the grip will not have to be changed as he assumes the weight of the limb and, with gravity eliminated, encourages the patient to move voluntarily with only a minimal assist. In this way the possibility of strain is eliminated, yet the facilitation of the proprioceptive reflexes, which are unstimulated when passive movements are employed, is permitted.

When the daily range of movement is completed the limb is returned to the splint again for 24 hours. Whatever method is employed the patient's tolerance must be carefully observed. An increase in pain or spasm for more than an hour or so after the exercise indicates an excessive amount of motion which must be reduced at the next treatment session.

Another form of exercise which can be practiced to advantage by the patient while the limb is in the splint is the "static" or isometric contraction of the muscles surrounding the affected joint. The muscle which has been relieved of spasm by splinting will tend to waste rapidly if not exercised. Duthie (9) has suggested that muscle wasting is in fact an innate feature of arthritic disease. There is ample reason to prevent wasting, since weakened muscles make rehabilitation in the stages of recovery more difficult. The patient should be encouraged to engage in static exercises for 2–3 min every hour of the day.

Exercise can be given for postural muscles in the same way, especially for the spinal and gluteal muscles—again, without exceeding the exercise tolerance.

As the patient's condition improves, the strength of the exercises, the frequency of repetition and the range of movement should be increased, provided there is no undue reaction as indicated by joint pain, adverse systemic changes and an elevated sedimentation rate. There is no advantage at this stage in progressing too rapidly, since a temporary relapse may result, with its inevitable lowering of the morale and a feeling of depression

The Subacute Stage

After a variable period of time with good anti-inflammatory drug therapy adjustment, the patient will often progress to a chronic stage of the disease in which the joint inflammation becomes quiescent and active measures of rehabilitation do not cause relapse. Between the acute and chronic phases there lies a period in which, although the joint condition will appear to have settled, overindulgence in joint strain or movement is followed by a flare-up of the arthritic symptoms. This is the subacute stage.

The three main aims in treatment in this stage are: the maintenance of general health, the prevention of further exacerbation, and the commencement of the correction of deformity.

This is the transition period between recumbency and gentle cautious movement and gradually progressive weight bearing and active exercises. Although at this time exercise plays a far greater part than in the acute stage, there is still need for general body rest even though this may be increasingly reduced in duration.

Local joint rest can be correspondingly reduced; the splints may be left off for increasing periods until they are used at night only. The use of night splints is of great value, and patients frequently find these offer relief long after they have passed into the chronic stage.

Progress is judged not only from improvement in the local joint condition but also from the patient's general health and attitude, the sedimentation rate, systemic temperature and hemoglobin level. Whatever form of drug treatment is being followed must be continued in full at the beginning of this stage. As the patient gradually improves, the medication can be correspondingly reduced as the exercise therapy is stepped up. There is an ever present need for caution, however, and the physician must be prepared to decrease the amount of exercise and increase the medication and bed rest at the least significant sign of deterioration. It is important that rest be provided before excessive fatigue has occurred; therefore, it is better to maintain two periods of bed rest during the day, with three periods of activity sandwiched between these two daytime rest periods and a long rest at night.

LOCAL MEASURES

More strenuous measures must be deferred until previous gains have consolidated, and it is preferable for each step in the progression to take 1 or 2 weeks. The eventual aim is a mobile joint, and, since stiffness and reduction in joint range develop during the period of rest, the first step is to increase mobility. For this purpose apparatus designed to assist the patient in performing movements in bed in the earlier stages is invaluable. A Guthrie-Smith (15) type of suspension frame is used extensively in Great Britain in this way, but any form of overhead framework to which slings or pulleys can be attached would be equally suitable.

When it is decided that the patient is ready to progress to more active treatment we use the following schedule:

Phase 1). The patient remains in bed receiving both active assisted exercises and isometric exercises.

Phase 2). The patient is taught to get into a chair at the bedside and continues the exercises, increasing the duration of the period gradually.

Phase 3). Standing exercises are begun. It is important to ensure that balance is well established before progressing further, and it may be necessary to prolong this period as much as ten days to two weeks.

Phase 4). Walking, either in a walker or with manual assistance, is begun. A useful and readily available piece of "apparatus" to assist in walking is a wheel chair. Patients who could not walk otherwise can frequently proceed quite satisfactorily supporting themselves on the chair back.

Phase 5). The next step is progress in walking with the assistance of crutches; our personal preference is for elbow crutches rather than the conventional axillary type. The former avoid any risk of crutch "palsy," which, when it occurs, is responsible for considerable delays in rehabilitation of patients with lesions involving the upper limbs. When there is severe involvement of the wrists, axillary crutches may have to be used.

The next step after crutches is canes. When starting a patient off on the full weight bearing required at this time it may be necessary to support the knees and ankles with bandages and splints. Ambulatory splints in the form of metatarsal bars for the foot, braces and T-straps for the ankles and light calipers for the knees will also be invaluable.

There is no point in following this routine exactly in every patient. Many, particularly those in the younger age groups, can satisfactorily omit one or two of the steps without handicap, provided the precautions mentioned earlier are observed.

Painstaking and sympathetic reeducation is very necessary in the weeks during which the patient passes through the subacute stage of arthritis. The steps of transition from complete immobilization, the building up of muscle control, the graduated development of active movement to the final stages of weight bearing and ambulation depend fundamentally upon the endeavors of the patient and not upon the magic of electricity, manipulative or other physical treatment.

The Chronic Stage

As the active phase of arthritis passes and the constitutional disturbance settles, it will be found that unless stringent precautions have been taken the patient will have almost certainly developed joint and postural contractures.

JOINT CONTRACTURES

In the course of arthritis, the patient may experience a vicious circle of joint pain, muscle spasm and immobility in the position of flexion. If untreated, this will eventually give rise to a condition in which the flexor muscles become hardened and thickened through continuous spasm. The corresponding extensor muscles become thin and wasted through disuse. Inflammatory products around the joints favor fibrous deposition, and the periarticular and articular layers of tissues become inextricably fused. It is possible for the ends of two bones to become so fused that the joint is completely effaced. This is more common in ankylosing spondylitis and other rheumatoid variants than in rheumatoid arthritis per se.

Flexion deformities are not the only contractures of chronic arthritis. There is often adduction spasm and, frequently, hypertonic flexion. The distal part of the extremities may develop the most bizarre types of muscle pulls, which result in many types of deformity so commonly seen in the rheumatoid arthritic, as pointed out by Charcot (4).

Various joints have different contractural tendencies. The cervical spine usually bends laterally and this may be so marked as to cause bedsores of the pinna; the shoulder joint often develops an upward subluxation of the humerus which prevents full or even adequate abduction; the bones, ligaments and soft tissues may eventually become fused, a condition first fully described by Howell (17).

When the elbow joint becomes the site of contracture it usually becomes fixed in partial flexion. This is occasionally associated with considerable bony changes involving the lower end of the humerus and upper part of the radius and ulna. The elbow joint may occasionally be fixed in an almost extended position, and when this deformity is bilateral the resulting disability is so great that the patient cannot raise his hand to his mouth or attend to his personal toilet.

Changes in the wrist joint produce a classical deformity of rheumatoid arthritis. It is surprising that despite the most marked changes very little disability results from lesions of this joint.

If patients with hip involvement are allowed to become immobile, the spasm of the flexor and adductor muscles will produce a flexion contracture of the hip with partial adduction and internal rotation; secondary flexion contractures of the knees also develop. These deformities tend to become progressive, and as a result the inner aspects of the knees approximate and press on each other with possible ulceration and necrosis.

The main deformity of the knee joint results from hamstring contractures which end in a joint flexion perpetuated by fibrosis. The patella eventually becomes fixed to the articular surface of the lower end of the femur and thereby renders extension even more unlikely and difficult.

The end stage of this type of deformity (seen occasionally) is a backward dislocation of the head of the tibia on the lower end of the femur, induced by extreme hamstring spasm. Once this develops, little short of radical surgery is of any value. It is also frequently accompanied by damage to the nerves and vessels in the popliteal fossa with a resultant edema of the foot and ankle which further complicates recovery.

Ankle deformities usually follow, as mentioned earlier, as a result of the muscle wasting and weakness which developed in the acute stages. A drop foot with external rotation results and occasionally becomes fixed by fibrosis. Other deformities which may occur in the foot include hammer toe, adduction of the great toe, flexion contracture of the toes and breakdown of the transverse arch. Walking may become so difficult as to require special shoes.

POSTURAL CONTRACTURES

These are consequent upon the maintenance of a flexed position in bed while the patient is at full bed rest and withdrawn from the world. The cervical spine flexes until the chin approximates to the chest, the dorsal and lumbar spine is fully flexed, the hips and knees are flexed and the ankles are extended. The patient in fact "curls up into a ball." The bones of such a patient, particularly in the aged, become osteoporotic and liable to fracture.

EXERCISES

Physical therapy is essential in the treatment of this stage to relieve muscular spasm and pain and to improve the circulation of blood and lymph in the neighborhood of the affected joint, with the expectation that the degenerative processes may eventually be reversed. This aim is best achieved by carefully planned and supervised exercise therapy. It is at this stage also that an attempt must be made to increase joint mobility to the greatest possible range and to increase muscle power.

Limitation of the range of movement impairs the function of a joint and the muscles that move it. Measures which increase the range of movement must, therefore, go hand in hand with those which build up sufficient muscle power to stabilize and control that movement. As instability and lack of control lead directly to further injury, it is essential that every degree of mobility gained can be controlled by muscular action. The development of range and power and the exercises required to increase these will be considered separately, but they should be practiced concomitantly.

Some form of heat treatment should precede a course of exercises to improve muscular relaxation and increase the blood supply of the affected part. Among effective forms of heat are heating pads, hydrocolator packs, paraffin baths, whirlpool baths, Hubbard tank, exercise pool, diathermy and ultrasound. In a series of patients suffering from arthritic joint contractures with gross bony deformities, Howell (18) found that 80% responded to ultrasound with an increased range of movement. Even more striking was the improved freedom of movement within this range and the fact that the affected joint retained this increase after treatment had ceased. Because ultrasound can break open cells and produce disolution of bone, this should be used carefully by one skilled in its use.

INCREASING JOINT MOBILITY

Increasing joint mobility after the development of contractures can prove a most difficult problem, since it requires sustained effort on the part of the physician, the physical therapist and, above all, the patient himself.

The exercises prescribed for a patient should be performed under supervision, but this is obviously impossible except in very few cases. Great attention should, therefore, be paid to the instruction of each patient in the aims of the exercise and the details of its performance.

It is far more valuable for a patient to repeat a few exercises for each affected joint daily than to spend one long period of exercise under supervision once or twice a week. It is usually convenient to have the

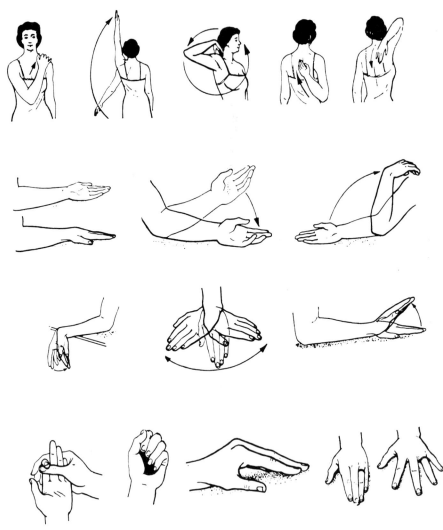

Fig. 23.1. Illustrated exercise charts are appreciated by patients. In this figure and the following figure are examples of illustrations used in the home exercise instructions given patients at the author's clinic for arthritis. Shoulder: 1, With your fingers pull you arm upward to your shoulder as far as it will go. 2, Try to touch you ear keeping your arm straight. 3, Circle you elbow several times in each direction 4, Put you hand into the small of your back, then push it as far as you can. 5, Push your hand as far down your back as you can. Elbow: 1, Turn your hand over and try to make your palm touch the table. 2, Straighten your elbow as far as possible. No attempt should be made to force your elbow straight with the other hand or with weights. 3, After pulling you hand back as far as you can, relax a little, then try again. Wrist: 1, Rest you forearm on a table with your elbow making a right angle. Lift your hand, relax, then lift again. 2, With your forearm and hand flat on a table, move your hand from side to side as far as you can. 3, Pull your hand back as far as you can

patient repeat each mobilizing exercise for each joint 2 or 3 times every day, if this does not overtax him or cause a recurrence. The repetition is increased to 6 or 8 times twice daily after 3–4 days and then to 10 times twice daily after another week. It is usually wisest not to increase mobilizing exercises beyond this number of repetitions in arthritic patients, for if they tire and lose muscular control over the movement the joint tends to "wrench" at the extremes of its range.

An exercise pool, where the buoyancy of the water reduces the gravitational force, is very helpful in gaining mobility.

Pendular movement is usually taught to increase the amplitude of ranges with "pressing" movements at the limit of range. A suggested system of regional exercises is printed on sheets together with illustrations describing exactly how they are performed. These are given to the patients so that they can check on their movements at home. Figures 23.1 and 23.2 reflect the instruction sheets used in our clinic (reproduced below).

Details of Range-of-Motion Exercises

I. Upper Extremities
Shoulder
1. Arms at side with elbow straight, bring arms forward – upward by ear.
2. Arms at side with elbow straight, take arm sideward – upward over head.
3. Arms at side, bend elbows to right angle and take hands apart.
Elbow
1. Bend elbow, touching fingers to top of shoulder.
2. Straighten elbow.
Forearm
1. Elbows bent, turn palm of hand and then back of hand toward face.
Wrist
1. Keeping forearm steady move wrist up and down as in waving.
2. Again hold forearm steady, move wrist up and down as in hand shaking.
3. Make circle with hands.
Hand and Fingers
1. Make tight fist.
2. Open fingers as wide as possible.
3. With hand open spread fingers away from each other and then together.
4. Touch tip of thumb to tip of each finger.
5. Bend thumb in toward palm of hand.
II. Lower Extremities
Hip
1. Pull knee to chest and return.
2. Keeping knee straight and toes pointed up, slide leg out to side.
3. Keep legs straight – roll legs in toward each other.
Knee
1. Slide heel up toward buttocks and back.

---

then relax a little and try again. Fingers: 1, Bend each finger joint individually then all simultaneously. 2, Try gripping a ball of wool tightly. 3, Try to arch your hand while keeping your fingers straight. 4, Put your hand flat on a table, separate your fingers, then squeeze them together again.

Ankle
1. Pull foot up and in, then push back down.
2. Make circle with foot.
3. Pull foot in toward other foot.
4. Pull foot to outside.

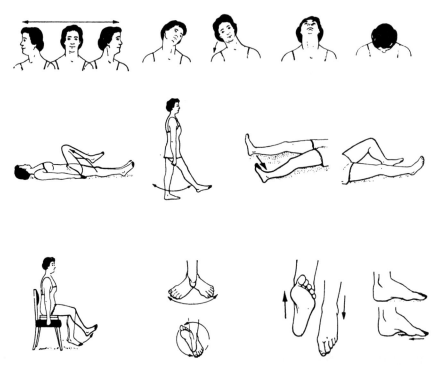

Fig. 23.2. Exercises for the neck: 1, In the sitting position, twist your head as far as possible in each direction. 2, Sit or stand with your hands on your hips. First circle your head clockwise, then counterclockwise. 3, In the sitting position, try to touch each shoulder with your head. 4, In the sitting position, look behind you as far as possible then look at your toes. For the back: 1, Sit up straight. The weight of you arms should turn your trunk around. 2, Try to place your head between your knees then slowly unwind yourself to the first position. This is a strenuous exercise and should be attempted only if specifically suggested by your physician. Hips: 1, Try to bend your knee to your chest; relax a little and try again. 2, Stand on your good leg and swing your other leg backward and forward from your hip. 3, Stretch your affected leg out to one side keeping it straight. 4, Lie on your back. Bend your knee and then move it from side to side across your body. Knee: 1, Sit with your feet off the floor. Lift your leg and then allow it to return to the bent position SLOWLY. Ankle: 1, Turn your foot inward and then outward as far as possible. 2, Circle your foot several times clockwise, then counterclockwise. Toes: 1, Sit with your legs crossed and your affected leg uppermost. Bend you ankle up and then straighten it, pointing your toe. 2, Stand upright and try to arch your foot while keeping your toes straight and pressed onto the floor.

Toes

1. Pull up on toes then curl toes under.

III. *Back Program*

Supine (with legs straight)

1. *Quad sets*: Tighten muscle above knee, hold for slow count of 5. Relax. Repeat (   ) times.

2. *Gluteal Sets*: Supine with legs straight tighten buttocks and hold for slow count of 5. Relax. Repeat (   ) times.

3. *Pelvic tilt*: Supine with knees bent, feet flat on surface, tighten abdominal and gluteal muscles forcing low back into surface. Relax. Repeat (   ) times.

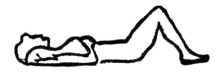

4. *Double knee to Chest*: Supine—bring both knees toward chest—Grasp knees with hands and gently stretch closer to chest—Maintain proper breathing pattern. Repeat (   ) times.

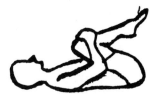

5. *Modified curl-up*: Supine with knees bent—feet flat without pillow with arms out-stretched, bring chin toward chest and attempt to sit up trying to touch knees with finger tips. Return slowly. Repeat (   ) times.

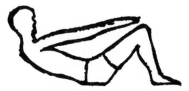

6. *Sitting stretch*: Sitting in chair, feet flat on floor spread about 2 feet apart. With arms crossed, bend forward allowing arms to pass between knees and gently stretch toward floor. Repeat (   ) times.

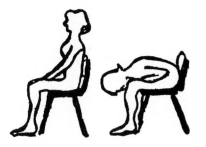

These exercises are all considered to be safe enough to be attempted by any patient without supervision at home, provided they have been well learned earlier. They are simple, and patients are told to repeat them only a very few times. It is more valuable for a patient to perform a simple series of exercises such as these than to "give up" after a few days because the schedule is too laborious or too complicated.

INCREASING MUSCLE POWER

At the same time that mobilizing exercises are practiced, a series of exercises must be included to develop power in the muscles that support the affected joint. As pointed out earlier, there is inevitably some degree of wasting of the muscles surrounding the joint, even though it be only minimally involved by an arthritic condition. It is a well established fact that the performance of muscles can be improved by systematic and voluntary exercises, although so far no agreement has been reached regarding the most effective way this can be achieved or the way in which the underlying functional and structural changes are altered (5). It has been recommended that different methods should be used to produce the desired results. For instance, it is said that an increase in strength is favored by heavy resistance work, whereas endurance is promoted by rapidly repeated contractions, and coordination, by light muscular work (1, 6, 9, 11, 21, 29).

It is also stated that different types of exercise induce different changes in the muscle. For instance, exercises of strength are said to cause hypertrophy, whereas those of endurance cause an increase in the capillary bed (28).

Although the size of muscle fibers may be increased by appropriate exercise, it is still not known how much this contributes to muscle strength, and it now seems fair to conclude that muscle bulk is not necessarily a reliable criterion of strength. Indeed, MacQueen (22) states that exercised muscle can increase in size, but not strength, or vice versa.

The object of strength-increasing exercises is, therefore, to ensure, as far as possible, the recovery of function rather than the restoration of normal muscle morphology.

It may be preferable, for instance, to reestablish muscle balance even though the strength of some muscles is below normal or even to encourage compensatory or "trick" movements when the prime movers cannot carry out their work effectively. It is most important to develop these exercises with relation to the patient's normal employment and encourage him to carry them out with this in mind. Only too frequently do we hear patients say, "But Doctor, I only do it that way during my exercises." It is probable, therefore, that these aims can be achieved by prescribing exercises designed to produce maximum activity of the involved muscles and thereby to maintain or restore their blood supply rather than by concentrating on the development of muscle bulk.

When prescribing exercises to develop muscle strength, it is obvious that there are many variables to be considered. First, should the object be to concentrate on isolated muscle groups or on mass movements; should the pattern resemble that normally occurring, or should the affected muscles be exercised in other ways? Second, should the exercises by isometric or isotonic? Third, in which position should the joint be exercised? Whichever type of contraction is decided upon, there are further factors to be considered: should resistance be applied, and, if so, what should its strength be; should the resistance be steadily increased, and, if so, how often: what should be the duration of the exercise period and the frequency of repetition? The most important principle in deciding on these problems is that the joint condition should not be worsened by the exercise. It is unwise, for example, to apply strong resistance in the early stages of treatment of a patient with an arthritic knee and a weak quadriceps muscle. If the weight to be lifted is too great or if the movement is repeated too frequently, the joint will become more painful and prevent further exercise. It is probably better that the patient should lift 10 lb 10 times every hour through the day than 10 lb 50–100 times, or 20 lb 20 times in the day. As mentioned earlier, if the joint is very painful, then the exercise must in the first instance be static and not dynamic. Brewerton (3) has shown quite clearly that when giving resistance exercises it does not matter which position the joint is in when it is being exercised providing there is no pain at some joint in the range. If there is, the resistance must be given in the least painful position.

Progressive resistance exercises can be graded from a little more than a few ounces to more than 100 lb. In the earlier stages of such exercise, gravity alone may be an adequate resistance.

A course of exercises must be designed for each patient, bearing in mind the stage of the disease and age, size and strength variations. Patients should be encouraged to acquire their own equipment and perform progressive exercises at home. It is surprising how well patients will push themselves in resistive exercise; they become so keen, in fact, that they should be told of the dangers of excessive exercise.

Exercise therapy in the various forms of arthritis must be correlated with other forms of treatment. In the acute stages it must fit in with systemic drug therapy and bed rest; in the subacute stage, with reeducation and ambulation; and in the chronic stage, with occupational and work therapy and the eventual return to work.

Three factors will always remain outstanding in the management of arthritics: physical therapists who are enthusiastic and understanding, a constantly prevailing optimistic atmosphere and a physician who deals not only with the patient's joints but also with his fears and social problems. There is nothing better than renewed confidence for restoring a man to health.

REFERENCES

1. ASMUSSEN, E. Training of muscular strength by static and dynamic muscle activity. Kongressen Föredrag. Stockholm, 1949.
2. BEECHER, E. K., KEATS, A. S., AND D'ALESSANDRO, G. L. A controlled study of pain. *J.A.M.A., 147:* 1761, 1951.
3. BREWERTON, D. A discussion. Evaluation of methods of increasing muscle strength. *Proc. R. Soc. Med., 49:* 1006, 1956.
4. CHARCOT, J. M. *Clinical Lectures on Senile and Chronic Diseases.* London, 1881.
5. DARCUS, H. D. Discussion. Evaluation of methods of increasing muscle strength. *Proc. R. Soc. Med., 49:* 999, 1956.
6. DELORME, T. L., AND WATKINS, A. L. Technics of progressive resistance exercise. *Arch. Phys. Med., 29:* 263, 1948.
7. DUNLOP, R., DAVIDSON, S., AND McNEE, G. *Textbook of Medical Treatments.* Edinburgh, 1946.
8. DUTHIE, J. J. R. Fundamental treatment of rheumatoid arthritis. *Practitioner, 166:* 22, 1951.
9. DUTHIE, J. J. R. Chapter, in (8).
10. EHRLICH, G. E. *Total Management of the Arthritic Patient.* Philadelphia, Lippincott, 1973.
11. ELKINS, E. C., AND WAKIM, K. G. Effects of artifically induced fever on the circulation in arthritis patients. *Arch. Phys. Med., 28:* 274, 1947.
12. FLETCHER, E. *Medical Disorders of the Locomotor System.* Edinburgh, 1947.
13. GOLDTHWAIT, J. E., BROWN, L. T., SWAIN, L. T., AND KUHNS, J. G. *Essentials of Body Mechanics in Health and Disease.* Philadelphia, 1952.
14. GULL, W., AND SUTTON, H. G. Cases of acute rheumatism. *Guy's Hosp. Rep., 12:* 509, 1866.
15. GUTHRIE-SMITH, O. *Rehabilitation, Re-education and Remedial Exercise.* London, 1947.
16. HOLLANDER, J. L. AND McCARTY, D. J., JR. (Eds.) *Arthritis and Allied Conditions,* Ed. 8. Lea & Febiger, Philadelphia, 1972.
17. HOWELL, T. H. *Med. Illustr., 4:* 385, 1950.
18. HOWELL, T. H. Joint contractures. *Proc R. Soc. Med., 50:* 70, 1957.
19. KNAPP, M. E. Rehabilitation of severe poliomyelitis. *J. Iowa Med. Soc., 43:* 369, 1953.
20. LICHT, S. AND KAMENETZ, H. L. (Ed.) *Arthritis and Physical Medicine.* Waverly Press, Inc., Baltimore, 1969.
21. LUNDERVOLD, A. J. *Sport and Health.* Olso, 1952.
22. MACQQUEEN, I. J. Recent advances in the techniques of progressive resistance exercise. *Br. Med. J., 2:* 1193, 1954.
23. MOSKOWITZ, R. W. *Clinical Rheumatology.* Lea & Febiger. Philadelphia, 1975.
24. REITER, H. Ueber eine bisher unerkannte Spirochateninfektion. *Dtsch. Med. Wochenschr., 42:* 1535, 1916.
25. RODNAN, G. P. (Ed). Committee of the American Rheumatism Association Section of the Arthritis Foundation. Primer on the Rheumatic Diseases. Reprinted from the *J.A.M.A., 224* (Suppl): April 30, 1973.
26. TIMBRELL FISHER, A. G. *The Rheumatic Diseases.* London, 1938.
27. TROUSSEAU, A. *Clinical Medicine.* London, 1871.
28. WAKIM, K. G. In *A.M.A. Handbook of Physical Medicine and Rehabilitation.* Philadelphia, 1950.
29. WATSON, T. In *The Principles and Practices of Medicine,* edited by C. H. Fagge. London, 1886.
30. WATSON-JONES, R. T. *Fractures and Other Bone and Joint Injuries.* Edinburgh, 1940.

24

Exercise in Peripheral Vascular Diseases

During the past few decades exercise has received only limited attention as a therapeutic agent in the management of disease of the peripheral vascular system. The chapter on the history of exercise lists only two references which relate to exercise in vascular disorders. This neglect is a reflection of the lack of enthusiasm for the diseases of the peripheral circulation on the part of medical practitioners. It is only in the past 40–50 years that interest in this area has grown, largely in the result of the pioneering work of Buerger (7), whose monumental treatise on peripheral vascular disorders was published in 1924, and of Brown of the May Group (2), who surrounded himself with young physicians, who subsequently became specialists in peripheral vascular diseases.

Another important cause for the lack of interest exhibited by the profession is that the term "peripheral vascular diseases" is probably one of the poorest choices of medical usage. "Peripheral vascular disease" is not a disease; it is a descriptive term used to designate a temporary or permanent impairment of the circulation in the extremities. More recently the term has been used to include diseases of all the vessels distal to the heart. As a result of this broadened definition, disorders of the lymphatic vessels have frequently been excluded, although consideration of lymph vessels is appropriate in the group of conditions encompassed in the term "peripheral vascular diseases."

Disorders of the peripheral circulation may be grouped into four major categories:

1. (a) Organic arterial obstruction, which may be divided into the acute and chronic types. Into the acute group fall embolism, acute thrombosis and acute trauma. In the chronic category are arteriosclerosis obliterans,

531

thromboangiitis obliterans, traumatic arterial disease and the various types of chronic arteritis. (b) Functional arterial disorders characterized primarily by spasm of the blood vessels. In this group are Raynaud's syndrome, traumatic arterial spasm, usually due to various occupational hazards (pneumatic drill hammers, etc.), and the disorders of reflex arterial spasm such as hyper-reactivity to cold, psychogenic factors, and so forth. (c) Combined disorders of organic and functional causes, such as thromboangiitis obliterans, Raynaud's disease and frost-bite.

2. Disorders of the venous circulation, including varicose veins, probably the most common form of peripheral vascular disturbance, and thrombophlebitis and phlebothrombosis.

3. Disorders combining arterial and venous involvement. Thromboangiitis obliterans is the most important in this group. Other conditions in this category are arterial spasm associated with thrombophlebitis and arteriovenous fistula.

4. Disorders of the lymphatic system, with lymphangitis and lymphedema the two most important conditions.

In the following discussion we shall confine ourselves to those disorders in which exercise as a therapeutic measure plays a significant role. In addition, the use of exercise in the diagnosis of peripheral vascular disorders will be touched upon briefly.

The Collateral Circulation

The aim of any form of treatment in occlusive arterial disease is improvement in the status of the circulation. In a number of instances this can be accomplished surgically: through embolectomies, endarterectomies and for the past two to three decades through advanced techniques of replacement and by-pass grafts. These procedures are of value only in diseases of the large vessels such as the aorta and the main stem vessels of the extremities. In a small number of instances nature achieves reestablishment of circulation through recanalization of a thrombus which had occluded the vessel. In a majority of instances, however, improvement in local circulation depends upon reestablishment of blood flow through collateral vessels. The manner by which such collateral circulation develops has interested investigators for many decades. Thoma (44) in 1884 published his investigations on the circulation in amputation stumps 1–31 months following surgery, comparing the vessels in the stump with those in the normal contralateral limb. He found that the diameter of the vessels in the stump was narrowed and that the lumen was narrowed by connective tissue proliferation in the intima, which he believed to be caused by the diminished blood flow required by the foreshortened limb. In experiments in which he ligated femoral arteries in three dogs, he found collateral circulation developing between the vessels proximal to the point of ligation and those distal to the ligation. He felt that circulation kept pace with demand on a mechanical basis. Several years later Nothnagel (34), attempting to establish the physiologic mechanism of the development of collateral circulation, came to the conclusion that the increased blood flow which occurred in the direct anastomotic branches between the vascular bed above the ligation and that below the ligation led to hypertrophy and hyperplasia of these anastomotic vessels and thus produced an adequate collateral circulation. Lewis (25) felt that collateral channels developed in response to local tissue needs and suggested that the growth of these vessels was controlled by a stimulus, probably chemical in nature, arising locally as a product of tissue metabolism and acting locally. Buerger (7) stated that there were several factors upon which the development of collateral circulation depended. He was the first to recognize that the status of the blood vessels beyond the point of blockage was of tremendous significance and that methods designed to produce collateral flow were not likely to succeed if a significant degree of occlusion in the distal arteries preexisted or developed following the major occlusion.

Extensive investigations of arteriovenous anastomoses led Reid (36) to the conclusion that such arteriovenous shunts were the most powerful stimulus to the development of collateral circulation, being greater even than that resulting from ligation of a vessel. This finding led for a time to the idea that the surgical establishment of arteriovenous anastomoses might be an effective method of treating circulatory embarrassment in the extremities. The error of this reasoning became apparent when Reid was able to establish by careful anatomical studies that the collateral circulation resulting from an arteriovenous shunt occurred primarily in the immediate vicinity of the fistula and that the arteries distal to the fistula were contracted and small, with the total circulation of the limb distal to such a shunt markedly impaired in spite of the increased collateral and capillary beds. It was his opinion that the diminished circulation of the distal segment of the limb was the result of impaired nutrition and atrophy of the vessel, caused by a lowering of the pulse pressure in the vessels distal to the arteriovenous anastomosis.

Effect of Exercise on Muscle Blood Flow

Buerger (7) stated that the function of the collateral circulation was the establishment of blood flow between an occluded vessel and the continuation of that vessel below the site of occlusion. He attempted to enhance the formation of such collaterals by a series of exercises which consisted of the following sequence: the limbs were supported in an elevated position at an angle of 60–90° for 30–180 sec or for the minimum time required to produce blanching. Following onset of blanching, the feet were permitted to hang down over the edge of the bed or table for from 2 to 5 min, or for as long as necessary to produce reactive hyperemia or rubor, plus 1 min, the total time not to exceed 5 min. Next the legs were placed in a horizontal position for 3–5 min. This cycle was repeated 6–7 times at a sitting, and the entire sequence was repeated several times during the course of the day. In the original description of this exercise Buerger also recommended placing an electric heating pad or hot water bag on the limbs during the 3–5-min interval while the limbs were in the horizontal position. The application of local heat was later abandoned when it became apparent that local heating increased metabolic demand by tissues which could not readily be supplied by the compromised circulation. This form of treatment, which was widely used for many years, was apparently based on the theory that blood vessels which were emptied and distended alternately would eventually accept an increased function in the transport of blood. This assumption remained unchallenged for many years, although some investigators (2) cast much doubt upon its efficacy. With time, Buerger's exercises were prescribed less frequently as other therapeutic measures came into vogue.

In 1936 Sylvan (42) described a method of mild resistive exercises which he administered to various muscle groups in both the upper and the lower extremities. These exercises were based on previous observations which had demonstrated that physical activity of muscles diverted blood from the viscera to the muscles. These exercises consisted of several repetitions against mild resistance of 12–20 muscle groups and were given with the thought that such exercises would strengthen the vasomotor center and thereby improve circulation in the impaired extremity.

Efforts to study muscle blood flow during exercise met with considerable technical difficulties. Using the venous occlusion plethysmograph, Grant (15) was able to demonstrate that following a single sustained contraction limb volume decreased at first, was followed three to five seconds later by a rapid rise in volume, reaching a maximum in about thirty seconds. This maximal rise was maintained for the duration of the contraction. A small additional rise was evident during the early recovery phase, followed by a gradual decline to the resting level. With refinement in instrumentation, Abramson (1) was able to measure the blood flow of a forearm or calf before and after rapidly repeated exercises. A marked increase in the rate of local blood flow occurred immediately after the exercise, followed by rapid partial subsidence with a slow return to resting levels. The duration of the recovery phase was directly proportional to the severity of the exercise. Abramson found that resting blood flow in muscle was 1.5 ml per 100 ml of limb volume, that blood flow rose rapidly to 12.7 ml immediately after exercise, with a rapid decrease to 4.5 ml within $3^{1}/_{2}$ min. This was followed by a slow decline in blood flow until resting levels were reached 15 min after cessation of exercise. Barcroft and Dornhorst (4) devised a method of measuring blood flow during rhythmic exercise of the calf, using venous occlusion plethysmography and correcting for venous outflow during active calf contraction as well as for collateral arterial inflow at rest and during contraction. They confirmed Grant's observation that during active contraction there was a decrease in blood flow, with rapid increase following cessation of the exercise. They found that with repeated exercise of moderate degree blood flow in muscle increased about ten times the resting value and about twelve times the resting value with moderately heavy exercise. However, immediately after cessation of exercise, flow increased to eighteen times the resting value with moderate exercise and to thirty times the resting flow following the heavier exercise. Although some doubt has been expressed about the accuracy of the figures presented by Barcroft and Dornhorst (4) on the basis of simultaneous skin blood flow changes, the results nevertheless indicate the magnitude of the augmented blood flow in muscle during and after exercise in the normal individual.

In a study on the visceral vascular effects of exercise, Lowenthal and co-workers (30) demonstrated that exercise of the muscles of an extremity resulted in no significant change in blood flow in an inactive, nonparticipating muscle group. Comparison of blood pressures in central arteries and peripheral arteries at rest and during exercise (21) revealed that during rest the blood pressure in the brachial, radial and femoral arteries was higher than in the aorta or subclavian artery but that during exercise of one leg blood pressure in the contralateral femoral artery fell below the level in the aorta or subclavian artery. This decrease in blood pressure was related to the decreased peripheral resistance following exercise, resulting in vasodilatation in the vascular bed of the femoral artery. Total blood flow studies, however, were not performed in this investigation.

Using the clearance of ^{24}Na from exercising muscles in control individuals and in patients with arteriosclerotic peripheral vascular disease, Wisham and associates (49) studied the effects of Buerger's exercises, of modified Buerger's, or so-called Buerger-Allen exercises, and of resistive exercises to the calf. After obtaining clearance values in the resting state, a group of normal volunteers and a group of patients with arteriosclerosis obliterans were subjected to the three types of exercises. Buerger's exercises were the original postural exercises described earlier in this chapter. In the modified Buerger's exercises the subjects performed the same postural exercises, and in addition active plantar and dorsal flexion of the ankle was carried out 30 times a minute while the leg was in the elevated and in the dependent position. No active exercise was performed during the third phase with the limb horizontally placed. In the third exercise the subject, while lying supine, actively dorsiflexed and plantar flexed the ankle at the rate of 30 repetitions a minute. A therapist exerted considerable manual resistance to active plantar flexion, while dorsiflexion was unopposed. Resistance was offered in a manner to permit full plantar flexion; exercise was carried out for 20 min. If muscle fatigue or intermittent claudication occurred, the subject was permitted to rest for a short period before exercise was resumed. The results of this study demonstrated what had been suspected for many years, namely, that postural exercises alone produced no increase in muscle blood flow during exercise or after exercise, both in normal individuals and in patients with obliterative arterial disease. Active exercise produced a significant increase in the clearance rate during the exercise in the normal and in patients with vascular disease, although the effect was of lesser magnitude in the patients with impaired circulation. In addition, a considerable increase in circulation was still evident five minutes after cessation of exercise both in the controls and in the patients. Resistive exercise was the most effective method of increasing blood flow in both groups of individuals, and a significant increase in muscle blood flow was evident 5 min after cessation of the exercise in the normals and in patients with occlusive arterial disease. The figures presented are in terms of increased clearance of radioactive sodium from the muscle. These values, unfortunately, cannot be interpolated into specific values of blood flow.

On the basis of these studies we must conclude that the postural exercises of Buerger are of no value in enhancing collateral circulation since they do not increase local muscle blood flow. Their clinical value in the management of peripheral vascular diseases is, however, not doubted by some observers (50). It is suggested that postural filling and emptying of veins and arteries might increase vascular reactivity, representing a form of training of an ischemic vascular tree (20). Buerger's exercises may, however, be of psychological value since they impress upon the patient the need for care of the circulatory problem. The time consumed in the performance of these exercises is great and probably not consistent with the benefits derived.

Active or resistive exercise is the most effective means of improving the circulatory status of a limb. Larsen and Lassen (23) conducted extensive studies on the value of exercise in intermittent claudication. They studied the clearance of xenon-133 from the gastrocnemius muscle during a standard walking test on a treadmill prior to instituting a therapeutic exercise regimen, with repetition of the test at 1-month intervals for the 6-month duration of the study. Patients were instructed to take a brisk walk of 1 hour's duration every day in addition to their normal physical activities. When stopped by pain they were to rest a few minutes and then resume brisk walking. At the end of the study period the exercised patient group increased walking ability an average of 3-fold, whereas a control group, treated with vasodilator drugs, showed no change in claudication time.

In the patient with peripheral arteriosclerosis obliterans who is bedfast or confined to a chair, such exercises should be administered in the form of progressive resistive exercise performed by a therapist or by a member of the family. The patient should be encouraged to perform exercises of all muscle group actively for 2–3 min in succession. If symptoms are not produced by this degree of activity, mild resistance increased within the patient's tolerance. Care must be taken at all times to observe the patient for evidence of cardiac or respiratory distress.

In the absence of rapidly progressive occlusive disease, a patient with intermittent claudication can derive tremendous benefit from an exercise program of this type. The value of such treatment is perhaps best illustrated by the following case history:

A 67-year-old white man was first seen on July 1, 1953, with the complaint of intermittent claudication after walking 5 blocks. Walking uphill or climbing stairs for a very short time produced considerable discomfort. The skin color, temperature and texture were normal. Both femoral pulses were present. Both popliteal pulses were faint, and all foot pulses were absent. The oscillometric indices were: below the knee on the right, 3; on the left, 1; at the right ankle, 2; on the left, 1.

The patient was given vasodilator medication by mouth and was placed on a regimen of walking exercises to the point of tolerance several times daily. Since the patient was employed at the time, this presented no problem. He was seen $3^1/_2$ months later, at which time he reported ability to walk 10 blocks or more, but at a slightly slower pace. Walking uphill and climbing steps still produced typical calf pain. Pulse palpations were essentially unchanged except that the posterior tibial pulse on the right was now faintly palpable. Oscillometric indices were: below the knee on the right, $4^1/_2$; on the left, 2; at the ankle on the right, $1^1/_2$; on the left, $1^1/_2$.

The patient was again seen 5 months later, at which time he stated that he was able to walk unlimited distances at a slightly slower pace than normal. He still, however, had pain on walking uphill. Both posterior tibial pulses were not palpable. The oscillometric indices were: below the knee on the right, 6; on the left, 2; at the right ankle, 3; on the left, $1^3/_4$. The patient, aged 71, returned for a follow-up examination on May 4, 1957. He had continued with walking exercises until shortly prior to the last examination when he accepted a position as civil engineer. He had no complaint on walking ability, although there was still some discomfort on climbing stairs. The skin of both lower extremities was entirely normal. Both posterior tibial pulses were still readily palpable, but the dorsalis pedis pulses had not be reestablished. The femoral and popliteal pulses were readily felt. Oscillometric indices were: below the knee on the right, 8; on the left, $2^1/_2$; at the right ankle, $3^1/_4$; on the left, $2^1/_2$.

In a period of 4 years, between the ages of 67 and 71, this patient had return of both posterior tibial pulses (previously absent); the oscillometric indices below the knee on the right rose from 3 to 8; on the left, from 1 to $2^1/_2$, and at the ankle they increased from 2 to $3^1/_2$ on the right and from 1 to $2^1/_2$ on the left. This marked improvement was accomplished entirely by an almost compulsive adherence to the exercise regimen without other significant change in the patient's mode of life. This patient, undoubtedly, showed a most favorable response to therapeutic exercise, but there is no doubt that tremendous benefits will accrue to many patients with intermittent claudication who will adhere to prescribed exercise therapy with even a moderate degree of regularity.

A word of caution is appropriate, however. Up to this point occlusive arterial disease was discussed without reference to etiological factors, and what has been said applies equally to arteriosclerosis obliterans and to thromboangiitis obliterans (Buerger's disease). But there is one important factor which will influence the course of thromboangiitis obliterans. Although cigarette smoking has been shown to be detrimental in all forms of peripheral arterial occlusive disease (18), it is particularly harmful in thromboangiitis obliterans. No matter what treatment may be prescribed — whether medical, pharmacological, or exercise — the signs and symptoms of thromboangiitis obliterans will progress relentlessly unless the patient gives up smoking completely. Failure to do so will most certainly nullify all therapeutic efforts. It is commonly stated that in medical practice there is no rule without exceptions; this is one rule to which all experts in vascular diseases subscribe unequivocally.

However, the picture with respect to thromboangiitis obliterans may be changing. Doubts have been expressed about the existence of the clinically recognized entity of thromboangiitis obliterans as described by Buerger. Wessler and co-workers (47) questioned the existence of this disease based on extensive pathological studies, expressing the view that the several clinical features of this disease are fully compatible with early onset atherosclerosis. Other notably experienced students of vascular disease (31) have just as strongly defended the existence of Buerger's disease. All are, however, agreed that the incidence of thromboangiitis obliterans has markedly decreased in the past 10–15 years and is becoming a rare disease, seen very infrequently even in active and busy peripheral vascular disease clinics. One may wonder whether the rapid decline in the incidence of this clinical and pathological entity in the recent past may not be directly related to the rapid proliferation of filter-type, low tar and low nicotine cigarettes which made their earliest appearance in the mid 1930s, began a rapid rise between 1952 and 1954, and in 1974 accounted for 86% of the total American cigarette output (17). One may justly speculate whether these relationships are not more than just coincidental.

The treatment of gangrene of the lower extremities has as a rule consisted of medical or surgical means and the interdiction of walking. It has always been felt that walking would result in additional trauma to the necrotic tissue, with spread of the lesion or the development of secondary infection, although some peripheral vascular disease clinics have not objected to the "ambulation treatment" of localized and demarcated gangrenous lesions (39). Recently Foley (14) described his results of walking in the treatment of gangrene of the feet and legs. He reported on 22 patients with localized gangrenous lesions of the legs or feet, which were treated by the usual medical and pharmacological means, but in addition the patients were encouraged to remain ambulatory, using protective dressing to prevent trauma to the involved parts. In this group were 5 patients with thromboangiitis obliterans, 1 with gangrene secondary to an embolus and 16 patients with gangrene secondary to arteriosclerosis obliterans with complicating diabetes and hypertension in some. Of these 22 patients, 21 went on to healing and 1 was subjected to amputation. The contraindications to this method of treatment are given by Foley to be severe debility, recent myocardial infarction or severe myocardial insufficiency, active thrombophlebitis, high fever and progressive gangrene or spreading cellulitis. The warning against this ambulatory treatment of gangrene in patients with myocardial insufficiency or myocardial infarction is in keeping with several studies. Donald et al. (8) showed that patients with cardiac impairment extract a greater percentage of oxygen from the blood returning from the extremities after exercise than do individuals with normal cardiac reserve. They also demonstrated (6) that skin circulation of the arm in the normal individual during leg exercise showed transient vasoconstriction, which was followed by vasodilatation during the remainder of the exercise period. In patients with cardiac insufficiency, however, there was a slightly delayed but far greater degree of vasoconstriction in the skin during exercise, and this vasoconstriction was sustained until the end of exercise (9). On the basis of these findings it is apparent that with impaired cardiac reserve the ambulatory treatment of gangrene is hazardous because of vasoconstriction in the skin during muscular activity. It would appear that ambulation is not contraindicated in patients with well demarcated gangrenous lesions of the lower extremities who are otherwise well compensated and whose lesions can be followed easily for signs of edema or progression. Edematous tissue may be an excellent culture medium for bacterial invaders, especially in the diabetic, and thus a well demarcated or separating necrotic lesion may become a spreading infectious gangrene. Patients with such lesions who are on "ambulation treatment" should be put to bed at once if edema, cellulitis or progression of the lesion is seen.

Exercise in Disorders of the Venous System

Since the introduction by Virchow in the nineteenth century of the concept of cellular pathology as the cause of disease, the use of rest in the treatment of disease has found an important place in medical practice; it has become an important therapeutic measure. When, in 1943, Newburger (33) suggested that the diminished venous return produced by long bed rest might be the most important single etiological agent in the pathogenesis of postoperative thrombosis in the deep veins of the leg and when he further suggested that this physiologic factor could be directly and favorably influenced by early activity and walking, he changed a method of treatment which had gone unchallenged for almost a century. He expressed concern over the lack of universal success in preventing postoperative complications by frequent changes of position of the patient and by exercises in bed and expressed the view that walking might actually minimize the development of venous thrombosis. Several years earlier, Smith and co-workers (40) had studied the effects of various physical agents on circulation time. They found that the circulation time from the ankle to the carotid sinus was decreased by elevation of the extremity and by active exercise of the leg with the patient in the supine position. On June 15, 1944, a new era in medical practice began. On that date a symposium was held at the 94th Annual Session of the American Medical Association on "The Abuse of Rest in the Treatment of Disease" (43). Extensive evidence was presented of the beneficial effects of exercise and ambulation in the prevention of postoperative thrombophlebitis and phlebothrombosis.

Venous return is influenced primarily by the subatmospheric pressure within the thorax, which has an important effect upon the flow of blood along the great veins of the thorax and abdomen. However, in the extremities the most important factor in the movement of blood is the intermittent pressure of the contracting limb muscles upon the venous structures. In addition, the veins are supplied with valves permitting flow of blood in only one direction, toward the heart, and preventing the full hydrostatic effect of the column of venous blood to be brought to bear upon the distal portions of the venous circulation. The muscles of the extremities and of the abdominal wall also support the vein walls directly and thereby prevent their distention, which would otherwise occur under the weight of the column of blood (5). The supporting effect of the muscles, the presence of valves and the intermittent contraction of the skeletal muscles are, then, the most important factors in the movement of blood against gravity. These factors are important considerations in the management of the patient with venous disease.

Phlebothrombosis, usually a complication of prolonged bed rest, is best treated prophylactically by avoiding the development of this complication whenever possible. A patient of whom absolute bed rest is required but who is permitted a mild degree of exercise in bed should be encouraged to turn from side to side several times a day, to lie on his abdomen for short periods of time several times daily and to elevate the lower extremities (from the hip) alternately to an angle of 60–75°, with active flexion and extension of the knees and ankles as permitted. The patient possessing the muscular strength and the cardiopulmonary reserve to perform these activities by himself should be encouraged to perform this exercise routine three to four times daily. For the patient in whom active exercise is prohibited for medical reasons, motion may be administered passively by a nurse or a therapist several times daily to speed venous flow and thereby prevent the stagnation of blood in the dependent pelvic structures. A patient who is too ill to have any type of exercise and in whom the threat of phlebothrombosis exists might best be treated by placing the foot of the bed on 6–8-inch shock blocks until such time as mild exercise may be initiated.

Exercise therapy is usually not advisable early in the treatment of acute thrombophlebitis because movement produces considerable pain and increases congestion of the venous channels. Drainage of the venous system should be promoted by proper elevation of the involved extremity until such time as the inflammation has subsided sufficiently to make motion permissible. At that point gentle passive motion of the involved extremity may be undertaken while the uninvolved extremities, including the uppers, are exercised actively (as previously outlined) to promote increased venous flow. Although some authors (2) have recommended the use of vigorous exercise as soon as the diagnosis of thrombophlebitis is established, there does exist a possibility that too vigorous exercise may increase the tendency to embolization. As soon as the inflammation has been brought under control, the patient should be permitted to ambulate actively, with an elastic bandage around the extremity if edema develops.

Thrombophlebitis of the superficial veins usually requires no special exercise. Simple elevation of the extremity and warm compresses are all the treatment usually required.

A less well known form of venous disorder requires consideration from the standpoint of exercise. Phlegmasia cerulea dolens, also known as acute massive venous occlusion, has been reported in the literature from time to time (16). In a number of instances the venous occlusion has become so extensive, involving not only the main channels but the lesser vessels as well, that eventual stoppage of arterial inflow by mechanical back pressure has occurred. If not corrected the condition frequently results in gangrene of the involved extremity without any associated arterial thrombosis or occlusion. In some of the reported cases visceral carcinoma was present as an associated finding (10). The causal relationship between neoplasm and venous thrombosis has never been clearly defined (19, 41). The prognosis is poor in patients with gangrene complicating massive venous thrombosis, particularly in patients in whom visceral neoplasm is also present. In the absence of known malignancy the condition may respond to vigorous and thorough exercise therapy. It is most essential that the correct diagnosis be established without delay. The symptoms which should lead one to suspect this condition are extensive edema, usually involving the entire extremity, associated with blanching of the skin in the early phases, followed rapidly by blue discoloration and coldness of the extremity. Severe pain may be sudden in onset or progressive. Arterial pulses are present early in the disease, but may disappear as edema progresses and as secondary arterial spasm or arterial stasis occurs.

In 1951, Veal and associates (45) reported 11 patients with massive venous occlusion from various causes and none with neoplasm. Nine of the 11 patients responded to a regimen of extreme elevation of the extremity and to vigorous rapid flexion and extension exercises of the ankle and knee. Later Moser et al. (32) described a patient with this condition who was successfully treated with exercise. The success of therapy in these patients has been so different from the usual outcome in patients previously reported that a detailed description of the treatment for this serious problem is given. As soon as the diagnosis is established, the involved extremity is elevated to an angle of 65-70° and maintained in that position by means of mechanical supports. Passive exercises of the ankles, knee and hip are carried out continuously for at least four hours. Since even slight motion may produce considerable pain, analgesics may have to be administered to control pain. Other medical measures such as anticoagulants (in the form of intravenous heparin) or the ganglionic blocking agent trimethaphan (Arfonad), or the peripherally acting sympatholytic drug dibenzylene, are administered. Following the period of passive exercise the patient must actively exercise the entire limb for 24–36 hours. With successful treatment cyanosis will usually subside in 8–10 hours, and the swelling and turgidity of the limb will slowly decrease in 20–24 hours. After subsidence of the acute manifestations treatment is continued as for thrombophlebitis. There is probably no other disorder of the peripheral circulation in which exercise therapy plays so vital a role as in acute massive venous occlusion.

Exercise in Disorders of the Lymphatic Circulation

The lymph vessels of the lower extremities are arranged in two systems, one superficial, the other deep. There is no communication between these two systems except through the popliteal and inguinal lymph nodes. The superficial lymph vessels of the foot and leg and some of the deeper vessels from the muscles of the leg terminate in the popliteal lymph nodes. All limb vessels eventually enter lymphatic trunks, which accompany the main femoral lymph vessels and drain into the large iliac nodes. The superficial lymph vessels of the upper extremity pass upward on the ulnar and radial sides of the hand and forearm, where they join to continue upward into the axillary nodes. The deep lymph vessels of the arm follow the large vessels and empty into the axillary lymph nodes. At the elbow the two systems are connected by the deep and superficial cubital lymph nodes.

Lymph vessels possess an unbroken endothelial lining and endothelial valves which prevent back flow of the lymph. The rate of flow of lymph depends on the intermittent external pressure supplied by the skeletal muscles and on the direction of the pressure gradient produced by the contracting muscles. Pressure in lymph vessels is very low, usually measured in millimeters of water. The pressure is greatly influenced by exercise, massage and inflammatory changes. White (48) demonstrated that the flow of lymph varied with the degree of physical activity by observing the rate of flow from the paw of a dog during walking and during rapid running. This massaging effect of the skeletal muscle is recognized as the normal mechanism for the promotion of lymph flow.

In a more extensive study, the variability of lymph flow in response to various stimuli was effectively demonstrated. Ladd (22) and associates measured the flow of lymph from a cannula inserted into the main lymph vessel of the foreleg of a number of dogs. The resting flow averaged 0.16 ml in 10 min. Electrical stimulation, producing an isometric contraction, resulted in an average flow of 0.75 ml in 10 min. Passive exercise caused an increased flow averaging 1.78 ml in 10 min, whereas massage produced a flow of 2.81 ml. Active exercise in an anesthetized animal produced by shivering in response to cooling resulted in a lymph flow equal in volume to that produced by massage. The effectiveness of active exercise and massage in augmenting flow in the lymphatic system is well documented.

Lymphangitis is usually the result of an acute infection associated with sudden onset and severe systemic reaction. Such inflammation is best treated with rest, moist local heat and specific antibacterial agents. Exercise is not indicated. Elevation of the extremity to promote improved lymphatic drainage is a valuable adjunct to treatment.

One of the major problems encountered in patients with chronic occlusive arterial disease is edema of the lower extremities. This is caused by a combination of edema secondary to venous stasis caused by dependency and muscle inactivity and also by lymph stasis. Patients who are confined to the wheel chair for vascular disease or for other medical or surgical reasons should be encouraged to contract the muscles of the foot and leg vigorously at frequent intervals and to maintain the involved extremity in a horizontal position by proper support of the limb in the wheel chair. In patients who are unable to exercise, massage may be effective in place of active exercise in diminishing venous and lymphatic edema.

Exercise is of doubtful value in the hereditary forms of lymphedema, in lymphedema secondary to malignancy, following surgical removal of lymph nodes, in compression of lymph channels and in fibrosis resulting from roentgen or radium therapy.

Exercise in the Diagnosis of Peripheral Vascular Disease

The syndrome of intermittent claudication produced as a result of exercise has been a controversial subject for several decades. It is generally agreed, and evidence has been presented earlier in this chapter, that exercise in an extremity produces increased blood flow in that extremity. Leary and Allen (24) studied 25 normal subjects and 8 patients with chronic occlusive arterial disease by means of oscillometry before and after exercise. In all cases the pulsations either remained unchanged or increased following exercise. They felt, however, that a decrease in pulsations after exercise would be indicative of some disease of the arteries. Lindqvist (26), in a study of 8 patients with intermittent claudication found variable responses to exercise by oscillometry. In some patients with arterial disease the oscillometric pulses decreased after exercise, while in others they increased. Similar discrepancies were found in patients with only mild involvement. The role of arterial spasm in the production of the symptom of intermittent claudication could not be determined. Subsequently Lindqvist (27) described a patient with intermittent claudication after exercise who demonstrated decreased oscillometric values and diminished pulses for a short period after exercise but who had normal pulses and normal oscillometric studies at rest. His case was followed for several years, and he was ultimately shown to have structural disease of the aorta (28).

Some investigators have concluded that the syndrome of the disappearing pulse after exercise is always associated with organic occlusion of the proximal arterial tree (12, 38), while others believe that it is caused by closure of the smaller arteries supplying the muscles, leading to loss of arteriolar and capillary branches by which the muscle fibers are supplied with blood (46). The phenomenon is probably not as uncommon as was previously believed (24). In a recent study of patients with arteriosclerosis obliterans observed in an ambulatory working population, 20% displayed this inverse reaction (29).

The mechanism of the disappearing pulse on exercise is not entirely clear. It has been suggested that a vasospastic component which would manifest itself for a short period only after exercise is involved (35). Current investigations tend to indicate that this inverse reaction is a manifestation of changes in blood flow distribution in an exercising extremity related to changes in the peripheral resistance in the presence of limited arterial inflow capacity (29).

In an effort to differentiate between pain in the extremities secondary to peripheral arterial disease and pain not related to vascular disorders, Ejrup (13) studied the fluorescence of histamine-induced intradermal wheals at rest and after exercise. He demonstrated that in the normal person fluorescence appeared at rest in 20–40 sec and after exercise in 15–35 sec; in patients with arteriosclerosis obliterans, fluorescence did not appear at rest until 40–60 sec, but after exercise (walking) fluorescence was delayed 1–18 min. There has been no confirmation of this work.

Determining a patient's walking ability and establishing the claudication time is undoubtedly the best means of assessing his vascular impairment with respect to muscle blood flow. The electrically driven treadmill or walking belt has been shown to have a high degree of reliability with an error of between 16 and 20% in three test runs (11). As an alternative, a simple clinical test has been found quite adequate if a treadmill is not available. The patient is asked to walk on level ground, accompanied by a therapist, at the rate of 3 miles per hour (120 steps per minute). The pace is maintained by the therapist, and the time and distance covered are noted when symptoms of intermittent claudication appear. It is important that the correct pace be maintained since symptoms of intermittent claudication can be delayed by slowing the pace. For this reason it is advisable to make several determinations for control. The test is not suitable for patients with diminished cardiac or respiratory reserve.

In patients in whom ligation or stripping of the superficial venous circulation is contemplated for extensive varicosities, it is essential that the patency of the deep circulation be determined before surgery is undertaken. This can be accomplished by radiography of the deep venous circulation by the intraosseous route (3, 37). A simple exercise test, however, will usually provide the physician with adequate information about the state of the deep circulation. The involved lower extremity is wrapped rather tightly with a rubber-reinforced elastic bandage up to the thigh. This will effectively occlude the superficial venous circulation. The patient is then asked to walk about with the bandage in place for several hours. If no discomfort is experienced and edema of the extremity does not develop, it may be assumed that the deep vessels are patent and that surgery of the superficial venous system may be safely undertaken. Should the patient experience severe discomfort due to swelling and tightness, this would indicate that the superficial circulation is essential for adequate venous drainage of the limb and must not be interrupted (Perthe's test). Ligation or stripping procedures should not be performed in a limb which has been the seat of deep thrombophlebitis within a year prior to contemplated surgery. This period will usually allow for formation of deep collateral venous channels or for recanalization of the deep veins.

REFERENCES

1. ABRAMSON, D. I. *Vascular Responses in the Extremities of Man in Health and Disease.* Chicago, 1944.
2. ALLEN, E. V., BARKER, N. W., AND HINES, E. A., JR. *Peripheral Vascular Diseases.* Philadelphia, 1955.
3. ARNOLDI, C. C., AND BAUER, G. Intraosseous phlebography. *Angiology, 11:* 44, 1960.
4. BARCROFT, H., AND DORNHORST, A. C. The blood flow through the human calf during rhythmic exercise. *J. Physiol., 109:* 402, 1949.
5. BEST, C. H., AND TAYLOR, N. B. *The Physiological Basis of Medical Practice.* Baltimore, 1955.
6. BISHOP, J. M., DONALD, K. W., TAYLOR, S. H., AND WORMWALD, P. N. The blood flow in the human arm during supine leg exercises. *J. Physiol., 137:* 294, 1957.
7. BUERGER, L. *The Circulatory Disturbances of the Extremities.* Philadelphia, 1924.
8. DONALD, K. W., WORMWALD, P. N., TAYLOR, S. H., AND BISHOP, J. M. Changes in the oxygen content of femoral venous blood and leg blood flow during leg exercise in relation to cardiac output response. *Clin. Sci., 16:* 567, 1957.
9. DONALD, K. W., BISHOP, J. M., AND WADE, O. L. Changes in the oxygen content of axillary venous blood during leg exercise in patients with rheumatic heart disease. *Clin. Sci., 14:* 531, 1955.
10. EBEL, A., KAUFMAN, M., AND EHRENREICH, T. Gangrene of an extremity secondary to venous thrombosis. *Arch Intern. Med., 90:* 402, 1952.
11. EBEL, A. AND KUO, J. C. Tolerance for treadmill walking as an index of intermittent claudication. *Arch. Phys. Med. Rehabil., 48:* 611, 1967.
12. EJRUP, B. Tonoscillography after exercise. *Acta Med. Scand.* (Supp. 211), *130:* 159, 1948.
13. EJRUP, B. Fluorescin after exercise; a method of investigation in peripheral arterial disease. *Angiology, 4:* 253, 1953.
14. FOLEY, W. T. Treatment of gangrene of the feet and legs by walking. *Circulation, 15:* 689, 1957.
15. GRANT, R. T. Observations on the blood circulation in voluntary muscle in man. *Clin. Sci., 3:* 157, 1938.
16. HAIMOVICI, H. Gangrene of the extremities of venous origin: review of literature with case reports. *Circulation, 1:* 225, 1950.
17. *Historical trends in the tobacco industry: fifty year summary.* The Tobacco Institute, Inc., Washington, 1975.
18. JUERGENS, J. L., BARKER, N. W., AND HINES, E. A., JR. Arteriosclerosis obliterans. *Circulation, 21:* 188, 1960.

19. KENNEY, W. E. The association of carcinoma in the body and tail of the pancreas with multiple venous thrombi. *Surgery, 14:* 600, 1943.
20. KRAMER, D. W. *Peripheral Vascular Disease.* Philadelphia, 1948.
21. KROEKER, E. J., AND WOOD, E. H. Comparison of simultaneously recorded central and peripheral arterial pressure pulses during rest, exercise and tilted position in man. *Circulation Res., 3:* 623, 1955.
22. LADD, M. P., KOTTKE, F. J., AND BLANCHARD, R. S. Studies of the effect of massage on the flow of lymph from the foreleg of the dog. *Arch. Phys. Med., 33:* 604, 1952.
23. LARSEN, O. A., AND LASSEN, N. A. Medical treatment of occlusive arterial disease of the legs. *Angiologica, 6:* 288, 1969.
24. LEARY, W. V., AND ALLEN, E. V. Intermittent claudication as a result of arterial spasm by walking. *Am. Heart J., 22:* 719, 1941.
25. LEWIS, T. The adjustment of blood flow to the affected limb in arteriovenous fistula. *Clin. Sci., 4:* 277, 1940.
26. LINDQVIST, T. Intermittent claudication and vascular spasm. I. *Acta Med. Scand., 121:* 32, 1945.
27. LINDQVIST, T. Intermittent claudication and vascular spasm. II. *Acta Med. Scand., 121:* 409, 1945.
28. LINDQVIST, T. Value of various examination methods in diagnosing arterial disease in extremities. *Acta Med. Scand.* (Suppl. 206), *130:* 162, 1948.
29. LIPPMANN, H. I. Personal communication.
30. LOWENTHAL, M., HARPUDER, K., AND BLATT, S. D. Peripheral and visceral vascular effects of exercise and postprandial state in supine position. *J. Appl. Physiol., 4:* 689, 1952.
31. McKUSICK, V. A., HARRIS, W. S., OTTESEN, O. E., GOODMAN, R. M., SHELLEY, W. M., AND BLOODWELL, R. D. Buerger's disease; a distinct clinical and pathologic entity. *J.A.M.A., 181:* 5, 1962.
32. MOSER, M., BABIN, S. M., COTTS, G. W., AND PRANDONI, A. G. Acute massive venous occlusion: report of a case successfully treated with exercise. *Ann. Intern. Med., 40:* 361, 1954.
33. NEWBURGER, B. Early postoperative walking. *Surgery, 14:* 142, 1943.
34. NOTHNAGEL, H. Ueber Anpassungen und Ausgleichungen bei pathologischen Zustaenden. III. Die Entstehung des Collateralkreislaufs. *Z. Klin. Med., 15:* 42, 1889.
35. PEARL, F. L. Angiospastic claudication with a report of six cases. *Am. J. Med. Sci., 194:* 505, 1937.
36. REID, M. R. Abnormal arteriovenous communications, acquired and congenital. *Arch. Surg., 11:* 25, 1925.
37. SCHOBINGER, R. *Intraosseous Venography.* New York, 1960.
38. SEMPLE, R. Diabetes and peripheral arterial disease. *Lancet, I:* 1064, 1953.
39. SILBERT, S. S. In, Lippmann (29).
40. SMITH, L. A., ALLEN, E. V., AND CRAIG, W. M. Time required for blood to flow from the arm and from the feet of man to the carotid sinuses; effect of temperature, exercise, increased intramuscular tension, elevation of limbs and sympathectomy. *Arch. Surg., 41:* 1366, 1940.
41. SPROUL, E. E. Carcinoma and venous thrombosis: the frequency of association of carcinoma in the body and tail of the pancreas with multiple venous thrombosis. *Am. J. Cancer, 34:* 566, 1938.
42. SYLVAN, F. Heilgymnastik bei Altersgangraen. *Fortschr. Med., 54:* 297, 1936.
43. Symposium: The Abuse of Rest in the Treatment of Disease. *J.A.M.A., 125:* 1075, 1944.
44. THOMA, R. Ueber die Abhaengigkeit der Bindegewebsneubildung in der Arterienintima von den mechanischen Bedingungen des Blutumlaufes. *Virchow Arch., 95:* 294, 1884.
45. VEAL, J. R., DUGAN, T. J., JAMISON, W. L., AND BAUERSFELD, R. S. Acute massive venous occlusion of the lower extremities. *Surgery, 29:* 355, 1951.

46. VEAL, J. R., AND McFETRIDGE, E. M. Vascular changes in intermittent claudication with a note on the value of arteriography in this symptom complex. *Am. J. Med. Sci., 192:* 113, 1936.

47. WESSLER, S., MING. S., GUREWICH, V., AND FREIMAN, D. G. A critical evaluation of thromboangiitis obliterans; the case against Buerger's disease. *N. Engl. J. Med., 262:* 1149, 1960.

48. WHITE, J. C., DRINKER, C. K., AND FIELD, M. D. On the protein content of normal flow of lymph from the foot of the dog. *Am. J. Physiol., 103:* 34, 1933.

49. WISHAM, L. H., ABRAMSON, A. S., AND EBEL, A. Value of exercise in peripheral arterial disease. *J.A.M.A., 153:* 10, 1953.

50. WRIGHT, I. S. *Vascular Diseases in Clinical Practice.* Chicago, 1948.

25

Exercise and the Heart

_____ CHARLES A. GILBERT

The use of physical exercise by physicians in caring for patients with various diseases of the heart has increased greatly in recent years. Many claims for the supposed benefits of regular physical activity (i.e., _training_) in certain cardiac patients have been made, but few of these claims have been proven by acceptable clinical studies. Conversely, exercise _testing_ of patients has been widely studied and its value and limitations have now been defined with some precision. It is the purpose of this chapter to outline the indications, usefulness, methods, and risks of the use of physical activity in dealing with patients who have heart disease or are suspected of having heart disease. The two major roles for physical activity in cardiac patients are 1) exercise testing and 2) physical training of cardiac patients. Before proceeding with these areas, though, it is necessary that a definition of certain terms be understood as well as an outline of some cardiovascular physiologic concepts.

At the beginning the type of physical exercise most useful in dealing with cardiac patients should be defined. In this chapter, exercise is intended to mean dynamic muscular exercise of large muscle groups such as is used in walking, jogging running, bicycling, and swimming. As contrasted with this type of isotonic exercise is isometric exercise in which muscular force is exerted but _no movement occurs_. One example of such isometric exercise is handgrip exercise which is known to evoke a proportionately greater rise in blood pressure and a smaller increase in heart rate. In contrast isotonic (or dynamic) exercise is a more potent stimulus to increase heart rate than it is to cause a rise of blood pressure. While handgrip exercise, a form of isometric exercise, is useful in cardiac practice for accentuating physical findings and inducing a cardiovascular stress which is physiologic and rapidly reversible it is reviewed elsewhere and a full discussion is beyond the scope of this chapter (1).

Physiologic Alterations with Dynamic Exercise

The cardiovascular physiologic alterations in humans with dynamic exercise have been extensively studied and recently reviewed (2, 3). Briefly, it is important to recall that heart rate and, to a lesser degree, blood pressure do increase with skeletal muscle exercise. Cardiac output increases 4–5 times as a normal human subject progresses from rest to maximal exercise on a treadmill or bicycle ergometer. At the same time significant shifts in blood flow distribution are made to supply working muscle with substrate and oxygen for energy production. The result of all of the cardiovascular and pulmonary changes is to allow oxygen consumption to increase 10–12 times in a normal human subject progressing to maximal exercise.

For therapists working with patients who have coronary atherosclerotic heart disease (CASHD) manifested by either angina pectoris or myocardial infarction the changes in demand for coronary blood flow with exercise are important. It is known that in normal human subjects coronary blood flow increases five fold as the subject exercises progressively to a maximal level (4, 5). In a clinical setting the relative *demand* for coronary blood flow can be estimated by using the "double product" of heart rate multiplied by systolic blood pressure. The greater the external work load, the greater will be the double product, and the coronary blood flow requirement. In a patient with a limited coronary artery delivery system, i.e., blocked or narrowed coronaries, the myocardium will become ischemic as the external physical work load increases. The point at which ischemia is expressed clinically either as angina pectoris and/or electrocardiographic (ECG) ST segment alteration can be noted and heart rate and blood pressure measured. For a given patient, the resultant double product at which myocardial ischemia occurs is relatively constant. Thus, drugs such as nitroglycerine or propranolol may increase the external work performed prior to the onset of angina pectoris, but the double product at the time of ischemia remains essentially constant (6–8). The same situation is true in most studies of physical conditioning in patients with angina pectoris or following myocardial infarction. That is, the patients can do more exercise before ischemia, but the double product at the time of symptoms is unchanged (9, 10). Drugs and physical conditioning only alter the relative *demand* for coronary blood flow, not the *supply*. Saphenous vein by-pass surgery, on the other hand, can allow a higher double product prior to symptoms or ECG signs of ischemia because more coronary blood flow is being delivered.

Exercise Stress Testing

Information obtained from a properly performed test in cardiac patients can guide therapeutic decisions, and help in assessing the results of that therapy. In presumed normal subjects, information from exercise testing can help uncover subclinical disease, assist in prescribing an appropriate physical conditioning program, and encourage participation in such a program. In summary, the indications for an exercise test are either to determine the functional, working capacity of a patient or to use the results of the test in making a diagnosis, of most commonly, coronary atherosclerotic heart disease.

Methods and Procedure

Equipment for dynamic exercise stress testing need not be elaborate and expensive. In an office or clinic, a measured hallway, standard Master's stairsteps, or a chair can be used to effect a repeatable exercise stress. In such a setting measurements should include resting and postexercise, blood pressure, and other clinical observations such as the timing and character of chest pain and the occurrence of excessive dyspnea. For more precise and quantifiable stress testing either a motor-driven treadmill or upright bicycle ergometer are used. The choice between the two instruments should be made on consideration of the planned use, available space and money, the experience of the physician and other personnel involved and local community practice.

Exercise testing requires environmental control of temperature and humidity, and for optimum reproducibility should be performed at a single time of day, i.e., between 8:00 a.m. and noon. For testing of cardiac function a light meal 1 or 2 hours prior to testing is allowable to aid in preventing exercise-induced nausea and possibly, vasovagal reactions. However, glucose ingestion can alter ECG repolarization and cause false positive ECG results. For this reason, when the test is for diagnostic purposes it should be after a 4-hour fast (11). Patients are advised to take their usual medications on the day of the test.

The patient should have the nature of the test explained. If anxiety and/or emotional distress is overpowering, the test should not be done. An informed consent is obtained in writing (12).

An interim cardiovascular history and physical examination should be performed immediately prior to the test to exclude subjects with new, changing or rapidly progressive or prolonged (greater than 15 min) chest pain patterns. Other contraindications to exercise testing are noted in Table 25.1.

Electrocardiographic Monitoring

Continual ECG monitoring of at least one lead (CM_5 or V_5) must be done by the responsible physician or delegate before, during and up to 5 or 10 min after exercise. Proper skin preparation, the use of commercially available "floating" ECG electrodes, and shielded, isolated and grounded ECG recording techniques should give an artifact-free ECG recording (13). If a single ECG lead is used during exercise, a complete 12-lead ECG can be obtained immediately, and at 2 and 5 min after exercise for added diagnostic discrimination. In addition to monitoring the continuous ECG on an oscilloscope, periodic recordings must be obtained for permanent

TABLE 25.1. *Contraindications to Exercise Testing*

1. Clinical evidence of myocardial infarction (MI) or acute coronary insufficiency within the previous 8 weeks.
2. Cardiovascular surgery within the previous 8 weeks.
3. Recent marked increase in frequency and severity of anginal episodes.
4. New ECG evidence either of MI or ST-T changes compatible with injury not present in the most recent ECG.
5. Newly acquired major conduction defect not present in previous ECGs.
6. Clinical evidence of overt left ventricular decompensation.
7. Any acute illness such as respiratory infection or gastrointestinal hemorrhage.
8. Failure to sign "informed consent."
9. Blood pressure greater than 180/110 mm Hg.

records and interpretation. The recording instrument must be properly grounded, electrically isolated from the patient, and have adequate low frequency capability down to 0.05 Hz (13).

Emergency Capability

Emergency equipment, drugs, intravenous tubing, fluids, and needles should be available in the exercise laboratory as well as a step-by-step emergency plan. A DC cardiac defibrillator should be part of the regular equipment of the laboratory. Physicians and other personnel should periodically review and gain practice in the use of this emergency setup.

Design of Exercise-Testing Protocol

A single workload applied for 3 min using standard stairsteps 9 inches high has been used for many years in Master's double two-step exercise test (14). A relative steady state of the cardiovascular system has probably been reached at the end of this test at an energy expenditure level of approximately six METs* or 20 ml/kg (min) oxygen consumption (15).

A series of gradually increasing workloads applied in a continuous fashion is the basis for many treadmill or bicycle exercise tests. The work periods in a continuous protocol should be at least three minutes long to allow a hemodynamic steady state to occur. Table 25.2 lists the speeds and grades of a multistage treadmill test of a continuous type (16).

End Points

In Master's double two-step test the end point is defined by the completion of the required trips in 3 min. The occurrence of angina pectoris or undue fatigue before the completion of the required number of steps for sex, age, and weight should terminate the test immediately.

In the "maximal" or symptom-limited test done on a treadmill (Table 25.2) or bicycle, the subject is asked to exercise until the onset of moderate fatigue or symptoms. Such "subjective end points" are angina pectoris, unusual fatigue or dyspnea, or pain in the legs. The responsible physician

---

* A MET is equal to the resting or basal oxygen consumption of about 3.3–3.5 ml/kg (min).

TABLE 25.2. *Multistage, Continuous Treadmill Exercise Protocol*[1]

Stage[2]	Speed	Grade
	mph	%
0	1.0	5
I	1.7	10
II	2.5	12
III	3.4	14
IV	4.2	16
V	5.0	18
VI	5.5	20
VII	6.0	22

[1] Source: Bruce and Hornsten (16).
[2] Each stage is 3 min long.

monitoring the test must be aware of "objective end points" to stop the test at any development with potential hazard to the patient (Table 25.3).

The submaximal or graded exercise test (GXT) uses 90% of an age-predicted maximal heart rate, adjusted for habitual physical activity, as an end point (14). Maximal heart rate decreases with age. For example, a sedentary 45-year-old man is asked to continue until a heart rate of 168 beats per minute is achieved. If symptoms or one of the objective end points occur before the required heart rate is reached, the test is stopped just as with the maximal or symptom-limited test.

If the above end points, safety precautions, emergency equipment and plan, and presence of a responsible physician are employed, the risk of exercise testing is minimal. A survey of exercise laboratories where submaximal or maximal testing on a bicycle or treadmill is carried out revealed a risk to the individual patient of 2.4 in 10,000 for serious events and 1 in 10,000 for death immediately associated with the test (18).

Measurements during Exercise Testing

The total time in minutes that a patient walks the numbered stages (Table 25.2) is noted as the treadmill duration score (TDS). For example, a patient walking 2½ min of Stage III (3.4 mph, 14% grade) would have a TDS of 8.5 min. Another patient developing angina pectoris and stopping after 1¼ min of Stage 1 (1.7 mph, 10% grade) would have a TDS of 1.25 min. The warm-up Stage 0, is not counted in determining the TDS, although there are some severely disabled patients who cannot proceed beyond this step in the test.

In addition to the TDS, measurements made during exercise testing to a maximal or symptomatic end point and to submaximal level as determined by heart rate (GXT) should include blood pressure (cuff) and ECG for heart rate, QRS wave form, ST segment, and arrhythmias.

Other measurements which can be made during exercise stress testing include oxygen consumption and peripheral blood lactate. These measurements do give added information concerning the patient's physiologic

TABLE 25.3. *Objective End Points for Maximal or Symptom-limited Exercise Testing*

1. Diagnostic ST-segment elevation or depression even without chest pain (≧2 mm).
2. Supraventricular tachycardia.
3. Premature ventricular beats which are precipitated by or increased with exercise and constitute 25% of beats.
4. Ventricular tachycardia (three or more ectopic ventricular complexes in a row).
5. Drop in blood pressure during exercise (17).
6. Excessive arterial blood pressure
   Systolic ≧260 mm Hg
   Diastolic ≧120 mm Hg
7. Signs of cerebral hypoxia (ataxia, head nodding, failure to answer questions or obey commands).
8. Signs of peripheral circulatory insufficiency (pallor, development of cyanosis, clammy skin).

adaptation to exercise and the highest work load attainable (19, 20). Since those measurements add expense and are not yet widely used clinically they will be mentioned only in passing.

Evaluation of Results of Exercise Testing

A quantitative functional assessment of overall cardiovascular performance can be obtained by evaluating the TDS (or peak load on a bicycle), heart rates, blood pressures, and symptoms obtained. A given subject or patient's response to exercise test should be compared to known normal values and an assessment of any disability made (19, 21). Factors other than cardiac or pulmonary disease that can alter working capacity are *age* (decreases with age), *sex* (women generally able to do less endurance physical work than men) *habitual state of physical activity* (endurance training increases working capacity) and *motivation* (22, 23).

Diagnostic information obtained in exercise testing is largely obtained from the ECG response to exercise. The classic ECG with exercise of 1–2 mm of horizontal or downsloping ST segment *depression* occurring in a patient with a normal or near-normal resting ECG has now been well correlated with significant, i.e., ischemia-producing, coronary artery atherosclerotic narrowing or occlusion (Fig. 25.1). In addition to horizontal or downsloping ST segment depression, other signs are highly suggestive of significant myocardial ischemia when standard ECG leads are used. These alternate "positive" signs include a depressed STJ point with slowly upsloping ST segment so that at 0.08 sec after the J point,* the ST segment is still 1.5 mm below the baseline (24). It is important to use the PQ segment of the ECG as the "baseline" or reference by which ST segments are measured. If the ST segment is upsloping and reaches the

---

* The J point is the take-off point of the ST segment at the end of the QRS complex; see Figure 25.1.

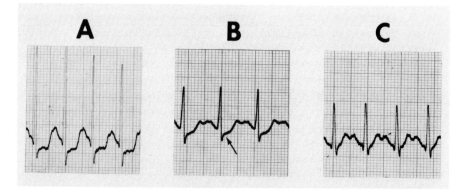

Fig. 25.1. Three common electrocardiographic responses to exercise are illustrated in different patients. All three have the same standardization of 1 mV equals 10 small blocks and all three are the bipolar lead CM_5. *Tracing A* shows a characteristic *horizontal* ST segment depression of 0.2–0.3 mV which indicates a "positive" or ischemic response.

Tracing B shows a 0.2–0.3 mV J point depression (*Note:* arrow pointing to J point at the beginning of ST segment) with a gentle upsloping ST segment. Eighty milliseconds (0.08 sec) after the J point, however, the ST segment is still 0.15 mV below the reference level (PQ segment). Note also that the T wave is starting 0.15 mV below the reference. These features define a "positive" or ischemic response.

Tracing C shows some J point depression but the ST segment is sharply upsloping and is certainly back to, or above the reference level by 0.08 sec. These features define a physiologic electrocardiographic response and this is a "normal ECG response to exercise."

baseline by 0.08 sec after the J point, then this is *not* a "positive" ECG response to exercise. This upsloping ST segment reaching the baseline quickly is the normal response expected in healthy subjects with no myocardial ischemia (24–26). Nonorthogonal, bipolar leads whose lead axis is oriented in a vertical direction should not be used because of much upsloping ST segment depression even in normal subjects (27).

Another significant but much less common ECG response to exercise is the ST segment *elevation* of 1 or 2 mm. If the resting ECG is normal, this ECG sign can indicate severe, transmural ischemia and should signal the end of the test (28, 29). In the setting of a previous old, transmural myocardial infarction, ST segment elevation is seen more commonly and can indicate the presence of ventricular wall abnormalities such as dyskinesia or akinesia (30, 31). Another important clue to probable myocardial ischemia is a drop of 20 mm Hg in systolic blood pressure, especially if this is associated with chest pain and significant ST segment alteration as previously defined (17). An important exercise testing rule is that the lower the external work load and the earlier in the exercise test that the ischemic changes occur, the more likely is it that the patient has significant two or three vessel coronary atherosclerotic disease (32). A second rule is that the deeper the ST depression (2, 3, or 4 mm), the more likely that the patient has important coronary disease of more than one vessel (33, 34). Therefore, for example, a patient with 3-mm horizontal depression after 2 min of Stage I (1.7 mph, 10% grade) should probably be considered for coronary angiography and the angiographer warned that left main coronary artery narrowing may be present (35).

Interpreting Exercise ECGs

Interpreting an exercise ECG requires that no drug or condition known to cause false positive results be present. Digitalis within 3 weeks may cause false positive results as do conditions which affect ventricular repolarization such as left ventricular hypertrophy, electrolyte imbalance, hypertension, rheumatic heart disease, ventricular conduction delays (left bundle branch block and, less often, right bundle branch block) and Wolf-Parkinson-White Syndrome. Vasoregulatory asthenia and pectus excavatum can also cause false positive results (28).

Cardiac dysrhythmias occurring during an exercise test are usually cause to stop the test. Dysrhythmias are not diagnostically significant, in and of themselves, but ventricular ectopic beats occurring in patients with known heart disease especially if the extrasystoles increase in frequency with exercise or emerge in couplets, triplets or runs of ventricular tachycardia can indicate a potential candidate for "sudden death" (27, 36, 37). A patient with such an exercise ECG response should be carefully evaluated and treated appropriately.

The standard by which exercise ECGs are judged in research studies is either coronary anatomy and pathology derived from coronary angiography, or it is the incidence of clinical events (sudden death, myocardial infarction, or angina pectoris) developing in a succeeding time period. Standard statistical calculations allow determination of sensitivity, specificity, predictive value, predictive error, and risk ratio (Table 25.4) in a given study group or defined population (38). The calculation of these values, however, cannot be separated from knowledge of the prevalence or incidence rate of coronary atherosclerotic heart disease in the study group or population (39). Bayes' theorem or rule states that any laboratory test will have a greater percentage of true positive results, fewer false results and a better predictive value if the population studied has a high proportion of the abnormality (39, 40). Therefore, in an asymptomatic, basically healthy, younger population (assume 5% have disease), exercise ECGs will tend to produce a high percentage of false results and have a low predictive value. Conversely, in a referral group of older patients with chest pain, (assume 50% have disease) exercise ECGs will score a high percentage of true positive results and a high predictive value. Currently the use of exercise testing ECGs in women is being studied (41–

TABLE 25.4. *Standard Statistical Calculations of Risk in Exercise ECGs*

Results of Exercise ECG	Results of Indicative Study[1]	
	Coronary atherosclerotic heart disease	No coronary atherosclerotic heart disease
Positive	A	B
Negative	C	D

$$\text{Sensitivity } (SE) \quad = \frac{A}{A + C} \times 100$$

$$\text{Specificity } (SP) \quad = \frac{D}{D + B} \times 100$$

$$\text{Predictive value } (PV)^2 \quad = \frac{A}{A + B} \times 100$$

$$\text{Predictive error } (PE) \quad = \frac{C}{C + D} \times 100$$

$$\text{Risk ratio} \quad = \frac{PV}{PE}$$

[1] May be coronary angiography or future appearance of clinical sign of disease: myocardial infarction, sudden death, angina pectoris

[2] *PV* is sometimes referred to as accuracy or predictive accuracy

43). It is possible that women may have a higher percentage of false positive results than men. The reasons for this may be related, in part, to Bayes' rule.

Use of Regular Physical Activity in Cardiac Rehabilitation

Cardiac rehabilitation seeks to restore and to maintain the highest level of physical, emotional, vocational, and psychological function to patients who have had a myocardial infarction, suffer from angina pectoris, or are recovered from coronary artery bypass surgery. An important element of cardiac rehabilitation is to attempt to decrease known risk factors for coronary atherosclerotic heart disease: hypertension, elevated blood cholesterol, cigarette smoking, and physical inactivity (44). It is not the purpose of the present chapter to review the early phases of a comprehensive cardiac rehabilitation program. The in-hospital and early post-hospital phases include graduated physical activity prescribed on the basis of the patient's medical progress and an educational program about risk factors, drugs, warning symptoms for coronary patients, and other information (44).

The long-term phase of cardiac rehabilitation usually begins about 8–12 weeks after a myocardial infarction or after coronary bypass surgery. At this time, if specific contraindications are not present (Table 25.5) patients are eligible for beginning a regular physical activity program which should be physician-prescribed and physician-monitored.

Why Physical Activity for Patients with Coronary Atherosclerotic Heart Disease?

An attractive, but unproven, hypothesis is that regular physical exercise will prevent or delay further progression of coronary atherosclerosis. The evidence now available *in humans* which bears in some manner upon this hypothesis can be divided into four separate categories: epidemiologic effects, coronary risk factor effects, coronary artery collateral effects, and other possible mechanisms whereby physical activity might favorably influence coronary atherosclerotic heart disease.

Among the epidemiologic data the pioneer study of J. N. Morris and his colleagues in 1953 was first to demonstrate that the more active London bus *conductors* had a statistically significant lower incidence of all coronary heart disease manifestations compared to less active bus *drivers* (45). Subsequently, dozens of epidemiologic studies have shown a lower incidence of coronary heart disease among groups of men who are more active in work or in leisure time activities compared to similar but more sedentary groups (46). It is of great interest but still an enigma that most of these studies show a decreased incidence of myocardial infarction but no difference in angina pectoris.

That the epidemiologic data do not prove the efficacy of regular physical activity in preventing further myocardial infarctions or death in patients who already have clinically manifestations of the disease should be apparent. None of the epidemiologic studies were intervention trials in defined populations with suitable controls. Other objections and problems are summarized elsewhere (46).

Coronary risk factors, especially the three major ones of hypertension, elevated cholesterol and cigarette smoking, are not importantly influenced by regular physical exercise. Early studies which appeared to demonstrate decreased cholesterol with active conditioning were not well controlled

TABLE 25.5 *Exclusions from Long-Term Cardiac Rehabilitation*

1. Significant coexisting cardiovascular disease, such as aortic stenosis (includes idiopathic hypertrophic subaortic stenosis), mitral valve disease, the presence of a prosthetic valve, or congestive heart failure.
2. Complete atrioventricular block with or without ventricular pacemaker.
3. Diastolic blood pressure measured in excess of 100 mm Hg at supine rest on multiple visits (despite drug therapy).
4. Coexisting disease such as metastatic carcinoma or chronic renal insufficiency which make long term survival unlikely.
5. Uncontrolled diabetes mellitus: insulin dependent with random blood sugars exceeding 250 mg/dl or with frequent episodes of hypoglycemia (more than one episode per week).
6. Physical and/or emotional impairments which are judged to preclude participation and adherence to physical activity programs, such as pulmonary disease, rheumatoid arthritis, cerebral vascular accident, alcoholism, or psychoses.
7. Failure to sign "informed consent."

with respect to diet or body weight (46). Triglycerides and high density lipoproteins may be importantly influenced by regular physical exertion, but the contribution of these changes to coronary heart disease risk remains to be shown. It may be that patients enrolled in a regular physical activity program with risk factor education sessions included will be more inclined to decrease smoking, alter diets, and take their antihypertensive medications, although this concept has not been subjected to controlled trial.

Recently, three separate studies have shown that at least 1 year of regular physical conditioning does not significantly enhance coronary artery collaterals (47–49).

A host of other possible mechanisms whereby physical activity might reduce the risk of coronary heart disease have been proposed. These include possible favorable alterations in such things as fibrinolytic capability, platelet stickiness, neurohormonal reactions, vulnerability to cardiac dysrhythmias, blood oxygen content, and tolerance to stress. It is also possible that sudden death may be less frequent among more physically active men. In this regard exercise-induced premature ventricular complexes were diminished in a group of high risk middle-aged men following a conditioning program (50). All of the above need more research before they can be definitely accepted as involved in decreasing coronary heart disease morbidity and mortality.

The National Exercise and Heart Disease Project (NEHDP), a cooperative, multicenter, randomized control study is currently investigating whether post myocardial infarction patients live longer or have fewer subsequent heart attacks if they exercise regularly (51). Results will not be available until 1981.

Just as there must be a scientific withholding of final judgment as to the usefulness of regular physical activity in decreasing coronary atherosclerotic heart disease morbidity and mortality, it is now clear that such exercise does provide two definite benefits. The first benefit is that of increased physical working capacity. For many cardiac patients, regular physical activity as described can lessen or eliminate cardiac symptoms because they are able to perform physical tasks at a lower heart rate times systolic blood pressure product, the "double product" (9, 10).

Hemodynamic changes in conditioned cardiac patients which allow such a benefit include, largely, alterations in the peripheral circulation and the training-induced bradycardia at rest and at sub-maximal exercise loads (52).

The second important benefit from regular physical conditioning is a psychological one. Patients state that they "feel better" when they are involved in an exercise program. Psychological testing indicates reductions in anxiety and depression and a more hopeful attitude toward the future (44, 53).

Writing an Exercise Prescription

The first step in beginning an appropriate patient in a conditioning program is to do an exercise test. The results of the exercise test are used in determining the intensity and duration of the prescribed exercise. The usual procedure is to recommend that the patient maintain his or her highest conditioning heart rate at 80–85% of the measured maximal or symptomatic heart rate on the exercise test for 15–20 min 3 times per week. Studies on normal, deconditioned subjects and preliminary data on patients with coronary atherosclerotic heart disease indicate that this level of intensity, duration and time of conditioning do provide measureable benefits in 6–12 weeks (54). Exercise testing for patients enrolled in a conditioning program should be repeated after the first 3 months and then every 6 months thereafter. Each new exercise test will check progress for the patient and physician. The exercise prescription is updated after the new test using the same formulation as given for the initial test, i.e., 85% of measured peak heart rate.

Physical Training of Patients with Coronary Atherhosclerotic Heart Disease

A basic premise of a physical activity program for cardiac patients is that it must be *safe* for the patient. It profits no one if a patient dies suddenly while exercising in an injudicious, unsupervised manner. Therefore, based on current knowledge, all such programs should be physician-prescribed and physician-monitored. This means that, for the most part, such activity programs are *group endeavors*. Groups of patients meet with a trained therapist who guides their activities individually and as a group. Each patient has an exercise prescription which states target heart rates to achieve, and other pertinent medical information such as current drugs, other risk factors and any arrhythmias on exercise test.

Patients eligible for such a program are usually at least 8–10 weeks after their most recent myocardial infarction. A postoperative patient recovered from saphenous vein bypass grafting is also eligible at 8–10 weeks after surgery. A baseline exercise test, a written referral from their physician who provides continuous, comprehensive care, and a signed consent form are required. Patients best excluded from cardiac conditioning programs are listed in Table 25.5.

The setting for cardiac conditioning programs may be almost any convenient location: a hospital physical therapy department, a community center or YMCA, or a school gymnasium after regular school hours (44, 55). Whatever the setting, emergency drugs, emergency equipment, intravenous apparatus, and a DC defibrillator need to be immediately available. Personnel involved in cardiac conditioning programs can also be diverse but may include physical/occupational therapists, physical educators, exercise physiologists, nurses, and physicians. At least two persons trained in cardiopulmonary resuscitation should be available on the site during the sessions. A physician, trained and capable of treating cardiac emergencies, should ideally be at the session also. If the physician is "on call" at some distance away, he should be able to respond within one or two minutes.

Most cardiac conditioning programs eventually do have a participant who develops ventricular fibrillation and requires immediate medical attention (56).

In Atlanta-based cardiac conditioning programs from 1971 to 1976 several hundred patients have been involved. Only two patients have suffered cardiac arrest and required emergency medical treatment. As is the case elsewhere when adequate emergency care is immediately available, the two patients referred to above suffered no myocardial infarction and were observed in the hospital for only 1 or 2 days (56). The patients are able to return to the conditioning program after appropriate medical consideration of their underlying disease and their proven propensity to develop cardiac dysrhythmias.

Cardiac Group Exercise Session Format

On arrival at the cardiac program site, suitably attired for exercise and climate, the patient must "check in" with the nurse or exercise specialist. The patient picks up his/her prescription card, has his/her blood pressure and pulse checked, and is asked about any unusual cardiovascular symptoms. The prescription card should have the target heart rate and the recommended number of repetitions for the calisthenics (55).

The format for the activity sessions is as follows (51):

1. *Warm-up Period:* This phase should include gross motor movements directed at maintaining range of motion (flexibility) about the joints (time = 5–10 min).
2. *Intermittent Physical Activity:* This phase is divided into two portions in which controlled, aerobic exercises are emphasized. *One part* consists of 15 min of continuous exercise aimed at keeping heart rates at target levels, i.e., 85% of measured peak exercise. This is usually walking, jogging, swimming, or bicycling. The *second portion* consists of games and skills which interest the group. This latter period (15–20 min) is quite important in maintaining adherence to a long term program. The single most popular activity for this period is cardiac volley ball. Rules are modified slightly to make it possible for different skill levels of players to participate. The game aspect which involves some competition has provided a great stimulus to regular participation while not causing excessive cardiac responses.
3. *Cool-down:* This phase includes light resistance activities or just walking for 3–5 min.

Patients take their own pulse rates and report any excessive rates or unusual symptoms. Groups ideally include 15–20 patients.

An alternative format for smaller groups (3–6) involves circuit interval training on 5 or 6 mechanical devices: treadmill, bicycle ergometer (legs), arm ergometer, stair steps, shoulder-arm resistance wheel, and rowing machine. The rowing machine, however, has been found to aggravate some low back conditions. After a warm-up period (see above), patients use the devices set to their own speed or resistance for 4 min at the end of which time their heart rates should be at the target heart rate level. Two minutes of rest follow and each one of the group rotates to another "station" or device. The 4- and 2-min, work-rest, pattern is continued until each has completed the 5 or 6 stations. A cool-down period ends the session (51).

Musculoskeletal Problems

In working with middle-aged or older cardiac patients who may have led sedentary life styles for years, it is important to plan a gradual progression of stress to ankles, knees and hips. Therefore it may not be possible nor wise to attempt to reach target heart rates in the first 6–8 weeks for a new participant. For some patients, at least that long will be required before muscles, joints, and tendons become adapted to the increased activity level. A cardiac patient should be deriving benefit from a physical activity program, not additional symptoms from such serious mishaps as a ruptured achilles tendon. If degenerative joint disease of knees or hips is symptomatic and appears to be progressing, then that patient should be excluded from further participation. There seems no reason to try to build better physical endurance if it is at the expense of progressive disability from hip or knee osteroarthritis. Swimming involves much less joint trauma and may be substituted for walking, jogging, and volley ball type activities.

Conclusion

This chapter has tried to show how physical exercise can be used in the testing and training of certain patients with heart disease and/or in middle-aged normal subjects with high risk factors for developing coronary atherosclerotic heart disease. In this, as in other areas of medicine, the precept of "do no harm" must apply. If properly used, physical exercise can benefit selected patients.

REFERENCES

1. NUTTER, D. O., SCHLANT, R. C., AND HURST, J. W. Isometric exercise and the cardiovascular system. *Mod. Concepts Cardiovasc. Dis., 41:* 11–15, 1972.
2. SMITH, E. E., GUYTON, A. C., MANNING, R. D., AND WHITE, R. J. Integrated mechanisms of cardiovascular response and control during exercise in the normal human. *Prog. Cardiovasc. Dis., 18:* 421–443, 1976.
3. VATNER, S. F., AND PAGANI, M. Cardiovascular adjustments to exercise: hemodynamics and mechanisms. *Prog. Cardiovasc. Dis., 19:* 91–108, 1976.
4. KLOCKE, F. J. Coronary blood flow in man. *Prog. Dis., 19:* 117–166, 1976.
5. KITAMURA, K., JORGENSEN, C. R., GOBEL, F. L., TAYLOR, H. L., AND WANG, Y. Hemodynamic correlates of myocardial oxygen consumption during upright exercise. *J. Appl. Physiol., 32:* 516, 1972.

6. SEALEY, B. J., LILJEDAL, J., ABLAD, B., AND NYBERG, G. The effects of intravenous alprenolol on exercise tolerance in patients with angina pectoris. *Pharmocol. Clin., 2:* 46-50, 1969.

7. DWYER, E. M., JR., WIENER, L., AND COX, J. W. Effects of beta-adrenergic blockade (propranolol) on left ventricular hemodynamics and the electrocardiogram during exercise-induced angina pectoris. *Circulation, 38:* 250-260, 1968.

8. GOLDSTEIN, R. E., ROSING D. R., REDWOOD D. R., BEISER, G. D., AND EPSTEIN, S. E. Clinical and circulatory effects of isosorbide dinitrate. *Circulation, 43:* 629-640, 1971.

9. DETRY, J-M., AND BRUCE, R. A. Effects of physical training on exertional ST segment depression in coronary heart disease. *Circulation, 44:* 390-396, 1971.

10. REDWOOD, D. R., ROSING, D. R., AND EPSTEIN, S. E. Circulatory and symptomatic effects of physical training in patients with coronary-artery disease and angina pectoris. *N. Engl. J. Med., 286:* 959-965, 1972.

11. RILEY, C. P., OBERMAN, A., AND SHEFFIELD, L. T. Electrocardiographic effects of glucose ingestion. *Arch. Intern. Med., 130:* 703-707, 1972.

12. KATTUS, A. A. (Chairman), American Heart Association Committee on Exercise: Exercise testing and training of individuals with heart disease or at high risk for its development: A handbook for physicians, American Heart Association, Dallas, Texas, 1975.

13. SHEFFIELD, L. T., AND ROITMAN, D. Stress testing methodology, *Prog. Cardiovasc. Dis., 19:* 33-49, 1976.

14. KATTUS, A. A. (Chairman), American Heart Association Committee on Exercise: Exercise testing and training of apparently healthy individuals: A handbook for physicians, American Heart Association, New York, 1972.

15. HELLERSTEIN, H. K., AND FORD, A. B. Energy cost of the Master two-step . *J.A.M.A., 174:* 1868-1874, 1957.

16. BRUCE, R. A., AND HORNSTEN, T. R. Exercise stress testing in evaluation of patients with ischemic heart disease. *Prog. Cardiovasc. Dis., 11:* 371-390, 1969.

17. THOMSON, P. D., AND LELEMEN, M. H. Hypotension accompanying the onset of exertional angina, a sign of severe compromise of LV blood supply. *Circulation, 52:* 28, 1975.

18. ROCHMIS, P., AND BLACKBURN, H. Exercise tests; a survey of procedures, safety and litigation experience in approximately 170,000 tests. *J.A.M.A., 217:* 1061, 1971.

19. GILBERT, C. A. Exercise Testing of Cardiac Function. In *The Heart,* Ed. 4, edited by J. W. Hurst, R. B. Logue, R. C. Schlant, and N. K. Wenger. McGraw-Hill, New York (in press).

20. MITCHELL, J. H., AND BLOMQVIST, G. Maximal oxygen uptake. *N. Engl. J. Med., 284:* 1018-1022, 1971.

21. FOX, S. M., NAUGHTON, J. P., AND GORMAN, P. A. Physical activity and cardiovascular health. *Mod. Concepts Cardiovasc. Dis., 41:* 17-29, 1972.

22. ASTRAND, P-O, AND RODAHL, K. *Textbook of Work Physiology,* pp. 277-315 and 453-484. McGraw-Hill Co., New York, 1970.

23. GERSTENBLITH, G., LAKATTA, E. G., AND WEISFELDT, M. L. Age changes in myocardial function and exercise response. *Prog. Cardiovasc. Dis., 19:* 1-21, 1976.

24. STUART, R. J., AND ELLESTAD, M. H. Upsloping ST segments in exercise stress testing. *Am. J. Cardiol., 37:* 19-22, 1976.

25. RAUTAHARJU, P. M., PUNSAR, S., BLACKBURN, H., WARREN, J., AND MENOTTI, A. Waveform patterns in Frank lead rest and exercise electrocardiograms of healthy elderly men. *Circulation, 48:* 541-548, 1973.

26. DAVIES, C. T. M., NEILSON, J. M. M., AND SAMMUELOFF, S. Electrocardiographic changes during exercise in Kurdish and Yemenite Jews in Israel. *Br. Heart J., 35:* 207-210, 1973.

27. FROELICHER, V. F., THOMPSON, A. J., WOLTHUIS, R., FUCHS, R., BALUSEK, R., LONGO, M. R., FRIEBWASSER, J. H., AND LANCASTER, M. C. Angiographic findings in asympto-

matic aircrewman with electrocardiographic abnormalities. *Am. J. Cardiol., 39:* 32–38, 1977.

28. KATTUS, A. A. Exercise electrocardiography; recognition of the ischemic response, false positive and negative patterns. *Am. J. Cardiol., 33:* 721–731, 1974.

29. DETRY, J.-M. R., MENGEOT, P., ROUSSEAU, M. F., COSYNS, J., PANLOT, R., AND BRASSEUR, L. A. Maximal exercise testing in patients with spontaneous angina pectoris associated with transient ST segment elevation. *Br. Heart J., 37:* 897–903, 1975.

30. HEGGE, F. N., TUNA, N., AND BURCHELL, H. B. Coronary arteriographic findings in patients with axis shifts or ST segment elevations on exercise-stress testing. *Am. Heart J., 86:* 603–615, 1973.

31. FORTUIN, N. J., AND FRIESINGER, G. C. Exercise-induced ST segment elevation. *Am. J. Med., 49:* 459–464, 1970.

32. ELLESTAD, M. H. Can stress testing predict the severity of coronary disease? *Chest, 69:* 708–710, 1976.

33. BARTEL, A. G., BEHAR, V., PETER, R. H., ORGAIN, E. S., AND KONG, Y. Graded exercise stress tests in angiographically documented coronary artery disease. *Circulation, 49:* 348–356, 1974.

34. GOLDMAN, S., TSELOS, S., AND COHN, K. Marked depth of ST segment depression during treadmill exercise testing. *Chest, 69:* 729–733, 1976.

35. KHAJA, F. -U., SHARMA, S. D., EASLEY, JR., R. M., HEINLE, R. A., AND GOLDSTEIN, S. Left main coronary artery lesions. *Circulation* (Suppl. II), *49–50:* II-136-II-140, 1974.

36. DOYLE, J. T. Mechanisms and prevention of sudden death. *Mod. Concepts Cardiovasc. Dis., 45:* 111–116, 1976.

37. MOSS, A. J., AND AKIYAMA, T. Prognostic significance of ventricular premature beats. *Cardiovasc. Clin., 6:* 274–298, 1974.

38. GALEN, R. A. Letter to editor: Predictive value of laboratory tests. *Am. J. Cardiol., 36:* 536–538, 1975.

39. VECCHIO, T. J. Predictive value of a single diagnostic test in unselected populations, *N. Engl. J. Med., 274:* 1171–1173, 1966.

40. REDWOOD, D. R., BORER, J. S., AND EPSTEIN, S. E. Editorial: Whither the ST segment during exercise. *Circulation, 54:* 703–706, 1976.

41. CUMMING, G. R., DUFRESNE, C., AND SAMM, J. Exercise ECG changes in women. *Can. Med. Assoc. J., 109:* 108–111, 1973.

42. SKETCH, M. H., MOHIUDDIN, S. M., LYNCH, J. D., ZENCKA, A. E., AND RUNCO, V. Significant sex differences in the correlation of electrocardiographic exercise testing and coronary arteriograms. *Am. J. Cardiol., 36:* 169–173, 1975.

43. LINHART, J. W., LAWS, J. G., AND SATINSKY, J. D. Maximum treadmill exercise electrocardiography in female patients. *Circulation, 50:* 1173–1178, 1974.

44. WENGER, N. K., AND GILBERT, C. A. Rehabilitation of the Myocardial Infarction Patient. In *The Heart,* Ed. 4, edited by J. W. Hurst, R. B. Logue, R. C. Schlant, and N. K. Wenger. McGraw-Hill, New York (in press).

45. MORRIS, J. N., HEADY, J. A., RAFFLE, P. A. B., ROBERTS, C. G., AND PARKS, J. W. Coronary heart disease and physical activity of work. *Lancet, 2:* 1053, 1953.

46. Fox, S. M., III, Relationship of Activity Habits to Coronary Heart Disease. In *Exercise Testing and Training in Coronary Heart Disease,* pp. 3–21, edited by J. P. Naughton and H. K. Hellerstein. Academic Press, New York, 1973.

47. FERGUSON, R. J., PETITCLERC, R., CHOQUETTE, G., CHANIOTIS, L., GAUTHIER, P., HUOT, R., ALLARD, C., JANKOWSKI, L., AND CAMPEAU, L. Effect of physical training on treadmill exercise capacity, collateral circulation and progression of coronary disease. *Am. J. Cardiol., 34:* 764–769, 1974.

48. KENNEDY, C. C., SPIEKERMAN, R. E., LINDSAY, JR., M. I., MANKIN, H. T., FRYE, R. L., AND MCCALLISTER, B. D. One year graduated exercise program for men with angina pectoris. *Mayo Clin. Proc., 51:* 231–236, 1976.

49. Conner, J. F., LaCamera, Jr., F., Swanick, E. J., Oldham, J. J., Holzaepfel, D. W., and Lyczkowskyj, O. Effects of exercise on coronary collateralization angiographic studies of six patients in a supervised exercise program. *Med. Sci. Sports, 8:* 145–151, 1976.

50. Blackburn, H., Taylor, H. L., Mamrell, B., Buskirk, E., Nicholas, W. C., and Thorsen, R. D. Premature ventricular complexes induced by stress testing. *Am. J. Cardiol., 31:* 441–449, 1973.

51. Common Protocol: The National Exercise and Heart Disease Project, A Collaborative Project, Second Edition, 1975; Coordinating Center: George Washington Universtiy Medical Center, 2300 Eye Street, N.W., Washington, D.C. 20037.

52. Froelicher, V. F., Jr. The Hemodynamic Effects of Physical Conditioning in Healthy Young, and Middle-aged Individuals and in Coronary Heart Disease Patients. In *Exercise Testing and Training in Coronary Heart Disease*, pp. 63–77, edited by J. P. Naughton and H. K. Hellerstein. Academic Press, New York, 1973.

53. Naughton, J., Bruhn, J. G., and Lategola, M. T. Effects of physical training on physiological and behavioral characteristics of cardiac patients. *Arch. Phys. Med. Rehabil., 49:* 131–137, 1968.

54. Fox, S. M., III, Naughton, J. P., and Gorman, P. A. Physical activity and cardiovascular health. *Mod. Concepts Cardiovasc. Dis., 41:* 21–29, 1972.

55. Fletcher, G. F., and Cantwell, J. D. Outpatient gym exercise program for patients with recent myocardial infarction. *Arch. Intern. Med., 134:* 63–68, 1974.

56. Bruce, R. A., and Kluge, W. Defibrillatory treatment of exertional cardiac arrest in coronary disease. *J.A.M.A., 216:* 563–658, 1971.

26

Exercise in Pulmonary Disease

_____ J. D. SINCLAIR

Patients with pulmonary disease benefit from specific breathing exercises, which involve a retraining of breathing patterns, and from general exercise programs which support normal daily activities. Breathing exercises have been used continuously since 1930; the widest recognition of their value arose with the advent of thoracic surgery; they have retained a respected place in the treatment of asthma, bronchitis, and emphysema. The value of general exercise in the support of the chronic respiratory invalid has been appreciated only recently as the role of physical exercise in rehabilitation has been more widely recognized.

After surgery, breathing exercises help restore maximum lung function at the earliest possible stage, help maintain posture, and shorten the period of convalescence. In chronic lung disease, where the precise contribution of any single form of therapy is notoriously hard to assess, an exact effect of breathing exercises has still not been positively identified. If clinical investigators remain uncertain, patients are consistently generous in praise of therapy while physicians with long experience maintain their faith in the benefits provided (24).

Therapeutic attempts to modify the pattern of breathing require a firm appreciation of thoracic mechanics, with regard to the physical characteristics which shape the lung and chest wall and the muscular actions which change these shapes to produce ventilation. There needs to be some regard, too, for the consequences of ventilatory change in terms of the primary function of respiration, the supply of oxygen to the body and the removal of carbon dioxide. An account of these aspects of respiratory physiology will therefore be given here before specific forms of exercise are detailed.

Mechanics of Breathing

Elastic Properties of Lung and of Thoracic Wall. The physical property of the lung which is most essential to its mechanical function is its elasticity. This term, used in its scientific sense, indicates a resistance to a change of shape. The lung resists distension, inclining to empty toward a gasless state. This property arises in part from the geometric arrangement of the alveolar mesh and in part from the specific property of elastic tissue, fibrous tissue, blood vessels, and bronchi. In abnormal states, some of the resistance to distension arises from the surface tension of the smallest alveolar bubbles. The inclination to minimize surface area would be a serious factor opposing inspiration if it were not for the secretion in alveoli of surfactant, a phospholipid which greatly reduces surface tension and thus stabilizes alveolar diameter.

The elastic behavior of the lung is measured as its compliance, the volume change per unit change of distending pressure. In an average adult breathing normally, the compliance of the lung is 100–200 ml per cm H_2O.

Balancing the inclination of the lung to empty, there is an inclination of the surrounding chest wall to distend. The "chest wall" here includes the thoracic wall and the diaphragm. If the pleural space is opened to air, the chest wall inclines to spring out toward the position of full inspiration. Again, this physical characteristic arises from the geometric arrangement of the ribs, intercostal muscles, and diaphragm.

In the normal state, therefore, the inclination of the lung to empty is opposed by the inclination of the thoracic wall to fill. If there is no muscle activity (as seen for example in the anesthetized patient given a muscle relaxant) the lung comes to a volume determined by the relative sizes of elasticities of lung and chest wall; a stiffer lung will empty to a smaller volume, a rigid chest wall will hold the lung at a greater volume.

This lung volume established passively by elastic properties is the functional residual volume of the lung, normally varying around 3000 ml.

It is important to appreciate that this is the volume to which the lung will return passively. A change of lung volume away from the functional residual volume requires active muscular effort.

Muscles of Respiration. The major respiratory muscles are the diaphragm, the intercostal muscles and the abdominal muscles. The important accessory muscles are the scalene muscles and the sternomastoids. The relative importance of the muscles was much argued when the evidence relied on anatomical dissections of past centuries. Recently, however, the refinements of electromyography have established a clear picture of the respiratory roles of the muscles and groups has been set out by Campbell, Agostoni, and Newson Davis (10). The separate actions of the muscles will be summarized here; then the general pattern of respiratory movement will emerge.

The Diaphragm. The major muscle of respiration, the diaphragm is characterized by anatomical and geometric features as complex as those of any muscle in the body. The muscle fibers of the diaphragm arise in three groups: from vertebrae and the surrounding fascia of psoas and quadratus lumborum, from the lower six ribs, and from the posterior surface of the xiphoid process of the sternum. All fibers converge on the central tendon. Innervation is by the phrenic nerve. There are few sensory organs, that is muscle spindles or Golgi tendon organs.

Contraction of the diaphragm decreases thoracic pressure and thus increases lung volume while simultaneously compressing the abdomen and increasing abdominal pressure. The unusual geometry of diaphragmatic muscle means, as well, that in most circumstances its contraction also distends the thorax. This occurs because in the usual end-expiratory position, the early phase of contraction lifts the ribs upward, and they swing outward. The lower ribs can be seen to do this in patients with transection of the spinal cord at the cervical level; in them, diaphragmatic breathing occurs in isolation from intercostal and abdominal. At higher lung volumes, this phenomenon ceases and the diaphragm tends to pull the ribs inward.

Although the action of the diaphragm is to produce inspiration, its electrical activity continues into expiration, presumably stabilizing movements. It is also active in expulsive efforts such as vomiting and defecation.

Voluntary control of diaphragmatic contraction can apparently be achieved by a small number of people. It was reported in one of three physical therapists studied by Stigol and Cuello (45). Often the impression of voluntary control obtained at fluoroscopy results from failure to study simultaneous movements of diaphragm and rib cage. Subjects appear to inspire without diaphragmatic contraction, and the diaphragmatic position remains constant; but this occurs because the thorax is lifted away from the diaphragm (46).

Measurements of electrical activity and transdiaphragmatic pressures show that contraction is occurring though the diaphragmatic position is constant.

The excursion of the diaphragm contributes two-thirds of the volume of air moved in respiration. The phrenic nerve may be stimulated electrically to maintain ventilation. Yet the loss of unilateral function produces only a temporary disturbance and respiration can be maintained without diaphragmatic contribution.

Intercostal Muscles. The external intercostals are of greater bulk than the internal muscles; the externals are dominantly posterior, the internals anterior; the externals slope forward from each rib to the rib below, the internals slope backward. Their innervation is by the segmental thoracic nerves. They are well supplied with muscle and tendon receptors.

After decades of controversy it is now clear that the external intercostal muscles act for inspiratory movements and the internal intercostal muscles act dominantly in expiration but have a minor part with inspiratory action.

The combined action of the intercostal muscles makes a rigid thoracic wall. Mead (28) suggests that this synergistic action enhances diaphragmatic function and thus has important secondary effects on breathing.

The Abdominal Muscles. These are the muscles of the ventral abdominal wall: the external and internal oblique, transverse abdominal and rectal muscles. They are supplied by the lower six thoracic and first lumbar nerves (T.7 to L.1). Their action is to compress the abdomen and to constrict the lower part of the rib cage.

Electromyographic studies show that the abdominal muscles do not act in quiet breathing or even in moderately increased breathing, in normal or diseased conditions. At high levels of ventilation, the power of the abdominal muscles operates increasingly to assist expiration.

The Accessory Muscles. The scalene muscles originate in the cervical vertebrae and are attached to the first and second ribs. They act to elevate the thorax, often in quiet breathing but consistently as breathing effort increases and upper chest movement increases.

The sternomastoid muscles similarly and visibly act in increased ventilation to elevate the sternum and clavicle. They are inactive in quiet breathing.

Movements of Breathing. Integration of individual muscle actions into a single pattern of respiratory movement is made complex by the many variations involved. At different lung volumes, the changing geometry means that muscle fibers may act in different directions. For example, the diaphragm acts to distend the thorax at low volume and to constrict it at high volume; with great lung inflation, the lowered mechanical advantage of the diaphragm and the intercostal muscles increases the relative effectiveness of the sternomastoid, which maintains its normal direction of action.

The following general picture has been established in careful studies of human subjects. In quiet, tidal breathing the diaphragm moves approximately 1.5 cm in the standing position and a little more in the supine. The rib cage circumference increases by 1 cm standing, 0.6 cm supine; the anterior posterior displacement is greater than the lateral. In breaths of maximum volume the rib circumference increases by 8 cm, the anteroposterior diameter by 3 cm, and the lateral diameter by 1.5 cm. The maximum diaphragmatic excursion is some 10 cm but at fluoroscopy only a 5-cm displacement is seen—the other 5 cm are obscured by active elevation of the rib cage away from the contracting diaphragm.

Linear displacement of the diaphragm accounts for approximately two-thirds of the change of lung volume.

Intrathoracic Pressure Distribution. Inspiration is achieved by the development of intrapleural pressure varying from 6 to 10 cm H_2O below atmospheric pressure in quiet breathing to 50–60 cm H_2O in deep breathing. Intrapulmonary pressure is also below atmospheric pressure by about 3–4 cm H_2O in quiet respiration and more in deep breathing.

During quiet, passive expiration, intrapleural pressure falls to a final level of 2 cm H_2O below atmospheric pressure in the normal, while the elastic contraction of lung produces a slightly positive pressure in the lung alveoli. In forced expiration, intrapleural pressures of 50–70 cm H_2O

may be attained, giving high intrapulmonary pressures. Much the same pressures are obtained by patients with lung disease.

Mechanical Effects on the Airways. Two forces oppose a change of lung volume. The first, the elastic properties which determine the distensibility of the lung and thorax, has already been discussed. The second is the resistance of the airways to gas flow along them; this is the resistance which increases in the common pulmonary diseases, it is the resistance which must be overcome by ventilatory work and energy.

Normally, the resistance of the airways is so low that an alveolar pressure of 0.5–1.5 cm H_2O will empty alveolar gas to the atmosphere at a flow rate of 1 L/sec. The airway resistance increases at low lung volumes when pulmonary distension and a low thoracic pressure no longer hold the airways open. Conversely, airway resistance decreases at high lung volumes. In pulmonary disease, important increases of airway resistance occur with bronchial muscle constriction, with mucosal congestion and with hypersecretion.

One factor is fundamental to retraining of breathing movement. The intrathoracic airways can be totally closed by active expiratory effort. Positive intrathoracic pressure tends to compress the airways, even in normal subjects, where total compression occurs at full expiration. The phenomenon accounts for "closing volumes" in lung, volumes of alveoli prevented from emptying by mechanical occlusion of their airways resulting from extrinsic compression. In the presence of bronchial disease, the increased resistance of distal airways lowers the pressure in proximal airways so that they are more easily compressed.

Thus increased airway resistance, even closure, is readily produced by overactive expiratory effort. Less forceful expiration may expel more air.

Energy, Work, and Efficiency of Respiration. During quiet respiration the oxygen consumption of the respiratory muscles is about 1 ml/minute/ liter of ventilation. The total O_2 requirement of respiration is thus 5–10 ml/minute. In hyperventilation the O_2 requirement may rise to 3 ml/ minute/liter of ventilation; at a ventilation rate of 75 L/minute, the O_2 requirement for respiration alone might be 200 ml/minute in a healthy subject.

In emphysema (16) the energy requirement for respiration is much higher; each additional liter ventilated may require an extra 4–5 ml of O_2 absorption. Any exercises which attempt to produce a higher minute volume might therefore be jeopardized, because the extra oxygen absorbed might, at least theoretically, be consumed by the respiratory muscles in their increased effort. This occurs in severe kyphoscoliosis (6).

The work done in inflating and deflating the lung can be measured by the product of tidal volume and intrapleural pressure changes. Intrapleural pressure changes can be recorded accurately by a suitable device in the esophagus. A narrow plastic catheter is used for the purpose, its tip lying in the lower third of the esophagus. Changes in esophageal pressure are conducted along this to a transducer (strain-gauge or capacitance manometer) whose output operates an electrical recorder (cathode ray or ink-writing oscillograph). It is comparatively easy to record the changes in tidal volume simultaneously. Corresponding points on these tracings may be plotted graphically as ordinate and abscissa, to give a loop such as that shown in Figure 26.1.

The work done during inspiration is the area $OIAN$, and consists of the area OAN, work done against the elastic resistance of the lung (which increases with the depth of breathing), and the area OIA, work done mostly against airway and tissue viscous resistance (which increases with the speed of air movement).

The work OAE done during expiration is normally carried out passively by the energy stored in the stretched lung. Only in the forced expiration of exercise, or with increased airway resistance, does expiration become active.

Perhaps the most important aspect of this work is the observation of McIlroy, Marshall, and Christie (26) that both normal and abnormal subjects, whether at rest or exercise, breathe at the rate and depth which demand the least work. This occurs because slow, deep respiration requires excessive work against elastic resistance, while rapid, shallow respiration requires excessive work against airway and tissue viscous resistance. Between the two extremes is an optimal level which is automatically chosen by the patient. Therefore, again, breathing exercises should not be designed to alter the respiratory rate and depth chosen by the patient when therapy has not changed the physical characteristic of his lungs.

The efficiency of any machine is the ratio:

$$\frac{\text{Mechanical work done}}{\text{Energy consumed}}.$$

For a steam engine, the efficiency is 7–20%, the greater part of the energy being lost as heat. For skeletal muscle, the efficiency varies from 20 to 30%.

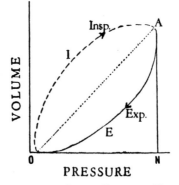

Fig. 26.1. A normal pressure-volume diagram. The line *AO* represents the elastic resistance of the lung, increasing directly with volume. The area of the loop represents the work done against viscous resistances of lung and airway.

The efficiency of respiratory movements is 5–10%. Thus only a small amount of the energy expended goes into useful work. This inefficiency is almost certainly exaggerated in emphysema. It follows that even a small increase in efficiency of effort would reflect an appreciable decrease in energy expenditure in respiration.

Disturbances of the Mechanics of Breathing. Disturbances can occur in the proximal and distal airways, in alveolar tissues and in the chest cage. Mechanical or microbial threats to the airway are dealt with in part by the secretion of mucus and by the cough reflex, mediated by the vagus nerve (35). In the distal airways, hypersecretion of mucus, bacterial infection, mucosal congestion, and smooth muscle contraction produce an increase of airways resistance, already discussed. Compression and even closure are produced by positive thoracic pressure. Tissue destruction reduces the elastic recoil of lung tissue; the tendency of the chest wall to distend leads to hyperinflation of lung. Growth of excessive fibrous or granular tissue may reduce the distensibility of lung; its stiffness reduces its static volume and may seriously impede respiration. In the chest wall, the rigidity of kyphoscoliosis and obesity may also impose an increased resistance to breathing.

Measurement of Breathing Functions

Measurements of vital capacity and residual volume are old and established. These are, respectively, the maximum volume of gas exhaled from full inspiration and the volume then remaining in the lungs. Largely from the work of Cournand and his colleagues (15), emphasis shifted by 1941 from these static measurements to dynamic measurement of ventilation, particularly the minute ventilation at rest or exercise, and the maximum breathing capacity, that is, the greatest volume breathed by voluntary hyperventilation, normally about 100 L/minute. Later tests have been well reviewed by Comroe et al. (14), Bates et al. (4), Bouhuys (8), Cherniack et al. (11), and Peters (36).

It is logical to group lung function tests according to this involvement with: 1) mechanics of respiration; 2) volumes ventilated: according to evenness of distribution of gas in the lung; 3) alveolar gas levels: according to: (a) efficiency of gas diffusion; (b) evenness of blood flow to well-ventilated areas; (4) arterial blood gas levels.

In these four major divisions, the following functions may be analyzed:

1. *Mechanics of Respiration*
    (a) Movements.
    (b) Intrathoracic pressure distribution.
    (c) Energy consumption.
    (d) Work done in respiration.
    (e) Mechanical efficiency of respiration.
2. *Volumes Ventilated ("Bellows" Function)*
    (a) Minute volume at rest.
    (b) Minute volume in exercise.
    (c) Maximum voluntary ventilation, or maximum breathing capacity.

 (d) Forced (or timed) vital capacity.
3. *Intrapulmonary Gas Mixing: Alveolar Gas Levels*
 (a) Mixing efficiency.
 (b) Analysis of alveolar gas samples.
4. *Diffusion; Evenness of Pulmonary Blood Flow, Arterial Blood Gas Levels*
 (a) Diffusing capacity.
 (b) Analysis of O_2 and CO_2 exchange.
 (c) Analysis of arterial blood gases.

Thus it is possible to measure with some accuracy the energy required for the respiratory movements and the work that is done by the lungs and thorax during these movements, which increases with increased pulmonary ventilation. The ratio of this work to the energy consumed gives a measurement of the mechanical efficiency of the system. Ventilatory volumes may be measured either at rest, during exercise or during voluntary maximal respiratory effort. Factors such as bronchiolar obstruction from spasm or mucus may cause the inhaled air to be distributed unevenly among the alveoli. Accordingly, different levels of alveolar oxygen and carbon dioxide may be attained in different parts of the lung. Increased ventilation of an alveolus raises the oxygen and lowers the carbon dioxide concentration in it. As long as gas transfer (or diffusion) is normal and pulmonary blood flow is distributed evenly to the ventilated areas, the alveolar gas levels determine the gas levels of the capillary blood, which are the final reflection of the efficiency of the cardiorespiratory system.

Such a scheme as this gives an overall view of the process of respiration. All the measurements named can be made during normal breathing, either at rest or at work. They are all good functional tests and are largely independent of physical maneuvers. For the study of the effect of breathing exercises, some will obviously be more useful than others; for example, since changes in the structure of alveoli or capillaries are not likely to be achieved, study of pulmonary blood flow or gas exchange is not likely to be rewarding. The factors which might be expected to improve will be discussed now in a little more detail.

Volumes Ventilated. The average volume of gas respired per minute by a normal patient at rest is about 5–8 L. If he breathes 16 times per minute at a tidal volume of 500 ml, about 150 ml of each inspiration fills the anatomical dead space of his airways. The remaining 350 ml at 16/minute ventilates his alveoli at 5.6 L/minute; this is the important figure in function. If his tidal volume becomes much smaller, say 300 ml, then only 150 ml enter his alveoli, and he would have to breathe much faster to achieve a satisfactory alveolar ventilation.

In fibrotic diseases of the lung, resting ventilation volumes increase. In early emphysema, they may do likewise, but later they become normal or low. In exercise, normal people may achieve ventilation rates of 60–100 L/ minutes. By maximum voluntary hyperventilation, measured as the maximum breathing capacity, they may achieve volumes of 80–200 L/

minute, with considerable variations according to age, sex, and body size. In emphysema, the ventilatory response to exercise may be normal, but invariably the maximum breathing capacity is low, sometimes as low as 15–20 L/minute. Such a dynamic measurement is clearly more significant than, say, measuring vital capacity.

Instead of recording maximum breathing capacity, laboratories now use tests based on a single forced expiration, the timed vital capacity (19) or forced vital capacity (20) (Fig. 26.2). In the last tests, the patient exhales as fast as possible. The volume exhaled in the first 1.0 sec is measured from the recorded tracing or some electronic device. This volume is closely related to the maximum breathing capacity. It is described as the forced expired volume (F.E.V. 1 sec).

Intrapulmonary Gas Mixing; Alveolar Gas Levels. From the inspired gas which passes the dead space, that is, the alveolar ventilation, each alveolus should ideally receive the same quota; the distribution or "mixing" of gas in the lung is then said to be ideal. However, when bronchial spasm or edema occurs, or when infection and mucus result in stenosis of bronchioli, normal parts of the lung remain well ventilated, while those beyond diseased airways become underventilated. Blood still flowing through these areas will then enter the pulmonary veins with the low oxygen and high carbon dioxide content of mixed venous blood. The unevenness of gas mixing is tested in various ways, mostly requiring rather more complicated apparatus (47).

Diffusion, Even Blood Flow, Arterial Blood Gas Levels. Gas transfer between alveolar gas and capillary blood depends on the resistance of the alveolar-capillary membrane (that is, its diffusing capacity) and on the pulmonary blood flow to the ventilated areas (14).

The final criterion of the adequacy of respiration is the maintenance of normal arterial gas levels, that is, oxygen saturation, carbon dioxide content and also pH. Blood gas electrode systems measure partial pressures of gases rather than their volumes. Normal values for arterial blood

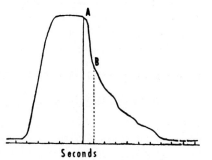

Seconds

Fig. 26.2. A tracing of a forced (or timed) vital capacity of a patient with emphysema. He exhales from the point a, but in the first second (to b) he exhales only 40% of his vital capacity (normal 70–80%). The step-and-stairs pattern results from sudden release of various volumes of "trapped" gas.

are:

O_2 saturation	95%
pO_2	95 mm Hg.
CO_2 content	45–55 vol %
pCO_2	40 mm Hg
pH	7.38–7.42

Any therapy which improves a patient's capacity to ventilate his alveoli should therefore produce an improvement in blood gas levels. Arterial samples can be taken perfectly easily. In emphysema they show, in early disease, a fall in oxygen saturation and, later, a rise in carbon dioxide content and a fall in pH as respiratory failure becomes more manifest. With exercise, the changes are accentuated.

Lung Function Tests in a Physical Medicine Clinic

Of the tests described, some require simple equipment only, while others can be done with expensive equipment which requires considerable technical knowledge. Details of both apparatus and technique, with adequate references, are given in *Methods in Medical Research* (13).

The basic requirement is a spirometer to measure the vital capacity. A good description of the uses and limitations of the vital capacity in a physical therapy clinic are given in Dail and Affeldt (17).

A large Tissot spirometer or Douglas bag, with suitable valves, is useful for collecting gas expired over a timed period of rest or exercise.

Next most useful, probably, is the estimation of arterial gas levels, either by the standard technique of sampling from the brachial artery or by the use of the ear oximeter.

Intrapulmonary gas mixing is measured either by the speed of nitrogen washout during oxygen breathing or by the speed of equilibration of helium in the lung when breathed from a spirometer, or, better, during a single expiration using a nitrogen meter or other rapid gas analysers to show the variations of expired oxygen, carbon dioxide, nitrogen, or helium.

Measurement of the work of breathing is feasible if suitable pressure-recording apparatus is available, esophageal pressures being transmitted through a small latex balloon on the end of a fine polyethylene tube. Pressure changes and tidal volume must be recorded simultaneously.

Asthma, Bronchitis and Emphysema: Diseases of Airway Obstruction

CLINICAL DEFINITIONS

Because of differences in emphasis and definitions, patients with chronic lung disease are likely to be diagnosed as asthmatic because of their wheeze, bronchitic because of their cough and sputum, or emphysematous because of their continuous dyspnea. Differentiation among the three diseases is often difficult and sometimes impossible.

Classical asthma, characterized by intermittent paroxysmal wheezing between intervals of normal health, should be separated from the others because of the importance of its better prognosis; many patients with this disease never develop complications and ultimately die with lungs that appear normal.

We may define chronic bronchitis as a disease with continual cough, productive of mucoid sputum, and complicated by episodes of acute infection. Again, many patients suffer no great deterioration with the passing of the years, though probably the majority eventually develop signs of emphysema.

Emphysema is usually defined in pathological terms as a disease in which the lungs show areas of tissue destruction and hyperinflation. In living patients, clinicians infer that these processes have occurred by the history of continuous dyspnea and the various signs of excessively aerated lungs in an overdistended chest.

PATHOLOGICAL ANATOMY

In asthma, as already mentioned, the lungs usually remain quite normal; only a minority of patients ultimately develop emphysema.

In bronchitis, Reid (41) has described hypertrophy of mucous glands in the trachea and bronchi, with a high proportion of goblet cells, which produce excessive mucus, obstructing the air passages. In the bronchioles there may be obstruction, with or without infection, leading to more severe consequences of abscess formation, stenosis, or obliteration. With this disruption of the peripheral part of the lung, nodules of nonfunctioning tissue are formed from obstructed bronchioli and alveoli. In parts there is tissue destruction and in parts inflation, maybe by "collateral ventilation" from adjacent alveoli, leaving the characteristic cyst or bullae. The extent of these irreversible changes of emphysema clearly limits the ultimate value of any form of therapy.

GENERAL EXERCISE TRAINING

Patients with obstructive lung disease may benefit from a simple exercise program, for example on an ergometer or treadmill or steps. The duration of the exercise is increased systematically. The fixed regime should be coupled with a daily walk, for example of 1/2–1 mile. The patient should be encouraged to exercise as part of his normal daily activity, for example by walking instead of driving short distances, by climbing stairs instead of using an elevator. The exact program and advice must be adjusted according to the circumstances of the individual patient.

Patients respond to exercise training with a renewal of self-confidence and they increase their exercise tolerance (31, 32). With the subjective improvement they show a fall of heart rate during exercise (3) and even those who are considerably restricted can increase their exercise levels and oxygen uptakes by 20% (12).

BREATHING EXERCISES

Specific exercise which aim at retraining in breathing, should be viewed in terms of what can be realistically expected from them.

1. The strength of respiratory muscles can be increased; but this will seldom be a relevant aim because excessive effort will compress the airways and increase breathlessness.
2. Inefficient use of muscles, especially accessory muscles, can be eliminated so that the oxygen cost of breathing is reduced.
3. Forceful breathing which actively compresses airways can be replaced by relaxed patterns in which opening of the airways is enhanced.
4. Gross hyperinflation of the lung can be reduced by increased expiration, so that inspiration is not required of a fully stretched lung.
5. Increased diaphragmatic excursion with reduced thoracic movements can reduce the neural input from muscle and joint receptors and so reduce the sensation of breathlessness (10).
6. Altered patterns can, at least theoretically, alter the distribution of inspired gas and so alter the efficiency of gas exchange.
7. The clearing and defence of the airways can be enhanced.
8. The patient can be given confidence in his ability to withstand breathlessness and to undertake the activities of everyday life.

Since much the same exercises are taught for asthma, bronchitis, and emphysema, their physical treatment will be considered together, with mention of the occasional modifications for one or other disorder.

Furthermore, while there are regional variations in methods used throughout the world, in the present account these will be condensed as much as possible to their common fundamentals.

The exercises date from the Asthma Research Council's recommendations in 1934 (2) and the account given by Livingstone and Gillespie (23) in 1935. The exercises were developed and modified by Miss H. Angove (1) and then, particularly, by the Misses W. Linton and J. Reed at the Brompton Hospital of London, which has been the teaching source of this therapy for many countries (39). Some innovation and modification for emphysema has been described by Miss M. Miller of the Johns Hopkins Hospital (29), while variations for asthmatics have been proposed by Bolton, Gandevia, and Ross of Australia (7, 42). A brief review is given by Dorinson (18). Scherr and Frankel (43) have described a broad program for asthmatic children. Orlava (34) has described exercises used in Russia for the treatment of pneumonia.

In general, treatment is aimed at: 1) physical and mental relaxation, 2) adoption of good posture, 3) lower rib respiration, 4) diaphragmatic respiration.

It is convenient to work at times with individuals and at other times with groups. It is essential that the physical therapist should have the patient's confidence, which usually requires at least one preliminary session of close individual attention. Later, the patients may gain by watching others, joining them in their endeavors, and taking heart from the more enthusiastic.

Relaxation. It is easy to perceive the tension of the patient with asthma or emphysema. He is anxious and worried at the best of times, as is readily appreciated, because of his continual efforts to avoid suffocation. This is reflected generally in various nervous habits, in the tremor of his hands and in the twitching of his closed eyelids (7). In his respiration, of which he is often extremely conscious, it may lead to any sort of movement pattern, especially when he is observed; particularly, he may show an increase of upper chest, shoulder, neck, and spinal movements, which represent continuous, wasteful and unproductive motions.

Many therapists now regard the teaching of physical relaxation as an essential preliminary to the teaching of exercise in the belief that the patients can then be taught more efficient breathing patterns. Their arguments are analogous to those of athletes and swimmers, who adopt a style of movement which combines maximal use of some muscles with minimal use of others. First, the therapist must show the patient the wasteful associated movements and absent abdominal movement of his breathing. The patient is told that he can learn a new way of breathing which will make fewer demands on him and will reduce both the frequency and the severity of his attacks of asthma. He must realize that the exercises are meant as a permanent change, not as pills to be taken morning and night. In conditions of greatest tension, when his asthma or breathlessness is worst, he needs to pay more attention to his manner of breathing, but at these times he can profit most from his new knowledge. Whenever possible, sources of worry should be eliminated by whatever social measures are practicable; even a man of obsessive personality can learn a little of the happy-go-lucky demeanor of his more placid fellows.

The personal element in this approach is obvious. The successful therapist will be the one with the right combination of understanding, tact, skill, and enthusiasm. Usually patients appreciate the points readily. They are glad to hear of a treatment that lies in their own hands, while their general nervous tension is partly relieved by the mere fact of receiving positive treatment, in contrast to the negative attitude that many of them have experienced previously.

Next, in as quiet an environment as possible, the patient is taught physical relaxation. This is often easiest if he lies on his back, with head and knees supported by pillows and with his arms resting comfortably. He is shown the difference between a contracted and a relaxed muscle and is then taught to tense and relax his muscles alternately, the relaxed phase lasting longer, until he relaxes them voluntarily and completely without the preceding contraction. This maneuver should begin in easily observed muscles, for example, the flexor of the elbow, and then continued in other groups affecting the shoulders, neck, face and abdomen. Success is measured as a neurologist measures tone, by the ease with which a limb drops back to its resting place after the examiner lifts it and allows it to fall.

When the patient has learned some relaxation of this type, he begins exercises aimed at stretching and relaxing the short, tight muscles of the shoulder girdle and upper chest. The various rhythmic swinging exercises designed for this purpose are best carried out in time with respiration. Some examples that have been proposed are:

1. Sitting, shrug shoulders, tighten all arm muscles, then slowly relax, the last phase lasting longer.
2. Sitting, let the head and shoulders fall forward until well lowered, then straighten first the back, then the neck and head. Breathe out during the first phase and breathe in during the second (Fig. 26.3a).
3. Sitting, with fingers on the shoulders, make circling movements with the elbows, moving them forward and upward in inspiration, back and down in expiration. Rest and repeat. The back should be held straight, and the patient should lean forward so that the movement is in the shoulders, not the spine.
4. Sitting with feet apart, back straight and hands on knees, throw the left arm sharply to the left and turn that way, then relax. Breathe in during the turn, breathe out while relaxing or recovering. Do not bend forward. Repeat with the other arm.
5. Standing with feet apart, lift the arms upward on inspiration; on expiration bend to the left and then forward, allowing the arms to swing easily out and down (Fig. 26.3b). Repeat to each side three or four times.
6. Standing with feet slightly apart, swing the arms forward to shoulder level during inspiration, then backward during expiration; gradually bend knees, hips and spine in time with the downward movement of the arms, until able to assume a semisquatting position by the end of expiration (Fig. 26.3c).

During these exercises the therapist works to eliminate unnecessary movement, especially of the shoulders and spine.

Posture. In asthma there is likely to be a reversible defect of posture

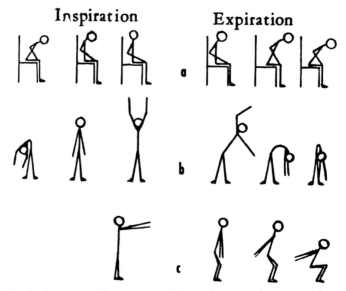

Fig. 26.3. A diagrammatic representation of some of the exercises used for muscle training and relaxation. Details are given in the text.

which is similar to the fixed abnormality seen in emphysema. The shoulders are hunched up high, there is a thoracic kyphosis and a compensatory lordosis below it, and there may also be individual abnormalities requiring separate treatment.

The defects should be convincingly demonstrated to the patient; a mirror may be helpful for this. He is then watched at rest and in various activities until he has learned to maintain a more correct habit of posture, particularly in association with his normal day-to-day routine. Ross et al. (42) point out the frequently bad sitting posture of asthmatics, important in children and office-workers. They also warn against overcorrection to the equally inefficient military posture of the "chin-in, chest-out, stomach-in" kind.

In older patients it is often desirable to give generalized exercises to increase mobility, especially of the articulations of the ribs between both the cervical and the thoracic vertebrae. Since there has been difficulty of expiration there is often a tightening of auxiliary muscles of inspiration. To stretch a shortened scalenus, have the patient hold his head to the side of tightness and push the head in the opposite direction. It may even be desirable to give vertical traction to the extended head to loosen tight scaleni. Exercises are also indicated to loosen the scapulae and shoulder girdle. Have the patient clasp his hands behind his back and then lift them.

Low Costal Respiration. Attention is next given to breathing movements. The patient is taught first to increase the excursion of his lower ribs. "Lateral basal expansion" is achieved by inhaling against pressure in the particular region. The patient, sitting, places his hands comfortably across his lower ribs, applies pressure, with one hand only, to assist deeper expiration, and then maintains some of this pressure to resist inspiration (Fig. 26.4). The exercise is repeated on the other side until unilateral control appears adequate when bilateral pressure is applied.

Pressure can be applied better with a wide belt round the lower ribs. It crosses in front of the body, and the ends are held by hand. A pull with the right hand then exerts a controlled pressure on the left ribs, while the left hand and arm are still relaxed (Fig. 26.5). Bilateral pull gives bilateral pressure.

When lower costal breathing is satisfactory it is integrated with diaphragmatic breathing.

Diaphragmatic Respiration. We now come to the most controversial aspect of breathing exercises, the teaching of voluntary control of diaphragmatic or abdominal respiration.* This is regarded as important in virtually all clinics, though with some differences of emphasis. Thus Miller (29) teaches such active deep diaphragmatic expiration that inspi-

---

* *Editor's note*: If weakened abdominal muscles interfere with respiration the patient should be taught to use his latissimus in the expiratory phase. This is aided by the use of an abdominal corset.

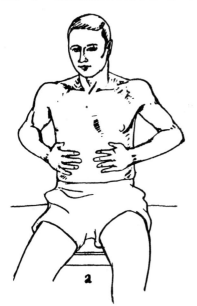
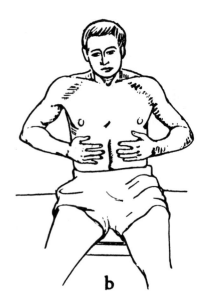

Fig. 26.4. Lateral basal breathing: (a) mild pressure with the right hand provides resistance to inspiration; (b) mild pressure ensures deep expiration. The left hand is relaxed. Bilateral breathing is taught when unilateral control appears satisfactory.

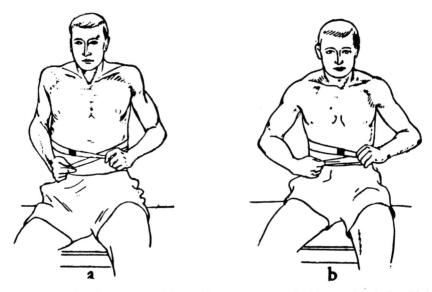

Fig. 26.5. Segmental breathing with pressure applied by a wide belt which should allow more relaxation of the arms, though in this figure the patient has tensed his shoulders: (a) inspiration; (b) expiration.

ration becomes passive from the rebound of the chest wall, while Bolton, Gandevia and Ross (7) concentrate on "diaphragmatic mobilization" in inspiration rather than expiration as is usual.

The patient is shown that the outline of his abdomen barely changes during respiration because of the abnormal mechanics of his movements, while his upper thoracic movement is accentuated.

Exercises to overcome this abnormal breathing pattern are best begun with the patient lying down, with bent knees supported by pillows, his hands resting on his lower front ribs. Attention is given first to the upper rib movement; he practices suppression of this until in quiet breathing it subsides toward a normal level. He then concentrates on abdominal movements, until his abdomen relaxes and distends in inspiration and tenses and retracts during expiration, which is usually taught to last up to twice as long as inspiration. He practices prolonging expiration until he can exhale for ten to fifteen seconds without losing control of his next inspiration, which should not be associated with gasping or with upper chest movement.

This exercise is sometimes learned more easily in various postures other than the supine. In patients having great difficulty in learning diaphragmatic breathing, it is sometimes helpful to use a rocker, so that the inspiratory fall of the diaphragm is assisted by synchronous tipping toward upright position. Some patients and therapists prefer the semi-prone position, the patient lying curled up a little and relaxed (Fig. 26.6). Another alternative is for the patient to rest on his hands and knees, when gravity again assists inspiration; he may also perform a full knee-bend to assist expiration.

Continuing from this, diaphragmatic expiration is encouraged during other body maneuvers. The patient may sit on a stool or chair, his feet apart and his arms relaxed. He leans forward as he expires, until his head is near or between his knees; at the same time he firmly contracts his abdominal muscles. He slowly uncoils during inspiration.

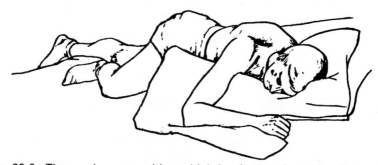

Fig. 26.6. The semiprone position which is often preferred for the teaching of diaphragmatic breathing. Patient should be well supported to allow full relaxation.

Next, the patient lies on his back with knees up, draws one knee up to his chin during expiration and lowers it again during inspiration. This is repeated first with the other knee, then with both knees being lifted together. The shoulders and arms are relaxed.

By this stage the patient should appear to control his breathing in relaxed positions so that there is a much more normal abdominal movement and much less upper thoracic movement. He is now taught to maintain this breathing pattern while sitting or standing and during some of the bending and swinging exercises practiced previously for relaxation. He should then maintain control during light activities such as stepping, walking, running-on-the-spot, climbing stairs, walking uphill, or weight lifting. Exercises should be chosen with special reference to the patient's occupation and the circumstances under which he suffers from dyspnea in his normal routine. He must not progress to a more complicated exercise unless his breathing is well controlled during revision of simpler exercises.

EXERCISES FOR CONTROL OF DYSPNEA OR ASTHMA

It is convenient at this stage to discuss exercises for the control of dyspnea or an attack of asthma. Asthmatic patients can be assured that proper breathing will make their attacks less frequent and, during an attack, will relieve their distress. The patients are taught to adopt a posture in which gravity assists inspiration. Suitable positions are: 1) sitting, leaning forward, with head on arms, the arms resting on a table or on pillows (Fig. 26.7); 2) lying semiprone, with arms and legs slightly

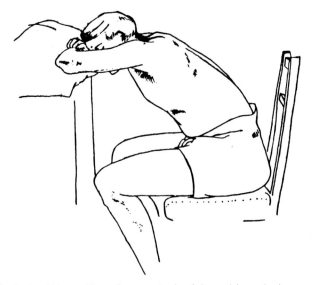

Fig. 26.7. A useful position for control of breathing during an attack of asthma.

bent and relaxed, body and limbs being well supported by pillows (Fig. 26.6). The previously described diaphragmatic breathing is too slow for a patient who is acutely breathless. For this condition, he is therefore taught short, quick respirations, in which again expiration is achieved by abdominal contraction and inspiration by abdominal relaxation. Ross, Bolton, and Gandevia (42) strongly urge that forced expiration should be abandoned, the patient being taught first to relax completely despite his asthma, and second to inspire by improved diaphragmatic descent.

The frequency and duration of the lessons in breathing will have to depend on the circumstances and progress of the patient. Generally in the early stages the more frequent the teaching, the better the result, while lessons can be reduced later to monthly intervals which ensure continued practice and attention by the patient. He should be reminded of the need to continue his new breathing pattern outside the physical therapy department and particularly when faced with any severe test of his capacity for exercise. Most patients appreciate this quite well.

During acute asthma or in the severely breathless patient with emphysema, physical therapy should be preceded by bronchodilator therapy. The use of nebulizers or the various inhalation techniques is recommmended, both in institutional and domestic therapy (37). Petty and Nett (38) have set out a simple account in a manual for patients.

ASSESSMENT OF THE EFFECTS

The most extensive investigation of the changes in lung function with physical therapy was that of Becklake (et al.) (5), who showed no consistent improvement in lung volumes, maximum breathing capacity, intrapulmonary gas mixing or arterial oxygen saturation, despite the patients' subjective improvement. This investigation was carried out after patients had received the full benefit of other orthodox therapy, and there were good control tests before breathing exercises began. Similar results were obtained by Sinclair (44), in whose 22 patients there was a slight improvement in most tests, for example, of 6 L/minute in maximum breathing capacity, the result of appreciable improvement in five patients who otherwise appeared similar to the rest. On the whole there was disappointingly little physiological change in comparison with the claims of subjective improvement. Campbell and Friend (9) found similar results; their patients achieved no more efficient lung ventilation during "exercise" breathing than during normal breathing. McNeill and McKenzie (27) found no improvement in the fast expiration of their patients. Miller (30), in contrast, found quite marked improvements in vital capacity, maximum breathing capacity and arterial oxygen and carbon dioxide levels. His patients were breathing with a much increased tidal volume after their treatment.

Bolton, Gandevia, and Ross (7) made a very careful survey of asthmatic patients before and after modified breathing exercises. They found a significant correlation between clinical improvements and the ability to breathe "abdominally." Miller (30) had noted increased diaphragm excursion in his patients after their course of treatment. Sinclair (44) found the same high degree of improvement in diaphragm excursion but with no increase in vital capacity. This apparent anomaly resulted from different mechanics of respiration, because by measuring the extent of "lifting" of the thoracic cage in the method of Wade (46), already discussed, he showed that true diaphragm movement remained constant. The appearance of increased movement, accompanied by "abdominal" breathing, reflected the diminished lifting of the thorax when the patient was taught to suppress wasteful movements of spine and shoulders.

The only close analysis of respiratory movements during treatment has been that of Campbell and Friend (9), who found that during "exercise breathing" respiration became slow and deep. Electromyography then showed increased activity in the abdominal muscles, especially in the obliques. There was only occasionally a reduction in the activity of the sternomastoid muscle. In exertion the patients were unable to continue their "exercise breathing" because the inspired volume became inadequate, so they reverted to natural breathing. The only worthwhile gain they noticed was an impression that patients recovered more quickly from dyspnea when breathing as they had been taught.

CONCLUSIONS AND INDICATIONS

In the light of these investigations and of the known processes of pulmonary physiology, we can summarize the effects of breathing exercises in asthma, bronchitis and emphysema and can decide which aspects of the exercises are of value.

First, it must be agreed that the exercises have no effect on the basic processes of the diseases. In emphysema, the exercises do not prevent the progressive deterioration of lung function which is associated with the disease for they produce no consistent improvement in vital capacity, in speed or efficiency of lung ventilation or, most important, in arterial oxygen and carbon dioxide levels. At best, a minority of patients may show a measurable benefit, but it is always hard to be sure whether the state of their disease is not showing a natural fluctuation toward improvement.

Observations of diaphragm excursion, however, show that the exercises produce an undeniable change, though this is not from the learning of true voluntary control of the diaphragm. In fact, the changed pattern of breathing which Wade (46) showed in normals, Bolton et al. (7) in asthmatics and Sinclair (44) in emphysema results from decreased lifting of the thoracic cage. Since this is a wasteful effort, not usually contributing to respiration, its suppression is in accord with the basic principles of the therapy. This significant change of movement is probably obtained in part by the teaching of relaxation and in part by the encouragement of low rib and abdominal movement while other movements are suppressed.

The theory of "diaphragmatic breathing" may be fallacious, but the practice still produces a worthwhile result. In asthmatics (7) it decreases the frequency and severity of attacks, while in emphysema it decreases the strained breathing movements which give the sensation of breathlessness.

Some of the exercises which have been advocated in various clinics are clearly unsound in their physiological concept. Possibly by misinterpretation of published work, therapists sometimes teach a slow, deep respiration that is quite impractical, since it diverges from the principles of economy in the work of breathing. It is possible to see patients who practice their breathing exercises for 5-10 min until they become so breathless they admit they must stop. Also somewhat fallacious is the forced expiration which is sometimes taught. Expiration may be prolonged within the limits of the respiration rate, but, if forced, it may obstruct air flow more than it assists it. In the patients in this group, relaxed, sighing expiration may, in fact, produce faster air flow than an expiration with maximum force behind it. Emphasis on unilateral lower costal breathing is also unlikely to be of great value since the appearance of control must result largely from some bodily distortion, probably a slight lateral twist of the spine.

We remain with a useful form of treatment which produces benefits which are psychological and physiological. The first is obvious. Many patients have had little positive therapy before they come for breathing exercises. At this point a confident approach with the right mixture of enthusiasm and understanding will relieve much of the patient's anxiety and worry. The participation in increasingly strenuous activity is especially relevant in the management of asthmatic children (43). The second benefit, the physiological, is the improvement of breathlessness by a mechanically more efficient pattern of respiration, which gives more comfortable breathing though the measurable results are the same as before. This benefit may be likened to the "second wind" of athletes, who travel at the same speed as before but feel better because of a better coordinated rhythmical movement.

Therefore, physicians faced with chronic and disabling chest diseases are justified in recommmending the breathing exercises that in the past they have considered a valuable stand-by. The function of the therapist is to obtain understanding and cooperation from the patient, to teach relaxation and economy of effort and to incorporate these, by preliminary use of the standard exercises, in the everyday activities of his patient.

The indications for the treatment remain somewhat general because it is not yet possible to show, in advance, which patients are more likely to benefit. The most positive value of the exercises is perhaps in young asthmatics, who are relieved of their symptoms and in whom a postural deformity should be prevented. In older patients, the group which seems to receive most advantage includes those whose wheeze or dyspnea is just becoming severe enough to interfere with their daily activities. Often they can be returned, at least temporarily, to reasonable employment or household duties. A few will improve greatly. In the worst cases—patients who are breathless at rest—therapists are working against overwhelming disease, yet both they and their patients frequently find that the breathing exercises produce enough benefit to be worthwhile.

Segmental Breathing and Other Exercises Associated with Thoracic Surgery

Perhaps the biggest demand for physical therapy in a chest unit is in conjunction with thoracic surgery. This is certainly so in England, where T. Holmes Sellors has been particularly encouraging and demanding toward his therapists. Developing the suggestions of a speech therapist, Cortlandt MacMahon (25), Miss Linton began work at St. Bartholomew's Hospital, London, under Mr. J. E. H. Roberts and later, in 1934, at the Brompton Hospital under Mr. T. Holmes Sellors. The localized breathing exercises, or segmental breathing, which she elaborated were accepted widely and won further acceptance in the treatment of chest injuries during World War II.

Once the methods were established, they were introduced in the treatment of tuberculous patients, until even preoperative exercises came to be accepted as normal in some units. Most of the surgery was at first thoracoplasty, which required much time of the therapists to prevent postoperative deformities. With the trend toward resection rather than collapse, this problem became less pressing, whereas the teaching of segmental breathing was required more frequently.

Physical exercises in surgery are designed mostly for two purposes: 1) to maintain body posture and limb movement; 2) to bring about reexpansion and function of the lung after thoractomy. They are used in conjunction with other maneuvers with the same object, for example, postural drainage and tipping, bronchoscopy, etc. In general, the exercises need to be taught for various periods before operation if the therapist is to obtain reasonable cooperation from the patient suffering the pain and discomfort of the postoperative period. Later, the patient can receive longer courses of treatment.

POSTURAL EXERCISES AND LIMB MOVEMENT

In the first days after operation, the therapist watches the patient's posture, correcting with pillows if a spinal curvature develops. When drainage tubes are removed and the patient is out of bed, the problem is easier. At the same time, stiffness of the shoulder on the affected side is prevented by shoulder girdle movements and by appropriate occupational therapy. Various preventive and corrective exercises have been proposed by Winston (48), Linduff (22), and Krout and Shires (21). They teach hip, shoulder and spinal movements to prevent scapulohumeral displacement.

Krout and Shires (21) advocate the use of active assistive exercises in all ranges of shoulder motion on the side of the operation, beginning the day after operation, in order to prevent "frozen shoulder." They add shoulder-wheel and pulley exercises to strengthen the middle and lower trapezius muscles and the rhomboids. They found that the movements most affected by surgery were active abduction and forward flexion. A comparison of function on the two sides, before and after surgery, demonstrated the good functional result of exercise therapy. The timing and the extent of the exercises need graduation according to the medical condition of the patient: this requires the cooperation of physician and surgeon with the physical therapist. In the degree of teamwork lies much of the success of the treatment.

SEGMENTAL BREATHING

This is the most commonly used treatment in current surgical cases, in which exercises are used to encourage full lung expansion after operation. The extent of modern chest surgery, the length of anesthesia and the severe nature of the disease in some patients combine to make the therapy so much in demand.

The technique of these localized breathing exercises has been mentioned briefly under "Low Costal Respiration" and "Diaphragmatic Respiration." It has been reviewed in detail by Reed (40). The exercises aim to produce expansion of local regions of the lung and chest (for example, upper costal, lower costal, posterior basal), while movement of other regions is voluntarily suppressed. Gradually the important movement is integrated into a normal, bilateral inspiration, while a normal posture is maintained.

The patient is most easily taught control of movement in a region by breathing against a light pressure there (Figs. 26.4 and 26.5). This can be applied by palms or knuckles over the lateral basal and upper lateral areas and by flat fingers in the pectoral and apical regions. The patient may be taught to use a broad belt, with its short ends crossed in front, to feel and control his lower costal movements. This is also most useful for posterior basal movements. The therapist or patient applies a little pressure at the end of expiration and maintains this steadily during expansion. During expiration, the pressure is relaxed. Unilateral movement is taught first, until overworking parts are relaxed. The rate of respiration should be dictated by the patient and will naturally vary greatly. When unilateral regional breathing is satisfactory, bilateral exercises are commenced.

The rationale of these exercises might seem somewhat doubtful in view of the previous discussion of the control of movements. This may be less so, however, than it appears, because movement which can be observed is more easily controlled, so that chest wall movement is more controllable than diaphragm movement; this was so in the studies of Wade (46). Also, patients in this group are different from those with chronic respiratory deficiency and may react more favorably. This is especially so in tuberculous patients, who sometimes show a remarkable increase in vital capacity in the circumstances where their physicians encourage expanding exercises (for example, before operation).

Nevertheless, the therapist needs to be careful that the appearance of good segmental breathing is not obtained falsely by a trick movement of spine or limb girdle. Experiences therapists are well aware of this substitution.

The benefits produced by the exercises are probably not susceptible to physiologic proof. However, most surgeons find them a valuable asset in the postoperative management of their patients. Perhaps this results in part from the attention the therapists give to the clearing of secretions, and perhaps the regional breathing causes mostly increased ventilation of all parts of the lungs, but the benefit, nevertheless, appears very real.

Nichols and Howell (33) have confirmed the high frequency of postoperative pulmonary complications after abdominal surgery. Prophylactic physical therapy did not reduce the frequency of complications in subjects without lung disease. It seems that subjects with lung disease, and cigarette smokers, should have a course of preoperative therapy if postoperative troubles are to be minimized.

Exercise and Heart Surgery

Therapeutic exercises have not established themselves in the medical treatment of heart disease where the disorders are not prone to physical treatment. With the advent of cardiac surgery, however, the management of the accompanying thoracotomy has brought new patients under the care of the physical therapist. His attention is needed for much the same reasons as in the case of lung surgery, except for the different general medical condition of his patients. The vigor of the exercises he encourages must be judged with care for the severity of the cardiac lesion; he must use a different approach for an older patient with mitral stenosis and heart failure from the one he uses with a fit youth with a patent ductus arteriosus. His duty is to assist in full recovery of lung function and to prevent postoperative deformity.

Before operation, patients are taught good posture, local and general breathing exercises and the act of coughing. Usually their mobility is encouraged and increased.

In the first days after operation, posture is emphasized, especially in the first day or so before the drainage tube is removed when the patients bend to that side. Assistance in coughing and postural drainage is helpful. Passive movements of the legs and feet may reduce the possibility of venous thrombosis.

After the patient leaves his bed, more extensive breathing exercises are given until normal respiration is maintained and normal posture is restored.

REFERENCES

1. ANGOVE, H. S. *Remedial Exercises for Certain Diseases of the Heart and Lungs.* London, 1936.

2. Asthma Research Council. Physical Exercises for Asthma. London, 1934.

3. BASS, H., WHITCOMB, J. F., AND FORMAN, R. Exercise training; therapy for patients with chronic obstructive lung disease. *Dis. Chest, 57:* 116, 1970.

4. BATES, D. V., MACKLEM, P. T., AND CHRISTIE, R. V. *Respiratory Function in Disease.* Philadelphia, 1971.

5. BECKLAKE, M. R., McGREGOR, M., GOLDMAN, H. I., AND BRANDO, J. L. A study of the effects of physiotherapy in chronic hypertrophic emphysema using lung function tests. *Dis. Chest, 26:* 180, 1954.

6. BERGOFSKY, E. H., TURINO, G. M., AND FISHMAN, A. P. Cardiorespiratory failure in kyphoscoliosis. *Medicine, 38:* 263, 1959.

7. BOLTON, J. H., GANDEVIA, B., AND ROSS, M. The rationale and results of breathing exercises in asthma. *Med. J. Aust., 43:* 675, 1956.

8. BOUHUYS, A. Breathing. In *Physiology, Environment and Lung Disease.* New York, 1974.

9. CAMPBELL, E. J. M., AND FRIEND, J. Action of breathing exercises in pulmonary emphysema. *Lancet, I:* 325, 1955.

10. CAMPBELL, E. J. M., AGOSTONI, E., AND NEWSOM DAVIS, J. The Respiratory Muscles. In *Mechanics and Neural Control.* London, 1970.

11. CHERNIACK, R. M., CHERNIACK, L., NAIMARK, A. *Respiration in Health and Disease.* Philadelphia, 1972.

12. CHRISTIE, D. Physical training in chronic obstructive lung disease. *Br. Med. J., 2:* 150, 1968.

13. COMROE, J. H. *Methods in Medical Research,* Vol. 2 Philadelphia, 1950.

14. COMROE, J. H., FORSTER, R. E., et al. The Lung: Clinical Physiology and Lung Function Tests. Chicago, 1955.

15. COURNAND, A., AND RICHARDS, D. W. Pulmonary insufficiency. I. Discussion of physiological classification and presentation of clinical tests. *Am. Rev. Tuberc., 44:* 26, 1941.

16. COURNAND, A., et al. The oxygen cost of breathing. *Trans. Assoc. Am. Physicians, 67:* 162, 1954.

17. DAIL, C. W., AND AFFELDT, J. E. Vital capacity as an index of respiratory muscle function. *Arch. Phys. Med., 38:* 383, 1957.

18. DORINSON, S. M. Breathing exercises for bronchial asthma and pulmonary emphysema. *J.A.M.A., 166:* 931, 1954.

19. GAENSLER, E. A. Analysis of ventilatory defect by timed capacity measurement. *Rev. Tuberc., 64:* 256, 1951.

20. GANDEVIA, B. AND HUGH-JONES, P. Terminology for measurements of ventilatory capacity. *Thorax, 12:* 290, 1957.

21. KROUT, R. M., AND SHIRES, E. B. Physical therapy in thoracic surgery. *Am. J. Phys. Med., 34:* 342, 1955.

22. LINDUFF, F. S. Physical therapy and chest surgery. *Physiother. Rev., 27:* 94, 1947.

23. LIVINGSTONE, J. L. AND GILLESPIE, M. The value of breathing exercises in asthma. *Lancet, II:* 705, 1935.

24. LIVINGSTONE, J. L., BREWERTON, D. A. AND DORNHORST, A. C. Breathing exercises; are they of value? *Ann. Phys. Med., 4:* 241, 1958.

25. MACMAHON, C. Prophylactic and remedial breathing and physical exercises. *Br. J. Tuberc., 28:* 184, 1934.

26. McILROY, M. B., MARSHALL, R., AND CHRISTIE, R. V. The work of breathing in normal subjects, in mitral stenosis and emphysema. *Clin. Sci., 13:* 127, 1954.

27. McNEILL, R. S., AND McKenzie, J. M. An assessment of the value of breathing exercises in chronic bronchitis and asthma. *Thorax, 10:* 250, 1955.

28. MEAD, J. Mechanics of the chest wall. In *Loaded Breathing*, edited by L. D. Pengelly, A. S. Rebuck, and E. J. M. Campbell, Edinburgh, 1974.

29. MILLER, M. E. Respiratory exercises for chronic pulmonary emphysema. *Bull. Johns Hop. Hosp.*, *92:* 185, 1953.

30. MILLER, W. F. Physiologic evaluation of the effects of diaphragmatic breathing training in patients with chronic pulmonary emphysema. *Am. J. Med.*, *17:* 471, 1954.

31. MILLER, W. F. Rehabilitation of patients with chronic obstructive lung disease. *Med. Clin. North Am. 51:* 349, 1967.

32. NICHOLAS, J. J., GILBERT, R., GABE, R., AND AUCHINCLOSS, J. H. Evaluation of an exercise therapy program for patients with chronic obstructive pulmonary disease. *Am. Rev. Respir. Dis.*, *102:* 1, 1970.

33. NICHOLS, P. J. R., AND HOWELL, B. Routine pre- and postoperative physiotherapy. *Rheumatol. Phys. Med.*, *10:* 321, 1970.

34. ORLAVA, O. E. Therapeutic physical culture in the complex treatment of pneumonia. *Phys. Ther. Rev.*, *39:* 153, 1959.

35. PAINTAL, A. S. Vagal sensory receptors and their reflex effects. *Physiol. Rev.*, *53:* 159, 1973.

36. PETERS, R. M. *The Mechanical Basis of Respiration.* Boston, 1969.

37. PETTY, T. L. *Intensive and Rehabilitative Respiratory Care.* Philadelphia, 1974.

38. PETTY, T. L., AND NETT, L. M. *For Those Who Live and Breathe.* Springfield, 1972.

39. REED, J. M. W. Notes on physiotherapy for medical and surgical chest conditions. *Brompton Hosp. Rep.*, *16:* 195, 1947.

40. REED, J. M. W. Localised breathing exercises in surgical chest conditions. *Br. J. Phys. Med.*, *16:* 111, 1953.

41. REID, L. M. Pathology of chronic bronchitis. *Lancet*, *I:* 275, 1954.

42. ROSS, M., GANDEVIA, B., AND BOLTON, J. H. The physiotherapy of asthma. *Austral. J. Physiother.*, December, 1957.

43. SCHERR, M. S., AND FRANKEL, L. F. Physical conditioning program for asthmatic children. *J.A.M.A.*, *168:* 1996, 1958.

44. SINCLAIR, J. D. The effect of breathing exercises in pulmonary emphysema. *Thorax*, *10:* 246, 1955.

45. STIGOL, L. C., AND CUELLO, A. C. Voluntary control of the diaphragm in one subject. *J. Appl. Physiol. 21:* 1911, 1966.

46. WADE, O. L. Movements of the thoracic cage and diaphragm in respiration. *J. Physiol.*, *124:* 193, 1954.

47. WEST, J. B. *Respiratory Physiology–the Essentials.* Baltimore, 1974.

48. WINSTON, H. R. Physical therapy and chest surgery. *Physiother. Rev.*, *26:* 227, 1946.

Index